# Public health nutrition in developing countries

# Public health nutrition in developing countries

Part - II

Edited by
**Sheila Chander Vir**

**WOODHEAD PUBLISHING INDIA PVT LTD**
New Delhi • Cambridge • Oxford • Philadelphia

Published by Woodhead Publishing India Pvt. Ltd.
Woodhead Publishing India Pvt. Ltd., G-2, Vardaan House, 7/28, Ansari Road
Daryaganj, New Delhi – 110002, India
www.woodheadpublishingindia.com

Woodhead Publishing Limited, 80 High Street, Sawston, Cambridge,
CB22 3HJ UK

Woodhead Publishing USA 1518 Walnut Street, Suite1100, Philadelphia

www.woodheadpublishing.com

First published 2011, Woodhead Publishing India Pvt. Ltd.


Woodhead Publishing India Pvt. Ltd. ISBN: 978-93-88320-35-1

Woodhead Publishing Pvt. Ltd. e-ISBN: 978-0-85709-004-1

Typeset by Sunshine Graphics, New Delhi
Printed and bound by Replika Press Pvt. Ltd.

Dedicated to my mother
Shanta Metre and father, Padma Bhushan W. B. Metre,
in fond memory of their love, blessings, inspiration and
encouragement.

# Contents

# Foreword

Public health nutrition has increasingly gained attention as an important subject in the field of development. It is recognized as a specialized discipline of nutrition that deals with expanding and integrating the understanding of nutrition issues across various levels – individual, family, community, national and global – geared towards solving nutrition problems of individuals and communities.

Malnutrition is known to contribute to approximately one-third of child deaths. High levels of malnutrition in developing countries is a major area of concern inhibiting achievement of the Millennium Development Goals (MDGs). Alleviation of malnutrition in developing countries poses to be a major challenge and needs urgent attention.

In the developing world, a total of 129 million children under the age of five years are underweight; 27 percent of these are in Asia and 21 percent in Africa. Stunting affects 195 million children under the age of five years in the developing world; and more than 90 percent of stunted children live in Asia and Africa. Many of these children have a poor start in life with 13 million infants being born with intrauterine growth restriction annually, resulting in low birth weight. Deficiencies of micro-nutrients, such as iodine, iron, vitamin A, folic acid and zinc, caused mainly due to inadequate dietary intake and frequent infections, affect the population in developing world.

There is immense hope in reducing malnutrition in a positive international development environment. The multiple causes of malnutrition are well known, new technologies are available and vast knowledge has been generated on effective interventions from programmes that have successfully accelerated reduction of malnutrition in countries such as Thailand, and more recently, Vietnam and Brazil. Experiences from successful programmes emphasize that political commitment and support, leadership and strategic capacity development, provision of basic and essential services, combined with community ownership for improving nutrition indicators are key ingredients for accelerated reduction of malnutrition. The enormous challenge for the developing world is the scaling up of malnutrition reduction programmes in order to achieve multiple MDGs. Adaptations of known effective interventions in the national and local context would save time and reduce the risk of implementing strategies that are unlikely to yield results. Understanding existing gaps and the key elements of successful programming are critical for formulating, implementing and evaluating effective programmes.

This book on Public Health Nutrition is timely and collates information on the current situation of malnutrition in the developing world. It not only presents recent technical developments in nutrition science but also highlights the application of proven sound recommendations for programme implementation. The book will be helpful to health and nutrition professionals, as well as, policy makers, programme designers and project implementers, in dealing with various nutrition issues effectively. The editor, taking into consideration the defined scope and focus of the book, has brought together authors who not only have in-depth technical knowledge of the subject but also have first-hand experience in planning and implementation of public health nutrition programmes. The book is reader friendly and the lessons learned from programmes are emphasized in box formats where appropriate. It also focuses on broader health and social issues that need to be addressed for achieving the goal of reducing malnutrition. Interestingly, the book also covers other issues of public health nutrition that relate to a wide variety of situations such as neonatal care, safe drinking water, diarrhoea and HIV. In addition, one section of the book concentrates on programming, with chapters on programme planning and implementation, communication, monitoring and evaluation, linking evidence-based research to programming. These chapters will enable practitioners to apply nutrition science to appropriate programme designing and its implementation.

The editor, Dr Sheila C. Vir, has over 25 years of experience working with UNICEF and has contributed significantly in the field of public health nutrition. The passion in the subject is evident from the effort put in by her for undertaking this monumental task of bringing together over thirty selected experts to contribute to this book. She should be congratulated for this exceptional publication in public health nutrition.

The book will be a very useful reference not only for nutritionists and public health specialist but also for pediatricians, development professionals, programmers and international agencies. It should be of interest to politicians, policy makers, bureaucrats, economists and agriculture scientists. Non-government organizations and civil society organizations will also find this book interesting, informative and thought provoking. It is hoped that this book will help adaptation of proven successful interventions from across the developing world and accelerate and scale up their implementation towards reducing malnutrition.

It is indeed my great pleasure and honour to write the foreword for this book.

10th October 2010
**Prof Emeritus Kraisid Tontisirin MD, Ph D**
*Chairman of the Policy Board,*
*The Thailand Research Fund, Bangkok*
*Formerly Director Nutrition and Consumer Protection Division,*
*Food and Agriculture Organisation of the United Nations (FAO), Rome*

# Preface

*Public Health Nutrition in Developing Countries* focuses on application of public health and nutrition sciences for formulating strategies and actions for preventing and solving the serious problem of malnutrition in developing countries. Presented are experiences, evidences and developments in addressing public health nutrition problems, over the last three to four decades. The lessons learnt from past experiences are highlighted to facilitate understanding of the basis of policy formulation, development of strategies, designing and implementation of programmes within a result-based framework. Along with these, a description of universally recommended processes and impact indicators is presented for measuring progress and outcomes of a wide range of public health nutrition interventions. In this context, the metabolism of a few selected nutrients are described to explain the rationale for the selection of a specific set of indicators in relation to specific nutrition intervention programmes.

This book presents an update on public health nutrition problems of developing countries along with a description of approaches used and efficacy of trials undertaken for addressing them. It highlights the experiences emerging from up-scaling intervention trials to programme models and elaborates on the principles of public health nutrition programme planning and implementation. The book covers emerging global experiences for a wide spectrum of public health nutrition issues, ranging from those addressing women and child undernutrition and micronutrient deficiencies, nutrition care in HIV, and management of nutrition in emergency situations. It therefore aims to provide not only an update on current knowledge but also to generate interest in upcoming challenges and scenarios for future programmes. Presentation of case studies from developing countries is incorporated to draw the attention of policy makers and programmers, and academics to actual experiences, processes, value additions, lessons learned and to potential challenges that remain to be addressed. The book intends to elaborate on the 'how' of addressing public health nutrition programming, to inform strategic planning, design and implementation of effective plans that would accelerate the reduction of malnutrition. Specific reference is made to policy formulation processes and programme experiences in India since the country has historically taken a global lead in launching various public health nutrition programmes.

The book highlights the emerging double-burden of undernutrition and overnutrition in developing countries. The association of malnutrition with the increasing challenge of communicable and non-communicable diseases has also been described. Additionally, the problem of nutrition of the aged population faced by many countries undergoing demographic transition is also dealt with. Separate sections are devoted to nutritional epidemiology, undernutrition in children and women and major micronutrient deficiency programmes such as iron, vitamin A, iodine and zinc. However, there is some intended overlap in micronutrient sections since different perspectives of similar subjects are addressed.

It is envisaged that this book, produced in two volumes, will provide public health experts, nutrition programmers, medical and nutrition graduates, nurses, programme managers with NGOs, or food industry and policy makers with information on technical and programmatic aspects of public health nutrition and thereby enhances skills in formulating and implementing appropriate solutions and actions.

I am indebted to innumerable women living in the developing world who greatly inspired me to address issues of public health nutrition with a new perspective. Women play a central role in influencing the nutrition status not only of children but of the entire family. This is well reflected in the profound statement of Swami Vivekananda, "there is no chance for the welfare of the world unless the condition of women is improved. It is not possible for the bird to fly on one wing". For improving nutrition situation in developing countries, we need to move beyond accessibility to food. Simultaneously, the social, educational and economic empowerment of women needs to be addressed. A multi-dimensional approach is essential for overcoming malnutrition.

As editor, I would like to acknowledge the contributors who are eminent scholars and leading programme specialists for their excellent contributions to this book. Their deep knowledge and vast experience has added immense value to the content of the book. I am particularly grateful to the authors for the colossal effort they have put in preparing the manuscripts. Furthermore, I would like to express my appreciation for the support provided by my team at the Public Health Nutrition and Development Centre (PHNDC), New Delhi. The invaluable assistance of Ms. Ritu Jain, Research Nutritionist, PHNDC, in reviewing literature and analyzing data, as well as, her continuous support in networking with the authors is appreciated. The support of Ms. Rachita Gupta, Research Nutritionist, PHNDC, in the final stage of this book is valued. I sincerely appreciate the contribution of Ms. Falguni Gokhale (Director, Design Directions) for the design of the cover page of this book.

I am deeply indebted to my mentor, late Professor A.H.G. Love, for his guidance during my doctoral work at the Institute of Clinical Sciences, Queen's University of Belfast, and for generating my interest in the subject of public health nutrition. The production of this book would not have been possible without the untiring love, care and support of my husband Dr. Chander Vir whose constant and unrelenting motivation helped me work towards my mission to promote public health nutrition issues in developing countries. My special thanks to my brother-in-law, Dr. Ishwar Dass, IAS, who constantly inspired and encouraged me to complete this book. The support, enthusiasm, patience and understanding of my daughters Parul and Anubha and my son-in-law Amit Garg is appreciated and acknowledged. I also sincerely appreciate and acknowledge the support, understanding and continuous encouragement from my extended family.

My special acknowledgement to the United Nations Children's Fund (UNICEF) with whom I have been associated for almost three decades, first as Project officer and now as a consultant. This association has provided me with the opportunity to learn in an ever evolving development environment.

This book could not have been produced without the cooperation of the publishers, Woodhead Publishing India Ltd. My sincere thanks to the publishing house team members—Mr. Ravindra Saxena and Mr. Sumit Aggarwal.

**Sheila C. Vir MSc Ph D**
Director,
Public Health Nutrition and Development Centre,
New Delhi, India
January 2011

# List of Contributors

Prof Bhattacharya Madhulika
Professor
Community Health Administration
National Institute of Health and Family Welfare(NIHFW)
New Delhi, India

Dr Bulusu Saraswati
Nutrition specialist,
UNICEF Field Office
Hyderabad, India

Dr Casanova Ines G.
Department of Nutrition and Health Sciences
Rollins School of Public Health
Emory University
Atlanta, USA

Dr Chaddha Ravinder
Associate Professor
Department of Food and Nutrition
Lady Irwin College
University of Delhi
New Delhi, India

Dr Chaudhary Deepika Nayar
Deputy Regional Director, Asia
The Micronutrient Initiative
New Delhi, India

Prof Das Tara Gopal
Director
Tara Consultancy Services
Bengaluru, India

Dr Dhingra Pratibha
Senior Research Scientist
Center for Micronutrient Research
New Delhi, India

Prof Dwivedi Shraddha
Professor and Head
Department of Preventive and Social Medicine
MLN Medical College
Allahabad, India

Ms Garg Aashima
Nutrition Specialist
UNICEF Field Office
Jaipur, India

Dr Gera Tarun
Consultant
Department of Pediatrics
Fortis Hospital
New Delhi, India

Prof Godbole Madan M
Professor and Head
Department of Endocrinology
Sanjay Gandhi Post Graduate Institute of Medical Sciences
Lucknow, India

Gulati Deepti
Senior Programme Associate,
Global Alliance for Improved Nutrition (GAIN)
New Delhi, India

Ms Jain Ritu
Research Nutritionist
Public Health Nutrition and Development Centre
New Delhi, India

Prof Kanani Shubhada
Professor
Department of Foods and Nutrition
Faculty of Home Science Maharaja
Sayajirao University of Baroda
Gujarat, India

Prof Kapur Deeksha
Professor
Department of Nutritional Sciences
School of Continuing Education
Indira Gandhi National Open University
New Delhi, India

Ms. Kathuria Ashi K.
Senior Nutrition Specialist
The World Bank
New Delhi, India

Dr Khanna Kumud
Director
Institute of Home Economics
University of Delhi
New Delhi, India

Dr Kotecha Prakash V
Country Representative
A2Z
USAID Micronutrient Project
Academy for Education Development
New Delhi, India

Dr Krishnaswamy Kamala
Former Director
National Institute of Nutrition
Hyderabad, India

Prof Kurpad Anura
Dean and Professor
Department of Nutrition
St. John's Research Institute
Bengaluru, India

Dr Lakshaman Anand
Coordinator, Planning and Knowledge Management
The Micronutrient Initiative (Asia office)
New Delhi, India

Dr Laxmaiah Avula
Deputy Director (Epidemiology)
Division of Community Studies
National Institute of Nutrition
Hyderabad, India

Dr Mathews Minnie
Former Senior Program Advisor
United Nations World Food Programme
New Delhi, India

Dr Menon Purnima
Senior Research Fellow
Division of Poverty, Health and Nutrition
International Food Policy Research Institute
New Delhi, India

Mr Mukherjee Ashish
Executive Director
Centre for Development Finance
Institute of Financial Management and Research
Chennai, India

Dr Nair K. Madhavan
Scientist and Head
Micronutrient Research Group
Department of Biophysics National Institute of Nutrition
Hyderabad, India

Prof Nandan Deoki
Director
National Institute of Health and Family Welfare (NIHFW)
New Delhi, India

Dr Nigam Arun K
Executive President
Institute of Applied Statistics & Development Studies
Lucknow, India

Dr Paintal Kajali
Nutrition Specialist
UNICEF
New Delhi, India

Prof Pandav Chandrakant
Head and Professor
Centre for Community Medicine
AIIMS
New Delhi, India

Dr Puri Seema
Associate Professor
Department of Food and Nutrition
Institute of Home Economics
University of Delhi
New Delhi, India

Dr Vijayaraghavan Kamasamudram
Former Head
Department of the Division of Community studies
National Institute of Nutrition
Hyderabad, India

Dr Raj Kamal
Emergency Nutrition Specialist
Child Nutrition & Development Section
UNICEF,
New Delhi, India

Dr Ramachandran Prema
Director
Nutrition Foundation of India
New Delhi, India

Dr Ramakrishnan Usha
Associate Professor
Hubert Department of Global Health
Rollins School of Public Health
Emory University
Atlanta, USA

Prof Ramji S
Professor
Department of Pediatrics
Maulana Azad Medical College
New Delhi, India

Prof Sachdev Harshpal S.
Senior Consultant
Pediatrics and Clinical Epidemiology
Sitaram Bhartia Institute of Research and Science
New Delhi, India

Dr Sankar Rajan
Regional Manager and Special Adviser in South Asia
Global Alliance for Improved Nutrition (GAIN)
New Delhi, India

Dr Sazwal Sunil
Associate Professor
Department of International Health
Program on Global Disease Epidemiology and Control
Johns Hopkins Bloomberg School of Public Health
USA

Prof Selvam Jerard M.
Professor and Head
Department of Epidemiology
The Tamil Nadu DrMGR Medical University
Chennai, India

Prof Seshadri Subadra
Senior Nutrition Consultant
Former Professor and Head at Department of Food and Nutrition
Faculty of Home Science Maharaja Sayajirao University of Baroda
Gujarat, India

Dr Seth Veenu
Associate Professor,
Department of Food and Nutrition
Lady Irwin College
University of Delhi
New Delhi, India

Dr Shah Dheeraj
Associate Professor
Department of Pediatrics,
University College of Medical Sciences
New Delhi, India

Dr Singh Padam
Head
Research & Evaluation
EPOS Health India
New Delhi, India

Dr Pandey Richa S.
Nutrition Specialist
UNICEF Field Office
Lucknow, India

Dr Swaminathan Sumathi
Research Supervisor
Department of Epidemiology and Statistics
St. John's Research Institute
Bengaluru, India

Dr Mannar M.G. Venkatesh
President
The Micronutrient Initiative
Ottawa, Canada

Dr Vir Sheila C.
Former Programme Officer ,UNICEF (India)
Director
Public Health Nutrition and Development Centre
New Delhi, India

Dr Wesley Annie S.
Senior Program Specialist
The Micronutrient Initiative
Ottawa, Canada

Dr Yunuss Shariqua
Programme Officer – Health and Nutrition
United Nations World Food Programme
New Delhi, India

Prof Zodpey Sanjay P.
Director, Public Health Education
Public Health Foundation of India and
Director, Indian Institute of Public Health, Delhi
New Delhi, India

* The content of the text presents views of the author and not necessarily reflect outlook of the organization.

# 23

# Metabolism of iron, folic acid and vitamin $B_{12}$

*K. Madhavan Nair*

**K. Madhavan Nair**, PhD in Biochemistry from Osmania University, Hyderabad, is a Scientist (E) and Head of the Micronutrient Research Division at the National Institute of Nutrition. He has received the Public Health Service International Research Fellow Award in1988 and ICMR's prestigious B.G.R.C. Silver Jubilee Oration Award for the year 1996 for his contributions in the field of Nutritional Hematology. His expertise includes basic, applied and population-based intervention programs in micronutrients. Dr. Nair has made significant contributions in understanding iron-induced free radical damage and its prevention by antioxidant supplementation and micronutrient food fortification.

## 23.1 Introduction

Iron along with folate and vitamin $B_{12}$ are by far the most important nutrients for cell proliferation. Major advances have been made in understanding the physiology of human iron metabolism. In addition to its role in cellular proliferation, it plays vital role in oxygen transport, oxidative metabolism and other physiological processes. Folic acid deficiency reduces the proliferative capability of rapidly dividing tissues of the body and a primary deficiency of vitamin $B_{12}$ can lead to a secondary deficiency of folic acid. There is a great deal of biochemical interdependence of iron, vitamin $B_{12}$ and folic acid in maintaining purine and pyrimidine supply to synthesize genetic material and maintain cell division. The scope of this chapter is to review the latest developments in the area of metabolism of these nutrients, highlighting their interactions in various metabolic pathways in order to provide a holistic understanding to improve public health nutrition.

## 23.2 Iron

Iron (Fe, atomic number 26, atomic weight 55.65) is the fourth most abundant element (O, Si, Al, Fe) and second most abundant metal in the earth's crust. In aqueous solution iron can exist as ferrous ($Fe^{2+}$) or ferric

($Fe^{3+}$) ions and is associated with a large variety of biological molecules. Iron is the most versatile of all biologically active metals owing to its ability to switch between the ferrous and ferric forms. It acts as a catalyst in redox reactions by donating or accepting electrons and participates in free radical chemistry by donating electrons to oxygen. It is the major hemopoietic factor [1].

Iron in the environment is almost exclusively in the $Fe^{3+}$ state. In spite of its abundance, iron deficiency anemia is the most common nutrient deficiency in the world today. It affects all age groups and both sexes. The prevalence of anemia is significantly higher especially in women of child-bearing age and infants. To a large extent the physiology of iron and the factors leading to iron deficiency are well defined. Healthy, non-anemic individuals have an optimum balance between iron intake and excretion [1, 2].

## 23.3 Distribution

Total iron content in an average adult man (60 kg) is estimated to be about 3.8 g, that in a woman (50 kg) is 2.3 g and in a new born it is about 70 mg per kg body weight or a total of 250 mg iron. The distribution of iron in the human body is conceptualized to exist in three main biological compartments; functional, transport and storage (Fig. 23.1). The *functional* compartment accounts for about 75% of total body iron and consists of hemoglobin (65–70%), myoglobin (3–4%) and enzymes (3%). The *transport* compartment corresponds to iron in circulation bound to plasma transport protein transferrin, contributing to less than 1% of body iron. The *storage* compartment contributes to the remaining 25%, and comprises iron stored in a nontoxic form as ferritin and hemosiderin proteins in liver, spleen and marrow. The storage compartment corresponds to iron absorbed in excess of that required for the functional compartment [1, 2].

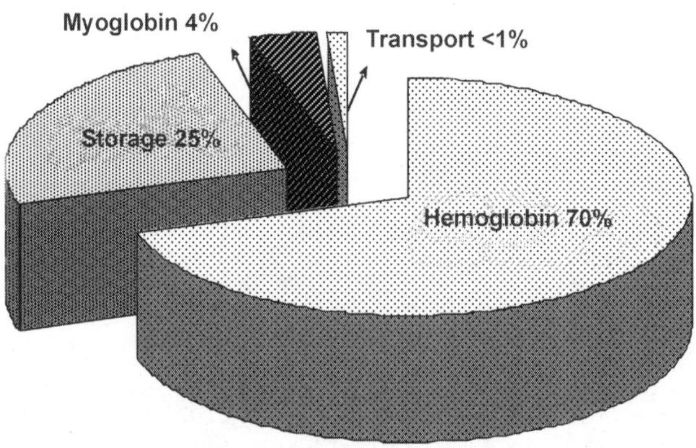


*23.1* Distribution of iron in man.

The three components are interlinked and coordinated to maintain systemic iron homeostasis. The transport compartment, estimated to turnover about 25 mg iron per day, links the storage and functional compartments by transporting iron to the functional compartment from the body stores [3].

## 23.4 Functional compartment

Iron containing proteins are conveniently grouped into two categories – heme and, non-heme proteins. The first category, heme-proteins, includes hemoglobin, myoglobin and certain enzymes involved in oxidative metabolism. The second category of non-heme iron proteins includes ferritin (iron storage), transferrin (transport) and certain enzymes containing the iron–sulphur cluster.

## 23.5 Heme proteins

Heme refers to a molecule that has a protoporphyrin IX ring with a ferrous ion coordinated to it (Figure 23.2). It thus consists of an organic component and an iron atom. Protoporphyrin IX is made of four pyrrole rings (tetrapyrrole).

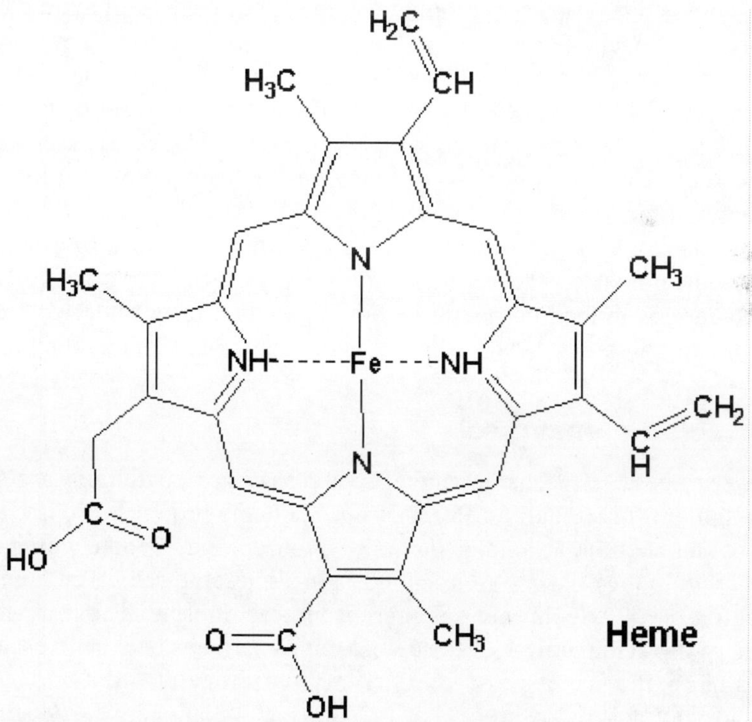


*23.2* Chemical structure of the Fe2+ protophorphyrin IX - heme group in hemoglobin and myoglobin.

The iron atom in heme binds to four nitrogens in the center of protoporphyrin ring. The ferrous ion can form two additional bonds, one above and one below the plane of the heme molecule. These bonding sites are termed fifth and sixth coordination positions respectively. There are a number of heme-containing proteins, most abundant are hemoglobin (Hb) and myoglobin (Mb). Hb is the oxygen carrier and plays a vital role in the transport of carbon dioxide and hydrogen ions. Normal hemoglobin concentration in humans ranges from 11 to 14 g/dl and is age and sex specific. Myoglobin, located in muscle, serves as a store of oxygen and facilitates the movement of oxygen within skeletal and cardiac muscles. The concentration of myoglobin is about 3–5 mg/g of muscle tissue.

The globin or protein component of Hb is made up of four separate chains and is hence called a tetrameric protein. In humans, four different types of globin chains are found, namely, $\alpha$ (alpha), $\beta$ (beta), $\gamma$ (gamma) and $\delta$ (delta). Human adult hemoglobin has a $\alpha 2$, $\gamma 2$ configuration and the chains are held together by non-covalent interactions. Each chain binds a heme molecule. The $\alpha$ and $\beta$ chains of hemoglobin closely resemble those of myoglobin, which is a monomeric heme protein. Hb can also have a $\alpha 2$, $\delta 2$ configuration called HbA2 and fetal Hb has a $\alpha 2$, $\gamma 2$ configuration. Myoglobin is a monomeric protein, meaning it has only one globin chain with a heme attached to it.

The capacity of hemoglobin and myoglobin to bind oxygen depends on the presence of the heme group, which also gives them the distinctive colour. The iron atom can be in the $Fe^{2+}$ or $Fe^{3+}$ oxidation state and the respective forms of hemoglobins are called ferrohemoglobin and ferrihemoglobin (methemoglobin). Only $Fe^{2+}$ oxidation state can bind oxygen. The, globin chain, in these molecules confers a distinctive microenvironment to the heme, enabling it to carry oxygen and this phenomenon is termed co-operative binding. When fully saturated, each gram of hemoglobin is capable of carrying about 1.34 ml of oxygen [4, 5].

## 23.6 Heme enzymes

Heme enzymes, as the name suggests, are enzymes containing a heme group and are functionally different from the heme proteins discussed in the previous section. Examples include cytochromes a, b and c which are present within the cristae of mitochondria in all aerobic cells. The highest concentration of cytochrome c is present in heart muscle. The iron atom present in the heme moiety of the cytochrome oscillates between $Fe^{3+}$ and $Fe^{2+}$ during the process of oxidative phosphorylation. Oxidative phosphorylation is redox process that results in cellular energy production in the form of adenosine tri phosphate (ATP). Given below is a non-exhaustive list of important heme-containing enzymes and their functions.

These examples illustrate the myriad functions of these enzymes in physiology and metabolism and thus underscore the importance of iron in systemic homeostasis [4].

Cytochrome b5 is a component of liver microsomal membranes where it probably provides energy for protein synthesis. It is also present within the cytoplasm of the red blood cells, where it functions as an intermediate in the reduction of methemoglobin. Cytochrome P-450 family of enzymes is involved in xenobiotic or drug metabolism and are located predominantly within the microsomal membranes of liver cells and also in the intestinal mucosa. Other heme enzymes, catalase, peroxidase, myeloperoxidase are part of the cellular antioxidant defense mechanism(s) and tryptophan pyrrolase is involved in tryptophan metabolism.

The other important heme enzymes are nitric oxide synthase (NOS) and prostaglandin synthase or cyclooxygenase (COX). Both these enzymes are important for initiating and propagating immune responses. The enzyme NOS catalyzes the formation of nitric oxide (NO) from oxygen, arginine, requires several cofactors and contains a heme group which is part of the catalytic site. NO is an important signaling molecule with major roles in neurotransmission, blood pressure control and blood clotting. (COX) converts arachidonic acid to prostaglandin $H_2$ ($PGH_2$), the precursor of eicosanoids. The enzyme contains two active sites, with the heme moiety having peroxidase activity. The eicosanoids, prostaglandins, prostacyclins and thromboxanes are known to be involved in reproductive functions, in inflammation, fever, and pain, associated with injury or disease; in the formation of blood clots and the regulation of blood pressure; in gastric acid secretion; and in a variety of other processes important in human health or disease [4, 5].

## 23.7 Non-heme iron proteins

In these proteins, the iron is present not as a heme moiety but in other forms such as iron-sulfur clusters, such as proteins of oxidative phosphorylation. The iron transport protein transferrin and storage proteins ferritin are the other forms of non-heme iron proteins and will be discussed in detail subsequently. Aconitase, ribonucleotide reductase, lipoxygenases, tyrosine hydroxylase, inositol oxygenase, proline and lysine hydroxylase, dehydrogenases, and xanthine oxidase are some of the important enzymes of this class.

*Aconitase* is an enzyme that catalyses the stereo-specific isomerization of citrate to isocitrate via *cis*-aconitate in the tricarboxylic acid cycle (TCA) that occurs within the mitochondria. Aconitase contains four iron atoms that are complexed to four inorganic sulfides as $[4Fe\text{-}4S]^{2+}$ cluster (iron–sulphur cluster) in its active site. These sulphide groups are provided by cysteine residues in the protein. The fourth iron atom of the $[4Fe\text{-}4S]^{2+}$

cluster, called the labile iron, is not coordinated by a sulphide but by water molecules. Thus the Fe–S cluster binds citrate (substrate) and participates in sequentially dehydrating and rehydrating the bound substrate. The aconitase protein is bifunctional in that it can function either as an active aconitase (enzyme), or as a RNA-binding protein which controls the expression of proteins involved in cellular iron metabolism. The cellular iron status enables the protein to switch between the enzyme form and the RNA-binding protein form. This phenomenon is called the 'aconitase switch' and is discussed in detail later in the chapter. This protein illustrates the possible role of iron in energy homeostasis.

*Ribonucleotide reductase* is essential for DNA synthesis and therefore cell proliferation. This enzyme catalyzes the de novo synthesis of deoxyribonucleotide diphsophates (dNDPs) from ribonucleotide diphosphates (NDPs). The dNDPs are in turn subsequently used for DNA synthesis. The active site of the enzyme contains an iron centre consisting of two ferric ions ($Fe3^{+}$), a tyrosyl free radical and two sulfhydryl groups. The free radical at the active site is stabilized by the two $Fe^{3+}$ ions connected to each other by an oxygen atom. The mechanism of catalysis is as follows. The hydroxyl group bonded to C-2 of the ribose ring is steriospecifically replaced by a H. This reduction is initiated by the free radical at the active site [6].

Actively dividing tissue such as the bone marrow requires a constant supply of dNDPs. This supply can be met only if ribonuclotides are not limiting, implying that NDPs also have to be continuously synthesized. However, NDP synthesis involves one-carbon transfer reactions carried out by methyl transferases. Most methyl transferases require methylated forms of tetrahydrofolate (e.g., $N^{10}$-formyl-tetrahydrofolate for thymidylate synthase) as the carrier of the transferable carbon. Deficiency of folate severely hampers NDP synthesis, thus inhibiting DNA synthesis and finally cell division. This pathway is a good example of why anemia, caused by iron deficiency or folate deficiency, has similar clinical manifestations. This example also highlights the importance of accurately identifying the etiology of anemia, as iron supplementation alone will not correct an underlying folate deficiency. It is for this reason that folic acid is given along with iron supplements for correcting anemia.

*Lipoxygenases* are iron-containing enzymes that catalyze the dioxygenation of polyunsaturated fatty acids. Products of lipoxygenases are leukotrienes which are involved in inflammatory pathways.

*Tyrosine hydroxylase* or tyrosine 3-monooxygenase catalyzes the conversion of the amino acid L-tyrosine to dihydroxyphenylalanine (DOPA). DOPA is a precursor for dopamine which in turn is a precursor for norepinephrine (noradrenalin) and epinephrine (adrenaline) all of which are important neurotransmitters.

Myo-inositol oxygenase catalyzes conversion of *myo*-inositol to D-glucuronate, initiating the only known pathway in humans for catabolism of the carbon skeleton of cell-signaling inositol (poly) phosphates and phosphoinositides.

*Proline and lysine hydroxylase enzymes.* Collagen contains 2 post-translationally modified amino acids hydroxyproline and hydroxylysine. The hydroxylase enzymes responsible for these modifications require $Fe^{2+}$ for activity. Ascorbic acid, acting as a reducing agent keeps the iron in the reduced $Fe^{2+}$ state. This is the reason why ascorbic acid deficiency causes scurvy [1–5, 11, 16].

Thus, from the above examples it is evident that depletion of iron in the functional compartment can adversely affect energy production, DNA synthesis, response to inflammation, neurophysiology and collagen integrity. The effects of iron deficiency are therefore manifested as anemia, impaired psychomotor development, impaired effort tolerance and adverse pregnancy outcome. The cited examples also provide a biochemical explanation to the observed multi-systemic manifestations of iron deficiency [5].

## 23.8 Storage compartment

The storage compartment is composed of intracellular iron storage proteins, ferritin and hemosiderin. In normal tissues, ferritin contains about 20% of iron. Stored iron serves as a reservoir of iron, primarily for the production of hemoglobin.

Ferritin is a high molecular weight (450kDa) protein produced intracellularly in response to iron. It is a polymer of heavy (H, acidic) and light (L, basic) chains arranged so as to form a hollow sphere or core. The core can accumulate about 4500 atoms of iron. Iron is stored in the $Fe^{3+}$ state as ferrihydrite, $[FeO(OH)]_8[FeO(H_2PO_4)]$. Cells release ferritin into the systemic circulation in a glycosylated, iron-depleted form. The circulating ferritin is directly proportional to cellular ferritin content and ranges between 12–200 ng/ml. Quantitatively it has been established that 1 ng/ml serum ferritin is equivalent to 10 mg storage iron and therefore serum ferritin is used as a measure of iron stores [7, 10].

The second iron-storage protein, hemosiderin is formed mainly in the spleen, marrow and the Kupffer cells of the liver and is found only in abnormal conditions such as repeated transfusions or iron overload. Hemosiderin may contain up to 35% iron by weight and is believed to be a partially denatured form of ferritin. Hemosiderin iron is available for heme synthesis but is mobilized at a rate slower than that of ferritin.

## 23.9 Transport compartment

The transport compartment represents the smallest pool of iron (<1%). Iron is transported in blood mainly bound to transferrin, the transport protein. Transferrin is a glycoprotein and each molecule can bind two ferric ions very tightly (affinity $10^{23}$ $M^{-1}$ at pH 7.4) but reversibly. Although iron bound to transferrin is less than 0.1% (34 mg) of the total body iron, dynamically it is the most important iron pool, with the highest rate of turnover at 25 mg per 24 h.

## 23.10 Recycling of iron in the body

Iron is derived from two major sources, viz. diet and destruction of RBC hemoglobin. As mentioned earlier, most of the iron in the body is located in the hemoglobin. When red blood cells reach a certain age (120 days, ageing RBCs), they are engulfed by macrophages in the spleen and bone marrow. In these cells, the internalized iron-containing hemoglobin is degraded; iron released and transferred onto circulating transferrin molecules in the blood. Most of the iron used for hemoglobin production comes from such iron recycling and is utilized for the synthesis of new RBCs in the bone marrow. Thus, iron is effectively recycled continuously for hemoglobin formation. It is because of this recycling phenomenon that it takes longer for iron deficiency anemia to develop in adult males when dietary iron alone is restricted. Further as presented in Figure 23.3, most of the iron is recycled efficiently within the body, the major factor affecting iron requirement is the amount of iron lost from the body [4, 8].

## 23.11 Iron losses

### 23.11.1 Obligatory (basal) iron losses

In an adult, basal iron loss from the gastrointestinal tract, skin and urinary tract is about 1 mg/day or 14 µg/kg/day. This is also the quantity of iron lost by an adult male. In women of child bearing age, the losses due to menstruation are about 16 µg/kg/day (15 mg totally or 0.5–0.6 mg/d). This must be added to the basal iron losses for estimating loss / day. The iron loss for normal menstruating women is therefore 30 mg/kg/day or about 1.5 mg iron daily for a 50 kg woman.

### 23.11.2 Iron loss during pregnancy and lactation

Although pregnancy is associated with a temporary cessation of menstruation, the overall cost to the mother in terms of iron balance is greater than in the non-pregnant stage. Total iron requirements include

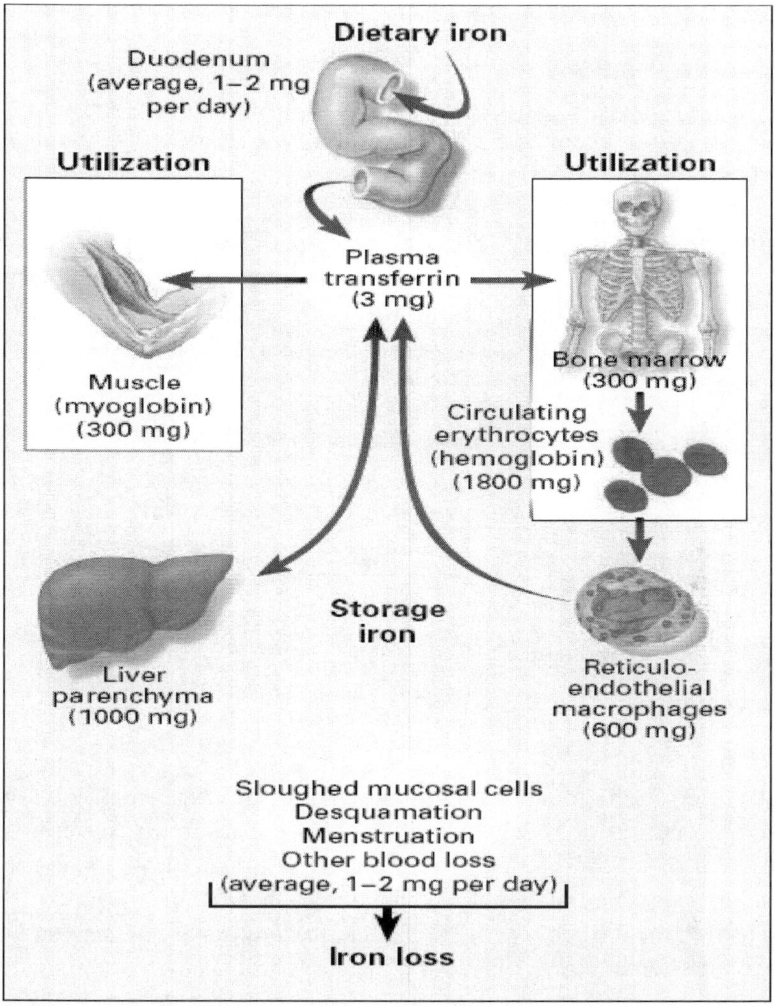


*23.3* Recycling and utilization of iron in man [1].

those necessary to replace basal losses, to allow for expansion of the maternal red cell mass and to provide for the needs of the growing fetus and placenta. The obligatory iron loss, in terms of actual quantity of iron used, calculated throughout pregnancy in a well-nourished woman of 55 kg, is approximately 230 mg. Increase in red cell mass requires about 450 mg of iron. The fetus at term contains 270–300 mg and the products of conception account for a further 50–90 mg. Thus, the total cost of pregnancy just about exceeds 1000 mg or approximately 20 mg/kg body weight. Therefore, pregnancy and parturition result in severe depletion of stored iron, necessitating mandatory iron supplementation [8, 10].

## 23.12 Dietary iron bioavailability

Bioavailability of dietary iron is defined as the proportion of iron that is actually available for absorption and utilization by the body. In the case of iron alone, absorption is synonymous with bioavailability, as there is no regulated excretion of iron. Variations in food iron bioavailability are determined by the dietary source of iron rather than the absolute amount of iron ingested. While the absorption of heme iron is unaffected by dietary promoters and inhibitors, non-heme iron is subjected to the interplay of dietary factors as shown in Fig. 23.4 [11].

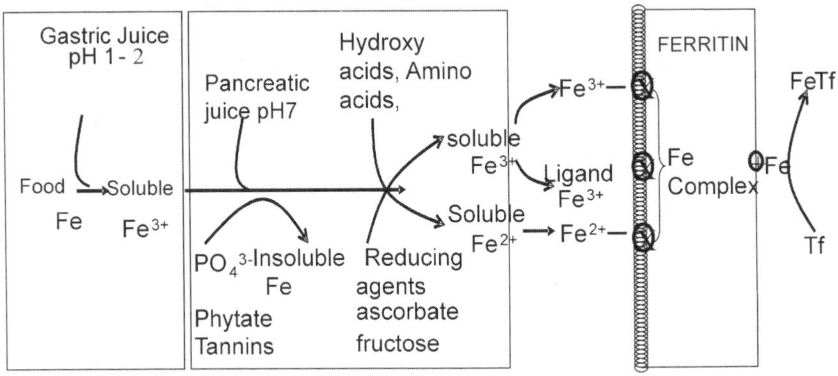


*23.4* Gastrointestinal digestion of dietary non-heme iron.

It is very well known that the food matrix can influence the solubility of iron in the gastric milieu before it reaches the absorptive surface of the intestinal mucosa. The majority of dietary non-heme iron enters the GI tract in the ferric form, which is soluble in the gastric milieu (pH 1–2) and reduced to the ferrous form. There are numerous dietary components that can render ferric iron to exist in its insoluble form (phytates, tannic acid, fiber) or to reduce it (ascorbic acid, organic acids) to the soluble ferrous form.

### 23.12.1 Promoters of non-heme iron absorption

The most powerful promoter of non-heme iron absorption is ascorbic acid. In the acid environment of the stomach, ascorbic acid forms a chelate with ferric salts which remains soluble even at alkaline pH of the duodenum. It also converts ferric iron to the ferrous state, which maintains its solubility in the alkaline environment of the upper gut. Meat has a two-pronged beneficial effect on iron nutrition. Not only is it an excellent source of bioavailable heme iron but it also promotes absorption of non-heme iron. The mechanism whereby meat facilitates non-heme iron absorption is not clear but may be related to the release of the amino acid cysteine and cysteine containing peptides during digestion.

### 23.12.2 Inhibitors of non-heme iron absorption

A number of factors have been identified, which limit non-heme iron absorption. These include polyphenols, phytates, the dietary fiber complex, calcium and phosphorus, and the dietary protein complex. High molecular weight polyphenols (tannins) present in beverages such as tea and the polyphenol content of individual vegetables are major inhibitors of food-iron absorption. Phytate is present in many cereals, nuts and legumes to about 1–2% by weight. A number of plant foods which have high complex-protein content, including soya beans, significantly inhibit iron absorption.

## 23.13 Other factors influencing iron absorption

The most important known stimuli to iron absorption are the rate of erythropoiesis and tissue iron stores. Accelerated red blood cell production, as in the case of bleeding, hemolysis or hypoxia, results in enhanced iron absorption. Conversely, diminished erythropoiesis due to starvation, blood transfusion or return to sea level from high altitudes decreases the absorption of iron. It has been postulated that an erythrocyte stimulating factor acts as a messenger to the gut to increase iron absorption. However, enhanced iron absorption continues in iron-deficient subjects long after the hemoglobin mass is restored to normal levels and persists until the body stores become normally replete with iron. Inflammation and inflammatory stimuli also determine iron absorption with iron absorption decreasing during inflammatory conditions. It has also been postulated that quantity of gastric acid secreted may play a significant role in iron absorption as patients with decreased gastric acid output have sub-optimal iron status [12, 13].

## 23.14 Recommended daily allowance (RDA)

The RDA for iron has been determined using the factorial approach. Obligatory losses of 1 mg for men and 1.5 mg for women, requirement for growth in children and losses during pregnancy are taken into account for calculating the requirement (Table 23.1). The above losses have to be made up by absorption of an amount equal to the loss. The percent of iron absorbed from typical meals was estimated from studies carried out during the 1980s to be 3% for men, children and adolescent boys; 5% for adolescent girls and non-pregnant women; and 8% for pregnant women [14]. These absorption figures have been employed by the expert group of Indian Council of Medical Research (ICMR) in 1989 to calculate iron RDA for Indians. Based on a more recent iron absorption values, the RDA for India has been recently revised [10].

## 23.15 Iron homeostasis

At the systemic level, iron homeostasis is maintained by three key organs: the intestine, the liver and the macrophages of the reticuloendothelial system (RES). The absorptive epithelial cells of the intestine (enterocytes) are responsible for absorption, the hepatocytes sense iron requirements and store excess iron, and the macrophages efficiently recycle hemoglobin iron from senescent RBC. In the absence of regulated iron excretion, homeostatic control occurs by limiting iron absorption to requisite levels at the intestine. The rate of absorption appears to respond to a variety of interdependent factors such as total iron stores, the extent to which the marrow is producing new red blood cells (erythropoiesis), the concentration of hemoglobin in the blood, oxygen content of the blood and inflammatory status of the individual. Iron absorption increases during hypoxia or enhanced "erythropoietic need" and in the presence of decreased stores; but decreases during chronic inflammation or in the presence of sufficient stores [4]. Therefore, the quantity of iron absorbed is determined by the net result of the above-mentioned stimuli. The molecular aspects of systemic iron homeostasis are discussed below.

*Table 23.1* Iron requirement during various physiological stages

| Group | | Body weight (kg) | Iron requirement µg/kg | Total daily mg/day |
|---|---|---|---|---|
| Adult | Man | 60 | 14 | 0.840 |
| | Woman | 50 | 30 | 1.500 |
| | Pregnant woman | 50 | 60 | 3.000 |
| | Lactating woman | 50 | 30 | 1.500 |
| Infants | 0-6 months | 4.5 | 70 | 0.315 |
| Children | 1-3 years | 12.2 | 29 | 0.354 |
| | 4.6 years | 19.0 | 29 | 0.551 |
| | 7-9 years | 26.9 | 29 | 0.780 |
| Adolescents 10-12 years | Boys | 35.4 | 29 | 1.027 |
| | Girls | 31.5 | 30 | 0.945 |
| 13-15 years | Boys | 47.8 | 26 | 1.243 |
| | Girls | 46.7 | 30 | 1.401 |
| 16-18 years | Boys | 57.1 | 26 | 1.485 |
| | Girls | 49.1 | 30 | 1.497 |

*Source:* Nutrient Requirements and Recommended Dietary Allowances for Indian, A report of the Expert Group of the Indian Council of Medical Research, National Institute of Nutrition, Hyderabad 1990.

## 23.16 Mechanism of intestinal absorption of iron at the enterocyte

### 23.16.1 Heme iron absorption

Most of the heme iron seems to enter the intestinal absorptive cell (enterocyte) as intact metalloporphyrin. Recent research suggests that a heme carrier protein (HCP), present on the apical surface of the enterocyte facilitates the uptake of the intact heme molecule. Subsequently iron is released from the porphyrin ring by the enzyme heme oxygenase, which then enters the circulation as transferrin-bound iron.

### 23.16.2 Non-heme iron absorption

Non-heme iron absorption occurs throughout the small intestine but mainly in the duodenum (proximal small intestine). The enterocytes are known to adapt to the current body requirements of iron, which in turn are the resultant of all the above-mentioned interdependent stimuli. Although the exact mechanisms regulating iron transport across the intestinal mucosa are still being worked out, many factors affecting iron absorption have been studied.

Unlike heme iron, only a small percentage of total non-heme iron from digested food or supplements is absorbed. To be absorbed, dietary iron must be in the ferrous ($Fe^{2+}$) form. A ferric reductase enzyme on the enterocyte brush border, duodenal cytochrome-b (Dcytb), reduces dietary soluble iron from $Fe^{3+}$ to $Fe^{2+}$. A protein called divalent metal transporter-1(DMT-1), which transports a spectrum of divalent metal ions into the body, then transports the iron across the enterocyte apical membrane into the cell (Fig. 23.5) [4, 9].

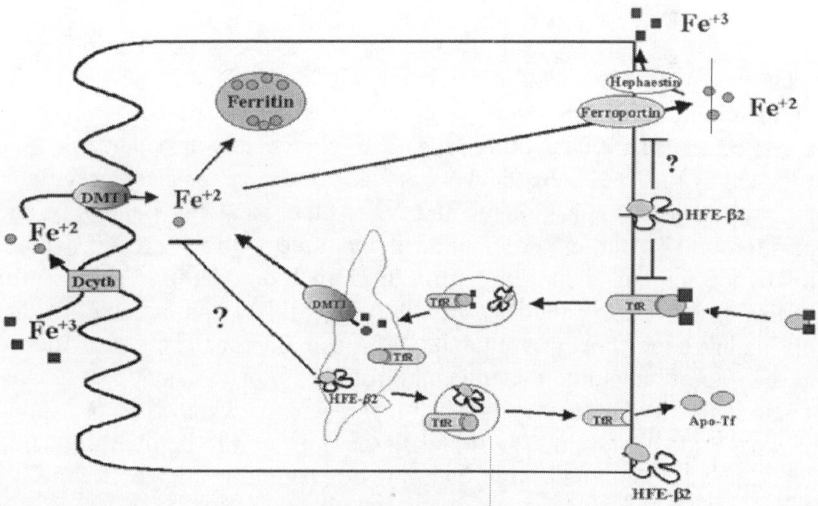


*23.5* Proposed mechanism of intestinal absorption of iron.

The enterocyte then transports acquired iron into circulation via the serosa through a protein called ferroportin-1 (FPN-1) located on the basolateral membrane. FPN-1 can transport only ferrous iron and not ferric iron, but transferrin can take up only ferric iron (Fig 23.6). This necessitates a ferroxidase. The exact mechanism by which iron in the cytosol of enterocytes is transferred to the blood is unknown and it is thought that circulating ceruloplasmin may be the ferroxidase. Recently, a basolateral membrane-associated ferroxidase, hephaestin protein, has been identified, which may also facilitate this process. Iron not transported to circulation is stored in the cell as ferritin, in which case the iron will leave the body when the cell exfoliates and is sloughed off into feces.

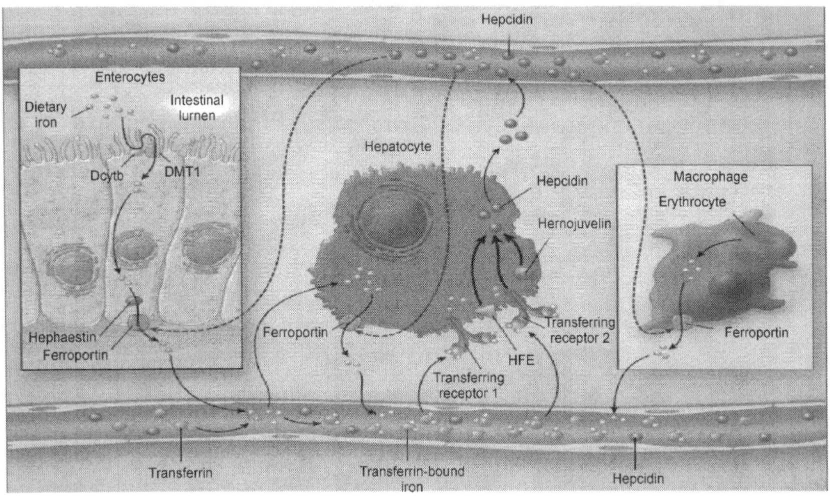


*23.6* Interplay of key proteins in iron homeostasis [9].

The body regulates iron levels by regulating each of these steps, viz. apical uptake and transfer to circulation. Hepcidin or LEAP-1 (liver expressed antimicrobial peptide), is a relatively recently discovered peptide produced by the liver (hepatocytes), that appears to be the master regulator of iron homeostasis in humans and other mammals. Independently, the antimicrobial properties associated with the same peptide were discovered, and hence named "hepcidin" (produced in liver "hep-", "-cidin" for "killing"). Now also called the iron hormone, this 25 amino acid residue peptide has been shown to regulate absorption of iron. The first evidence for the role of hepcidin in anemia and iron metabolism came from studies in patients with liver tumors who had severe anemia which did not respond to iron supplementation. The tumor tissue appeared to be overproducing hepcidin, and contained large quantities of hepcidin mRNA. Removing the tumors surgically cured the anemia. Taken together, these discoveries suggested that hepcidin regulated the release of iron in the body. The current scientific evidence suggests that hepcidin is a central regulatory hormone and its main action is to regulate systemic iron homeostasis. Circulating hepcidin levels vary with iron status, hypoxia, and inflammatory stimuli such as IL-6 (cytokine) levels. While Dcytb and DMT-1 are unique to iron transport across the duodenum, FPN-1, which is the basolateral iron export protein, is present on all cells which store iron, viz. enterocytes, hepatocytes and macrophages. More recent discoveries have shown that hepcidin directly binds with FPN-1, causing it to be internalized into the cell. The internalized protein is subsequently degraded thus preventing iron transport into systemic circulation (Fig. 23.5). Regulation of FPN-1 activity is the main pathway of regulating the amount of iron in circulation [9, 15, 16].

## 23.17 Mechanism of iron uptake in cells other than enterocytes

Each transferrin molecule has the ability to carry two iron ions in the $Fe^{3+}$ form. All cells need iron and obtain the same from diferric transferrin circulating in blood. As iron is tightly bound to transferrin, cells throughout the body have receptors for transferrin-iron complexes on their surfaces called transferrin receptor (TfR). These receptors bind diferric transferrin, the complex is engulfed (endocytosis) into vesicles called lysosomes. The lysosome is acidic (pH~4), causing transferrin to release its iron ions. The released iron is transported out of the lysosome and can be utilized in the functional compartment or be stored as ferritin. The receptor is then transported through the endocytic cycle back to the cell surface, ready for another round of iron uptake [3].

## 23.18 Molecular regulation of cellular iron

Cells have advanced mechanisms for sensing their own need for iron (Figure 23.7). In human cells, the best characterized iron-sensing mechanism involves translational regulation of mRNA. The mRNA sequence (also called transcript) of proteins involved in cellular iron metabolism such as transferrin receptor, ferritin contain a special sequence called the Iron Responsive Element (IRE). The IRE is actually a short self-complimentary sequence of about 5–7 nucleotides. This sequence enables the mRNA to acquire a loop-like structure at that point, called a 'stem-loop' structure. Certain proteins called IRE-binding proteins (IRE-BPs) bind specifically to these stem-loop structures to regulate the translation of the proteins in iron metabolism. The ends of any mRNA transcript are designated as the 5' and 3' end. The 5' end is the beginning of the transcript while the 3'end is the end of the transcript. The IRE structures can be present either in the 5' or 3' end.

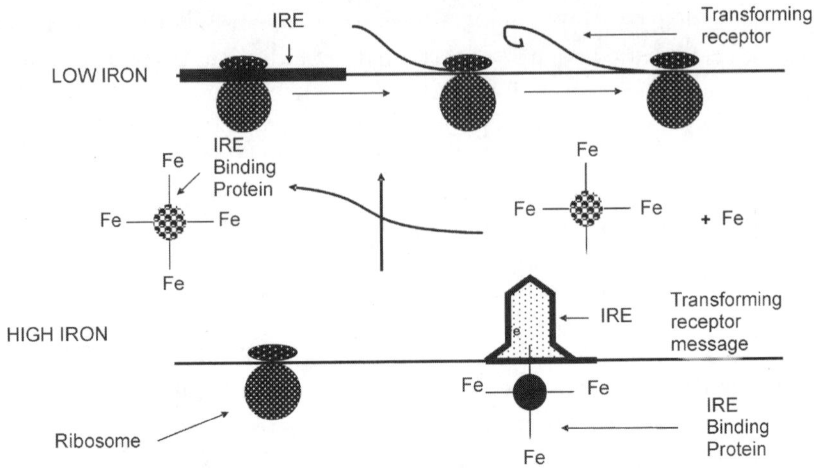


*23.7* Molecular regulation of iron metabolism. The synthesis of either ferritin or transferrin receptor depends on the iron status of the cell.

The type of translational regulation of the proteins depends on whether the IRE is present on the 5' or 3' end [17].

To understand the mechanism of such translational control, consider the following example. The ferritin mRNA has an IRE in the 5' end while the transferrin receptor mRNA has the IRE in the 3' end. The IRE–BPs can sense the level of iron in the cell. If the cells are iron depleted, the IRE–BPs bind to the IRE; but cannot bind to IRE if the cells are iron replete. Therefore, when the cells are depleted of iron, the IRE–BP binds to the 5' end of the ferritin transcript. This binding prevents the translation of the protein and prevents iron incorporation into ferritin, making iron available for cellular functions. However, when the IRE–BP binds to the 3' IRE of the transferrin receptor transcript, it actually prevents the transcript from being degraded. These results in increased protein synthesis for a longer time, enabling the cell to acquire more iron to fulfill its needs as there are more number of TfR molecules on the surface of the cell. Essentially, the reverse occurs when the cells are iron replete. IRE–BP cannot bind IRE under iron-replete conditions. Without IRE–BP binding, the ferritin mRNA is translated and the excess iron is incorporated into the newly synthesized ferritin. In the absence of IRE–BP binding, the TfR transcript is degraded and no more TfR is synthesized. Thus the cells cannot acquire anymore iron as there are less number of TfR molecules on the cell surface [17]. This phenomenon is called reciprocal regulation and is vital to maintain cellular concentrations of iron (Fig. 23.6). Cellular iron is tightly regulated as excess iron is toxic, capable of free-radical generation through Fenton chemistry.

Central to this reciprocal regulation is the fact that the IRE–BPs can sense cellular iron status. The mechanism by which they sense cellular iron is as follows. Recall that aconitase is an enzyme that assembles a 4[Fe-S] cluster and one iron atom is called a labile iron. When the cell is iron-deplete, aconitase loses the labile iron atom and subsequently loses the cluster too. Upon such cluster disassembly, the aconitase is converted to IRE–BP and is capable of binding to IRE. When the cells are iron replete, the iron–sulfur cluster is reassembled, cannot bind to IRE and the protein functions as aconitase. Thus the IRE–BP sense cellular iron levels and co-ordinate cellular iron acquisition and storage.

This mechanism of reciprocal regulation is operational in all cells in the body. We now consider the same in enterocytes and macrophages. Enterocytes acquire iron only through DMT-1 and the DMT-1 transcript has a 3' IRE, similar to that of TfR. Ferroportin on the other hand has a 5' IRE, thus enabling efflux of excess iron from enterocytes and macrophages.

The significance of this exquisite molecular control of cellular iron is evident when considered in the light of systemic iron homeostasis. Hepatocytes sense body iron concentrations through the transferrin-TfR system and produce ferritin in response to excess iron. Depending on various stimuli such as iron status, erythropoietic need, inflammatory status and Hb, hepatocytes synthesize and secrete hepcidin. Hepcidin in turn controls iron transfer from enterocytes and macrophages, thus controlling systemic iron homeostasis [3, 15, 16].

## 23.19 Assessment of iron status

Nutritional iron deficiency is commonly regarded as a state of insufficient iron supply to meet the need for functional iron after iron stores have been depleted. At the cellular level, iron deficiency can also result from insufficient release of storage iron despite sufficient iron stores, e.g. anemia of chronic disease. Physiologically, in iron deficiency there is a reduction in all iron-dependent functions, most importantly, the reduction in oxygen carrying capacity of hemoglobin and myoglobin resulting in lowered physical work capacity. Therefore, it is very important to understand the sequence of events leading to frank iron deficiency anemia. Various iron biomarkers are currently in use to define iron status [18–22].

## 23.20 Stages in the development of iron deficiency and iron status parameters

Three overlapping stages in the development of iron deficiency are defined, each of which is associated with certain abnormalities in the indicators of iron status (Table 23.2). The first stage, referred to as *deficient iron stores*, iron reserves are depleted although there is sufficient iron for erythropoiesis. This stage is recognized either by the absence of stainable iron on bone marrow examination or by a serum ferritin level below 12 μg/L. Serum ferritin is particularly valuable in nutritional surveys because of its high specificity. Quantitative phlebotomy studies have demonstrated that in normal adults, 1 μg/L serum ferritin is roughly equivalent to 10mg stored iron [18]. Expressed on a body weight basis, for a 50 kg adult, this is equivalent to 2.4 mg/kg body weight.

In the second stage of iron deficiency, referred to as *iron deficient erythropoiesis*, there is a curtailment in iron supply for erythropoiesis. As serum iron decreases and total iron binding capacity increases with iron deficiency, the most useful index is transferrin saturation, which is the ratio of serum iron to total iron binding capacity. Although transferrin saturation has been employed extensively in prevalence surveys, there are several limitations like susceptibility to iron contamination, diurnal variation and variations due to inflammation.

*Table 23.2* Diagnostic criteria for iron deficiency*

| Stages/ Parameter | Iron overload | Normal | Iron depletion | Iron deficient Erythropoiesis | Iron deficiency anemia |
|---|---|---|---|---|---|
| RE marrow Fe | 4+ | 2-3+ | 0-1+ | 0 | 0 |
| Serum ferritin (μg/L) | >300 | 100 ± 60 | 20 | 10 | <10 |
| Transferrin Saturation (%) | >60 | 35 ± 15 | 30 | <15 | <15 |
| RBC protoporphyrin (μg/dL) | 30 | 30 | 30 | 100 | 200 |
| TIBC (μg/dL) | <300 | 300 ± 30 | 360 | 390 | 410 |
| Serum iron (μg/dL) | >175 | 115 ± 50 | 115 | <60 | <40 |
| Serum transferrin Receptor (mg/dL) | Less than normal | 5.36± 0.82 | More than normal | 13.9±4.6 | Higher than iron deficient erythropoiesis |
| Erythrocyte Morphology | Normal | Normal | Normal | Normal | Microcytic/ hypochromic |
| Hematocrit cut-off value 0.35 (female) 0.40 (male) | Above cut-off | Above cut-off | Above cut-off | Above cut-off | Below cut-off |
| Hemoglobin (g/L) cut-off value 120 (female) 130 (male) | Above cut-off | Above cut-off | Above cut-off | Above cut-off | Below cut-off |

*A report of the INACG 1985, Nair et al 2004

Another laboratory measurement that can be used to detect iron deficient erythropoiesis is erythrocyte protoporphyrin. In contrast to the transferrin saturation, the erythrocyte protoporphyrin is a more stable index of marrow iron supply because elevation occurs only after several weeks of iron deprivation and the return to normal level is similarly slow following the start of iron therapy. One disadvantage of erythrocyte protoporphyrin, particularly in children, is that the level increases with lead poisoning.

Serum transferrin receptor (sTfR) is released from the cells into blood depending on the iron requirements after the stores have been exhausted. The concentration of sTfR is therefore increased in the second stage of iron deficiency. It is however less sensitive indicator than ferritin but more sensitive than Hb [22].

The third and final stage is *iron deficiency anemia.* This stage is characterized by a reduction in circulating hemoglobin high enough to be recognized as anemia. A decline in circulating hemoglobin equivalent to several hundred milligrams of iron is usually required before anemia can be identified clinically.

The optimal measurement or combination of measurements to detect iron deficiency anemia in a given situation depends on several factors. WHO/CDC have recommended that a combination of hemoglobin, serum ferritin, sTfR and indicator of infection such as c–reactive protein (CRP), be used as the best indicators to measure iron status [20].

## 23.21 Iron toxicity

A peculiar aspect of iron metabolism is the lack of a specific mechanism to eliminate excess iron. Excess iron, especially free iron, is toxic as it participates in free radical generation and the possible harmful consequences at the cellular level, have also been reported in numerous studies. It has been suggested that it is the difference in levels of stored excess iron that accounts for the gender difference observed in the mortality statistics of ischemic heart disease in developed countries. An epidemiologic study carried out in Finnish men showed a 2.2-fold increased incidence of acute myocardial infarction during the 3-year follow-up in men whose serum ferritin levels were high (>200 μg/L) at the beginning of the study. The authors hypothesized that free radicals induced by free iron caused increased peroxidation of low density lipoprotein and thereby contributed to atherogenesis. It was also observed in experimental studies that men who had higher levels of transferrin saturation had a greater incidence of cancer mortality. However, this type of relation was not observed in females [23].

Iron deficiency is also equally potent in promoting carcinogenesis in animal models. The iron deficient intestine is also susceptible to iron-mediated oxidative damage. Iron could also enhance oxidative stress by interfering with antioxidant system components of the intestine during repletion with high doses of iron. However, when preconditioned with a combination of antioxidant vitamins C and E or simultaneous administration of zinc, almost all the intestinal oxidative stress is reduced. Therefore, daily administration of therapeutic doses of iron should be accompanied by foods rich in these vitamins or minerals [24, 26].

## 23.22 Folic acid

Folic acid is chemically, pteroyl glutamate, consisting of a pteridine ring attached to *p*-aminobenzoic acid and glutamic acid. Mammals cannot synthesize *p*-aminobenzoic acid or attach glutamic acid to aminobenzoic acid and therefore depend on folic acid derived from microbial and plant sources.

## 23.23 Chemistry

Folate is the generic term for compounds that have vitamin activity similar to that of pteroylglutamic acid, are anti-anemic and growth factors. Folates may have one or more glutamic acid residues (polyglutamates, $PteGlu_n$) and exist in many chemical forms. Naturally occurring folates, called food folate and referred to as $PteGlu_n$, are present both in animal and plant foods. The naturally occurring forms, namely dihydrofolates ($H_2$) and tetrahydrofolates ($H_4$) are reduced forms of folate. Tetrahydrofolate is the biologically active molecule and can carry various one-carbon units, which include 5-formyltetrahydrofolate, 10-formyl-tetrahydrofolate, 5-methyl-tetrahydrofolate, 5.10-methenyl-tetrahydrofolate, 5.10-methylene-tetrahydrofolate (MTHF) and formimino-tetrahydrofolate (Figure 23.8). Normally, only trace amounts are found in human tissues. Intracellular folates generally are $PteGlu_7$

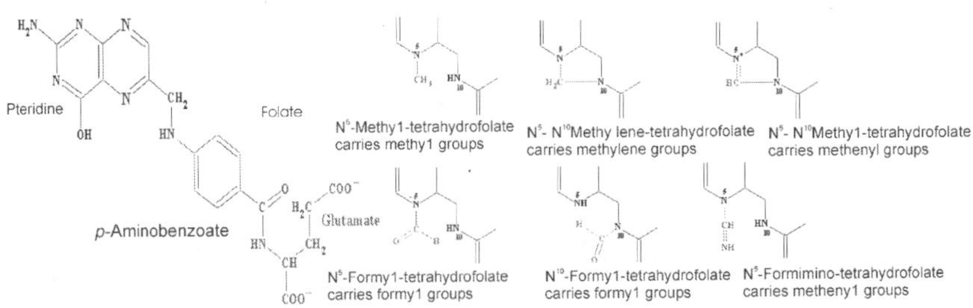


*23.8* Structure of tetrahydrofolate and conversion of one carbon units attached.

or $PteGlu_{11}$. In contrast, extracellular folates are monoglutamates. The basic folate compound, $PteGlu_1$, is used therapeutically because of its stability [5, 6, 27].

## 23.24 Dietary sources and recommended intake

Organ meats such as liver and egg yolk are good sources of folate and in the vegetarian context the major sources are whole grain cereals, legumes and green leafy vegetables. The recommended dietary allowance (RDA) of folic acid as folate equivalent for Indian adults is 200 μg/day. The intake of folate based on NNMB diet survey shows more than 60% of Indians obtain folate nutrition from cereals and pulses (Figure 23.9) [28].

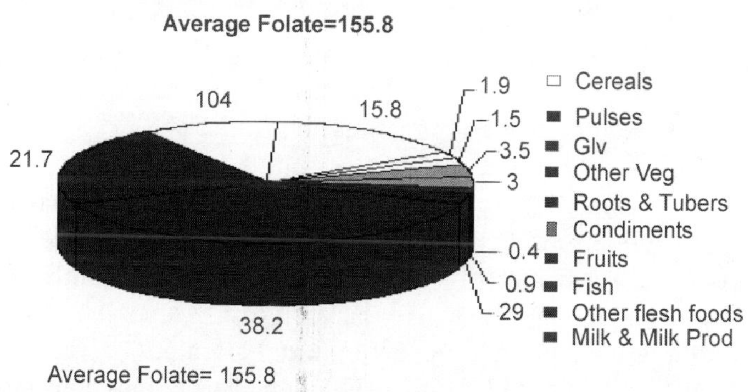


*23.9* Folic acid distribution from different Indian food stuffs ( g/CU) [19].

## 23.25 Availability of food folate

All naturally occurring folates are unstable to varying degrees, due to the presence of an endogenous enzyme, pteroylpolyglutamyl hydrolase, which removes glutamic acid residues but leaves an active compound, $PteGlu_1$. Heat, oxidation and ultraviolet light cleave the folate molecule, rendering it inactive. Reducing agents in food such as ascorbic acid provide greater stability to the vitamin. Germination, however, increases food folate availability. Information on the availability of food folate is fragmentary. Folate availability generally varies widely among foods with maximum availability found in egg yolk (72.2%) followed by cow's liver (55.7%) and low availability from vegetables (3–6%). The absorption of folate from foods varies from 25% to 70%. Synthetic folic acid is considered to be more bioavailable than natural folate. The bioavailability of folic acid supplements under fasting conditions is close to 100% [28–30].

Currently, there are many accurate methods of estimating the food folate level and their bioavailability. Folate content is expressed in terms of dietary folate equivalent (DFE) and is the amount derived after complete hydrolysis of food folate [31]. The term "free" folate has been used to designate the forms measurable by its ability to support the growth of a folate-dependent organism, *Lactobacillus casei,* without hydrolysis [14].

## 23.26 Food folate – digestion and absorption

Dietary folates, most of which are $PteGlu_n$ derivatives, undergo hydrolysis in the gut to $PteGlu_1$ before absorption across the intestinal mucosa. An intestinal enzyme known as folate conjugase (glutamate carboxypeptidase) found in the brush border, catalyses this rate limiting step in the process of luminal digestion of $PteGlu_n$. This enzyme is an exopeptidase and is activated by zinc. A second enzyme, an intracellular hydrolase, is found in the lysosomes of intestinal cells, has a pH optimum of 4.5 and is an endopeptidase. The function of this enzyme is still unknown.

Reduced $PteGlu_1$ are better absorbed (88–98 percent) than PteGlu(n) as the former are less acidic comparatively. In the absence of protecting agents such as ascorbic acid and reduced thiols, many labile folates may be lost during residence in the acid peptic milieu of the stomach. Other food constituents also affect action of the intestinal hydrolases.

The intestinal absorption of folate, as $PteGlu_1$, predominantly occurs in the duodenum and jejunum by active transport in a saturable, pH-dependent process. Monoglutamates are present in portal circulation, which is taken by the liver and converted to polyglutamate derivatives and stored or released into the blood. In plasma, methyltetrahydrofolate (MTHF) is bound to albumin, but about $1/3^{rd}$ circulates unbound.

Cellular transport of folate is mediated through a number of different folate transport systems. Most of them use the folate receptor or the folate carrier protein. Intracellular transport into organelles is only poorly understood, although it is known to be saturable [28–30].

## 23.27 Functions

Many vital steps in nucleic acid metabolism involve the addition of one carbon building blocks. Folate acts as a co-enzyme in several single carbon transfers in the biosynthesis of purine and pyrimidine nucleotides. These one carbon units are derived from the breakdown of serine and glycine and carried by the coenzyme tetrahydrofolate in different chemical forms. Each of these forms participates in different biochemical reactions. 10-formyl THF and 5,10-methylene THF donate the C2 and C8 carbons of purines, respectively. 5,10-methylene THF is also the cofactor for thymidylate synthase which methylates the uracil base (UMP, uracil monophosphate) of RNA to thymidine (dTMP, thymidine monophosphate) of DNA (Figure 23.9). It is for this reason that rapidly growing and multiplying cells require an adequate supply of folate. Folate deficiency therefore diminishes and compromises the cell's ability to synthesize these nucleic acids, resulting in decreased cell division. This effect is most pronounced in the rapidly dividing cells of the bone marrow which are RBC precursors, thus causing megaloblastic anemia [33].

The one carbon fragments can be oxidized and reduced while bound to the coenzyme and inserted into the receiving molecules as formyl groups (most oxidized), hydroxymethyl or methyl groups (most reduced). The immediate methyl-group donor in most reactions is S-adenosyl methionine and S-adenosyl homocysteine is the end product. This homocysteine (Hcy) is converted back to methionine through a series of reactions that requires methyl-THF as the one-carbon donor. Methyl-THF is formed by the reduction of 5,10- methylene-THF and is an irreversible process (Figure 23.8). The enzyme that catalyzes the conversion of homocysteine to methionine (methylation of Hcy) is methionine synthase. This enzyme requires $B_{12}$ as a cofactor and $B_{12}$ deficiency drastically reduces the activity of this enzyme. During this reaction, tetrahydrofolate, the biologically active form of folate, is regenerated from $N^5$-methyl-tetrahydrofolate. In the absence of this reaction, all the tetrahydrofolate will eventually end up trapped as $N^5$-methyl-tetrahydrofolate, as $N^5$-methyl-THF has no other biological fate. Thus a primary vitamin $B_{12}$ deficiency leads to a secondary folate deficiency. This phenomenon is called the folate trap [5, 6, 8, 33].

## 23.28 Folic acid and anemia

Folic acid deficiency reduces the capacity of proliferating cells to make dTMP thus inhibiting cell division. This effect is most pronounced in the rapidly dividing erythroid precursor cells in the bone marrow leading to cells being larger than normal. Macrocytosis (increased size) of RBCs ensues resulting in increased MCV (mean corpuscular volume) and progresses to decrease in Hb and PCV (packed cell volume). Generally, no change in MCHC (mean corpuscular Hb concentration; Hb/PCV) is observed as both Hb and PCV decrease. This condition is called megaloblastic anaemia. Where iron deficiency is the central problem, the restoration of adequate iron nutriture rapidly replenishes normal red cell mass. As the requirements for synthesis of a new deoxynucleic acid base for rapid cell proliferation place additional demands for folic acid, iron supplements have conventionally been combined with an adjunctive dosage of folic acid [12, 31–32].

Pernicious anaemia, due to primary deficiency of vitamin $B_{12}$, leads to secondary deficiency of folic acid because all the folate ends up trapped as $N^5$-methyl-tetrahydrofolate (folate trap, explained above).

During pregnancy, given the increase in blood volume and growth of the foetus, both of which require rapid cell division, folate deficiency has serious consequences. During early pregnancy folic acid is required for the closure of the neural tube which occurs around the 28th day of pregnancy. Incidence of neural tube defects (spina bifida and anencephaly) is reduced by 400 μg folic acid supplement/day before conception and during the first month of pregnancy [10, 31, 34].

## 23.29 Assessment of folate status

Biochemical assessment of folate nutritional status is most commonly done by measuring serum and RBC folate levels. Serum folate essentially reflects recent intake and red cell levels represent long-term tissue stores. It is generally accepted that serum folate above 14 nmol/L (6 ng/mL) or RBC folate above 360 nmol/L (159 ng/mL) are considered satisfactory; those between 7 and 14 nmol/L (3–6 ng/mL) serum folate and 320–360 nmol/L (141–159 ng/mL) RBC folate are considered to be low and suggestive of risk. Values lower than these indicate clear deficiency of folate. Normal body stores are estimated as 5–10 mg, half of which is in the liver. The turnover rate is estimated to be less than 1% per day [36]. The measurement of plasma concentrations of homocysteine is shown to be a good indicator of folate status. A striking negative correlation between serum folate and protein bound homocysteine is reported [35].

## 23.30 Vitamin $B_{12}$

Vitamin $B_{12}$ (Cobalamin) has been a challenging problem in biochemistry and medicine since the discovery by George Minot and William Murphy in 1926 that pernicious anemia can be treated by feeding the patient large amounts of liver. Cobalamin was first purified in 1948 and crystallized by Dorothy Hodgkin, who elucidated its complex three-dimensional structure in 1956 [5].

## 23.31 Chemistry

The core of cobalamin or vitamin $B_{12}$ consists of a corrin ring with a central cobalt atom (Figure 23.10). The corrin ring has four pyrrole rings and is similar to the porphyrin ring. The cobalt atom is bonded to the four pyrrole nitrogen atoms. The fifth substituent is a derivative of dimethylbenzimidazole that contains ribose 3-phosphate and aminoisopropanol. One of the nitrogen atoms of dimethylbenzimidazole is linked to cobalt. The sixth substituent of Co atom can be $-CH_3$, $OH^-$ or 5' deoxyadenosyl unit. The cobalt ion can be in the +1, +2 or +3 oxidation states. In the +1 oxidation state, it forms the coenzyme $B_{12}$ molecule which is the only biological compound known to have a carbon-metal bond [5].

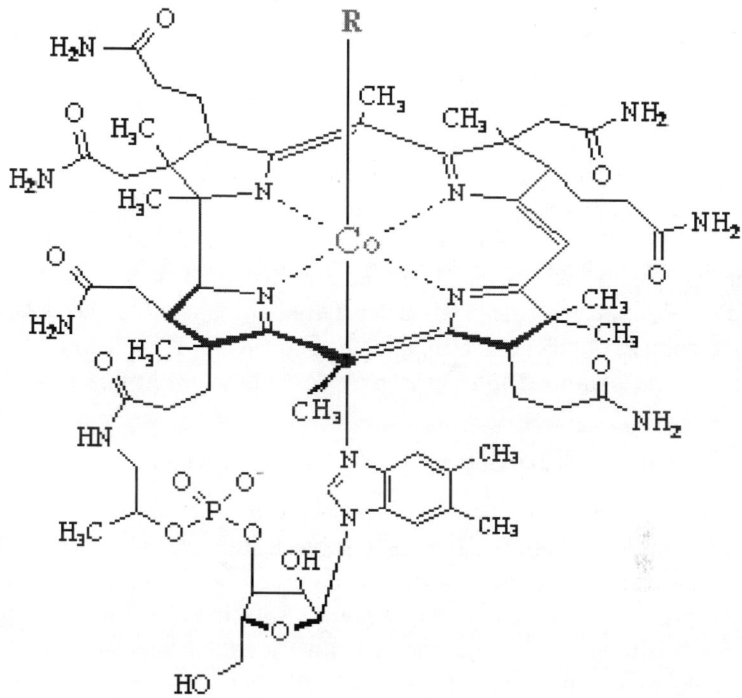


*23.10* Structure of vitamin $B_{12}$.

## 23.32 Dietary sources and recommended intake

All higher animals require the vitamin in their diet and cereals, vegetables and fruits do not contain measurable amounts of the vitamin unless "contaminated" by soil or water containing vitamin $B_{12}$. In nature, vitamin $B_{12}$ is largely produced by bacteria, fungi and algae. Animals get it from their natural gut bacterial flora or by eating other animals. Therefore, foods of animal origin (including meat, liver, fish, milk, milk products and eggs) constitute the main dietary source for humans. Vegetarians are at risk of $B_{12}$ deficiency unless they consume large quantities of fermented foods. The recommended dietary intake is 1.0 µg/day [10, 31, 35, 37].

## 23.33 Absorption and transport

Much of the vitamin $B_{12}$ in food is present in bound form and must be released by cooking or acid-peptic and/or tryptic digestion before it is available for absorption. The free vitamin then binds with salivary haptocorrin. Intrinsic factor (IF), a mucoprotein like substance present in gastric juices is essential for the utilization of vitamin $B_{12}$. The haptocorrin-$B_{12}$ complex is digested by proteases and the released vitamin $B_{12}$ combines with the intrinsic factor. The intrinsic factor-vitamin $B_{12}$ complex attaches to receptors in the ileal enterocyte is internalized and subsequently dissociated. The released vitamin $B_{12}$ binds to a specific $B_{12}$ binding protein called transcobolamin (TC II) and is actively transported across the ileal basolateral membrane into the bloodstream [35].

When a physiological dose of radioactive cyanocobalamin is given orally, normal people absorb a mean 72% of 0.5 μ dose or 56 percent of a 1 μg dose. Since the absolute amount absorbed depends on the amount of intrinsic factor and the number of receptors available, the percent absorbed decreases as the amount of the vitamin administered increases within the physiological range.

## 23.34 Bioavailability of dietary vitamin $B_{12}$

There is relatively little information on the bioavailability of different dietary forms of vitamin $B_{12}$. In normal subjects, the vitamin in liver, mutton and chicken appears to be absorbed as completely as a similar amount of cyanocobalamin administered in aqueous solution. On the other hand, vitamin $B_{12}$ in eggs or crystalline vitamin $B_{12}$ added to eggs is relatively poorly absorbed. The nature of the inhibitory factor(s) in eggs is not known. There is some evidence that the vitamin $B_{12}$ in food may not be as readily available to individuals with decreased gastric acid secretion (without pernicious anemia) as it is to normal subjects [35].

## 23.35 Body content

Vitamin $B_{12}$ is stored mainly in the liver in amounts (in omnivorous about 3–5 mg) sufficient to last a couple of years.

In humans, the liver contains up to 80 percent of the body's total store of vitamin $B_{12}$. At birth, the full-term infant has 25–30 μg of the vitamin which is stored in the liver. As the individual grows, vitamin $B_{12}$ is accumulated and in vegetarians the body content is much lower compared to omnivorous adults [10, 31].

## 23.36 Dietary deficiency of vitamin $B_{12}$

Dietary deficiency is a widespread problem in the Indian subcontinent due to vegetarian diet. Infants born to vitamin $B_{12}$ deficient vegan mothers are at high risk of developing the deficiency [37].

## 23.37 Malabsorption of vitamin $B_{12}$

Pernicious anemia (PA) is a specific autoimmune disease occurring with increasing age or when antibodies are formed in either the parietal cells or to gastric intrinsic factor or both.

## 23.38 Biochemical function

Vitamin $B_{12}$ is required for the recycling of a critical nucleotide base (deoxythymidine) essential for the rapid synthesis of DNA during cell replication. Hence it is indispensable for the proliferation of all of the hematological cell lines in bone marrow, especially the precursors of the myeloid lineage. The absence of vitamin $B_{12}$ allows these cells to enlarge, but not divide into generations of daughter cells, leading to hypo-proliferative anemia with giant, immature, macrocytic red cells in the circulation.

Vitamin $B_{12}$ is a cofactor for three enzymes, viz. methylmalonyl CoA mutase, leucine aminomutase and methionine synthase. Methylmalonyl CoA is an intermediate in valine catabolism and is produced upon carboxylation of propionyl CoA during the catabolism of isoleucine and cholesterol. Methylmalonyl CoA undergoes a rearrangement to succinyl CoA so as to enter the normal metabolic pathways. This rearrangement is catalyzed by methylmalonyl CoA mutase whose activity is greatly diminished during $B_{12}$ deficiency. This leads to an accumulation of methylmalonyl CoA which is reflected as increased serum and urine methylmalonyl CoA [35].

Methionine synthase causally links the biochemical basis of megaloblastic anemia of folate and vitamin $B_{12}$ deficiencies (Fig. 23.11). As mentioned previously, 5,10-MTHF is a cofactor for the very important enzyme, thymidylate synthase, and is responsible for the conversion of the uracil type base found in RNA to the thymine type base which is characteristic of DNA. The reduced rate of cell division results in nuclei that are larger and more poorly differentiated than normal. Identical megaloblastic anemia occurs in vitamin $B_{12}$ deficiency. The biochemical basis for this is as follows. Recall the folate trap phenomenon explained earlier. Methionine synthase uses the folate cofactor $N^5$-methyl-tetrahydrofolate ($N^5$-M-THF) as part of the methylation cycle. The enzyme that synthesizes $N^5$-MTHF from $N^{5,10}$-methylene tetrahydrofolate, $N^{5,10}$- methlyene tetrahydrofolate reductase (MTHFR) is known to be irreversible. Methionine synthase, during methylation of homocysteine, converts $N^5$-MTHF to THF and requires vitamin $B_{12}$ (Fig. 23.11). The activity of this enzyme is severely compromised in vitamin $B_{12}$ deficiency, thus leading to all folate accumulating as 5MTHF. This creates a pseudo folate deficiency with similar clinical manifestations. As methionine synthase is inhibited, homocysteine accumulates which is reflected as increased serum homocysteine [5, 6, 8].

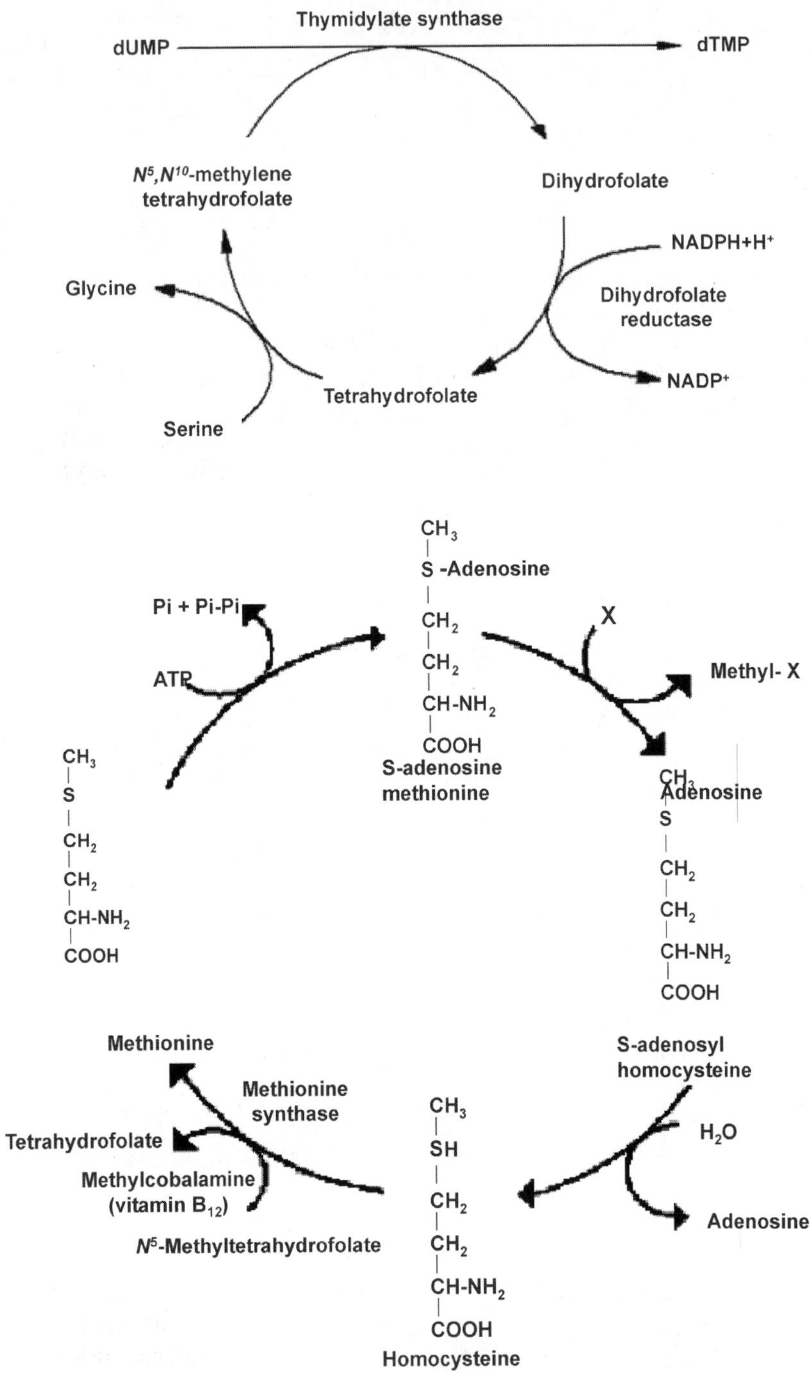


*23.11* Interrelationship between folic acid and vitamin $B_{12}$ .

Due to the above explained metabolic relationship, a moderately high intake of folic acid is not toxic but might mask an underlying vitamin $B_{12}$ deficiency that only becomes apparent once the irreversible neurological disorders set in. Folate and vitamins $B_6$ and $B_{12}$ are essential components in the metabolism of homocysteine, which occurs through remethylation to methionine or trans-sulfuration to cysteine [6].

## 23.39 Neurological manifestations

Vitamin $B_{12}$ deficiency leads to demyelination of CNS fibers. Peripheral nerves also show axonal degradation without demyelination. The biochemical basis for this is unknown but is attributed to decreased activity of methionine synthase. The myelin sheath is a continually regenerating tissue which would require a continuous supply of methionine. The fully developed neuropathy of $B_{12}$ deficiency is called subacute combined degeneration; however, not all $B_{12}$ deficiency presents with neuropathy. On a similar note, it would be expected that folate deficiency would also lead to neuropathy but it is not so as the nervous system preferentially accumulates folates [38].

## 23.40 Assessment of vitamin $B_{12}$ status

Serum vitamin $B_{12}$ level is a specific test for deficiency. Serum vitamin $B_{12}$ should possibly be considered a screening test, with high levels ruling out a vitamin $B_{12}$ deficiency, levels between 150 and 350 pmol/L (203–473 pg/mL) requiring confirmation, and levels lower than 150 pmol/L (200 pg/mL) probably not needing confirmation. Serum vitamin $B_{12}$ levels decline 18–28 pmol/L (24–38 pg/mL) annually in a normal elderly. There may be a marked increase in MCV (normal = 80–96 fL) to 110–140 fL, with no change in MCHC. Serum methylmalonic acid (MMA) and serum homocysteine are two valuable markers for vitamin $B_{12}$ deficiency as these are only two biochemical pathways that utilize this vitamin in humans. Homocysteine and a 24-hour urine collection for testing MMA can also be performed. Serum levels for homocysteine and MMA may be more specific, elevated levels of MMA are accurate as an indicator for cobalamin deficiency. Therefore if both homocysteine and MMA levels are elevated and the serum vitamin $B_{12}$ is low or borderline, vitamin $B_{12}$ deficiency exists. If the homocysteine level is the only elevated metabolite and the red blood cell folate level is not low, vitamin $B_{12}$ deficiency also may be indicated. Since elevated levels of homocysteine may also indicate a folic acid deficiency, red blood cell folate levels should be determined before vitamin $B_{12}$ replacement is begun. It is important to ensure there is no vitamin $B_{12}$ deficiency before starting folic acid replacement, as this therapy may worsen the associated neurologic symptoms [32, 37, 39].

## References


1. BEARD JL, DAWSON H, PINERO DJ (1996). Iron metabolism: A comprehensive review. *Nutrition Reviews*, **54**, pp. 295–317.
2. BOTHWELL TH, CHARLTON RW, COOK JD, FINCH CA (1979). *Iron Metabolism in Man.* Oxford, Blackwell Scientific Publications.
3. FLEMING RE and BACON BR (2005). Orchestration of Iron Homeostasis. *New Engl J. Med*, **352**, pp. 1741–44.
4. ANDREWS NC (1999). Disorders of iron metabolism. *New Engl J. Med,* **341**, pp. 1986–1995.
5. BERG JM, TYMOCZKO JL and STRYER L (eds.) (2007). *Biochemistry*. Sixth Edition, W.H. Freeman and Company, New York.
6. BOHNSACK BL and HIRSCHI KK (2004). Nutrient regulation of cell cycle progression. *Annu. Rev. Nutr.* **24**, pp. 433–453.
7. HALLBERG L and ASP NG (1996). *Iron Nutrition in Health and Disease*, John Libbey & Company, England.
8. MURRARY RK, GRANNER DK, MAYES PA, RODWELL VW (eds.) (2003). *Harper's Illustrated Biochemistry*, Twenty sixth Edition, McGraw-Hill, International Edition.
9. DOMENICO ID, WARD DM and KAPLAN J (2008). Regulation of iron acquisition and stotage: consequences for iron-linked disorders. *Nature*, **9**, pp. 72–81.
10. Nutrient Requirements and Recommended Dietary Allowances for Indians (A report of the Expert Group, 2009 Draft document), National Institute of Nutrition, Indian Council of Medical Research, Hyderabad.
11. RAO BSN (1981). Physiology of iron absorption and supplementation. *Brit Med Bull,* **37**, pp. 25–30.
12. KRAEMER K and ZIMMERMANN M (eds.) (2007), *Nutritional Anemia,* Sight and Life Press, Basel, Switzerland.
13. NAIR KM and IYENGAR V (2009). Iron content, bioavailability and factors affecting iron status of Indians. *Indian J. Med Res*, **130**, pp. 634–645.
14. Nutrient requirements and recommended dietary allowances for Indians (1990). A report of the expert group of the ICMR. New Delhi: Indian Council of Medical Research.
15. KEMNA EHJM, TJALSMA H, WILLEMA HL, SWINKELS D (2008). Hepcidin: from discovery to differential diagnosis. *Haematologica*, **93**, pp. 90–97.
16. NEMETH E and CANZ T (2006). Regulation of iron metabolism by hepcidin. *Annu Rev Nutr.* **26**, pp. 323–342.
17. MUEKENTHALER MU, GALY B and HENTZE MW (2008). Systemic iron homeostasis and the iron responsive element/iron regulatory protein (IRE/IRP) regulatory net work. *Annu. Rev. Nutr.* **28**, pp. 197–213.
18. Measurement of iron status (1985). A report of the International Nutritional Anemia Consultative Group. INACG Secretariat, The Nutrition Foundation, Inc. Washington.
19. WHO (2001). Iron Deficiency Anaemia Assessment, Prevention and Control — A guide for programme managers.
20. Joint WHO/CDC technical consultation on assessment of iron status at population level. Geneva, 2004, April 6–8.
21. SIVAKUMAR B and NAIR KM (1997). An appraisal of the iron status indicators. *ICMR Bulletin*. **27**(10).
22. NAIR KM, BHASKARAM P, BALAKRISHNA N, RAVINDER P, SESIKERAN B (2004). Response

of hemoglobin, serum ferritin and serum transferrin receptor during iron supplementation in pregnancy. *Nutrition*, **20**, pp. 896–899.

23. STEVENS RG, JONES DY, MICOZZI MS, TAYLOR PR (1988). Body iron stores and the risk of cancer. *New Engl J. Med,* **319**, pp. 1047–1052. Joint WHO/CDC technical consultation on assessment of iron status at population level. Geneva, 2004, April 6–8.
24. NAIR KM (2001). Alternate strategies for improving iron nutrition: lessons from recent research. *Brit J. Nutr,* **85** (Suppl 2), p. S187.
25. SRIGIRIDHAR K and NAIR KM (2000). Supplementation with alpha-tocopherol or a combination of alpha-tocopherol and ascorbic acid protects the gastrointestinal tract of iron deficient rats against iron induced oxidative damage during iron repletion. *Brit J Nutr*, **84**, pp. 165–173.
26. SREEDHAR B, NAIR KM (2007). Concurrent repletion of iron and zinc reduces intestinal oxidative damage in iron-and zinc-deficient rats. *World J Gastroentrol,* **13**(43), pp. 5707–5717.
27. COSSINS EA (1984). Folates in biological materials. In: *Folates and Pterins.* Blakley R.L, Benkovic, (ed.), New York: John Wiley and Sons Inc., **1**, pp. 1–60.
28. KRISHNASWAMY K and NAIR KM (2001). Importance of folate in human nutrition. *Brit J. Nutr,* **85**(2), p. S115.
29. PRINZ-LANGENOHL R, BRÖNSTRUP A, THORAND B, HAGES M, PIETRZIK K (1999). Availability of food folate in humans. *J. Nutr*, **129**, pp. 913–916.
30. GREGORY JF (1997). Bioavailability of folate. *Eur J. Clin Nutr*, 1997; 51: S54–S59.
31. WHO/FAO. Vitamin and mineral requirements in human nutrition, 2nd Edition, WHO, Geneva, 2004.
32. SELHUB J, MORRIS MS, JACQUES PF and ROSENBERG RH. Folate–vitamin B-12 interaction in relation to cognitive impairment, anemia, and biochemical indicators of vitamin $B_{12}$ deficiency. Am J Clin Nutr 89: 702S–706S, 2009.
33. KOURY MJ and PONKA P. New insight into erythropoiesis: Roles of folate, vitamin $B_{12}$, and iron. Annu. Rev. Nutr. 2004; 24: 105–131.
34. CUSKELLY GJ, MCNUTTY H and SCOTT JM (1996). Effect of increasing dietary folate on red cell folate: implications for prevention of neural tube defects. *Lancet*, **347**, 657–659.
35. BOWMAN BA, RUSSELL RM. (eds.) (2006). Present knowledge in nutrition. International Life Sciences Institute, ILSI Press, Washington, D.C.
36. KANG SS, WONG PWK and NORUSIS M (1987). Homocysteinemia due to folate deficiency. *Metabolism*, **36**, pp. 458–462.
37. STABLER SP and ALLEN RH (2004). Vitamin $B_{12}$ deficiency as a world problem. *Annu Rev Nutr*, **24**, pp. 299–326.
38. DAWSON DN and WATERS HM (1994). Malnutrition: folate and cobalamin deficiency. *Brit J. Biomed Sci*, **51**, pp. 221–227.
39. QUINLIVAN EP et al. (2002). Importance of both folic acid and vitamin $B_{12}$ in reduction of risk of vascular disease. *The Lancet*, **359**, January 19, 2002, pp. 227–28 (research letter).

# 24

# Iron deficiency and iron deficiency anemia in young children

*Sheila C. Vir* and *Prakash V. Kotecha*

**Sheila C Vir,** MSc, PhD, is a senior nutrition consultant and Director of Public Health Nutrition and Development Centre, New Delhi. Following MSc (Food and Nutrition) from University of Delhi, Dr Vir was awarded PhD by the Queen's University of Belfast, United Kingdom. Dr. Vir, a past secretary of the Nutrition Society of India, is a recipient of the fellowship of the Department of Health and Social Services, UK, and Commonwealth Van den Bergh Nutrition Award. Dr Vir worked briefly with the Aga Khan Foundation (India) and later with UNICEF. As a Nutrition Programme Officer with UNICEF for twenty years, Dr. Vir provided strategic and technical leadership for policy formulation and implementation of nutrition programmes in India.

**Prakash V. Kotecha**, MD, is country representative with A2Z, the USAID Micronutrient Project. Prior to joining USAID, he was the Professor and the Head of Department of Community Medicine at Medical College Vadodara India for over ten years. Besides MD degree in Community Medicine, he has a diploma in Public Health from M.S. University of Baroda and Masters Degree in Community Health from London School of Hygiene and Tropical Medicine, London University, United Kingdom.

## 24.1 Iron deficiency and iron deficiency anemia in young children

### 24.1.1 Prevalence of iron deficiency and iron deficiency anemia in young children

Deficiency of iron is the most common nutrition disorder in the world [1, 2]. In public health terms, iron deficiency is the primary cause of nutritional anemia worldwide. Folic acid deficiency is less widely spread and is in fact observed often along with iron deficiency. Vitamin $B_{12}$ deficiency is comparatively uncommon. From the public health point of view, prevalence of anemia is taken as a proxy indicator for iron deficiency. It is estimated that when prevalence of iron deficiency anemia of 40% is reported, the prevalence of iron deficiency will be around 100% (Figure 24.1) and when anemia prevalence is 20% iron deficiency is estimated to exist in 50% of the population [3].

The prevalence of anemia as a public health problem is categorized as follows: <5% no public health problem, 5.0–19.9% mild public health problem, 20–39.9% moderate public health problem, ≥40% severe public health problem [3]. Table 24.1 presents an overview of the situation of anemia as a public health problem in WHO member states. In 69 of the 192 countries, anemia is a severe public health problem. Only two countries with a low prevalence of anemia are excluded from the public health problem category [4].

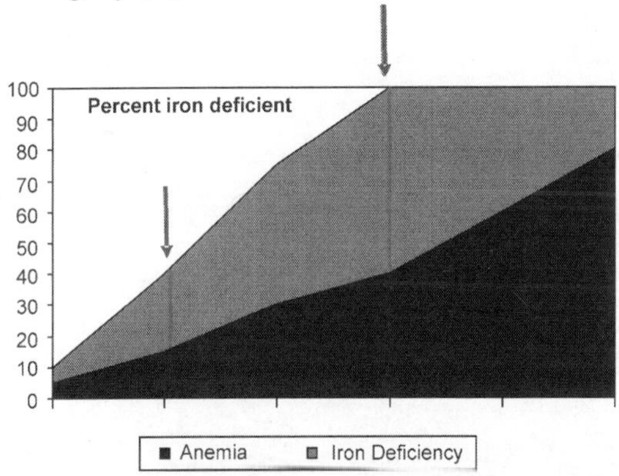


*24.1* Prevalence of iron deficiency based on prevalence of iron deficiency anemia [3]

*Table 24.1* Anaemia as a public health problem[(a)] in WHO member states [4]

| *Level of public health problem* | *Pre-SAC[(b)] Number of countries* | *Pre-SAC[(b)] Total population 1000s (%)[(c)]* | *PW Number of countries* | *PW Total population 1000s (%)* | *NPW Number of countries* | *NPW Total population 1000s (%)* |
|---|---|---|---|---|---|---|
| None | 2 | 20570 (3.3) | 0 | 0 (0.0) | 1 | 4171 (0.3) |
| Mild | 40 | 40921 (6.6) | 33 | 11156 (8.3) | 59 | 647857 (41.7) |
| Moderate | 81 | 208472 (33.7) | 91 | 46162 (34.2) | 78 | 441285 (28.4) |
| Severe | 69 | 348322 (56.3) | 68 | 77466 (57.5) | 54 | 459518 (29.6) |
| | 192 | 618285 | 192 | 134783 | 192 | 1552831 |

(a) The prevalence of anemia as a public health problem is categorized as follows: <5%, no public health problem; 5.0–19.9%, mild public health problem; 20–29.9%, moderate public health problem; ≥40%, severe public health problem.

(b) Population groups: pre-SAC, pre-school aged children (0.00–4.99 years); PW, pregnant women (no age range defined); NPW, non-pregnant women (15.00–49.99 years)

(c) This is the percentage of pre-school-aged children who live in countries where anemia presents this level of a public health problem.

An analysis of anemia status region wise of WHO member countries, representing 99.8% of global population, reveals that 47.4% preschool children or 293.1 million preschool child population are anemic [4]. Table 24.2 presents the region-wise situation of anemia. Asia, with 170 million anemic children, has the largest number of anemic pre-school children.

*Table 24.2* Anemia in pre-school-aged children, pregnant women and non-pregnant women globally and by region [4]

| *Area* | *Pre-SAC*[a] | | *PW* | | *NPW* | |
|---|---|---|---|---|---|---|
| | *Prevalence (%)*[c] | *Number affected (millions)* | *Prevalence (%)*[c] | *Number affected (millions)* | *Prevalence (%)*[c] | *Number affected (millions)* |
| Global | 47.4 (45.7–49.1) | 293.1 (282.8–303.5) | 41.8 (39.9–43.8) | 56.4 (53.8–59.1) | 30.2 (28.7–31.6) | 468.4 (446.2–490.6) |
| UN region[b] | | | | | | |
| Africa | 64.6 (61.7–67.5) | 93.2 (89.1–97.4) | 55.8 (51.9–59.6) | 19.3 (18.0–20.7) | 44.4 (40.9–47.8) | 82.9 (76.5–89.4) |
| Asia | 47.7 (45.2–50.3) | 170.0 (161.0–178.9) | 41.6 (39.0–44.2) | 31.7 (29.7–33.6) | 33.0 (31.3–34.7) | 318.3 (302.0–334.6) |
| Europe | 16.7 (10.5–23.0) | 6.1 (3.8–8.4) | 18.7 (12.3–25.1) | 1.4 (0.9–1.8) | 15.2 (10.5–19.9) | 26.6 (18.4–34.9) |
| LAC | 39.5 (36.0–43.0) | 22.3 (20.3–24.3) | 31.1 (21.8–40.4) | 3.6 (2.5–4.7) | 23.5 (15.9–31.0) | 33.0 (22.4–43.6) |
| NA | 3.4 (2.0–4.9) | 0.8 (0.4–1.1) | 6.1 (3.4–8.8) | 0.3 (0.2–0.4) | 7.6 (5.9–9.4) | 6.0 (4.6–7.3) |
| Oceania | 28.0 (15.8–40.2) | 0.7 (0.4–1.0) | 30.4 (17.0–43.9) | 0.2 (0.1–0.2) | 20.2 (9.5–30.9) | 1.5 (0.7–2.4) |

(a) Population groups: pre-SAC, pre-school-aged children (0.00–4.99 years); PW, pregnant women (no age range defined); NPW, non-pregnant women (15.00–49.99 years)

(b) WHO member states are stratified by United Nations regions: Africa, Asia, Europe, Latin America and Caribbean (LAC), North America (NA), and Oceania

(c) 95% CI

In terms of percentage of anemia in various regions of the world, Africa has the largest percentage prevalence of anemia in the pre-school-age group. In fact the percentage prevalence of anemia is higher in pre-school children as compared to pregnant and non-pregnant women in all the regions except Europe and Oceana. On the basis of data profile of vulnerable groups (Table 24.2), it has been proposed that figures for the prevalence of anemia in infants and for very young children in a region is often very similar to those among pregnant mothers when precise data is not available [5]. These surveys provide information only on anemia but iron deficiency is presumed to be the main cause of anemia.

A link between anemia prevalence and stage of country's development is evident [6, 7] when anemia prevalence rate of developing and developed countries is compared. Pre-school children in developing country are at a much higher disadvantage than in the developed world (Figure 24.2).

Within the pre-school-age group, iron deficiency and anemia prevalence in children 6–24 months of age is higher than in over two years. This is attributed

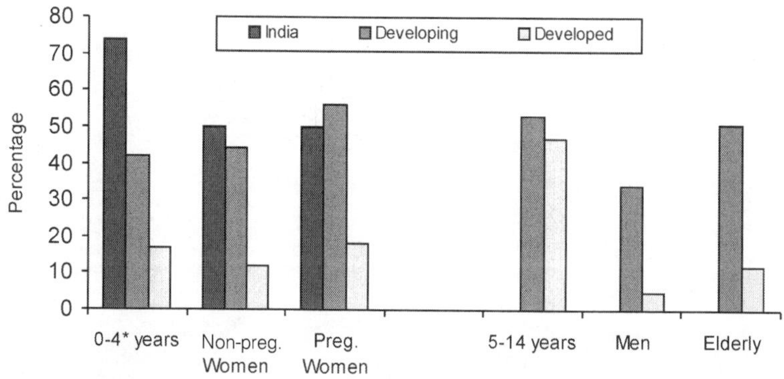


*24.2* Comparison of prevalence of anemia in India, developing and developed countries [7].

to rapid growth in this phase of life resulting in much wider gap between requirement for iron and dietary iron consumed. Additionally, complementary food consumed by young children in developing countries has low bioavailability of iron since it is often cereal dominated and has low or nil animal food content. It is observed that the prevalence of IDA in children peaks around 18 months of age and thereafter the prevalence tends to decrease as there is often an increase in iron intake through complementary foods. In France, iron deficiency and iron deficiency anemia affect 29% and 4% children younger than 2 years, while in the USA, only 2% children between 1 and 2 years have iron deficiency anemia [3]. Figure 24.3 indicates that the prevalence of anemia in India is 77–78% for under 2 years and about 71% for >2–5 years [8].

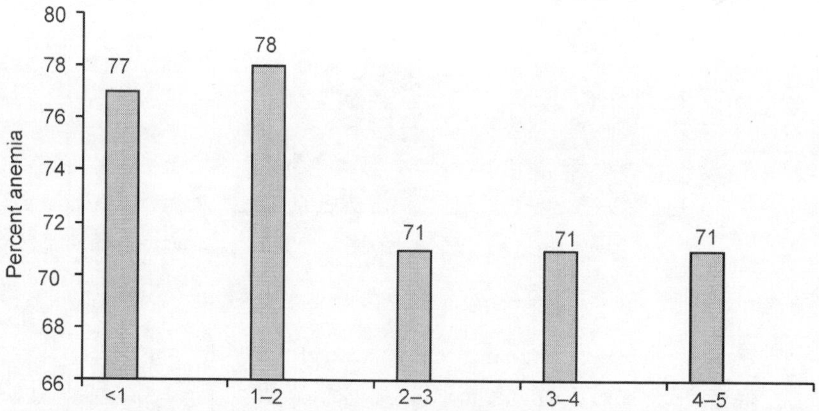


*24.3* Age-wise percentage prevalence of anemia in pre-school children of India [8]

## Box 24.1 The problem of anemia in pre-school children in India.

Anemia in preschool children is a major public health problem in India. The figures of anemia reported by the Indian Council of Medical Research (ICMR) and the national survey data show no difference in the last two decades [8,9] An analysis of anemia in children in different period between 1950-2001 indicates that the situation has in fact not changed in the last 30 years [2]. Anemia in young children in India has remained stagnant despite a reduction in IMR and decrease in clinical cases of severe malnutrition as well as vitamin A deficiency (Figure 24.4).

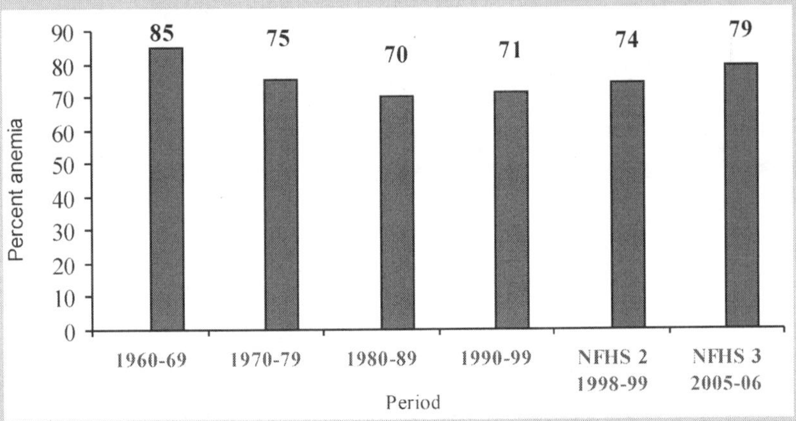


*24.4* Anemia (percentage) among children in different period [2, 6, 8]

Severity of anemia in preschool children 6–35 months, presented in Figure 24.5 [6, 8], indicates that nearly 8 out of 10 children below three years suffer from varying degrees of anemia and every second child suffers from moderate to severe anemia.

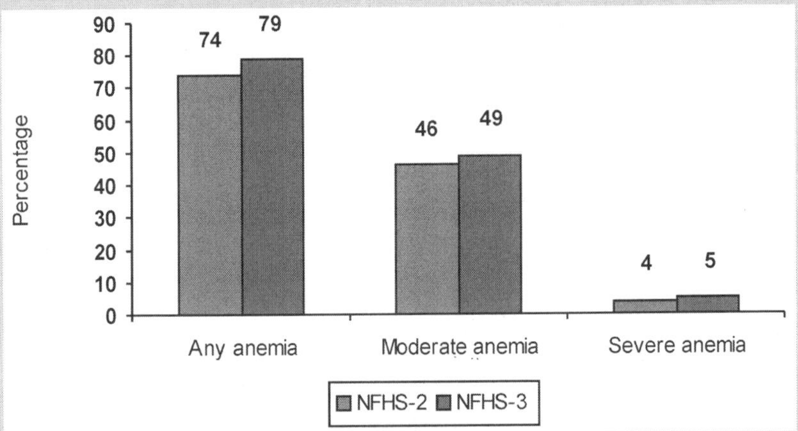


*24.5* Anemia (percentage) prevalence in children of age 6–35 months [6, 8]

State-wise analysis of prevalence of anemia in India (Figure 24.6) indicates a wide variation with only one state (Goa) is reported to have an anemia prevalence marginally below 40 percent and while three other states have anemia prevalence between 40% and 50% (Manipur, Mizoram, Kerala). Anemia prevalence of over 70% is reported from 8 out of the 28 states and UTs surveyed in 2005–06 [8]. These findings confirm that iron deficiency anemia is a public health problem in each and every state of India.

| *Anemia prevalence* | *State* |
|---|---|
| ≥70% | Bihar (78%), Madhya Pradesh (74.1%), Uttar Pradesh (73.9%), Haryana (72.3%), Chhattisgarh (71.2%), Andhra Pradesh (70.8%), Karnataka (70.4%) Jharkhand (70.3%) |
| >40 to <70% | Manipur (41.1%), Mizoram (44.2%), Kerala (44.5%), Himachal Pradesh (54.7%), Arunachal Pradesh (56.9%), Delhi (57.0%), Jammu & Kashmir (58.6%), Sikkim (9.2%), West Bengal (61.0%), Uttaranchal (61.4%), Tripura (62.9%), Maharashtra (63.4%), Tamil Nadu (64.2%), Meghalaya (64.4%), Orissa (65.0%), Punjab (66.4%), Assam (69.6%), Gujarat (69.7%), Rajasthan (69.7%) |
| <40 % | Goa (38.2%) |

*24.6* State-wise anemia prevalence [8]

## 24.2 Anemia, iron deficiency and iron deficiency anemia

Anemia is the most common indicator used to screen for iron deficiency. However, it is important to distinguish the terms "anemia", "iron deficiency", and "iron deficiency anemia" which are often used interchangeably.

### *(a) Anemia*

A pathological quantitative lower level of hemoglobin than WHO-acceptable level is defined as anemia. Iron deficiency is the most common but not the only cause of anemia. Other nutrition causes of anemia include folic acid and vitamin $B_{12}$ deficiency, chronic infections (particularly malaria), hereditary haemoglobinopathies and red cell diseases. Multiple causes coexist in an individual or in a population and contribute to the severity of anemia.

### *(b) Iron deficiency (ID)*

Iron deficiency is a reduction in body iron to the extent that the cellular storage iron required for metabolic/physiological function is fully exhausted with or without anemia. Iron deficiency is usually the result of inadequate bio-available dietary iron, increased iron requirement during rapid growth and blood loss due to any reason. There are no current estimates of total ID cases but based on anemia as an indicator, it is estimated that most pre-school children in developing counties are iron deficient [10].

### *(c) Iron deficiency anemia (IDA)*

IDA is defined as iron deficiency with low hemoglobin or anemia. Anemia is the result of inadequate availability of iron for hemoglobin formation. Some functional consequences may be observed in individuals who have iron deficiency without anemia but cognitive impairment, decreased physical capacity, and reduced immunity are commonly associated with iron deficiency anemia. In severe iron deficiency anemia, the capacity to maintain body temperature may also be reduced. Very severe anemia is life threatening.

The World Health Organization defined criterion for anemia [10] is for sea level only and will be higher at high altitude for the physiological increase in hemoglobin. Table 24.3 presents the details of hemoglobin and hematocrit cut-offs used to define anemia in people living at sea level. Anemia severity increases as haemoglobin concentration or hematocrit values decrease below the range for the healthy reference of the same age and sex as set by WHO (Table 24.4).

*Table 24.3* Haemoglobin and hematocrit cut-offs used to define anemia in people living at sea level [10]

| *Age or sex group* | *Haemoglobin below (g/dl)* | *Hematocrit below (%)* |
|---|---|---|
| Children 6 months to 5 years | 11.0 | 33 |
| Children 1–5 years | 11.5 | 34 |
| Children 12–13 years | 12.0 | 36 |
| Non-pregnant women | 12.0 | 36 |
| Pregnant women | 11.0 | 33 |
| Men | 13.0 | 39 |

*Table 24.4* Classification of anemia in children, based on haemoglobin levels [10]

| | Anemia measured by haemoglobin (g/dl) | | | |
|---|---|---|---|---|
| | Anemia | Mild | Moderate | Severe |
| Children 6–59 months | <11.0 | 10.0–10.9 | 7.0–9.9 | <7.0 |
| Children 5–11 years | <11.5 | 10.0–11.4 | 7.0–9.9 | <7.0 |
| Children 12–14 years | <12.0 | 10.0–11.9 | 7.0–9.9 | <7.0 |
| Non pregnant women above 15 years | <12.0 | 10.0–11.9 | 7.0–9.9 | <7.0 |
| Pregnant women | <11.0 | 10.0–10.9 | 7.0–9.9 | <7.0 |
| Men (above 15 years) | <13.0 | 12.0–12.9 | 9.0–11.9 | <9.0 |

## 24.3 Iron balance in children

Iron status can be considered as a continuum, which results from long-term negative iron balance when iron stores are progressively lost. Total iron in an adult man is 3.5–4.0 g – 73% of the body's iron is incorporated into hemoglobin, 12% is in the storage complexes ferritin and haemosiderin, and a very important 15 per cent is incorporated into a variety of other iron-containing compounds, some of them enzymes of vital importance. The heme iron compounds include myoglobin, cytochromes, catalases, and peroxidases. Infants and young children are prone to be affected by iron deficiency since the requirements for iron is high during this stage of rapid growth and development.

Almost all iron compounds in the body are continuously broken down and re-synthesized and iron that is released is very efficiently conserved and reutilized. An important consequence of this recycling is that very little iron is lost from the body on a daily basis that is required to be replenished in adult men with normal iron losses in the feces, sweat, and sloughed cells amounting to about 0.9 mg/day, equivalent to <0.1% of iron stores. However, women in their reproductive years need to absorb an average of 1.3 mg/day to make up for the additional iron loss in menstrual blood [11]. In case of infants and children, a large amount of iron is required for growth, i.e. substantially more iron must be absorbed than is lost from the body. For example, a 1-year-old infant loses about 0.2 mg of iron/day, calculated on the basis of body surface area from values measured in adults. The amount needed for growth averages roughly 0.6 mg. Consequently, about 75 % of the 0.8 mg of absorbed iron needed per day during this period is required to meet the needs of accelerated growth.

## 24.4 Patho-physiology of anemia in children under three years of age

Hemoglobin concentrations are normally higher on birth than at any other time of life as a result of the adaptation of the fetus to the hypoxic environment of the uterus. In addition, at full term neonatal reserves of storage iron are relatively generous. Consequently, most newborn infants are well supplied with iron. Between birth and 4 months of age, there is almost no change in total body iron in the term infant. The need for exogenous iron is therefore modest during this period. The abundant iron stores present at birth help to provide for synthesis of hemoglobin, myoglobin, and enzyme iron during the first 4 months. Additional iron from hemoglobin breakdown is also made available to meet iron needs because the concentration of hemoglobin declines from a mean of 17.0 g/dl at birth to a low of 11.0 g/dl at 2 months of age. This low point is also referred as "the early anemia of infancy" and is distinguished from the "late anemia of infancy" because it is unresponsive to iron treatment.

After about 4 months of age, a gradual shift occurs from an abundance of iron to the marginal iron reserves that characterize the period of continued rapid growth. The transition from feast to famine in respect to iron is primarily due to the large amount of iron required to maintain a near constant mean hemoglobin concentration of 12.5 g/dl within a rapidly expanding blood volume between 4 and 12 months. A large amount of iron, about 0.8 mg/day, needs to be absorbed from the diet during this period.

Mild maternal iron deficiency and anemia have few significant repercussions on iron status of the newborn, but severe maternal anemia does have a strong influence. The risk of infant developing iron deficiency is further increased if the umbilical cord is clamped before the appropriate stage [12]. Both these risk factors are high in developing countries.

In the first two months of life, there is minimal dietary iron absorption and stores are mobilized to meet the iron requirement. Thereafter, dietary iron absorption needs to supply enough iron to facilitate the increased need for more red cell mass. By about 6 months of age, iron stores are usually depleted and diet then becomes the vital source for iron. A low birth weight baby has less iron store and therefore not only such an infant requires extra iron but also needs additional amount of iron intake to be ensured at an earlier age.

The overall rapid growth of infancy between 6 and 24 months, include a significant increase in red cell mass and tissue volume. At this stage, requirement for iron is proportionality nearly as high as that for pregnant women. This increase in requirement is difficult to meet through breastfeeding practices or complementary feeding alone unless specific measures are taken to increase iron consumption. Therefore the most common reason for iron deficiency anemia in infants and children is the inadequate supply of iron in the diet. The risk of iron deficiency is high during infancy because only about 50% of the normal iron requirement of a normal six-month old can be obtained from breast milk and by this age the iron stores at birth are likely to have been used up towards providing support for body functions and growth even in children born at term to well-nourished mothers. In case a mother is anemic or a child is of low birth weight (LBW), the stores are depleted much earlier. Continued breastfeeding after six months will provide half of infant's iron need while the remaining half, approximately 0.4 mg/day, must come from complementary food or iron-containing supplement or use of iron-fortified foods for preventing deficiency of iron and iron deficiency anemia [13].

The risk factors that contribute to IDA in infants are low or non-iron fortified formula or breast-fed through the later months without supplementation of iron, premature infants or low birth weight (LBW), early cord clamping, maternal anemia, gastrointestinal blood loss due to infection (*Helicobactor pylori* and helminth infections), limited access to other nutrients that enhance the incorporation of iron into hemoglobin. Additionally, reduced absorption of iron in gastrointestinal disease due to chronic infections, recurrent diarrhea, celiac disease or an intestinal parasite infestation contributes to iron deficiency. However, the most common factor for ID and IDA in infants and children is the low intake of iron in the diet during the rapid growth spurt. Therefore, the two main reasons for IDA in children are (1) increased requirement for iron during rapid growth stage of infancy and early childhood that is between 6 and 24 months; and (2) insufficient intake of iron or poor bio-availability of iron consumed, related to low consumption of absorption enhancers and a high consumption of absorption inhibitors of iron in the second year of life. The situation is aggravated with increase in prevalence of worm infestation.

## 24.5 Consequences of iron deficiency and iron deficiency anemia in children

Anemia is a public health concern and is the most common cause of morbidity. Anemia, like fever, is a manifestation and not a disease per se. Anemia is most often a hidden problem with few overt symptoms [14]. Children with anemia are denied their rights to optimum physical and mental development before they ever reach a classroom. Anemia in children adds to the burden on health systems, affects learning and school performance, and reduces adult productivity. The massive economic cost of childhood anemia is often underestimated by policy makers while service providers often fail to recognize the "invisible" significant serious health consequences from anemia. The fact that anemia in young children can result in permanent cognitive deficits resulting in children being denied their rights to optimum physical and mental development makes childhood anemia a serious public health concern.

The various stages of iron deficiency are presented in Fig. 24.7 [15]. The first stage of iron depletion does not result in functional changes. In the second stage, stores are exhausted and tissues begin to have insufficient iron resulting in iron deficiency. In this stage when there is no outright anemia, negative effects include cognitive impairment, decreased physical capacity, and reduced immunity and these effects are more serious in the last stage of iron deficiency anemia [16].

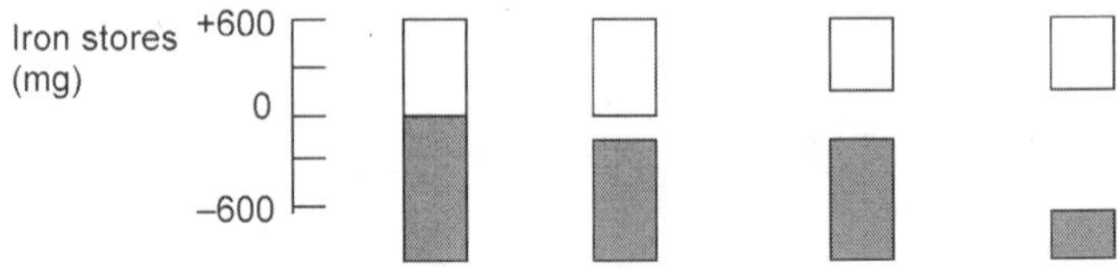


| | Normal iron stores | Iron depletion | Iron deficiency erythropoiesis | Iron deficiency anemia |
|---|---|---|---|---|
| Plasma ferritin (µg/L) | 60 | <12 | <12 | <12 |
| Transferrin saturation (%) | 35 | 35 | <16 | <16 |
| RBC protoporphyrin (µg/dL) | 30 | 30 | <100 | <100 |
| Hemoglobin (g/dL) | >12 | >12 | >12 | >12 |

*24.7* Iron status in relation to iron stores [15]

It is estimated that at least 200 millions of under-five children globally fail to reach their cognitive and socio-emotional development due to undernutrition including iron deficiency and inadequate stimulation [17]. In children less than two years, the most significant negative consequences of IDA are impairment in motor and mental development, which may be irreversible in later life [18, 19]. Poor iron status negatively impacts cognitive as well as motor and social development [20]. Significant adverse effects between 6 and 24 months include decrease in responsiveness and activity as well as increase in body fatigue.

Anemia during childhood is serious since it affects cognition and the effects that are observed in first six months of life could often lead to permanent brain damage. Moderate and severe deficiency impairs cognitive performance at any age. In general these effects are corrected with iron supplements but if moderate to severe iron deficiency occurs in infancy during the phase of brain development, the effects on cognition may not be reversible [13]. According to Lozoff et al [21], depending on the age when anemia occurs, some of the development deficits can be improved or even corrected with iron treatment but with iron deficiency in infancy some cognitive and social differences can remain permanent. Box 24.2 [22] presents details of results of a longitudinal study reported on the impact of iron deficiency on cognitive development. An anemic child is likely to remain vulnerable to infections and continues to have lower immunity towards infection. Anemia results in lowering appetite and sets up a vicious cycle which perpetuates to a series of events that need to be corrected and if no corrective action is taken could result in impaired development of mental and physical coordination skills. In older children, iron deficiency leads to impaired scholastic achievement [23].

**Box 24.2 Iron deficiency below age 2 years and cognitive score [22]**

Children between the ages 1–2 years were enrolled in a study and followed up over a period of 18 years; Anemia was corrected with iron supplements for those children in the intervention group. Children underwent cognitive test in early childhood and at ages 5–8 years, 11–14 years, 15–18 years and 19 years. Bayley tests were used in infancy and age appropriate Wechsler Test and other cognitive tests were applied for later ages. Anemic and non-anemic children were compared, irrespective of being in the intervention or control group. The results revealed that children from the middle socio-economic status (SES) with adequate iron stores scored 8–9 points higher than those who remained anemic in early childhood. This difference was maintained up to 19 years of age. In the lower SES group, children with adequate iron stores had 10 points higher in early childhood. The gap, however, widened substantially with increase in age and a difference of 25 points was noted at the age 19 years. These results indicate that iron deficiency below two years does influence cognitive ability and with such gaps in cognitive score it is expected to adversely influence schooling and earning capacity in future.

While it is well-established that iron deficiency anemia among children is responsible for higher morbidity and subsequent mortality, systemic studies to quantify them are practically difficult for a number of epidemiological reasons and therefore are not available. However, a study as early as 1920s from London has reported impact of iron supplement to infants on reducing bronchitis and gastroenteristis [24]. Infants receiving formula fortified with iron and vitamins were reported to have about 50% less respiratory infections than infants receiving unfortified version of the same formula [25]. Iron deficiency has been reported to be associated with increased diarrhoeal and respiratory diseases [26] while meningitis has been observed to be fatal among those who were anemic [27]. There are other studies which have found no such effect. Interactions of iron and infection reviewed in 2000 concluded that some issues related to iron deficiency and infection remain unresolved [28, 29].

Iron deficiency anemia rarely exists in isolation and to disentangle the role played by anemia from malnutrition and other precipitating factors is difficult to be obtained at the community level.

## 24.6 Measures for preventing iron deficiency and anemia

One of the goals of the World Summit for Children was reduction in IDA in women by one-third of the 1990 levels by 2010 [30]. There was no reference to address IDA in children in the World Summit Goal since knowledge on impact of ID or IDA on mental development was then not well-appreciated. Since 2000, there is increased concern to address anemia in preschool children with research highlighting the fact that even mild anemia in infants and young children can impair intellectual development and such damage by deficiency of iron to a young child's brain may not be reversed later in life [22, 31] and therefore priority needs to be accorded to the prevention of iron deficiency in this early stage of life [32].

Iron deficiency anemia can be prevented at low cost, and the benefit/cost ratio of implementing preventive programs is recognized as one of the highest in the realm of public health. Economic cost of achieving a reduction in nutritional anemia through iron fortification and iron supplementation indicate benefit to cost ratio of 6:1 in case of fortification while economic benefits of supplementation are indicated to far exceed the cost of intervention [33]. Effective and practical interventions are available and poor implementation rather than non-availability of the interventions is the constraint. Anemia-prevention strategies involve synchronized efforts to increase iron intake through supplements to high risk group of population of pre-school children combined with concurrent efforts to provide vitamin A supplements, access to fortified staple cereal or other food items, increasing iron levels in complementary food by promoting use of multi-nutrient mixes as "home fortificants" [34, 35], as well as by implementing measures to reduce parasitic infections and control malaria.

### 24.6.1 Iron–folic acid supplements

Traditionally, for over the last three decades, the IDA programme has focused on iron–folic acid (IFA) supplements to pregnant mothers and comparatively very little attention has been given to address ID or IDA in children, especially for under-two years. Iron deficiency anemia has been viewed merely as "women's problem" [36]. However, it needs to be recognised that rapidly growing infants need relatively high iron intake. Infants who do not have low birth weight are normally born with sufficient iron but beyond six months of age, iron content of milk is not sufficient.

It is virtually impossible for infants over six months to meet the iron needs through diet alone. Higher needs through diet may be met only in situations when the diets contain sufficient amount of fortified foods and heme iron from animal foods or if the iron stores of infant since birth or woman at the start of pregnancy is adequate. With evidence of serious implications of iron deficiency anemia in young children, it has been recommended by INACG/WHO/UNICEF [37] that "in situations where iron-fortified complementary foods are not widely or regularly consumed by young children, all infants should receive iron supplements after six months of age". In regions where the prevalence of anemia is below 40%, the duration of supplementation for normal birth infants should be from six months to until 12 months of age [3]. However, as presented in Table 24.5, in areas where the prevalence is 40% and above, it is recommended to continue supplementation up to 24 months of age [37].

*Table 24.5* Guidelines for iron supplementation to children 6–24 months of age [37]

| Prevalence of anemia in children 6–24 months | Dosage | Birth–Weight Category | Duration |
|---|---|---|---|
| <40% | 12.5 mg iron + 50 µg folic acid daily | Normal | 6–12 months of age |
| | | Low birth weight (<2500 g) | 2–24 months of age |
| $^{3}$40% | 12.5 mg iron + 50 µg folic acid daily | Normal | 6–24 months of age |
| | | Low birth weight (<2500 g) | 2–24 months of age |

The most practical iron supplement for use in infants and young children is an aqueous solution of a soluble ferrous salt, such as ferrous sulfate, or a ferric complex, such as iron polymaltose. A single, safe and effective dose for all children under-2-year old that can be easily dispensed by all mothers (literate and non-literate) is required. For the many past decades, oral ferrous sulphate syrup has been the primary strategy to control IDA in infants and young children [38]. However, compliance is adversely influenced due to a combination of factors: the syrup has an unpleasant metallic after taste, leaves dark stains on teeth and high doses cause abdominal discomfort [39]. Additionally, there are technical disadvantages associated with liquid iron such as short shelf-life and practical programme constraint such as high transportation costs due to weight of bottles, and difficulty in adequately dispensing the drops, especially among illiterate population as the care giver is required to measure decimal volume from a dropper [40, 41].

Requirement of iron dosage through supplements for prevention and treatment of IDA depends on the following factors:

- The level of iron stores of the child at the time of birth, which in turn depends on the iron status of the mother during pregnancy.
- Whether the child born is low birth weight or normal birth weight.
- Whether the child is on the breastfeeding which is exclusive or along with other foods that contain iron-absorption inhibitors and/or iron-absorption promoters or food consumed is fortified with iron-poor micronutrients.
- The quantity of the food consumed and whether the bio-availability of iron from it is poor (5%) or good (up to 15%).
- Level of anemia and the additional factors which contribute to anemia such as infection, worm infestation etc.

For therapeutic purposes, an adequate and safe hematological response to oral iron intake can be achieved in 4–6 weeks with 3 mg elemental iron per kg body weight/day [42]. However, in a prophylactic program, between 1 and 2 mg of iron per kg body weight/day is appropriate. Assuming 5 percent iron absorption, which is a very conservative estimate of absorption [43], 12.5 mg iron dose is equivalent to 2.5 mg iron per kg body weight for a 6-month-old child with an average weight of 5 kg. The same dose of 12.5 mg iron is adequate in case of 12 month-old infant weighing 8 kg, 1.6 mg iron per kg body weight and for an 18-month-old infant weighing 12 kg, 1.2 mg iron per kg body weight [37]. Table 24.5 presents the guidelines for iron supplementation to children 6–24 months of age [37]. If compliance is poor and children consume iron supplement dose equivalent to consuming the recommended dose only every other day, between 35 and 45 percent of the iron requirement would be available from the iron supplement alone.

Iron supplement administration to infants younger than six months of age is recommended in situations where mothers of infants are severely anemic during pregnancy resulting in lower iron stores at birth or infants who are born low birth weight (LBW). In such situations, iron status may be poor in infants at age younger than six months, resulting in adverse impact on growth and development. In poorly nourished populations, 20–30 percent newborns are LBW and these newborns have low levels of iron stores based on lower overall tissue and blood volume at birth. These facts, compounded with increased iron needs associated with rapid weight gain of low birth infants, are the basis for WHO and UNICEF recommendation that LBW babies receive iron supplement beginning at two months of age and the supplementation be continued up to 24 months of age [37, 44, 45].

Operational issues regarding demand, supply and logistics, communications and social mobilization, monitoring, building partnership with private sector needs to be given increased attention for effective implementation of iron supplementation programme for children. Operational feasibility needs to be well-defined following implementation of iron supplement administration programme on a large scale.

In India, the revised policy for anemia control includes iron supplementation to children in the form of syrup and small tablets. However, specific guidelines for distribution and monitoring are being finalised. Box 24.3 presents details of iron folic acid supplement programme evolvement in India.

## Box 24.3 Prevention and control of anemia in young children in India

Government of India's 10th five-year plan [46] goals for anemia control for children include

1. Screening of children for anemia wherever required and appropriate treatment of those found anemic.
2. Reducing the prevalence of anemia by 25% and moderate and severe anemia by 50% in children.

In India, the National Nutritional Anemia Prophylaxis Program (NNAPP) has been in existence since 1970 [47]. The Prophylaxis programme at the beginning included provision of iron folic acid (IFA) tablets to pre-school children besides pregnant women. Pre-school children with haemoglobin levels over 8 g percent were recommended to be included in the prophylaxis programme while children with hemoglobin less than 8 g percent were recommended to be put on anti-anaemic treatment. The programme was later revised to include children of 1–10 years and administration of supplements was changed to 100 days instead of six months. The supplement containing 20 mg of elemental iron (ferrous sulphate) and 100 μg of folic acid for children was provided in two forms – small tablets and 2 ml syrup liquid. The programme was evaluated by ICMR in 1988 [48] and this was followed by a meeting organized by the Government of India at Nirman Bhavan on 21–22nd Sept in 1989 [49]. The recommendations were reviewed by a core group of experts. The following major policy decisions were taken:

(a) The nomenclature of the programme was re-designated as National Nutritional Anemia Control Programme. (NNACP) since it was noted that over 80 percent pregnant mothers were reported to be anemic .It was agreed that the focus of the programme should be on control of anemia rather than on prevention alone.
(b) Program priority should be given to vulnerable sections of the population namely pregnant and lactating women, intrauterine device (IUD) users as well as children in the 1–5-year age group. The composition of "big tablet" for pregnant mothers/women in reproductive age was modified with one tablet containing 100 mg elemental iron instead of 60 mg. The amount of folic acid was retained at the dose of 500 μg. The dosage for prophylaxis and treatment was defined – one tablet per woman per day including pregnant women for a minimum of 100 days and two tablets per day for women with severe anemia.
(c) Taking into consideration the high cost of syrup recommended for children earlier, usage of syrup in the public health programme was discontinued and only "small IFA tablets" for children between 12 and 59 months was recommended. Each small tablet contained 20 mg elemental iron and 100 μg of folic acid which was recommended to be consumed for a minimum of 100 days in a year by young children.
(d) Iron-folic acid tablets were recommended to be supplied not as open tablets in bottles but in a packaged form. Blister packaging was recommended.

Based on the above recommendations, a Policy on National Nutrition Anemia Control Programme (NNACP) was formulated in December 1991 [50]. Small "IFA" tablets continued to be supplied under this programme. The NNACP programme was included in the Child Survival Safe Motherhood (CSSM) Programme of the Government of India in 1992 and later as a part of Reproductive Child Health (RCH) programme [51]. In 1998, the NNACP was reviewed at a National Consultation on Anemia organized by the Government of India and UNICEF [52]. No special additional recommendation was made for preschool children. Since

1992, the NNACP program has continued to be implemented as part of CSSM and later RCH I and RCH II package. The programme is being implemented through the existing health system with support of the Integrated Childhood Development Scheme (ICDS) Programme. However, the focus in implementation has been primarily on pregnant women and not on pre-school children. [53]

A nation wide study on usage of IFA supplements was undertaken during early 2000 by the National Nutrition Monitoring Bureau (NNMB) covering 2178 children of the age group one to five years from 8 states (Kerala, Tamil Nadu, Karnatka, Andhra Pradesh, Maharashtra, Madhya Pradesh, Orissa, West Bengal) [54]. The findings highlighted that only 3.8% of children received Iron Folic Acid (IFA) tablets (small iron folic acid tablets) and half of the children received the IFA tablets from the ICDS frontline workers while the remaining half received the supply of the supplements from the multipurpose health worker female. The number of children who received IFA tablets ranged from 0% to 5% in different states except in one state (Maharashtra) where the percentage of children receiving iron folic acid tablet was reported to be almost 12 per cent. In 2002, a technical consultation on "Strategies for Prevention and Control of Iron deficiency Anemia Amongst Under Three Children in India" was organized [54]. Based on the finding of the study as well as the recommendations of the 2002 consultation meeting [55], a consensus was reached that iron and folic acid tablet being supplied to young children under the age of three years is not well-accepted and it was recommended that IFA in the form of syrup should be supplied to children. Iron folic acid supplement was recommended to be administered from six months of age.

The above recommendation was endorsed in the Government Policy in the year 2007 [56]. As per 2007 Policy, it was recommended that the NNACP should cover infants aged 6–12 months. The Policy recommends that all children 6–60 months to be given iron folic acid supplements for a minimum of 100 days in a year. The composition of one millilitre of syrup or one small tablet is 20 mg elemental iron and 100 µg folic acid. For safety reasons it was recommended that each bottle of IFA syrup must be supplied with a dispenser that allows only one millilitre to be drawn at a time. Introduction of dispersible tablets has also been proposed. As per these recommendations, both IFA syrup and tablets are being supplied for children in Kit A under the National Rural Health Mission (NRHM) [57].

The Policy guidelines for addressing the public health problem of childhood anemia were revisited at a workshop organized by the Government of India in early 2008 [58]. It was recommended that for children with low birth weight, the IFA supplementation should start from 2 months of age rather than 6 months. It was also recommended that all children should receive the supplement since screening of children for anemia is not considered practical and not recommended. The experts at the meeting agreed that the Government of India guidelines regarding duration of administration of IFA for a minimum period of 100 days, presented in the national guidelines on Integrated Management of Childhood Illness (IMNCI), should be followed [59]. IFA supplementation has been recommended to be discontinued during active episode of illness. Details of delivery and monitoring system have been proposed with emphasis on use of existing health and ICDS systems.

Periodic deworming is simple and safe and has been reported to have significant effect on nutritional status, including iron status. The impact of deworming on nutritional status has been reported from Tanzania where deworming resulted in significant impact on anemia in children less than two-years old whereas the impact of supplementation with iron was not reported to be significant [60].

In severe malnutrition, supplementation of iron is hazardous [61]. Adequate iron status is essential for preventing and overcoming infections. On the other hand, pathogenic organisms also require iron for their growth and reproduction. In severe malnutrition, the immune system is compromised and iron supplements enhance the growth of pathogenic organism before immunity is restored since the body is not able to continually maintain its overall supply of iron in the forms that are not usable by pathogens or are not free to form compounds that can result in cellular and other damage. Therefore, iron supplementation given to severely malnourished children with impaired immunity can benefit the replication of pathogen before the immune system is rebuilt and restored. Parental iron administered to children with Kwashiorkor has been reported to result in serious illness and death [62]. According to Jackson 2007 [61], "an assumption that anemia found in malnourished individual is a simple consequence of poor or inadequate dietary intake of iron, without a critical consideration of the broader context, gives rise to the potential for serious error in care with inappropriate intervention".

In areas where *P.falciparum* malaria is hyperendemic, public health recommendations for implementation of a practical low-cost intervention package to correct iron deficiency anemia and promote healthy iron status among infants and young children remains unresolved [14]. The findings from the study in Zanzibar, Tanzania indicate that in the region with stable, perennial, and intense transmission of malaria, iron supplementation administered to children who were iron replete, with or without zinc, resulted in increased morbidity and mortality [63]. Subsequently, WHO consultation recommends that universal iron supplementation should not be used in areas of high malaria transmissions [14].

### 24.6.2 Obstetric care – delayed cord clamping

Cutting-off of the pulsating umbilical cord before iron rich cord blood is transferred to the newborn also results in lower iron in the infant at birth. Delayed clamping of the umbilical cord (most trials defined delayed clamping being soon after cessation of cord pulsation or at 3 minutes after birth) is an effective prophylactic measure for prevention of iron deficiency and anemia. Compared to early cord clamping (defined as immediately after birth or within 10 seconds of birth), delayed clamping results in increase in iron endowment of the child at birth by 50 per cent. The result of delayed clamping is higher blood flow to vital organs in the first week after birth and less cases of anemia at two months of age in full-term infants [64]. A systematic review has confirmed that a higher levels of hemoglobin is observed at 2–3 months of age in children in developing and industrialized countries where the practice of delayed clamping at birth is followed. The impact is noted to be higher when mothers are anemic [65]. Delayed clamping is recommended as one of the important measures for prevention of childhood anemia [66].

### 24.6.3 Fortification and home fortification

Food-based approach for increasing iron intake sufficiently to meet the very high requirements for iron for the highest risk group – children under two years and pregnant the mother – has been challenging. Effort is continuously on-going for the fine tuning of technology for iron fortification of traditional staple food, water and beverages, food sauce, table salt as well as commercial foods. A new technology and strategy of adding a fixed amount of fortificant mixture to an individual's portion of food is referred as "home fortification", is being experimented since mid-1990s [34, 35]. The concept of fortification of complementary food for young children has gained momentum since it has been noted that availability and use of commercial foods fortified with iron and other essential micronutrients in North America have historically been noted to have resulted in disappearance of IDA problem in children [67]. This decrease in IDA in children in western world is recognised as a successful public health accomplishment although specific groups of infants and children, such as infants born prematurely, remain at risk of IDA.

Since the use of commercially fortified food for young children is not easily available at affordable cost as well as the fact that regular administering supplements in syrup and drop had not been effective, the concept of home fortification was initiated in 1996 to address childhood IDA [41]. Home fortification pertains to sprinkling of a fixed amount of powder or mixture containing iron and selected micronutrient to cooked food served to a child at home level. One such formulation is Sprinkles. According to Zlottkin and Tondeur (2007) [18], who have pioneered this technology, "In Sprinkles, the iron in the form of ferrous fumarate is encapsulated within a thin lipid layer to prevent the iron from interacting with food, thereby limiting changes to taste, colour or texture of the food. Caregivers are instructed to add the entire content of sachet daily to any semi-solid food prepared for their infant or young child in the household, immediately before serving. Other micronutrients including zinc, iodine, vitamin C, D, A and folic acid may be added to Sprinkles sachets". The microencapsulate (an edible vegetable-based lipid) masks the taste of iron and prevents colour change by forming a barrier which does not allow an interaction between iron and food to which the Sprinkle is added. Table 24.6 [18] presents the composition of nutritional anemia-prevention formulation in Sprinkles; while Table 24.7 [18] presents the complete micronutrient formulation. The anemia formulation includes ascorbic acid to enhance iron absorption, folic acid to prevent megaloblastic anemia and zinc and vitamin A to enhance vitamin A status.

*Table 24.6* Composition of nutritional anemia formulation Sprinkles [18]

| *Micronutrient* | *Amount* |
|---|---|
| Iron | 12.5 mg |
| Zinc | 5 mg |
| Folic acid | 160 μg |
| Vitamin A | 300 μg RE |
| Vitamin C | 30 mg |

*Table 24.7* Composition of multi-micronutrient formulation Sprinkles [18]

| *Micronutrient* | *Amount* |
|---|---|
| Vitamin A | 400 μg RE |
| Vitamin C | 30 mg |
| Vitamin D | 5 μg |
| Vitamin E | 5 mg TE |
| Vitamin B1 | 0.5 mg |
| Vitamin B2 | 0.5 mg |
| Vitamin B6 | 0.5 mg |
| Vitamin B12 | 0.9 μg |
| Folic acid | 150 μg |
| Niacin | 6 mg |
| Iron | 12.5 mg |
| Zinc | 4.1 mg |
| Copper | 0.56 mg |
| Iodine | 90 μg |

Efficacy trials with anemic children using Sprinkles has demonstrated that the effect on anemia cure rate were comparable to that of standard iron drops [67]. In a period of two months, 58% children who received Sprinkles shifted from anemic to non-anemic stage. A follow-up study also showed that in most children who have been successfully treated for anemia, further intervention was not needed at 12 months post-intervention [18]. Box 24.4 presents the details of efficacy trial undertaken in India [68].

The feasibility and acceptability of Sprinkles has also been studied in a large scale trial in Mongolia between 2001 and 2004. The findings demonstrated that usage of Sprinkles in public health programme was feasible. Sprinkles have been successfully used in a wide range of settings ranging from community settings in Bangladesh [69] to emergency setting in Haiti [70]. Adherence and acceptability of Sprinkles has been positive and the only consistently reported side effect is darkening of infants stools. Pilot projects are being scaled up to national level in nine countries in South Asia and Latin America [68].

**Box 24.4 Low-dose Sprinkles – an innovative approach in India to treat IDA in infants and young children [68]**

In Maharashtra, a state of west India, effectiveness of flexible administration of Sprinkles delivered through existing Integrated Child Development Scheme (ICDS) for reducing the prevalence of anemia in children of age 6 months to 6 years was undertaken. A total of 17,126 children participated in the study where Sprinkles Plus comprising iron and other micronutrients (presented in Table 24.7) was given to children either at the ICDS centre or at home by caregivers/mothers. About 170 ICDS frontline workers were trained to participate in this project. The compliance of flexible administration of 60 sachets of Sprinkles Plus for over 120 days to these children was monitored either under the supervision at ICDS centre or by mother of children who were not attending ICDS centres. Compliance card was maintained by Anganwadi worker/mother.

Baseline Hb levels (random sample of 1500 children) was studied while end line Hb levels were estimated on fresh random sample of 1500 children. Sprinkles administration was reported to be well-accepted by mothers and children. Overall anemia reduced from 50.8% to 33.7% and compliance both at ICDS centre and at home was reported to be over 90 percent from the records of ICDS functionary while mothers reported a lower compliance of 56.4%. It was concluded that Sprinkles, flexibly administered through anemia prevention/control program is highly effective in reducing anemia in young children. It was also recognised that the challenge is to establish system to monitor and ensure proper use of Sprinkles and monitor compliance.

## 24.7 Conclusion

The significance of even mild anemia on intellectual development of infants and young children is of increased concern among the public health experts [32]. There is a need to urgently address the public health problem of anemia in young children, with special focus on under 2 years.

## References

1. WORLD HEALTH ORGANIZATION (2008). Global Burdon of Diseases 2004 update, World Health Organization, 20 Avenue Appia, 1211 Geneva 27, Switzerland.
2. CHAUDHARY P (2009). Micronutrient and Child Health Workshop, 20–23rd October, AIIMS, New Delhi.
3. UNICEF/UNU/WHO (2001). Iron deficiency Anemia: assessment, prevention and control. A guide for programme managers. WHO/NED, Report no 01.3.
4. MCLEAN, E et al. (2007). Worldwide prevalence of anemia in preschool aged children, pregnant women and non-pregnant women of reproductive age. In: *Nutritional Anemia*, Eds Kraemer, K and Zimmermann, M.B. Sight and Life Press.
5. WHO/UNICEF/UNU (1996). Indicators for assessing iron deficiency and strategies (draft based on a WHO/UNICEF/UNU consultation 6–10 Dec, 1993). WHO, Geneva.
6. National Family Health Survey (NFHS) 2, (1998–99). International Institute of Population Sciences, Mumbai.
7. Fourth Report on the World Nutrition Situation (2000). UN.

8. National Family Health Survey (NFHS) 3, (2005–06). International Institute of Population Sciences, Mumbai.
9. INDIAN COUNCIL OF MEDICAL RESEARCH (ICMR) (1989). Evaluation of the National Nutritional Anemia Programme, ICMR.
10. WHO/UNICEF/UNU (2001). Iron deficiency anemia: assessment, prevention and control: A guide for program managers, World Health Organization.
11. DALLMAN PR (1989). Review of Iron Metabolism, Dietary Iron Birth to years edited by L. J. Filter, Raven Press, Ltd., New York.
12. GUPTA R and RAMJI S (2002). Effect of Cord Clamping on iron Stores in Infants Born to Anemic Mothers: A Randomized Controlled Trial. Indian Pediatrics, *Journal of the Indian Academy of Pediatrics*, **39**(2), p. 130, New Delhi.
13. GLEASON G and SCRIMSHAW NS (2007). An overview of functional significance of Iron Deficiency, In: *Nutritional Anemia* edited by K. Kraemer and M.B Zimmermann, Sight And Life Press, pp. 45–58.
14. IDPAS (2001). (Iron Deficiency project Advisory Service) – CD Rom. International Nutrition Foundation.
15. DEMAYER EM (1989). Preventing and Controlling Iron deficiency Anemia through primary health care: a guide for health administrators and programme managers, Geneva, WHO.
16. UNICEF/UNU/WHO/MI (1998). Preventing Iron def in women and Children, Technical Consensus on key Issues. UNICEF/UNU/WHO/MI Technical Workshop, 7–9th October 1998, Boston and Ottawa, International Nutrition foundation and the Micronutrient Initiative.
17. JOLLY R (2007). Early Childhood Development: the global challenge. *Lancet*, **369**, pp. 8–9.
18. ZLOTKIN SH and TONDEUR MC (2007). Successful approaches: Sprinkles. In: *Nutritional Anemia*, Eds Kraemer, K and Zimmermann, M.B. Sight and Life Press.
19. GRANTHAM-MCGREGOR S and ANI C (2001). A review of studies on the effect of iron deficiency on cognitive development in children. *J Nutr*, **131**, 649S –685S; discussion 666s–668S.
20. LOZOFF B (2003). Iron Deficiency in Infancy: Impact on behaviour and development UN SCN annual Meeting Chennai, India, 3–7 unpublished presentation.
21. LOZOFF BH, MOLLEN E and WOLF A (2000). Poorer Behaviour and development outcome more than 10 years after treatment for iron deficiency in infancy. *Paediatrics*, **105**, p. 11.
22. LOZOFF B, JIMENEZ E, SMITH JB (2006). Double burden of Iron deficiency in infancy and low socio-economic status: a longitudinal analysis of cognitive test scores to 19 years. *Arch pediatr Adolesc Med*, **160**(11), pp. 1108–1113.
23. GRANTHAM-MCGREGOR S, ANI C (2001). A review of studies on the effect of iron deficiency on cognitive development in children. *J Nutr*, **131**, pp. 649S–685S.
24. MACKAY HM (1928). Anemia in infancy: its prevention. *Arch Dis Child*, **3**, p. 117.
25. ANDELMAN MB and SERED BR (1966). Utilization of dietary iron by term infants. A study of 1,048 infants from a low socio-economic population. *Amer J. Dis. Child*, **111**, pp. 45–55.
26. BROWN CV, BROWN GW, BONRHILL B (1967). Iron deficiency and its functional consequences. *Alaska Med*, **9**, pp. 93–99.
27. FORTUINE R (1966). Acute purulent meningitis in Alaska natives: epidemiology, diagnosis and prognosis. *Can Med Assoc J*, **94**(1): pp. 19–22.

28. BEARD J, STOLZFUS R (eds.) (2001). Iron Deficiency. *J Nutr.*, 131S; Supplement II2001:131S.
29. OPPENHEIMER SJ (2001). Iron and its relation to immunity and infectious disease. *J Nutr.,* **131**, pp. 616S–635S.
30. United Nation's Report of the 27th Session of the UN General Assembly Special session on Children, 2002.
31. LOZOFF B, JIMENEZ, R, EOLF AW (1991), Long term development outcome of infants with iron deficiency. *N Engl J Med*, **325**(10), pp. 687–94.
32. UNICEF Facts for Life, New York. UNICEF/WHO/UNESCO/UNFPA/UNDP/UNAIDS/WFP/World Bank 2002: 153.
33. ALDERMAN, H. and HORTON S (2007). The economics of addressing nutritional anemia. In: *Nutritional Anemia* edited by K. Kraemer and M.B. Zimmermann.
34. NESTEL P, et al. (2003). Complementary food supplements to achieve micronutrient adequacy for infants and young children. *J Paediatr Gastroenter Nutr,* **36**, pp. 316–328.
35. ZLOTKIN SH, SCHAUER C, CHRISTOFIDES A, SHARIEFF W, TONDEUR MC, HYDER SMZ (2005). Micronutrient sprinkles to control childhood anemia: A simple powdered sachet may be the key to addressing a global problem. *PLoS Medicine*, **2**(7); Internet: www.plosmedicine.org
36. MGV MANNAR (2007). The case for urgent action to address nutritional anemia In: *Nutritional Anemia* edited by K. Kraemer and M.B. Zimmermann, Sight and Life Press.
37. STOLTZFUS RJ, DREYFUSS ML (1998). Guidelines for use of iron supplements and to prevent and treat iron deficiency anemia. Washington, DC: INACG /WHO/ UNICEF.
38. ANDREWS NC (1999). Disorders of iron metabolism. *New Engl J Med*, **341**, pp. 1986–1995.
39. GALLOWAY R, MCGUIRE J (1994). Determinants of compliance with iron supplementation: supplies, side effects, or psychology? *Soc Sci Med*, **39**, pp. 381–390.
40. DEMAEYER EM, DALLMAN P, GURNEY JM, HALLBERG L, SOOD SK, SRIKANTIA SG (1989). Preventing and controlling iron deficiency through primary health care: a guide for health administrators and programme managers. Geneva World health organization.
41. NESTEL P, ALNWICK D (1997). Iron/multi-micronutrient supplements for young children. Summary and Conclusion of consultation held at UNICEF. August 19–20, 1996, Copenhagen Washington DC, ILSI.
42. REEVES JD, YIP R, LONNERDAL B, KEEN CL, DALLMAN PR (1985). Does iron supplementation compromise zinc nutrition in healthy infants? *American Journal of Clinical Nutrition*, **42**(4), pp. 683–687.
43. FAO/WHO (Food and Agriculture Organization/World Health Organization). (1988). Requirements of vitamin A, vitamin $B_{12}$. FAO, Rome, Italy: Food and Nutrition Series 23.
44. LLEWELYN–JONES D (1965). Severe anemia in pregnancy as seen in Kuala Lumpur. *Aust N Z J Obstet Gynaecol*, **5**, pp. 191–197.
45. BEISCHER NA, HJOLSMAN M, KITCHEN WH (1968). Relation of various forms of anaemia to placental weight, *Amer J gynae Obstet Gyn*, **101**, pp. 801–809.
46. Government of India (2002). Tenth Five Year Plan, Planning Commission, Government of India.

47. Prophylaxis against nutritional anaemia among mothers and children, family planning programme, fourth five year plan, maternal and child health, technical information: MCH No. I.
48. ICMR (1989). Evaluation of National Nutritional Anaemia prophylaxsis programme, An ICMR Task force study, ICMR, New Delhi.
49. Ministry of Health and Family Welfare, Government of India, New Delhi and UNICEF New Delhi (1989). Report of the meeting on Prevention and Control of Nutritional anaemia.
50. Policy on control of nutritional anemia (1991), Ministry of health and Family Welfare, Government of India.
51. VIR S (1998). Control of iron deficiency anaemia – A public health programme priority. Proceedings XXXI Nutrition society of India meeting, 26–27th Nov 1998.
52. National consultation on control of nutritional anaemia in India (16–17th October, 1997), Government of India, Department of Health and Family Welfare, New Delhi, 1998.
53. Government of India (2007). Eleventh Five Year Plan, Planning Commission, Government of India.
54. NNMB (2003). National Nutrition Monitoring Bureau: Prevalence of Micronutrient Deficiencies: NNMB Technical Report No. 22, National Institute of Nutrition, Indian Council of Medical Research, Hyderabad, India.
55. KAPIL U (2002). Technical Consultation on Strategies for Prevention and Control of Iron Deficiency Anemia amongst Under Three Children in India. *Indian Pediatrics*, pp. 640–647.
56. Government of India (2007). Notification no Z.28020/50/2003-ch dated 23rd April 2007.
57. National Rural Health Mission – Mission document. www.nihfw.nic.in
58. Child Anemia workshop, 6th February, 2008, National Institute of Health And Family Welfare, New Delhi.
59. IMNCI Guidelines.
60. STOLTZFUS RJ, et al. (2004). Low dose daily iron supplementation improves iron status and appetite but not anemia whereas quarterly anti-helminthic treatment improves growth, appetite and anemia in Zanzibari preschool children. *J Nutr*, **134**, pp. 348–356.
61. JACKSON AA (2007). Anemia in severe undernutrition (malnutrition). In: *Nutritional Anemia* pp. 215–230 edited by K Kraemer and MB Zimmermann, Sight and Life Press.
62. MURRAY MJ, MURRAY AB, MURRAY CJ, MURRAY MB (1978). The effect of iron status on Nigerian mothers on that of their infants at birth and six months, and on the concentration of breast milk. *Br J. nutr.*, **39**, pp. 627–630.
63. SAZAWAL S, et al. (2006). Effects of routine supplementation with iron and folic acid on admission to hospital and mortality in preschool children in a high malaria transmission setting: community based randomized, placebo controlled trial. *Lancet*, **367**, pp. 133–143.
64. MERCER J and ERICKSON-OWENS D (2006). Delayed cord clamping increases infants iron stores, *Lancet*, **367**, pp. 1956–1958.
65. VAN RHEENEN P, BRABIN BJ (2004). Late umbilical cord clamping as an intervention for reducing iron deficiency anemia in term infants in developing and industrialized countries: a systematic review. *Ann of Trop. Paediatr*, **24**, pp. 3–16.

66. BHUTTA ZA, et al. (2008). For the Maternal and Child Undernutrition Study Group; Maternal and Child Undernutrition 3, What Works? Intervention for Maternal and Child Undernutrition and Survival. *Lancet Series I.*

67. ZLOTKIN S, ARTHUR P, ANTWI KY, YEUNG G (2001). Treatment of anemia with microcapsulted ferrous fumerate plus ascorbic acid supplied as sprinkles to complementary (weaning) foods. *Amer. J. Nutr.*, **74**, pp. 791–795.

68. HIRVE S. Micronutrient and Child Health Workshop, 20–23 October, AIIMS, New Delhi.

69. HYDER SM, HASEEN F, RAHMAN M, ZLOTKIN SH (2005). The effectiveness of flexible administration of sprinkles in anemic and non-anemic infants and young children in Bangladesh. *Proceedings of Federation of American Societies for Experimental Biology (FASEB).* San Diego (abstract).

70. DE PEE S, MOENCH PFANNER, R, MARTINI E, ZLOTKIN S, DARTON-HILL I, BLOEM MW (2007). Home fortification in emergency response and transition programming: experiences in Aceh and Nias Indonesia. *Food nutr Bulletin.*

# 25

# Iron and multiple micronutrient supplementation in children: evidence from systematic reviews

*Tarun Gera*

**Tarun Gera**, MD, is a consultant in the Department of Pediatrics, Fortis Hospital, New Delhi. Following completion of MD (Pediatrics) from Maulana Azad Medical College, University of Delhi, Dr. Gera has been extensively involved in the field of evidence-based medicine and nutrition. He has published seven systematic reviews pertaining to the field of micronutrients.

## 25.1 Introduction

Anemia is one of the most common nutrient deficiencies in the world. Recent estimates suggest that as many as two billion people are affected by this affliction globally [1]. The problem is especially severe in the South Asian region, particularly India, and more so amongst the children and pregnant women [2]. This is probably because of a combination of factors including inadequate dietary intake, poor dietary patterns, increased requirements and physiologic losses. It has been estimated that more than half the children and as much as 90% pregnant women in India are anemic [3].

Iron deficiency is the main cause of anemia in most settings. The association between the two is strong that anemia is often considered the most common indicator of iron deficiency. However, it is the more severe forms of iron deficiency which contribute to anemia. Iron has a number of other important roles in the developing human's physiology apart from hematopoiesis. The ill effects of 'subclinical' iron deficiency are gradually being recognized and these are often categorized as *functional consequences* of iron deficiency in the literature. These include poor neurocognitive development, somatic growth and physical or work capacity.

In the last decade a lot of research has also focussed on the functional consequences (growth, development, and anemia) of other micronutrients' deficiencies other than iron, in children. The most well-studied include zinc, vitamin A, folate, vitamin $B_{12}$, vitamin D and vitamin E. It is also argued that multiple micronutrient deficiencies usually coexist largely due to poor quality of the diet and low intake of food from animal sources, mostly in the lesser developed countries. From a pragmatic and economic perspective, it might make sense to combine iron supplementation programs (which are already operational in a number of countries including India) with multiple micronutrient supplementation simultaneously, in order to address the problem of these deficiencies with a unified programmatic approach. Although, such an approach of simultaneous supplementation with multiple micronutrients may seem attractive, there is a strong possibility that there may not be any additional benefit to iron supplementation alone because of the possible negative interactions they may have on each other *in vivo*. Policy formulation in developing countries, like India, would need convincing documentation of the enhanced benefit of such an approach over isolated iron supplementation.

The objective of this chapter is to assess the evidence available in the scientific literature of the advantages of use of multi micronutrient supplement vis-à-vis isolated iron supplementation on anemia, and other functional consequences.

## 25.2 Iron and multiple micronutrient supplementation and anemia

Anemia continues to be the most well studied outcome of iron deficiency and combating iron deficiency is considered the most important way to control anemia. Several randomized controlled trial conducted in children, with iron being supplemented through either the medicinal route or fortification of food products, have shown a positive beneficial effect in reducing the prevalence of anemia. However, in spite of the fact that iron supplementation programs have been operational in many developing countries, similar reduction in anemia prevalence has not been seen on a public health scale. A possible reason for this apparent lack of effectiveness may be poor compliance and acceptance, low supplies and inadequate penetration of health infrastructure in populations that need them the most.

The earlier assumption that iron supplementation might control anemia to a major extent is being increasingly questioned [4, 5]. In a recent meta-analysis (Box 25.1) evaluating the effects of iron supplementation on anemia in developing countries, the authors concluded that 'there is a suggestion in the data, not well documented except in a couple of studies, that something other than iron may be operating to limit hemoglobin response and anemia control' [4]. In another meta-analysis of randomized controlled trials (RCTs), the increase in hemoglobin with iron supplementation alone was modest (0.74 mg/dl), the response being even

**Box 25.1 Meta-analysis**

In statistics, a meta-analysis combines the results of several studies that address a set of related research hypotheses. Resulting overall averages when controlling for study characteristics can be considered meta-effect sizes, which are more powerful estimates of the true effect size than those derived in a single study under a given single set of assumptions and conditions. Meta-analysis provides a systematic overview of quantitative research which has examined a particular question and is helpful in providing insight into the overall effectiveness of interventions, the relative impact of independent variables, and the strength of relationship between variables.

poorer in malaria endemic regions [6]. Projections from this analysis suggest that in under six children, on an average between 37.9% and 62.3% (mean 49.2%) anemia is responsive to iron therapy; the corresponding figures for malarial regions being 5.8% and 31.8% (mean 22.2%).

A probable reason for this is that apart from iron, several other micronutrient deficiencies can cause anemia [7–9]. For example, it is now established that vitamin A deficiency can cause anemia. Riboflavin, folate, ascorbic acid, zinc and vitamin $B_{12}$ deficiencies are also known to impair hemoglobin synthesis.

A number of randomized controlled trials have been done to assess the impact of multiple micronutrient (including iron) supplementation on hemoglobin levels and anemia prevalence in children. The data from these trials has been synthesized in two large systematic reviews to help one arrive at an intelligible conclusion. Allen et al. [10] extracted data from 26 studies that studied the effect of multiple micronutrient supplementation on hemoglobin levels and showed that it had a significant positive effect on the hemoglobin levels (Effect Size = 0.39 mg/dL; 95% CI 0.25, 0.53; $p<0.001$) (Figure 25.1). Younger children and studies using fortification as the method of supplementation showed better improvement in the hemoglobin levels. The reduction in point prevalence of anemia was reported in fewer studies and ranged from 10% to 40%. The reduction in anemia prevalence was greater in children with lower baseline anemia and in those who received a higher amount of iron in the supplement.

The most important lacunae in this systematic review was that it failed in making distinction in the composition of the supplement provided. Thus studies that provided multiple micronutrients with iron were combined with those who did not. Similarly, the placebo groups included iron as well as placebo controls. Thus, the review failed to assess the additive effect of multiple micronutrient supplementation on hemoglobin over and above the hematinic effect provided by iron supplementation alone.

These issues were addressed by a more comprehensive review [11]. Randomized controlled trials evaluating change in Hb levels with interventions that included Fe and multiple-micronutrient supplementation in comparison

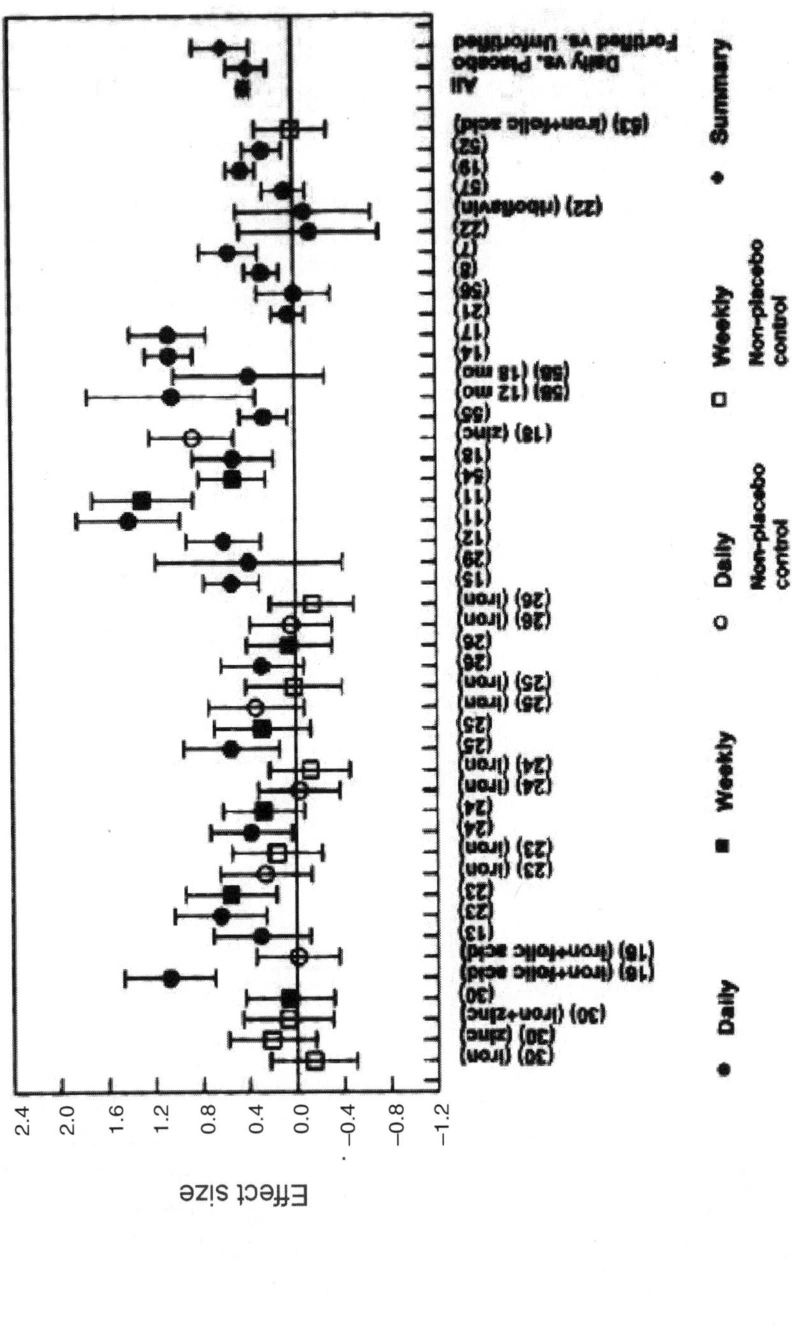


*25.1* Effect of multiple micronutrient supplementation on Hb levels in children [10]

to placebo alone or Fe alone were analysed in two separate systematic reviews. Twenty-five trials were included in the review comparing Fe and micronutrient supplementation with placebo. The pooled estimate (random effects model) for change in Hb with Fe and micronutrient supplementation (weighted mean difference) was 0.65 g/dl (95% CI 0.50, 0.80, P<0.001). Lower baseline Hb, lower height-for-age Z score, non-intake of "other micronutrients" and malarial non-hyperendemic region were noted to be significant predictors of greater Hb response and heterogeneity. These results were similar to a systematic review that had evaluated the effect of iron supplementation alone on hemoglobin levels in children [6]. Thirteen trials were included in the review comparing Fe and micronutrient supplementation with Fe alone. The pooled estimate for change in Hb with Fe and micronutrient supplementation (weighted mean difference) was 0.14 g/dl (95% CI 0.00, 0.28, P= 0.04) (Figure 25.2). Stratified analyses suggested at the possibility of a decremental response in hemoglobin with some micronutrients.

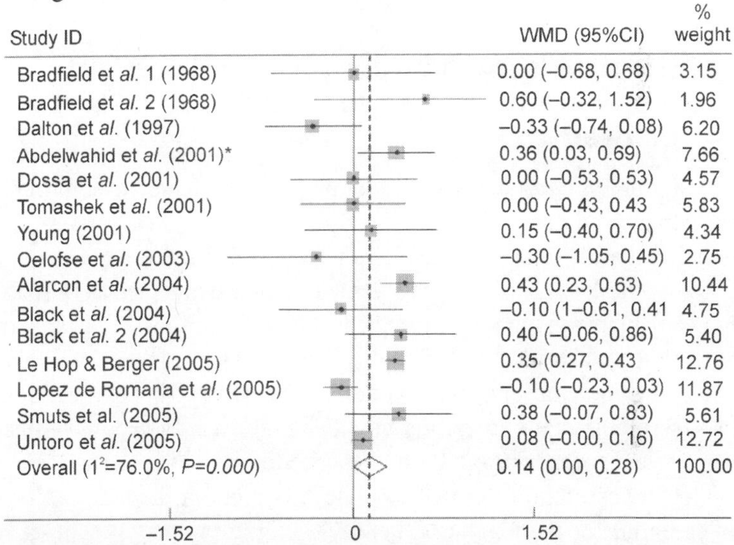


*25.2* Effect of iron and multiple micronutrient supplementation versus iron alone on hemoglobin levels in children [11].

From these two meta-analyses [6, 11], it may be postulated that the effect size of the change in hemoglobin is not likely to alter much with addition of multiple micronutrients to iron supplementation. Similar reductions in the prevalence of anemia in children may be expected (37–62% in non-malarial endemic areas and 5–31% for malarial endemic areas) despite the addition of multiple micronutrients to the iron supplement. These analyses indicate that an unselected addition of multiple micronutrients to iron supplementation will not result in a significant improvement in hemoglobin response in children.

The interaction of many of these micronutrients is still poorly understood. The possibility of negative and unpredictable interactions with co-administration of several micronutrients may therefore exist. This possibility is suggested by a decremental hemoglobin response with addition of "other micronutrients".

In conclusion, synthesized evidence available at present does not indicate that an unselected addition of multiple-micronutrients to iron supplementation will result in a significant improvement in hemoglobin response in children. There is a suggestion that some micronutrients may even have a negative effect on the hematinic effect of iron. Routine addition of unselected multiple micronutrients to iron therefore appears neither appropriate nor justified for nutritional anemia control programs. There is an urgent need to evaluate the interactive effect of individual micronutrients with iron on the hemoglobin response to provide programmatic direction.

## 25.3 Effect of iron and multiple micronutrient supplementation on mental development in children

The role of single micronutrients on cognitive performance of children has been investigated in many nutrition interventions. From these studies, it can be concluded that there is strong evidence for a beneficial effect of iron and iodine on cognition, while evidence for other micronutrients such as B-vitamins and zinc is plausible given their biological role in brain function [12]. Iron is required for proper myelination of the spinal cord and white matter of cerebellar folds, and it is a cofactor for a number of enzymes involved in neurotransmitter synthesis (serotonin, norepinephrine and dopamine) [13, 14]. Iodine is needed for the production of the thyroid hormones triiodothyronine (T3) and thyroxin (T4), which are essential for growth and development of the fetal brain [15]. Zinc is essential for neurogenesis, neuronal migration, and synaptogenesis and its deficiency could interfere with neurotransmission and subsequent neuropsychological behaviour [16]. B vitamins have a role as coenzymes in numerous metabolic processes, including formation of neurotransmitters (communication in the brain), neural tube formation, and synthesis of myelin basic protein (myelination of nerves) [12].

Amongst all these the strongest evidence of benefit of supplementation through well conducted RCTs and systematic reviews is restricted to iron and iodine supplementation. In a systematic review assessing the effect of iron supplementation on mental and motor development in children, the authors showed that iron supplementation did have a significant positive effect on mental development, albeit modestly [17]. The positive effects of iron were more pronounced in older and iron deficient, anemic children.

The mental development in children less than 2 years of age and the motor development were not affected by supplementation, indicating an irreversible effect of iron deficiency in this subgroup. There is a possible preventive role of iron supplementation in preventing cognitive deficits even in children who are apparently iron replete.

Previously conducted qualitative reviews have shown multiple micronutrient supplementation to be beneficial in neurocognitive development of children [18]. Recently a systematic review assessing the effect of multiple micronutrient supplementation on cognitive performance in children was conducted by Eilander et al [19]. This review synthesized data from 20 RCTs and concluded that there was a marginally positive effect of multiple micronutrient supplementation on fluid intelligence in children (statistically not significant) and no effect on crystallized intelligence. There was a statistically significant effect on academic performance in older children but the number of studies (four) found to be too few to derive any intelligible conclusions. These conclusions were very much in agreement with previously conducted reviews that had focussed on individual domains of mental development [18].

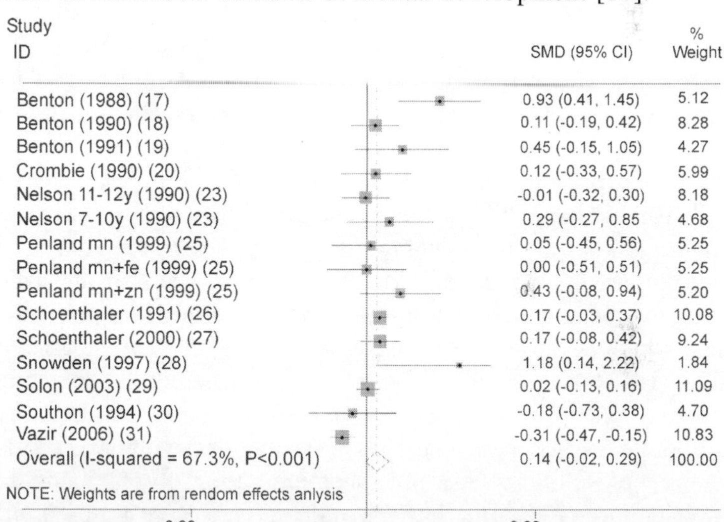


*25.3* Effect of multiple micronutrient supplementation on fluid intelligence in children [19].

Looking at the currently available data, there is definitely a case for iron supplementation in improving mental and motor development, more so, as preventive therapy. However, no robust evidence links routine multiple micronutrient supplementation with improvement in cognitive performance in children so as to suggest recommendation for supplementation as a public health measure.

## 25.4 Iron and multiple micronutrient supplementation in children and growth

Given the widespread prevalence of stunting and wasting in the world, especially in South Asia and Sub-Saharan Africa, its appropriate management has occupied many a scientific minds. It is obvious that the most needed therapies would include ensuring adequate protein and caloric intake, and access to health care for timely treatment of morbidities. However, despite addressing these concerns in large public health interventions has not always yielded the expected results. This led to two major interventions apart from the ones already stated – exclusive breastfeeding and micronutrient supplementation. Regarding the latter, a large number of trials have been conducted globally that have assessed the effect of both individual micronutrient and multiple micronutrient supplementation on growth in children, and these have been followed by meta-analyses as well that have tried to synthesize the available information quantitatively.

The most widely cited meta-analyses was the one conducted by Brown et al [20] that showed zinc supplementation to be associated with a beneficial effect on the linear growth in children. Systematic reviews on the same topic with reference to iron and vitamin A, however, failed to show any such benefit. In fact, one of these reviews even indicated at the possibility of a negative effect of iron supplementation in iron replete children and with longer duration (>6 months) of iron supplementation [21, 22]. One meta-analysis suggests the possibility of a beneficial effect with multiple micronutrient supplementation [10].

Some of these systematic reviews are more than 5 years old and a number of trials have been conducted on this topic since then, the most notable amongst which is the International Research on Infant Supplementation Initiative (IRIS) trial which is a large multicentric trial that evaluated the effect of multiple micronutrient supplementation in young children. In order to incorporate the new data available, a systematic review was conducted on the effect of individual and multiple micronutrient supplementation on growth in children [23]. The findings of this review were almost similar to the previously conducted reviews. Iron (27 trials) and vitamin A (17 trials) had no effect on physical growth. Zinc supplementation (43 trials) had a small positive effect on WAZ (weight for age) scores but no effect on linear growth, in contrast to the Brown meta-analyses. Multiple micronutrient supplementation was associated with an improvement in height but the effect size was very small.

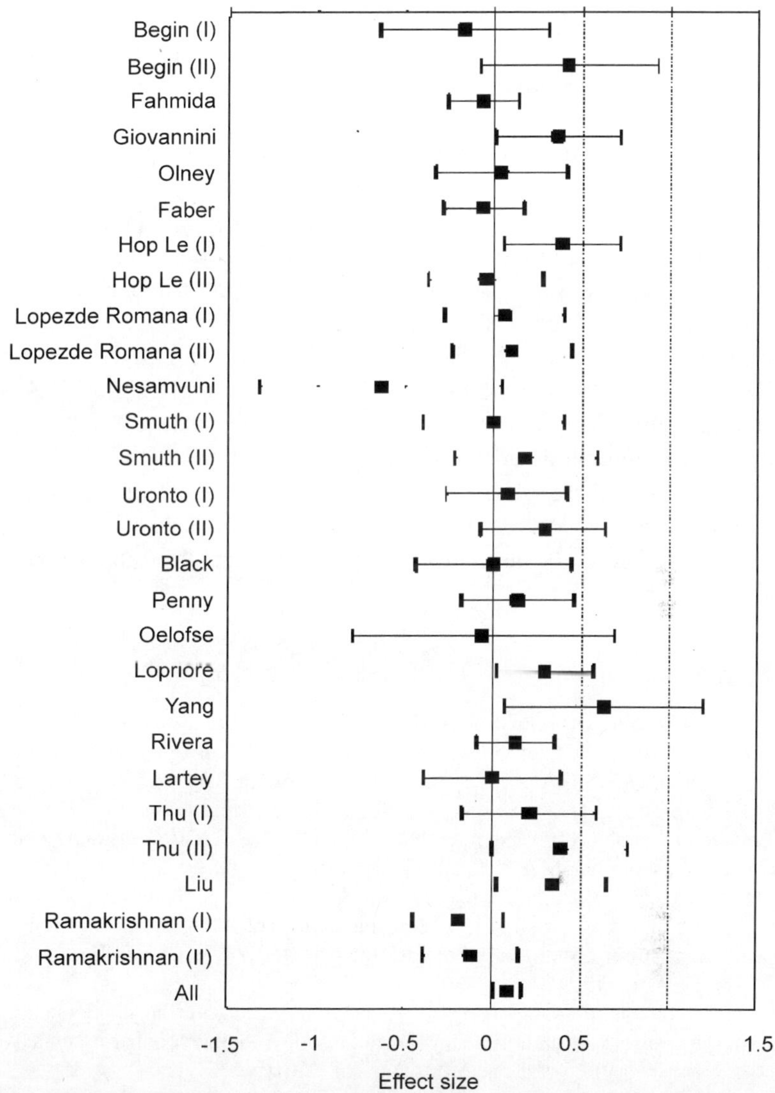


*25.4* Effect of multiple micronutrient supplementation on height gain in children [23]

The results from these reviews suggest that though micronutrient interventions (single and multiple) may have a marginal effect on anthropometric parameters, the effect on height is small.

The series of systematic reviews conducted so far suggest that iron supplementation alone has a positive effect on hematological parameters and mental development in children. The effect on growth and anthropometry is minimal. This, to a certain extent, justifies the need for mass scale iron supplementation programs for amelioration of anemia and to achieve optimal mental development, albeit with realistic expectations.

However, the addition of multiple micronutrients does not seem to offer any additional benefit as far as the specific outcomes on anaemia, mental development and growth is concerned. Furthermore, in some cases indiscriminate addition of micronutrients may even have a deleterious effect. This may be attributed to a number of reasons – the limited number of studies that differentiate between a therapeutic and preventive effects of supplementation, short duration of most of the supplementation trials, lack of uniformity of the composition of the combination of micronutrients used, variation in the settings in which the trials were conducted, the lack of understanding of the physiologic role of some of the micronutrients in developing human body and the interactions that occur in vivo when a number of micronutrients are given simultaneously, and the limiting role of other factors like poor complementary feeding, poverty and lack of food security, infections and infestations, inadequate stimulation etc. A better understanding of these issues and a clearer elucidation of micronutrient interactions is required. Presently, there is no scientific basis to support routine multiple micronutrient supplementation in children as a public health measure.

## References

1. United Nations Administrative Committee on Coordination Sub-Committee on Nutrition (ACC/SCN) (2000). Fourth Report on the World Nutrition Situation. Geneva: ACC/SCN in collaboration with International Food Policy Research Institute.
2. MASON JB, et al. (2001) The micronutrient report: Current progress and trends in the control of vitamin A, iodine, and iron deficiencies. Ottawa, The Micronutrient Initiative (Accessed at http://www.micronutrient.org on September 8, 2004).
3. SINGH P and TOTEJA GS (2003). Micronutrient profile of Indian children and women: summary of available data for iron and vitamin A. *Indian Pediatr*, **40**, pp. 477–479.
4. BEATON GH and MCCABE GP (1999). Efficacy of intermittent iron supplementation in the control of iron deficiency anaemia in developing countries: an analysis of experience. Ottawa, The Micronutrient Initiative.
5. SCHOLL T and HEDIGER M (1994). Anaemia and iron deficiency anaemia: compilation of data on pregnancy outcome. *Am J Clin Nutr.* **59**, pp. 492S–500S.
6. GERA T, SACHDEV HP, NESTEL P, SACHDEV S (2007). Effect of iron supplementation on haemoglobin response in children: systematic review of randomised controlled trials. *J Pediatr Gastroenterol Nutr.*, **44**(4), pp. 468–486.
7. HODGES RE, et al (1978). Hematopoietic studies in vitamin A deficiency. *Am J Clin Nutr,* **31**, pp. 876–885.
8. CAMPBELL TC, BRUN T, JUNSHI C, ZULIN F, PARPIA B (1990). Questioning riboflavin recommendations on the basis of a survey in China. *Am J Clin Nutr*, **51**, pp. 436–445.
9. BAKER SJ (1981). Nutritional anemias. Part 2: Tropical Asia. *Clinical Haemat.* **10**, pp. 843–871.

10. ALLEN LH, PEERSON JM, OLNEY DK (2009). Provision of multiple rather than two or fewer micronutrients more effectively improves growth and other outcomes in micronutrient deficient children and adults. *J Nutr*, **139**, pp. 1022–1030.
11. GERA T, SACHDEV HP, NESTEL P (2009). Effect of combining multiple micronutrients with iron supplementation on Hb response in children: systematic review of randomized controlled trials. *Public Health Nutr*, **12**(6), pp. 756–773.
12. BRYAN J, et al (2004). Nutrients for cognitive development in school aged children. *Nut Rev*, **62**, pp. 295–306.
13. BEARD JL, CONNOR JR, JONES BC (1993). Brain iron: location and function. *Prog Food Nutr Sci,* **17**, pp. 183–221.
14. BEARD JL, CONNOR JR, JONES BC (1993). Iron in the brain. *Nutr Rev*; **51**, pp. 157–70.
15. MELSE-BOONSTRA A, JAISWAL N (2010). Iodine deficiency in pregnancy, infancy and childhood and its consequences for brain development. *Best Pract Res Clin Endocrinol Metab*, **24**(1), pp. 29–38.
16. BOURRE JM (2006). Effects of nutrients (in food) on the structure and function of the nervous system: update on dietary requirements for brain. Part 1: micronutrients. *J Nutr Health Aging*, **10**, pp. 377–385.
17. SACHDEV HPS, GERA T, NESTEL P (2005). Effect of iron supplementation on mental and motor development in children. *Public Health and Nutrition*, **8**(2), pp. 117–132.
18. BENTON D (2001). Micro-nutrient supplementation and the intelligence of children. *Neurosci Biobehav Rev,* **25**, pp. 297–309.
19. EILANDER A, GERA T, SACHDEV HS, TRANSLER C, VAN DER KNAAP HC, KOK FJ, OSENDARP SJ (2010). Multiple micronutrient supplementation for improving cognitive performance in children: systematic review of randomized controlled trials. *Am J Clin nutr*, **91**, pp. 115–130.
20. BROWN KH, PEERSON JM, RIVERA J, ALLEN LH (2002). Effect of supplemental zinc on the growth and serum zinc concentrations of prepubertal children: a meta-analysis of randomized controlled trials. *Am J Clin Nutr*; **75**, pp. 1062–1071.
21. RAMAKRISHNAN U, ABURTO N, MCCABE G, MARTORELL R (2004). Multimicronutrient growth: results of 3 meta-analyses. *J Nutr,* **134**, pp. 2592–2602.
22. SACHDEV H, GERA T, NESTEL P (2006). Effect of iron supplementation on physical growth in children: systematic review of randomised controlled trials. *Public Health Nutr*, **9**, pp. 904–920.
23. RAMAKRISHNAN U, NGUYEN P and MARTORELL R (2009). Effects of micronutrients on growth of children under 5 y of age: meta-analyses of single and multiple nutrient interventions. *Am J Clin Nutr*, **89**, pp. 191–203.

# 26

# Nutritional anemia during pregnancy, early childhood and adolescence: the critical development periods

*Subadra Seshadri*

**Subadra Seshadri** MSc, MS, PhD, a senior nutrition consultant, was formerly Professor and Head of the Department of Foods and Nutrition at M S University of Baroda. She is the recipient of Dr S G Srikantia Memorial Lecture Award 2005 of the Nutrition Society of India. Her significant research contributions to nutritional anemia, especially iron deficiency anemia and cognition, are widely recognized. Dr Seshadri has served as a technical expert on micronutrient research and development to WHO, UNICEF and others.

## 26.1 Introduction

Nutritional anemia is a major public health problem worldwide, affecting an estimated 2 billion people, most of them in the developing world [1–2]. Given the impact that nutritional anemia has on psychological and physical development, behavior and work performance, it is a problem of serious public health significance.

Iron deficiency is by far the commonest cause of nutritional anemia [3–4]. Iron deficiency occurs when an insufficient amount of iron is absorbed to meet the body's requirements. This insufficiency may be due to inadequate iron intake from the diet, to reduced bioavailability of the dietary iron, or to increased needs of iron as occurs during infancy and pregnancy. Only when iron deficiency is prolonged does it lead to anemia, a condition in which hemoglobin level in the blood falls below normal for a given age and sex group. Iron deficiency is usually diagnosed with the help of several laboratory tests. These include serum iron, iron binding capacity, transferrin saturation, serum ferritin, transferrin receptors and erythrocyte proto porphyrin concentration in blood. In iron deficiency anemia, in addition to the changes in the above parameters, there is a gradual fall in blood hemoglobin level below normal resulting in different degrees of anemia from mild to moderate to severe.

While iron deficiency is the most common cause of anemia in India and the other developing countries, other nutritional deficiencies such as low intake of folic acid, vitamin $B_{12}$, riboflavin, vitamin A and vitamin C can all influence the etiology of anemia [3, 5, 6]. Important among these is folic acid deficiency. Combined folate and iron deficiency is especially common in women in the second half of pregnancy, in India [7]. Anemia is common in children suffering from severe protein energy malnutrition. Vitamin $B_{12}$ deficiency in strict vegetarians leads to anemia which is usually megaloblastic (the red cells are larger than normal in size) as against the microcytic anemia of iron deficiency (the red cells are smaller in size compared to normal). Folate deficiency also manifests as a megaloblastic anemia. If iron, folate and vitamin $B_{12}$ deficiencies co exist, the latter will become apparent only after iron deficiency has been corrected, thus making it necessary to use laboratory tests other than hemoglobin and red cell morphology for the diagnosis of these deficiencies. Besides folate and vitamin $B_{12}$ deficiencies, two other nutrient deficiencies involved in the causation of anemia, are riboflavin and vitamin A. Thus, multiple nutrient deficiencies may be involved in the pathogenesis of anemia. However, it is important to appreciate that iron deficiency is the major cause of anemia in the developing world, with some recent studies suggesting that 50% of all the anemias may be estimated to be due to iron deficiency. Additionally, there are a similar number of people manifesting iron deficiency without anemia, thus placing iron deficiency as the most common public health nutritional deficiency the world over [3].

### 26.1.1 Definition of nutritional anemia

Nutritional anemia in general is defined as a condition that results in a lowering of hemoglobin (Hb) levels below what is considered to be normal for specific demographic groups regardless of the underlying nutritional deficiencies that may be the cause. A WHO group of experts in 1971 defined normal hemoglobin concentration in the following terms:

"It is recognized that there is a homeostatic mechanism that sets the hemoglobin level in each individual. Whereas it is not known whether this is the optimum level for health it is accepted as 'normal' for the individual.The distribution of such normal values in the population should be derived from a representative sample of healthy persons in whom the presence of nutritional deficiencies has been excluded by specific laboratory determinations or by prior administration of hematinics.This distribution of normal values is likely to be the same throughout the world when allowance is made for factors such as age, sex, pregnancy and altitude" (WHO, 1972).

Nutritional anemia is thus defined "as a condition in which the hemoglobin level is below the level that is normal, for a given individual due to deficiency of one or more of the nutrients required for hemopoiesis and conversely as a condition in which the hemoglobin concentration can be raised by increasing the amount of nutrients absorbed".

"In a community in which there is no anemia, the frequency distribution curve of hemoglobin concentration follows a nearly normal distribution, but in a community with a high prevalence of anemia the frequency distribution curve will be skewed to the left" [8].

The criteria for determining the presence of nutritional anemia, was first recommended by WHO in 1968. A subsequent WHO committee has recommended that 11.5 g/dl be considered as the cut-off for anemia for school children aged 5–11 years. In addition, there is also defined hemoglobin cut-off values for various degrees of anemia. Moderate anemia is defined as hemoglobin levels below 10 g/dl and severe anemia as hemoglobin levels below 7 g/dl in individuals and population groups.

*Table 26.1* Hemoglobin values below which anemia is likely to be present in populations living at sea level as proposed by WHO in1968 [9] and modified for 5–11 year-old children later in 1998 [10]

| Groups | Hemoglobin level below which anemia is considered to be present (g/dl) |
|---|---|
| Children 6 months to 6 years | 11.0 |
| Children 5–11 years | 11.5 |
| Children 12–13 years | 12.0 |
| Adult males | 13.0 |
| Adult females (non-pregnant) | 12.0 |
| Adult females (pregnant) | 11.0 |

Additionally, epidemiological criteria for assessing the severity and the magnitude of nutritional anemia in populations [11] have also been proposed.

Population prevalence for defining the severity of the problem

| Parameters | Magnitude | | |
|---|---|---|---|
| | High | Moderate | Low |
| Percent of population with Hb level less than the above cut-off points | >40 | 10–39 | <10 |
| Percent of population with Hb level less than 7 g/dl especially women and children | >10 | 1–9 | <1 |

While the causes of anemia have been known for a long time, the multiple adverse functional effects of anemia have been brought to light only recently. Physical work capacity, mental functions and cognitive development, immune functions and pregnancy outcome are all affected adversely in iron deficiency anemia [12–17], thus contributing to the erosion of human resources in a country like India, making it imperative to have clear policies and programs for the prevention and correction of anemia. This chapter would first outline the global prevalence of anemia in different age, sex and physiological groups, followed by prevalence in India. The various factors in the etiology of nutritional anemia will then be discussed, followed by iron requirements of different age groups and physiological conditions, focusing on why some demographic groups are much more vulnerable to anemia than the others. This is followed by methods for assessment of anemia, indicators of iron, folic acid and $B_{12}$ deficiencies and the functional consequences of anemia. In the final section public health approaches for the prevention and control of anemia will be discussed. Through out this chapter, the term anemia is used to refer to nutritional anemia, i.e. anemia caused by nutritional deficiencies directly through inadequate diets or indirectly through conditions that increase the iron requirements. Anemias of other etiology, such as genetic anemia, are not within the scope of this chapter.

## 26.2 Prevalence of anemia: global and the Indian population

### 26.2.1 Global prevalence of anemia

Global and regional prevalence of anemia has been reported recently in a WHO publication for preschool-age children (<5 years) and for pregnant and non pregnant women [1]. These figures represented in the Table 26.2 below show that globally the prevalence of anemia is the highest in pre school age children, 47.4%, followed by pregnant women, 41.8% and lowest in non pregnant women, 30.2%. The prevalence figures are reported for 6 regions, namely Africa, Asia, Europe, Latin America, North America and Oceania. Highest prevalence in all the three groups is seen in Africa which is followed by Asia.

*Table 26.2* Global and regional prevalence of anemia [1]

| Area | Preschool age children | | Pregnant women | | Non-pregnant women | |
|---|---|---|---|---|---|---|
| | Prevalence % | Number in millions | Prevalence % | Number in millions | Prevalence % | Number in millions |
| Global | 47.4 | 293.1 | 41.8 | 56.4 | 30.2 | 468.4 |
| Africa | 64.6 | 93.2 | 55.8 | 19.3 | 44.4 | 82.9 |
| Asia | 47.7 | 170.0 | 41.6 | 31.7 | 33.0 | 318.3 |
| Europe | 16.7 | 6.1 | 18.7 | 1.4 | 15.2 | 26.6 |
| Latin America | 39.5 | 22.3 | 31.1 | 36.0 | 23.5 | 33.0 |
| North America | 3.4 | 0.8 | 6.1 | 0.3 | 7.6 | 6.0 |
| Oceania | 20 | 0.7 | 30.4 | 0.2 | 20.2 | 1.5 |

However within Asia, the prevalence of anemia is quite high in South and South East Asia as seen from the 5th Report of the World Nutritions situation by the ACC-SCN, 2004 [18] (Table 26.3).

*Table 26.3* Prevalence of anemia in women (15–45 years) (5th Report of the World Nutrition Situation, ACC-SCN, 2004) [18]

| Regions and countries | Mild anemia (%) | Moderate anemia (%) | Severe anemia | Any anemia (%) |
|---|---|---|---|---|
| **Sub-Saharan Africa** | | | | |
| Benin, 2001 | 40.7 | 21.8 | 1.8 | 64.3 |
| Mali, 2001 | 39.1 | 20.8 | 2.8 | 62.7 |
| Uganda 2001 | 22.1 | 7.5 | 0.7 | 30.4 |
| **North Africa West Asia/ Europe** | | | | |
| Armenia,2000 | 10.2 | 2.0 | 0.3 | 12.4 |
| Egypt,2000 | 22.7 | 4.6 | 0.3 | 27.7 |
| **Central Asia** | | | | |
| Kazhakhastan 1999 | 26.6 | 7.7 | 1.2 | 35.5 |
| Krygez Republic, 1997 | 27.7 | 9.0 | 1.5 | 38.1 |
| Turkmenistan, 2000 | 37.8 | 8.4 | 1.1 | 47.3 |
| **South and south east Asia** | | | | |
| Cambodia,2000 | 44.8 | 12.7 | 1.3 | 58.8 |
| India 1998–99 | 35.0 | 14.8 | 1.9 | 51.8 |
| **Latin America and Caribbean** | | | | |
| Bolivia, 1998 | 20.7 | 5.6 | 0.9 | 27.1 |
| Haiti, 2000 | 36.3 | 15.8 | 3.0 | 55.1 |
| Peru, 2000 | 25.4 | 5.9 | 0.3 | 31.6 |

Mild anemia women: Hb 10–10.9 g/dl for pregnant women; Hb 10–11.9g/dl for non pregnant
Moderate anemia: Hb 7–9.9 g/dl; Severe anemia: Hb <7 g/dl

Nationally representative data on iron deficiency and iron deficiency anemia has been reported for adolescents by the National Health and Nutrition Examination Survey III (NHANES-III) in the USA [19]. Iron deficiency was defined as having an abnormal value for at least two out of the three laboratory tests of iron status (erythrocyte protoporphyrin, transferrin saturation, or serum ferritin); and iron deficiency anemia was defined as iron deficiency plus low hemoglobin. Prevalence was determined based on the 5th percentile value of these parameters in the NHANES III data.

Nine to eleven percent of adolescent girls and women of childbearing age were iron deficient; of these, iron deficiency anemia was found in 3% and 2–5%, respectively. Iron deficiency was found in no more than 1% of adolescent boys and young men. Among women of childbearing age, iron deficiency was more likely in those who were minority, low income, and multiparous.

*Table 26.4* Prevalence of iron deficiency and iron deficiency anemia in adolescent males and non-pregnant females [19]

| Gender and age (years) | Iron deficiency (%) | Iron deficiency anemia (%) |
|---|---|---|
| Females | | |
| 12–15 | 9 | 2 |
| 16–19 | 11 | 3 |
| Males | | |
| 12–15 | 1 | <1 |
| 16–19 | <1 | <1 |

As against this situation in US, an example of a well developed country, the prevalence of anemia in India among all demographic groups is high.

## 26.2.2 Prevalence of anemia in India

Prevalence of anemia in India, in the different demographic groups is shown in Table 26.5.

*Table 26.5* Prevalence of anemia in India

| Group | Reference | Prevalence (%) |
|---|---|---|
| Pregnant women | ICMR 1989 [20] | 87 |
| | ICMR 2001 [21] | 85 |
| | NFHS II 1988–89 [22] | 50 |
| | NFHS III, 2006–07 [23] | 58 |
| Early childhood to pre-school | NFHS II, 1998–99 | 74 |
| Children (6 to 35 months) | NFHS III, 2006–7 | 79 |
| Adolescent girls | SESHADRI, 1999, Rural Gujarat [24] | 62 |
| | SESHADRI, 1999, Urban affluent [25] | 22 |
| | ICMR, 2001, Rural India | 90 |
| Adult women | | |
| Ever married women (15–49 years) | NFHS II 1998–99 | 52 |
| Ever married women (15–49 years) | NFHS III 2006–07 | 56 |

### *Pregnant women*

Nationally representative data on prevalence of anemia in pregnant women in India were generated in the year 1989 through a country wide evaluation of the anemia control program that was launched in 1975 but had not been evaluated since then. For the study of hemoglobin by the cyanmethemoglobin method, 4775 pregnant women at or beyond 20 weeks of gestation from 10 states and the union territory of Delhi were examined. The prevalence of anemia defined as Hb less than 11 g/dl was 87%. Other large scale studies since then have found the prevalence to be quite high, in the range of 80% and above [21]. However, the National Family Health surveys II and III [22, 23] have reported a somewhat lower prevalence of anemia which is attributed to a different method used for assessment of Hb rather than a fall in the prevalence rates.

*Early childhood*

Studies prior to 1985 in India gave an average prevalence rate of 68% in pre-school children [26]. More recently ICMR carried out a prevalence survey of anemia in preschool children from four regions of India. The NFHS II and III have also carried out Hb assays in a large sample of pre school children. The prevalence rates in children remain high, above 70 % and have shown no decline since the last four decades. See Table 26.4 for details.

*Adolescent females*

The prevalence of anemia in adolescent girls has been reported by a number of studies recently in India and all of them point to high prevalence, in the range of 60–90% in girls aged 11–18 years (Table 26.5), much higher than the 20% population prevalence cut-off for non-pregnant women in reproductive age group that was identified by WHO to classify the problem as one of public health significance. Thus there is enough evidence to establish that anemia is a major public health problem among adolescents also in India and needs to be tackled by appropriate public health measures.

## 26.3 Causes of nutritional anemia

While the major cause of nutritional anemia in India and the world over is related to dietary inadequacies, often these dietary inadequacies are aggravated by environmental factors such as poor sanitation leading to helminthic and protozoal infestations and infection with malarial parasites. Therefore, dietary factors as causative agents will have to be seen in conjunction with the other environmental factors while talking of preventive public health approaches.

### 26.3.1 Deficiency of several nutrients involved in etiology of anemia

Dietary deficiency of several micro nutrients can lead to anemia. These include, iron – a major dietary factor in the causation of anemia while other nutrient deficiencies such as folic acid, vitamin A [27–29], riboflavin [30] and vitamin $B_{12}$ [31] contribute in a secondary manner.

The cellular events in iron deficiency that eventually lead to anemia are well documented.

Iron is needed for the synthesis of hemoglobin, the main oxygen carrier in the blood; for the synthesis of myoglobin that serves as a ready source of oxygen for the oxidative processes in muscle, and for the synthesis of heme and non-heme proteins involved in cellular processes. Deficiency of iron results in impaired production of these molecules eventually leading to low hemoglobin levels and anemia.

### 26.3.2 Low dietary intake of iron – a major cause of anemia in India

Several dietary intake studies have been carried out in India, using a diet history, a 24 h dietary recall or weighed food intakes. Such larger studies have been done as a part of the National Nutrition Monitoring Bureau surveys [32–34]. In general, these studies indicate that iron intakes as a percent of the recommended dietary allowances set by the ICMR in 1989 is no more than 50. Thus low intakes are the order of the day. Even on these low intakes, the anemia prevalence figures need not be so high if the dietary iron bioavailability is high. Unfortunately, the iron bioavailability from Indian diets is one of the lowest in the world.

### 26.3.3 Low iron bioavailability is another major cause of anemia in India

Bioavailability of iron is defined as the fraction of the dietary iron absorbed and utilized for specific functions such as the synthesis of hemoglobin, heme containing enzymes and other iron containing functional proteins [35]. It is dependent on a variety of dietary factors such as the chemical form in which iron is present in foods, i.e. heme iron versus non-heme iron, its solubility in the gastro intestinal tract and the various iron absorption promoters and inhibitors in the foods which decide what fraction of the dietary iron will be absorbed and utilized [36].

There are two major chemical forms of iron in a mixed diet, and each is absorbed by a different mechanism. Heme, containing iron in a porphyrin ring structure is found in hemoglobin and myoglobin and accounts for nearly 40% of the iron present in animal tissue including fish and poultry [37]. Because of the porphyrin ring structure the iron in heme containing molecules is protected from the action of complexing agents present in the meal and is taken up by the mucosal cells as the intact protoporphyrin complex. Absorption of heme iron is therefore high averaging 15% in iron replete individuals to 35% in those lacking iron stores [38]. Once absorbed by the cell, iron in the heme molecule is split by a specific enzyme, xanthine oxidase. After this, the iron from the heme and non-heme sources form a common pool with in the cell.

The other chemical form of iron, namely non-heme iron is present largely in foods of vegetable origin and in non cellular animal foods such as eggs and dairy products. In addition, approximately half of the iron in meat, fish and poultry is non heme. The specific rate of non heme iron absorption depends upon other dietary constituents ingested concomitantly as well as the iron status of the individual [36]. Hence absorption of non-heme iron ranges widely from 2% to 20% depending on the above two determinants [38].

The various dietary factors affecting non heme iron bioavailability are shown in Table 26.5 below. The two major enhancers of iron absorption are: ascorbic acid and flesh foods like meat, poultry and fish, where as the inhibitors far outnumber the enhancers, especially in the Indian dietaries.

*Table 26.6* Food components affecting dietary non heme iron bioavailability [36]

(Potency is indicated in terms of + signs. The sign +++ indicates highest positive effect for enhancers and highest negative effect for inhibitors. For example tea has a most potent inhibitory effect on iron absorption while ascorbic acid is a very potent enhancer of iron absorption.)

| Food Components – The Enhancers and Inhibitors | Potency |
|---|---|
| ENHANCERS | |
| Ascorbic acid | +++ |
| Animal tissue | +++ |
| INHIBITORS | |
| Tea | +++ |
| Soy products | +++ |
| Coffee | ++ |
| EDTA | ++ |
| Calcium/Phosphate salts | ++ |
| Eggs | |
| Yolk | ++ |
| Albumen | ++ |
| Wheat bran | +++ |
| Phytate | + |
| Fiber | + |

Ascorbic acid has been shown to be a powerful enhancer of iron absorption. Several in vivo studies have been carried out using crystalline ascorbic acid as well as ascorbic acid from food sources [39–42]. The major findings that emerge from these studies are:

1. Ascorbic acid enhances iron absorption from both low and high bioavailability meals, when added as crystalline ascorbic acid or from food sources.
2. The magnitude of increase is much higher in the low availability non heme iron containing meals than in the high availability heme iron containing meals.
3. The increase in absorption that occurs with ascorbic acid is influenced by the ascorbic acid to iron molar ratio, larger the ratio, higher the absorption.
4. Further the ascorbic acid effect has also been shown to be dose dependent, up to a level of 1000 mg. However, the enhancing effect of ascorbic acid at lower dose level is much higher than the enhancing effect at higher levels.

Thus although dose dependent, it is not necessary in practical diets to have high levels of ascorbic acid to bring about a significant increase in absorption of iron. In vivo absorption studies have shown that 30 mg of ascorbic acid can increase the iron absorption twofold while 50–75 mg can bring about 3–5 fold increases in iron absorption. In other words within the range of physiological intakes, iron absorption especially from typical non heme iron containing diets can be increased very significantly, a finding that needs to be translated into dietary practices much more vigorously.

Ascorbic acid operates in multiple ways to increase iron absorption, by forming a soluble complex at the acidic pH in the stomach that remains soluble as the pH rises in the small intestine, by reducing the ferric to more readily absorbed ferrous ions, by preventing the formation of insoluble complexes with the inhibitors and by preferentially donating its iron to the brush border receptors to increase iron uptake by mucosal cells.

Meat and flesh foods in addition to containing better bioavailable iron, also possess the ability to enhance non heme iron absorption from primarily vegetarian diets [43–44]. The potency of 100 g of cooked meat in enhancing iron absorption has been graded as equal to that of 100 mg ascorbic acid [37].

Given the economic constraints to the consumption of flesh foods, the only enhancer of significance in the predominantly vegetarian Indian dietaries is ascorbic acid. The inhibitors of iron absorption on the other hand far outnumber the enhancers, as is evident from Table 26.5.

In general, the enhancers form soluble complexes with non-heme iron which readily give up their iron to iron binding proteins present on the microvilli of the intestinal lumen that in turn facilitate absorption across the lumen into the mucosal cells. On the contrary, the inhibitors form insoluble complexes with non-heme iron that remain insoluble and do not release the iron for absorption. Extensive studies on iron absorption from typical diets have shown that the Indian vegetarian diet high in cereals and pulses and low in fruits and vegetables, accompanied by tea, has the lowest iron bioavailability. Table 26.7 shows iron bioavailability in some typical meals estimated in vivo.

*Table 26.7* Iron bioavailability in some typical meals [45–49]

| S. no. | Type of meal | Ingredients | Bioavailability In vivo | Reference |
|---|---|---|---|---|
| 1. | Indian wheat break fast | Wheat flour, oil, potato Onion, tea, milk and sugar, | 1.8 | 45 |
| 2. | Indian rice lunch | Rice, red gram dhal, potato, onion, brinjal, oil, milk | 4.5 | 45 |
| 3. | Indian Ragi breakfast | Ragi, potato, onion, brinjal, oil, tea, milk, and sugar | 0.9 | 45 |
| 4. | Indian break fast | Sorghum, potato, onion, brinjal, oil Tea, milk and sugar | 0.8 | 45 |
| 5. | Hamburger meal | Commercial product containing minced meat, bread, onion sauce, Brussels sprouts | 38.8 | 46 |
| 6. | Latin American meal | Potatoes, maize, black beans, rice, | 3.2 | 47 |
| 7. | South East Asian rice and fish meal | Rice, cat fish, spinach, fish paste, beans and spices | 12.0 | 48 |
| 8. | Venezuelan breakfast | Maize, butter, cheese, oats, milk | 1.3 | 49 |
| 9. | Venezuelan lunch | Maize, black beans, fish paste, plantain, tomato, potato, carrot, meat | 3.9 | 49 |
| 10. | Venezuelan lunch | Maize, rice, plantain, fish, avocado, tomato, onion, water melon | 6.7 | 49 |
| 11. | Venezuelan supper | Maize, milk, plantain, fish, pumpkin, papaya, coffee, sugar | 11.1 | 49 |

In addition to the dietary factors, iron status of the individuals also plays a crucial role in determining the amount of iron absorbed. Iron deplete individuals absorb more iron from the same meal compared to iron replete individuals. The molecular basis of iron absorption is discussed under the section on iron homeostasis.

Thus to summarize, the chemical form of iron, the balance of the enhancers and inhibitors of iron absorption in the diet and the iron status of the individual are the three major factors that influence the amount of iron absorbed and transported to the body for specific functions which is defined as iron bioavailability. Given that the predominant chemical form of iron in the Indian dietary is non-heme iron and the inhibitors far outnumber the enhancers, in addition to the intake of enhancers being highly seasonal and very low most of the time, the absorption of iron is considered to be not more than 3–5% in most regional diets in India [50].

### 26.3.4 Parasitic infestations

Parasitic infestations aggravate the already existing states of nutritional deficiencies, especially iron, and may push the affected individuals into overt anemia. In this context, hook worms (*Ancylostoma duodenale* and *Necator Americanus*) are the most deleterious followed by whip worms (*Trichuris Trichuria*), both of which cause blood losses. Blood loss due to hook worms may vary from 2 ml to 100 ml per day [51] according to the severity of infestation. In a population whose iron status is already compromised by low dietary intake of iron and poor bioavailability, a small load of hook worms can precipitate anemia. Over a period of time, even small hookworm loads can cause blood losses sufficient to deplete iron reserves, placing these individuals at high risk of developing anemia. For example, blood loss of 1ml per day equivalent to 0.347 mg of iron at a Hb level of 10 g/dl can cause a loss of 250 mg of iron over two years which approximates the total body iron stores in an adult woman in India.

The reported prevalence of hook worm infestation increases with age in children. Therefore the greatest effect of hook worm infestation is seen in school aged children and adults. Approximately 20% of the world's population is reported to be infected by hook worms [52] Further some work places are particularly prone to hookworms such as the tea plantations where the moist unsanitary conditions coupled with walking bare foot makes the workers contract the infestation easily [53].

The other parasites like round worms (*Ascaris lumbricoides*) act by impairing absorption, the effect not confined only to iron but extend to other nutrients such as vitamin A; severe round worm infestation is reported to act by reducing the appetite and food intake. Poor sanitary and environmental conditions, over crowding and illiteracy, all favor the spread of helminthic infestations.

### 26.3.5 Chronic recurrent infections, malaria and human immunodeficiency virus

Chronic recurrent infections could also be one of the causes of anemia. A trend towards lower hemoglobin levels is reported in infections and inflammatory processes. Malaria is a major factor causing severe anemia in pregnancy and infancy, common in African countries [52, 54]. Malaria is thought to be the primary cause of severe anemia in at least 50% of subjects living in malaria endemic areas. A recent study in Tanzania confirmed malaria as the largest contributor to severe anemia in infants, 60% severely anemic due to malaria as against 30% due to iron deficiency [55]. Anemia associated with malaria is caused by hemolysis of the red blood cells, suppressed erythropoiesis, and secondary folate deficiency due to increased folate requirement consequent to acute hemolysis [52].

Longitudinal studies have shown that pregnant women are more susceptible to malarial parasites, compared to non pregnant women. A group that appears to have particularly lowered immunity to malaria in endemic areas is women in their first pregnancies [56].

Malaria in pregnant women is associated with low birth weight, pre mature deliveries and still births. Although a direct effect of malaria on these adverse effects cannot be ruled out, it appears that for the most part, these effects are due to the severe anemia caused by malarial parasitosis [57]. Malaria chemoprophylaxis is shown to be effective in abolishing parasitemias and in prevention of anemia, in pregnant women and young children living in malaria endemic areas [52]. However, the chemoprophylaxis for pregnant women should be given only after 19th week of pregnancy [57]. Malaria induced hemolysis increases the requirement for folic acid and results in megaloblastosis that can be corrected by chemoprophylaxis.

HIV infection is another cause for concern in the anemia situation, particularly in Africa [52]. A WHO report on severe anemia recommends that when anemia is associated with leucopenia (an abnormal lowering of white cell count) and thrombocytopenia (an abnormal drop in the number of blood cells, called platelets, involved in forming blood clots), the possibility of HIV infection must be suspected [57] .

Cytopenias (low count of different types of blood cells) of all major blood cell lines are common in Acquired Immune Deficiency Syndrome (AIDS). In one early series of patients with AIDS, anemia was noted in approximately 70 percent, lymphopenia in 70 percent, neutropenia in 50 percent, and thrombocytopenia in 40 percent [58]. The incidence of the various cytopenias correlates directly with the degree of immunosuppression.

Anemia is the most common hematologic abnormality associated with HIV, affecting 60 to 80 percent of patients in late stage disease. While it may be a mere laboratory abnormality in some individuals, in others typical symptoms may be present – fatigue, dyspnea, reduced exercise tolerance, and diminished functional capacity – that are directly related to a reduction in hemoglobin. In a review of more than 32,000 patients infected with HIV, the yearly incidence of developing anemia was reported to increase with disease progression, affecting 3% of all patients with asymptomatic HIV infection, 12% of asymptomatic patients with $CD_4$ cell counts below

200/μL, and 37% of patients with an AIDS-related illness [59]. Another source reports that up to 70% of people with AIDS are anemic [52].

Anemia of HIV is multifactorial. HIV infection per se causes anemia. Other common causes are anemia of chronic disease as a result of opportunistic infections secondary to HIV, suppression of the bone marrow by anti retroviral therapy and hemolytic anemias induced by oxidant drugs [60].

Treating reversible causes of anemia including treatment of opportunistic diseases, correcting deficiencies in vitamin $B_{12}$ or folic acid, changing myelosuppressive medications if feasible and appropriate, may all improve anemia in the appropriate setting. Effective antiretroviral therapy administered to all patients is expected to correct the anemia substantially if not completely.

## 26.4 Iron homeostasis

Iron homeostasis is maintained in the body by internal factors primarily by modulating iron absorption. Unlike other nutrients, iron is unique as once absorbed it is held within the body tenaciously with no physiological mechanism for its excretion. Excess iron accumulation within the body results in iron overload which is toxic while iron deficiency results in anemia of varying severity and causes several functional impairments. Both these are averted under normal conditions by a set of internal factors that regulate body iron stores primarily through regulation of iron absorption. Iron status of the individuals plays a very crucial role in determining the amount of iron absorbed. Iron deplete individuals absorb more iron from the same meal compared to iron replete individuals. The molecular basis of iron absorption and the different factors involved in the regulation of iron absorption are briefly reviewed.

Iron absorption involves the uptake of iron from the lumen of the intestine into the enterocytes and transfer across the baso lateral membrane into the portal blood circulation. Each step involves the participation of a transmembrane transporter coupled to an enzyme that changes the oxidation state of iron. Several key proteins are needed for the absorption and transport. These are duodenal cytochrome b (Dcytb), divalent metal iron transporter 1 (DMT 1), hephaestin and ferroportin [61].

Dcytb is a ferri reductase attached to the micro villi on the outer surface of the enterocytes. It reduces the ferric ions into the more readily absorbable ferrous ions and forms a tiny door way for the passage of iron into the body of the enterocyte. DMT 1, a divalent metal ion transporter is a brush border transmembrane transporter for several divalent cations including iron, copper and zinc. It pumps iron into the enterocyte by an active proton coupled transport mechanism requiring energy. DMT 1 transports only ferrous ions and so reduction of ferric ions to ferrous ions by Dcytb is a pre requisite. The amount of DMT 1 in the apical membrane is regulated by body iron requirements.

Once inside the enterocytes iron can take one of the two path ways .It may be incorporated into ferritin and stay within the enterocytes until the enterocytes are sloughed off and the iron is lost from the body. Alternately the iron may be taken to the baso lateral membrane across which it is transported into the blood stream by means of a specific iron carrier protein, ferroportin. It is then oxidised by a membrane bound ferroxidase, hephaestin, yielding ferric ions that are bound by plasma transferrin for distribution around the body via the blood.

Expression of DMT1, ferritin and ferroportin mRNA's is post-transcriptionally controlled by the IRP/IRE system to protect enterocytes from iron excess or depletion while allowing efficient iron flux across these cells. The mRNAs which code for these proteins have a region (iron responsive element, IRE) which can bind to iron regulating protein (IRP). The extent of binding will up or down regulate the production of DMT 1, ferritin or ferroportin. In iron excess, DMT 1 and ferroportin are down regulated while ferritin is up regulated resulting in removal of iron from the body along with the senescent enterocytes. In iron deficiency, the converse occurs resulting in greater absorption of iron into the blood stream [62].

Ferroportin as well as hephaestin are under the control of hepcidin, a peptide hormone secreted by the liver in response to three major stimuli: (1) body iron stores, (2) demand for erythropoiesis, and (3) hypoxia. The expression of hepcidin, the principal hormone involved in iron regulation, offers a unified mechanism to account for changes seen in iron deficiency, hereditary hemochromatosis and in chronic inflammatory disorders.

When body iron stores tend to fall or demand for erythropoiesis is increased, hepcidin is down regulated, with its secretion falling to low levels. When body iron stores are adequate and or demand for erythropoiesis is reduced, hepcidin is upregulated, resulting in increased secretion of the hormone. Hepcidin acts by binding to ferroportin and blocking the transport of iron across the baso lateral membrane, thus regulating the amount of iron absorbed depending on the iron status of the individual. Hepcidin expression is under the control of at least three genes, HFE (hemo chromatosis gene), TFR 2 (Transferrin receptor 2) and HJV (hemo juvelin). The molecular mechanism of action of these is yet to be unraveled [61].

Figure 26.1 provides a schematic representation of the regulation of iron absorption by the various proteins involved and by hepcidin.

Heme iron absorption is less well understood. Heme is taken into enterocytes by a carrier mechanism. A folate transporter, PCFT (also called HCP1) may contribute to this process. Heme is degraded in enterocytes by heme oxygenase releasing iron ions for efflux via ferroportin.

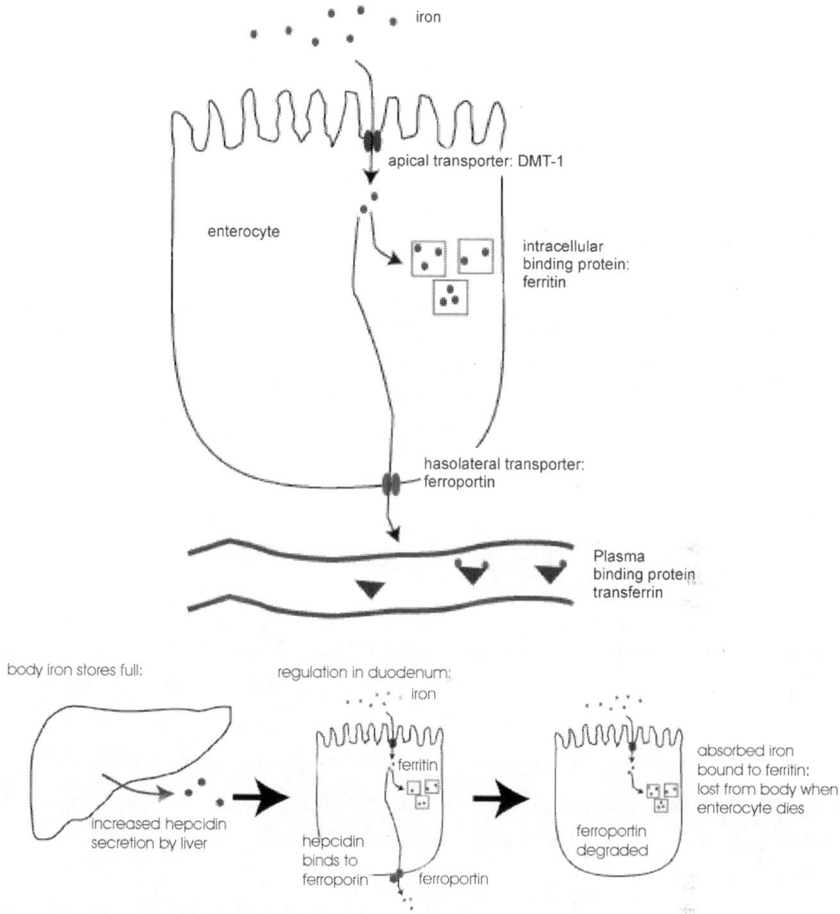


*26.1* Schematic representation of iron absorption.

## 26.5 Iron requirements

In addition to the factors discussed under the causes of anemia that contribute to the high prevalence in the Indian population, increased iron requirements during pregnancy, early childhood and adolescence and the inability of the habitual diets to meet these increased requirements are also responsible for the high prevalence of anemia in these groups.

### 26.5.1 Iron requirements in pregnancy

Studies on normal healthy pregnant women have shown that there is hardly any increase in iron requirements in the first trimester of pregnancy. However, during the second and third trimesters, there is an increase in maternal blood volume and transfer of iron to the fetus that impose a high demand for iron that cannot be met by the existing diets. The total iron cost of a pregnancy has been worked out to be 1100–1200 mg [63–65].

*Table 26.8* Iron cost of pregnancy

| Requirements | Iron (mg) |
|---|---|
| Fetus (at term) | 280 |
| Expansion of red cell mass | 450 |
| Placenta and umbilical cord | 90 |
| Maternal blood loss during delivery | 150 |
| Obligatory loss (wear and tear) | 230 |
| Total iron cost | 1200 |
| 15 m of amenorrhea saves | 240–480 |

If the iron saved due to amenorrhea is taken into account, the net requirement of iron for a pregnancy is about 700–850 mg, which translates into an iron requirement of 4 mg/d over the last two trimesters. Since it is difficult to obtain the entire requirement through the diet, iron supplements need to be provided during pregnancy. It is the practice in developed countries like US to provide supplements of 30 mg iron per day while under the National Anemia Control Program in India, pregnant women are provided 100 mg elemental iron and 0.5 mg folic acid daily for at least 100 days during the second and third trimesters of pregnancy.

## 26.5.2 Iron requirements in infancy and early childhood

During the first two years of life, there is rapid physical growth and brain development that increases the demand for tissue iron deposition. Iron content of breast milk is low (0.78 mg/l); however the iron in breast milk is well absorbed to the extent of 50% [70]. In a normal birth weight infant, this level of iron absorption from the breast milk ensures adequate amount of iron if the infant is exclusively breast fed.

However, the iron stores of a healthy normal birth weight infant are exhausted by 6 months; while the iron requirement continues to remain high. With complementary feeding remaining very inadequate, infants from 6 months to 2 years are particularly highly vulnerable to anemia. A critical aspect of iron nutrition in infancy, as compared to adults, is the greater dependency of the infant on external sources of iron for red cell production. It has been calculated that in a 10kg, one year old infant the diet must provide 30% of the iron needed for hemoglobin turn over as against only 5% in an adult [66].

Estimated requirements of absorbed iron for infants in the first year and for children 1–8 years is shown in the Table 26.9 below. As seen, total absorbed iron requirements for 6–12 months old infants is 0.9 mg, which at the rate of an average bioavailability of 5% translates into 20 mg iron per day. It is evident that either supplemental iron will be needed or the dietary iron bioavailability should increase if the iron requirements of infants are to be fully met in developing countries. Beyond 1 year the total absorbed iron requirement drops to about 0.8 mg per day.

*Table 26.9* Estimated requirements of absorbed iron for children (mg/day) [66]

| Age | 0–6 months | 6–12 months | 1–2 years | 2–8 years |
|---|---|---|---|---|
| Requirements for growth | 0.25 | 0.53 | 0.29 | 0.23 |
| Iron losses | 0.24 | 0.37 | 0.46 | 0.56 |
| Total requirements | 0.49 | 0.90 | 0.75 | 0.79 |

One third of all infants born in India are of low birth weight (LBW), defined as birth weight less than 2500 g. Low birth weight occurs due to premature birth, pre term delivery, i.e. before 37 w of gestation, or full term birth but small for gestational age due to intra uterine growth retardation. Thus LBW includes a heterogeneous group of infants. Very low birth weight infants are defined as having birth weights less than 1500 g, including mostly premature births.

Low birth weight infants have poorer stores of iron, exhaust their iron stores before 6 months of age; in some cases as early as two months, but their iron requirements remain high. Low birth weight infants are much more vulnerable to anemia due to these factors.

Most of the data on iron requirements of LBW infants are derived from studies on pre term births. Pre-term and full-term infants have on an average 74 mg iron per kg body weight at birth, about 75% of it is in the circulating hemoglobin, constituting a true iron reserve. Pre term infants birth weight however is low to very low, thus total body iron in a pre term infant at birth may only be one fourth of that in a full term infant. For instance, one of the studies by Siimes (1984) [67] showed that a very LBW infant with a body weight of 0.8 kg had a total body iron of only 50 mg. Pre term infants often become anemic a few months after birth. The iron stores in a pre term infant gets depleted by two months with the result that most such infants become anemic by two months or soon after that. A full term normal birth weight infant increases body weight from 3.2 kg at birth to 10 kg at 1 year. At the same time the total body iron content increases from 210mg to 365mg. Thus the estimated increase in iron content is about 50% although the body weight triples during this time. As against this, very low birth weight infants may increase their body weight up to 5–10 fold by one year, with an accompanying fivefold increase in body iron during this period. The following Table 26.10 shows the available data on increase in growth and iron content of pre-term and full-term infants.

*Table 26.10* Influence of growth on estimated iron needs of pre-term and full-term normal weight infants [67]

| Initial birth weight (kg) | Increase in body weight over 12 months | Increase in body iron over 12 months | Ratio – iron/weight (mg/kg) |
|---|---|---|---|
| 0.8 | 7.2 | 210 | 29 |
| 1.6 | 7.9 | 215 | 27 |
| 3.2 | 6.8 | 155 | 23 |

As seen from the above Table 26.10, the need for iron is higher per kg body weight gain in pre term infants compared to full term normal birth weight infants. This is considered applicable to all low birth weight infants as well. The current recommendation is to supplement all low birth weight infants with oral iron, in the form of ferrous fumarate or ferrous gluconate at the level of 2–3 mg/kg body weight per day from 6 to 8 weeks of age until 12 months [68].

## 26.5.3 Iron requirements of adolescent boys and girls

Adolescence is characterized by a large growth spurt. During this period iron requirements are increased dramatically in both boys and girls, and this occurs due to expansion in blood volume, increase in muscle mass, and in girls due to onset of menstruation. Overall the iron requirements nearly double in boys, from 0.7 to 0.9 mg per day to 2.2 mg/d, as they move from preadolescent to adolescent stage and the increase is even higher in girls, especially if they are heavily menstruating. [65]. These increased requirements are associated with the timing and size of the growth spurt as well as sexual maturation and the onset of menses.

The available data on iron intakes in adolescents suggest that adolescent girls are unlikely to acquire substantial iron stores during this time period because intakes tend to be low. The bioavailability from diets in developing and industrialized countries indicates a negative iron balance is likely in many female populations. The low iron stores in these young women of reproductive age will make them susceptible to iron deficiency anemia during pregnancy because dietary intakes alone are insufficient, in most cases, to meet the requirements of pregnancy.

Iron losses in adolescents through different routes such as urinary, bile and desquamated gastro intestinal cells are assumed to be similar to the losses in adults as there are no clear data to indicate otherwise, once body size is considered [69].

Iron requirement for expansion in blood volume is estimated to be 0.18 mg/d for boys and 0.14 mg/d for girls. Increase in total body essential iron pool is estimated as 0.55 mg/d for boys and 0.33 mg/d for girls. To this must be added the increase due to increase in hemoglobin levels. In girls allowances should be made for menstrual losses of blood. Overall, the requirement for absorbable iron in boys is estimated to be 1.8 mg/d and for girls 2.1 mg/d. [65]

Taking into account the predominantly cereal pulse based diets of Indians and the bioavailability of these diets, the Indian Council of Medical Research has proposed the following as iron requirements for different age and sex groups in its most recent revision [70].

The earlier ICMR expert committee in 1988 [71] used three levels of iron absorption, 3% for adult men, children and adolescent boys, 8% for pregnant women and 5% for all other women including girls above 10y to determine the dietary iron requirements for these groups. Recent studies on iron absorption in Indians using stable isotopes have indicated that iron absorption on habitual diets may not be as low as 3–5%. With a typical rice-based diet, iron absorption was found to be 17.5% in iron deficient adult women and 7.3% in normal women [72]. Therefore the present committee revised the absorption figures upwards and have used only two levels, 5% for men, and for children below the age of 18 both boys and girls and 8% for women including pregnant and lactating [70]. The principles of estimating the requirements for different age groups remain the same as described in earlier ICMR reports.

*Table 26.11* Daily iron requirement of Indians (ICMR, 2009) [70]

| Group | Male/Female/ Age group | Body weight Kg | Iron requirement Mcg/kg/d | Iron requirement Total mg/d | Dietary iron requirement Mg/d |
|---|---|---|---|---|---|
| Adult M (5%) | Man | 64 | 14 | 0.89 | 18.0 |
| W (8%) | Woman | 58 | 30 | 1.74 | 22.0 |
| Pregnant women (8%) | | 58 | 47 | 2.72 | 34.0 |
| Lactating women (8%) | | 58 | 22 | 1.27 | 16 |
| Infants | 0–6 months | 5.5 | 46 | 0.23 | [a] |
| | 6–12 months | 8.4 | 48 | 0.40 | [a] |
| Children (5%) | 1–3 years | 13.7 | 28 | 0.38 | 8.0 |
| | 4–6 years | 18.1 | 35 | 0.63 | 13.0 |
| | 7–9 years | 25.2 | 32 | 0.80 | 16.0 |
| Adolescents (5%) | 10–12 years | | | | |
| | Boys | 34.3 | 30 | 1.03 | 21.0 |
| | Girls | 35.3 | 37 | 1.30 | 26.0 |
| | 13–15 years | | | | |
| | Boys | 47.4 | 32 | 1.51 | 30.0 |
| | Girls | 46.6 | 29 | 1.35 | 27.0 |
| Adolescents | 16–18 years | | | | |
| | Boys | 56.2 | 22 | 1.23 | 25.0 |
| | Girls | 52.0 | 25 | 1.30 | 26.0 |

[a] *Note* – Data are insufficient to establish RDA for iron for infants from birth through 6 months of age and therefore recommended iron intake for this group is based on the average intake of healthy infants fed breast milk. Iron enriched solid food should complement breast milk from 7 to 12 months of age [70].

## 26.6 Assessment of anemia

### 26.6.1 Estimation of hemoglobin levels

By definition, anemia is a condition in which hemoglobin levels are lower than the normal for a given age, sex and physiological state. Therefore most assessments of anemia are based on hemoglobin levels. However hemoglobin level per se does not tell us anything about the causes of anemia. In order to have information on the cause of anemia, other parameters need to be defined. The major cause of anemia is iron deficiency either due to dietary deficiency or increased requirements due to growth or specific conditions like infections, blood losses, etc. Unlike hemoglobin which can be estimated with relative ease in the field situation, parameters of iron deficiency are dependant on laboratory facilities and are not practical or feasible in many settings especially in the developing countries. Fortunately the proportion of anemia that is due to iron deficiency can be estimated in many situations by assessing the hemoglobin response to iron therapy, provided that no other supplements are given during this period and that the diet does not change substantially.

Thus hemoglobin has been the major criterion for determining anemia, both due to all cause as well as iron deficiency. Methods of estimating hemoglobin can be broadly divided into qualitative and quantitative [73]. The qualitative methods provide information on broad range of hemoglobin values. Generally these are based on comparing the color of a drop of blood on a filter paper strip with standard color charts. Alternately a drop of blood is allowed to fall into a solution of copper sulphate of known specific gravity and observed to note if the drop floats or sinks for the first 10–15 seconds, indicating the specific gravity of the blood is lower or higher than that of the copper sulphate solution. A series of copper sulphate solutions of different specific gravities corresponding to defined hemoglobin levels are used in the estimation.

The third qualitative method does not require blood samples but depends on clinical symptoms of pallor. While the skill required for conducting these tests is low to medium, the accuracy and precision are low, making them unsuitable for assessing prevalence of anemia. However for deciding whether an individual should be placed on a therapeutic or preventive iron supplementation at the field level they are quite useful.

The quantitative methods use either undiluted whole blood or diluted blood samples. Although different diluting agents and different technologies are available, four of these are credited with high level of accuracy and precision. One of these four involves centrifugation of whole blood to determine the volume of the red cells expressed as hematocrit. This is seldom used in the field condition in India as it does not give a direct estimate of hemoglobin. Of the other three, the cyanmethemoglobin and the oxyhemoglobin methods are based on dilution of a very small amount of blood and require high level of skill and training. The hemocue uses a drop of whole blood and does not require carefully calibrated amount; nor does it need dilution. Therefore it calls for low levels of skill but the cost of instrument and the cost per estimation is high. Most anemia assessments in India have used the standard cyanmethemoglobin method using calibrated amount of blood diluted in a suitable agent, while the large scale surveys of NFHS II and III have used the hemocue.

Unfortunately the data obtained by the hemocue are not comparable with those of the cyanmethemoglobin method, based on dilution of the blood sample. It is now well established that the hemocue overestimates hemoglobin levels and therefore the method provides an under estimation of the anemia levels.

Thus we have to balance the high level of skill needed for the standard cyanmethaemoglobin method that calls for dilution of blood with the high cost of hemocue that under estimates anemia levels. A field level adaptation of the cyanmethemoglobin method has been used in situations where laboratory facilities are severely limited. In this method, a calibrated amount of blood is collected on a whatman filter paper circle of specified dimension, allowed to dry and transported to a lab within a week for elution and estimation. The difference between this and the standard laboratory method has been shown to be low and is of little consequence in assessing anemia prevalence.

### 26.6.2 Indicators of iron, folate and vitamin B12 deficiencies

Iron deficiency is considered to occur in three stages [74]. When the intake of iron is insufficient to meet the daily iron losses and the need for growth, iron reserves start getting depleted. In the first stage referred to as the iron deficient stores, iron reserves are essentially absent but the supply to erythroid marrow is not yet curtailed. This is reflected in the absence of 'stainable iron' in the bone marrow and a reduction in serum ferritin levels. Iron lack is the only condition in which there is a reduction in serum ferritin levels and therefore this parameter is highly specific for iron deficiency. However, inflammatory conditions produce an increase in serum ferritin making it difficult to interpret serum ferritin values in the presence of infections. Studies have shown that 1 mcg per liter of serum ferritin is equal to 10 mg of storage iron. More recently, transferrin receptors in blood have been shown to be a more sensitive indicator of iron stores as this parameter is not affected by infections and inflammation. Unlike serum ferritin, transferrin receptors are increased in iron deficiency, as a response to bind more of the serum iron so that it can be delivered to the bone marrow and other tissues.

In the second stage of iron deficiency referred to as iron deficient erythropoiesis, there is a reduction in iron supply to the erythroid marrow. Serum iron is reduced and total iron binding capacity is increased in this stage. The more useful index of stage 2 deficiency is the transferrin saturation (TS) which is the ratio of serum iron to total iron binding capacity. When the transferrin saturation falls below 15%, hemoglobin production in the developing red cells is curtailed. Transferrin saturation, however, suffers from three major limitations as an indicator of iron deficiency. First, serum iron measurement in the laboratory is highly susceptible to iron contamination, particularly with manual methods, resulting in erroneously high serum iron values if contamination is not scrupulously avoided. Secondly, the diagnostic ability of TS is reduced because of wide diurnal variations of serum iron in normal subjects, and finally the level of TS falls within hours of onset of even mild inflammation, leading to erroneous interpretation.

Erythrocyte protoporphyrin is another measurement that can be used to detect iron deficient erythropoiesis. When the iron supply to the bone marrow is curtailed, protoporphyrin in its free form increases in the erythrocytes, i.e. protoporphyrin not bound with iron and the protein globin. An advantage of the erythrocyte protoporphyrin is that it is a more stable index of iron supply to the bone marrow as elevation occurs only after several weeks of restricted iron supply to the bone marrow. A disadvantage of this indicator especially with children is that the level increases with lead poisoning.

The third and final stage of iron lack is iron deficiency anemia in which there is a fall in hemoglobin levels, below what is normal for the individual. The parameters for diagnosing iron deficiency with normal and abnormal values are portrayed in the Table 26.12 below.

*Table 26.12* Stages of iron deficiency and the normal and abnormal range of values for the indicators [74].

| Stage if iron deficiency/ indicators | Normal iron stores 600 mg | Depleted iron stores | Restricted supply of iron to erythroid marrow | Anemia |
|---|---|---|---|---|
| Plasma ferritin µg/L | 60 | <12 | <12 | <12 |
| Transferrin saturation (%) | 35 | 35 | <16 | <16 |
| RBC Protoporphyrin µg/dl | 30 | 30 | >70 | >70 |
| Hemoglobin (g/dl) | >12 | >12 | >12 | <12 |

In addition, values indicative of iron excess have also been defined. Serum ferritin in excess of 300 mcg/l and transferrin saturation in excess of 60% are indicatives of iron over load [75–76].

The concurrent presence of folate and vitamin $B_{12}$ deficiencies may be identified by the red cell folate, serum folate and serum vitamin $B_{12}$ levels. Red cell folic acid level below 100 nanogram per ml; serum folic acid levels below 3 nanogram per ml; and serum vitamin $B_{12}$ level below 100 pico gram per ml are all indicative of deficiencies of these vitamins [8].

## 26.7 Functional effects of anemia

Although nutritional anemia may result due to deficiencies of several nutrients, the focus of research has been on anemia due to iron deficiency as this is a major cause of anemia world over. The aspects discussed in the next section pertain mainly to iron deficiency anemia, as all studies have addressed the reversibility of the adverse effects of anemia on functional effects with iron therapy.

### 26.7.1 Anemia, iron deficiency and physical performance

Iron in the body plays an essential role in oxidative energy production; this iron is known as functional iron as against iron that serves as a reserve which is known as storage iron. Functional iron is found in hemoglobin in red cells, myoglobin in muscles, iron dependent enzymes and respiratory chain proteins in the mitochondria. Table 26.13 below summarizes their functions in energy production, which make it apparent that iron deficiency and anemia produce a range of impairments in oxidative energy production that gets reflected in impaired physical performance and working capacity [76].

*Table 26.13* Role of iron in energy production

| Name of protein | Functional site | Major function |
|---|---|---|
| Hemoglobin | Red blood cells | Oxygen transport |
| Myoglobin | Cytoplasm of muscle cells | Diffusion of oxygen to the mitochondria |
| Oxidative enzymes | Mitochondrial membrane | Oxidation of substrates |
| Respiratory chain proteins | Mitochondrial membrane | Electron transfer |

Studies in human adults have shown that iron deficiency and anemia, both limit physical capacity measured by tests of aerobic capacity and endurance tests. Anemia, with lower hemoglobin levels reduces oxygen delivery to the tissues and impairs primarily the aerobic capacity. Iron deficiency on the other hand, by reducing tissue oxidative capacity is considered to have a major adverse effect on the endurance capacity especially at sub maximal work loads. Iron deficiency anemia by virtue of low Hb levels and tissue iron deficiency affects both aerobic capacity and endurance. Endurance tests typically involve sub maximal work loads and time to exhaustion is determined under standard conditions, while aerobic capacity is measured either in a treadmill or a bicycle ergo meter at maximum exertion levels.

A recent review [12] which evaluated nine laboratory studies in human adults that were either unblinded or double blind randomized placebo controlled trials, found that both severe and moderate iron deficiency anemia impaired aerobic capacity. The impairment could be corrected by increasing hemoglobin concentration.

Iron deficiency without anemia was not found to affect aerobic capacity but had a significant adverse effect on endurance capacity in adults. The lack of effect of iron deficiency without anemia on aerobic capacity was attributed to the strong dependence of maximum oxygen consumption ($VO_2$ Max) on oxygen delivery which in turn is affected only when hemoglobin levels are reduced.

Several field studies in male and female tea pickers have shown strong positive association between anemia and aerobic capacity, measured either as heart rate during a step test or during tread mill tests [77–79] .These studies also demonstrated that work time and work load were proportional to hemoglobin. Most importantly, increases in various measures of aerobic capacity were found with increase in hemoglobin.

Impaired physical performance can adversely affect productivity, especially in income earning activities that are dependent on physical efforts. Most consistent data comes from tea and rubber plantation workers in whom productivity could be quantified. These studies in India, Indonesia and Sri Lanka have shown that there is a fall in productivity in anemic subjects that shows up in income earned as well as in the quality of the diets [80–82]. Economic losses expected due to iron deficiency is estimated to be 1.47% of the GDP in India which when translated into absolute terms is equivalent to 4294 million US dollars, a huge loss indeed [83].

Most laboratory and field studies of anemia versus physical performance have focused on adults with only a few that has investigated this aspect in children. The results of these studies have indicated that both aerobic capacity and endurance were impaired in anemic children, consistent with the observations on adults [84–85].

Animal studies provide extra ordinarily consistent data. Most severely anemic rats have the lowest aerobic capacity, severity of anemia directly proportional to decline in aerobic capacity from hemoglobin levels of 140 to 80 g/l [86]. A similar finding was also reported from tea pickers in Sri Lanka [77].

Taken together, these data provide clear evidence of compromised physical performance in adults while more studies are indicated in children [87].

Reduced ability to engage in physical activities in children can have other ramifications such as an adverse effect on learning due to limited scope for exploratory activities and the lack of activity stimulus for optimum development of motor skills.

In anemic adults, impaired physical work capacity, lower productivity, lower earnings, and poor quality of diets can set up a vicious cycle that result in severe losses at the national and individual level. Iron supplementation to correct anemia results in a significant improvement in physical capacity as well as in income earned [80–82, 88] and has the potential to reverse the huge losses in GDP.

## 26.7.2 Anemia and cognitive functions in children

In the last four decades several studies have addressed the issue of anemia versus cognitive development in children. While these studies in general are consistent in indicating impairment in cognitive development due to anemia in young infants and children, the reversibility of this with nutritional therapy, chiefly with iron has been conclusively shown only for older children, i.e. above the age of two years.

The first indication that cognitive development may be compromised in iron deficient anemic children came from co relational studies that showed a significant association between tests of cognitive development and hemoglobin levels, the anemic children performing poorly on a wide range of psychological tests compared to the non anemic children [89–91].

Several longitudinal observational studies that have tried to link cognitive development or school achievement in later childhood with anemia in infancy or early childhood have been consistent in showing that formerly anemic children continued to be at a developmental disadvantage at one or more of the follow up assessments, even after adjusting for some social background variables such as gender and birth weight. Deficits were noted in formerly anemic children in pre school skills, fine and gross motor skills, and visual motor integration [13].

Randomized supplementation trials provide final convincing evidence linking anemia with poorer cognitive development and the promising prospect of reversal of the adverse effects with nutritional therapy. The studies reported in the literature have measured a wide variety of cognitive functions in older children. These have included visual perception, memory, concentration, problem solving skills and discrimination learning.

Almost all the studies have shown poorer performance of the anemic children and a significant improvement after iron supplementation or iron and folic acid supplementation to correct anemia. The poorer performance in a variety of tests was seen in infants as well as in older children. However, the reversal of the adverse effects with iron supplementation was demonstrated convincingly only in the older children, i.e., in children above the age of two years [13, 92–94]. This has raised two questions in relation to the younger children: one that iron deficiency anemia when it occurs at a very young age (i.e. in the first year of life) may leave a permanent deficit that may not be corrected by supplementation later in life and the second relates to the tests used that they may not be sensitive enough to detect the improvements. Available evidence appears to indicate that the former rather than the latter may be the case which underscores the importance of effective public health measures to prevent anemia in the young children.

### 26.7.3 Effects of anemia on pregnancy outcome

An association between anemia and adverse pregnancy outcome has been found in many studies. Birth weights have been reported to be lower at both ends of hemoglobin, the relationship being U shaped [95]. Unfavorable pregnancy outcomes consequent to anemia have included lower mean birth weight, lower gestational duration, and increased perinatal mortality [96]. Oral iron supplementation during pregnancy increases weight at birth and reduces the incidence of low birth weight [97–98]. Accumulating evidence suggests an association between maternal iron status during pregnancy and iron status of infants post partum. Although anemia, especially severe anemia has been reported as an associated cause of maternal mortality in several countries around the world, prospective trials are lacking. Other effects of anemia such as maternal morbidity, well being and infant health also need further documentation [95].

### 26.7.4 Lowered cellular immunity and increased morbidities

Anemia has been shown to result in impairment in cell mediated immunity and lymphocyte proliferation response to mitogens in pregnant women that is corrected by iron therapy [99]. In young children, both cell mediated immune response and bactericidal activity of leucocytes, was found to be impaired in anemia, especially when hemoglobin levels fell below 10 g/dl [100] both of which were corrected by iron therapy [101]. The effect of anemia on morbidities is less clear [102].

### 26.7.5 Impaired thermo regulation

There are some studies to show that ability to withstand cold temperatures is compromised in iron deficient and anemic women. It appears likely that this effect is mediated by thyroid hormone. Lack of iron may result in a lack of adequate stores of thyroid hormone which curtails increased cellular metabolism on exposure to cold, leading to increased intolerance [103].

### 26.7.6 Child growth deficits

Only a few studies have investigated the effect of anemia on child growth [104, 105]. These have reported a positive effect of iron supplements on growth which will need to be pursued further to clearly document if child growth can be improved with iron supplements in anemic young children [106].

## 26.8 Approaches for the prevention and control of anemia

There are broadly two approaches for the control of iron deficiency anemia: one is to increase the amount of absorbable iron by one or more of the following means: (a) fortifying common foods with iron; (b) increasing the bioavailability of the dietary iron by increasing the enhancers in the diet and reducing the inhibitors; (c) by providing iron through medicinal supplementation; the other is one of controlling infestations and infections that cause lowering of hemoglobin. While food based strategies may be adequate in areas where anemia prevalence is less than 10% in the population, medicinal supplementation in addition to food fortification will be needed in areas of high prevalence, i.e. more than 40%. In new borns, umbilical cord clamping, delayed for at least two minutes after birth, can increase body iron stores of the infant at birth and improve iron status in the first few months. Therefore it is an important additional measure specific to this age group for prevention of iron deficiency anemia

### 26.8.1 Food fortification

Food fortification refers to the addition of iron to foods over and above what is naturally present in them. Food fortification can take many forms; mass fortification refers to the fortification of foods consumed widely by the general population; targeted fortification is the fortification of foods consumed by specific sub population groups such as complementary foods meant for young children; and market driven fortification where the food manufacturer voluntarily fortifies foods with nutrients, an example is the wheat atta fortified with iron and marketed by private food companies [107]. Besides these, bio fortification of staple foods, i.e. breeding and genetic modification of plants so as to improve their nutrient contents and or absorption of the nutrients is a novel approach that is currently being researched. The golden rice is an example of genetically modified rice grains containing beta carotene. Much more work is needed in this area before the foods can become a part of our daily diet.

For food fortification to be successful, the food vehicle chosen should be consumed by a vast majority of the needy population, it should be possible to fortify the entire required quantities in a few places to assure quality, the selected fortificant should have a high bioavailability and must not react with other foods when cooked or mixed, and the fortified food must be consumed in fixed amounts daily so that wide variations do not occur in intakes. Staple foods like rice and wheat and others such as salt, soy sauce and fish sauce have been developed as food vehicles for iron fortification [107]. Among these, salt is a good vehicle for iron in the developing countries for the general population. Efforts to fortify salt with iron and iodine has been successful in India and else where.

The double fortified salt developed by the National Institute of Nutrition in India, using a low cost technology, provides 1mg iron and 100 mcg iodine per g salt, i.e. 1000 ppm of iron and 40 ppm of iodine. The average daily salt consumption by adults in India is estimated as 8 g which, at the level of fortification described above provides 8mg iron /d. The bioavailability of the iron in the DFS has been shown to be good, 6.1% [108]. The stability, safety and acceptability at the community level have all been satisfactorily demonstrated. Impact data on residential school children who consumed the double fortified salt for two years showed a decline in anemia prevalence from 42% to 30% [109]. Currently, production of double fortified salt has been floated in India in some of the southern states [110].

### 26.8.2 Increasing bioavailability of dietary iron

There are basically two ways in which the bioavailability of iron in the diets can be improved. The first is by increasing the enhancers, namely ascorbic acid and, meat, fish and poultry (MFP) in the diet and the other is to reduce the content of inhibitors in the diet. A large body of literature is available which demonstrates convincingly that under controlled conditions, MFP and ascorbic acid increase the absorption of non heme iron in humans [36–39, 111]. As little as 10 mg of ascorbic acid can increase the absorption of iron two fold. There are many foods in the Indian context that are high in ascorbic acid. These are usually the fruits and vegetables. It is important to note here that ascorbic acid is easily lost at high temperatures and in the presence of oxygen. Therefore, the fruits should be consumed in fresh uncooked forms for best effects and immediately after the meals. The important fruits that are good sources of ascorbic acid are citrus fruits of any kind, guavas, papaya, and among the vegetables all green leafy vegetables, cauliflower, Indian gooseberry are all good sources of ascorbic acid.

The typically vegetarian Indian dietary is known for its high content of inhibitors of iron absorption. These are phytic acid present in whole grain cereals and flours, fiber in wheat bran, tannins in tea and ragi, calcium in milk, soya bean products, and egg yolk. The inhibitors reduce iron absorption by forming insoluble complexes with iron that get precipitated in the alkaline environment of the small intestine which do not release the iron for absorption.

Reduction of inhibitors of iron absorption such as phytic acid, concomitantly with an increase in ascorbic acid content of foods, by processes such as germination and fermentation have also been shown to result in increased bioavailability of iron.

There are two approaches by which these can be integrated into a public health policy and program. One is to augment the production of fruits and vegetables which are good sources of ascorbic acid so that access and availability of these foods to the general population is increased. The other is to promote, through nutrition education and counseling, the consumption of these fruits and vegetables and processes at the household level such as germination and fermentation that can reduce the inhibitors in the diet. Germination and fermentation are traditional food processing methods extensively used in India at the household level until recently but are showing a decline in the current period. Thus it is important that diet practices at the household level are preserved/modified in a manner as to allow for better iron absorption and improved iron bioavailability.

### 26.8.3 Nutrient supplements

This approach involves provision of the missing nutrient as a supplement to the population at risk. Iron and folic acid supplements have received the most attention as these are two nutrients that contribute to the high prevalence of anemia. Far fewer studies have been done with other nutrients such as vitamin A or vitamin $B_{12}$. Many developing countries have used iron folic acid supplementation as the main public health approach to control anemia, although with only limited success [20,112], primarily due to several limitations in the implementation of the program.

The current recommendations by WHO [76] for iron supplementation are shown in Table 26.14.

The anemia control program in India provides iron-folic acid supplements (IFA) consisting of 100 mg iron and 500 μg folic acid daily for a minimum of 100 days to pregnant women, starting as early in pregnancy as possible and continuing for the rest of pregnancy. The same dosage and tablets are provided to lactating women in the first three months post partum. Young children receive 20 mg iron and 100 μg folic acid.

*Table 26.14* Guidelines for the use of iron supplements to prevent anemia

| Age groups | Indications for supplementation | Dosage schedule | Duration |
|---|---|---|---|
| LBW infants | Universal supplementation | Iron: 2 mg/kg body weight per day | from 2 to 23 months of age |
| Children 6–23 months of age | Where anemia prevalence is above 40% | Iron: 2 mg/kg body weight per day | From 6 to 23 months |
| Children 24–59 months of age | Where anemia prevalence is above 40% | Iron: 2 mg/kg body weight per day up to 30 mg | 3 months |
| School-age children above 60 months | Where anemia prevalence above 60 months is above 40% | Iron: 30 mg/d Folic acid : 250 μg/d | 3 months |
| Women of child bearing age | Where anemia prevalence is above 40% | Iron: 60 mg/d Folic acid: 400 μg/d | 3 months |
| Pregnant women | Universal supplementation | Iron: 60 mg/d Folic acid: 400 μg/d | As soon as possible after gestation starts – no later than the 3rd month – and continuing for the rest of pregnancy |
| Lactating women | Where anemia prevalence is above 40% | Iron: 60 mg/d Folic acid 400 μg/d | 3 months post partum |

Adolescents are prescribed the same adult tablets as for pregnant and lactating mothers. However, bi-weekly administration of the adult supplement is recommended for adolescent girls and women in the reproductive age.

Recently the World Health Organization has issued a position statement on weekly supplementation of iron for reproductive age women. This position statement is based on the consensus of a World Health Organization (WHO) Global Consultation on Weekly Iron and Folic Acid Supplementation [113]. While recommending that the strategies to combat iron deficiency and anemia should be integrated, the consultation recognized that weekly iron folate supplementation (WIFS) is an important strategy for the prevention of iron deficiency, improvement of pre-pregnancy iron reserves and the improvement of folate status in women. In population groups where anemia prevalence is above 20% in women of reproductive age and in the absence such data where anemia prevalence is above 40% in pregnant women, the consultation recommended that WIFS should be considered.

The weekly supplement should contain 60 mg iron in the form of ferrous sulfate ($FeSO_4.7H_2O$) and 2800 mcg folic acid, although the dose level recommended for folic acid is supported by very limited evidence. Since folic acid supplementation may reduce the efficacy of anti malarial treatment, it may be prudent to use iron only as a weekly supplement in this setting. Upon confirmation of pregnancy, the dose schedule mentioned in Table 26.12 for pregnancy should be followed.

It is intended that WIFS programs will be integrated with other efforts to control iron deficiency and anemia and will be planned in such a way that it will become a self sustaining long term program that the women of reproductive age will use during their child bearing years.

### 26.8.4 Parasite and malaria control

As hookworms and malaria contribute to anemia and iron deficiency in a significant way, especially in pregnant women [114] and in young children, deworming using appropriate drugs will be the choice, until such a time when sanitary conditions can be improved.

Albendazole and Mebendazole are reported to be effective against most of the helminthic infestation seen in the south Asian region. They are also considered relatively safe if administered in the 2nd or 3rd trimester of pregnancy and in children above 1 year of age. These drugs are not to be given in the first trimester of pregnancy.

The dosages as recommended by the WHO[10] are: for pregnant women in endemic areas (prevalence 20–30% or more), a single dose of albendazole (400 mg) or mebandazole (500 mg) is considered effective and safe if given in the 2nd trimester. It is recommended that this be repeated in the 3rd trimester if the women live in highly endemic areas (prevalence of helminthes more than 50%).

If *plasmodium falsiparum* malaria is endemic and transmission of infection is high, the women in their first or second pregnancies should be given curative anti malarials on the first pre natal visit, followed by prophylaxis as per local recommendations.

Single dose albendazole (400 mg) or mebendazole (500 mg) twice a year is recommended for children above 5 years in endemic areas.

Malaria prophylaxis is reported to improve hemoglobin levels, reduce prevalence of anemia and improve birth weights in the first and second pregnancies in malaria endemic areas. Malarial prophylaxis and anti malarials should be administered as per the local recommendations [10].

## 26.9 Summary

Nutritional anemia is a major public health problem in the world affecting an estimated 2 billion people of which 90% are in the developing countries, especially in South East Asia and Africa. Dietary iron deficiency and low availability are the two major causes of anemia on such a wide scale; however other nutritional deficiencies such as vitamin A, folic acid, vitamin $B_{12}$ and riboflavin may contribute to the prevalence of anemia in certain settings. It is estimated that on a world wide basis, iron deficiency accounts for 50% of the total anemia in the population and where prevalence is high, iron deficiency would account for a much higher percentage of the total anemia seen in the population.

Dietary iron exists in two chemical forms; heme iron present in flesh foods and non heme iron present in foods of vegetable origin. Diets in developing countries comprise predominantly of non heme iron that is absorbed poorly compared to heme iron. Three major factors influence the amount of iron absorbed and transported to the body for specific functions which is defined as iron bioavailability. These are the chemical form of iron, the balance of enhancers and inhibitors of iron absorption in the diet and the iron status of the individual. Given that the predominant chemical form of iron in the Indian dietary is non-heme iron and the inhibitors far outnumber the enhancers, the absorption of iron is about 5% in most regional diets in India. Increased iron needs during pregnancy, early childhood, and adolescence make these population groups particularly vulnerable to anemia, especially in a situation of dietary deficiency and poor bioavailability.

Regulation of iron absorption at the intestinal level is the chief mechanism for iron homeostasis, as there is no physiological mechanism for excretion of iron once it is absorbed into the body. Iron homeostasis is a complex process that involves several proteins, hepcidin secreted by the liver being the principal hormone involved in iron regulation.

Assessment of anemia is usually done by measuring hemoglobin level in the blood. However, the relative role of different nutrients in the causation of anemia calls for other laboratory investigations of iron, folate and vitamin $B_{12}$ status.

Anemia is of grave public health concern in view of its wide ranging adverse functional consequences that include impaired physical work capacity and a resultant reduced productivity and income in adults; impaired cognitive functions in children with the possibility of a permanent deficit in children below the age of one year; adverse pregnancy outcomes that include low birth weight, increased pre mature births and higher perinatal mortality. Maternal mortality is significantly higher in anemic pregnant women. Other functions affected by iron deficiency anemia include the ability to mount an appropriate immune response to infections, poor thermo regulation and possibly impaired growth in young children.

The serious consequences of anemia require that there is a need for a clear public policy in support of integrated efforts for the control of anemia in all developing countries, which should focus on appropriate food fortification, methods to improve iron availability, nutrient supplements, and control of infections and infestations.

## References


1. BENOIST DE B, MCLEAN E, EGLI I, COGSWELL M (eds.) (2008). Worldwide prevalence of anemia 1993–2005: WHO global database on anemia. Geneva, WHO and CDC.
2. DEMAEYER E and ADIELS-TEGMAN M (1985). The prevalence of anaemia in the world. *World Health Statistics Quarterly*, **38**, pp. 302–316.
3. HURRELL RF and HESS SY (2004). Role for micronutrient interactions in the epidemiology of micro nutrient deficiencies: Interactions of iron, iodine and vitamin A. In: *Micronutrient Deficiencies During the Weaning Period and the First Years of Life*. Pettifor JM, Zlotkin S (eds). Basel (Switzerland): Nestle Nutrition/Karger, pp. 1–19.
4. WHO (2002). The World Health Report: Reducing risks, promoting healthy life: overview. World Health Organization, Geneva (WHO/WHR/02.1).
5. FISHMAN SM, CHRISTIAN P, WEST KP (2000). The role of vitamins in the prevention and control of anemia. *Public Health Nutrition*, **3**, pp. 125–150.
6. ALLEN LH, CASTERLINE-SABEL JE (2004). Prevalence and causes of nutritional anemias. In: *Nutritional Anemias*. Ramakrishnan U. (ed.). Boca Raton FL: CRC Press, pp. 17–21.
7. RAMAN L, SUBBALAXMI PV, VASUMATI N, RAWAL A, VASANTHI G, PARVATHI CH, ADINARAYANA K, RAO KV (1989). Iron and folic acid nutritional status of women in slum. *Nutr Rep Internat* **39**, pp. 73–80.
8. BAKER SJ and DE MAEYER EM (1979). Nutritional anemia: its understanding and control with special reference to the work of the World health organization. *Am J Clin Nutr*, **32**, pp. 368–417.
9. WHO (1968). Technical Report Series No 405, Nutritional Anemias, Geneva.
10. STOLTZFUS RJ and DREYFUSS ML (1998). Guidelines for the use of iron supplements to prevent and treat iron deficiency anemia. Geneva: International Anemia Consultative Group/ UNICEF/WHO.
11. FAO/WHO (1992). International Conference on Nutrition: Major issues for Nutrition Strategies. Italy: Food and Agriculture Organization and World Health Organization, Theme paper No 6, p. 12.
12. HAAS JD and BROWNLIE T (2001). Iron deficiency anemia and reduced work capacity: A critical review of the research to determine a causal relationship. *J Nutr*, **131**, pp. 676S–690S.
13. GRANTHAM MC, GREGOR S, ANI C (2001). A review of studies on the effect of iron deficiency on cognitive development in children. *J Nutr*, **131**, pp. 649S–668S.
14. SESHADRI S (2005). The persistent problem of iron deficiency anemia and its consequences: A life cycle approach is critical for its control. *Proc Nutr Soc India*, **52**, pp. 19–36.
15. OPPENHEIMER SJ (2001). Iron and its relation to immunity and infectious disease. *J Nutr*, **131**, pp. 616S–635S.
16. PREMA K, NEELA KUMARI S, RAMALKASHMI BA (1981). Anemia and adverse obstetric outcome. *Nutr Rep Internat*, **23**, pp. 637–643.
17. ALLEN LH (2000). Anemia and iron deficiency: Effects on pregnancy outcome. *Am J Clin Nutr*, **71**, pp. 1280S–1284S.
18. ACC/SCN (2004). 5th Report on the world nutrition situation – Nutrition for improved development outcomes. Geneva: ACC/SCN/WHO, p. 20.

19. National Health and Nutrition examination Survey (NHANES) III (1998). Recommendations to prevent and control iron deficiency anemia in the United States. *Morb Mortal Wkly Rep*, **47**, pp. 1–29.
20. INDIAN COUNCIL OF MEDICAL RESEARCH (ICMR) (1989). Evaluation of the National Nutritional Anemia Prophylaxis Programme. A Task Force Study. ICMR, New Delhi.
21. INDIAN COUNCIL OF MEDICAL RESEARCH (ICMR) (2001). Micro Nutrients Deficiency Disorders in 16 Districts of India. Report of an ICMR Task Force Study. ICMR, New Delhi.
22. NFHS II (2000). National Family Health Survey of India, 1998-99, International Institute of Population Sciences, Bombay.
23. NFHS III (2008). National Family Health Survey of India, 2006-07. International Institute of Population Sciences, Bombay.
24. SESHADRI S (1999). Oral iron supplementation to control anemia in adolescent girls: Community trials of effectiveness of daily versus weekly supplementation. Department of Foods and Nutrition and WHO collaborating Center for nutritional anemia, M S University, Baroda.
25. SESHADRI S, IYER U, SANGHVI A (1999). Studies on nutritional anemia in pre adolescent and adolescent children (6–15 y) from upper income group public schools in Baroda. Department of Foods and Nutrition, and WHO collaborating Center for Nutritional anemia, M S University, Baroda.
26. SESHADRI S (1998). A data base on iron deficiency anemia: Prevalence, etiology, consequences, and strategies for control. A Task Force Report. Department of Women and Child Development, New Delhi.
27. HODGES RE, SAUBERLICH HE, CANHAM JE, WALLACE DL, RUCKER RB, MEJIA LA, MOHANRAM M (1978). Hematopoietic studies in vitamin A deficiency. *Am J Clin Nutr*, **31**, pp. 876–885.
28. THURNHAM DI (1993). Vitamin A, iron and hemopoiesis. *Lancet*, **342**, pp. 1312-1313.
29. SEMBA RD and BLOEM MW (2002). The anemia of vitamin A deficiency: Epidemiology and pathogenesis. *Eur J Clin Nutr*, **56**, pp. 271–281.
30. POWERS HJ (1995). Riboflavin-iron interactions with particular emphasis on the gastrointestinal tract. *Proc Nutr Soc*, **54**, pp. 509–517.
31. SOOD SK, RAMACHANDRAN K, MATHUR M, GUPTA K, RAMALINGASWAMY V, SWARNABAI C, PONNIAH J, MATHUR VI, BAKER SJ (1975). WHO sponsored collaborative studies on nutritional anemia in India: The effects of supplemental oral iron administration to pregnant women. *Quart J Med (New Series)*, **54**, pp. 241–258.
32. NNMB (1999). Report of Second Repeat Survey: Rural 1996-97, National Nutrition Monitoring Bureau, National Institute of Nutrition, Hyderabad.
33. NNMB (2003). Prevalence of micro nutrient deficiencies. Technical Report No 22, National Nutrition Monitoring Bureau, National Institute of Nutrition, Hyderabad.
34. NNMB (2006). Diet and nutritional status of population and prevalence of hypertension among adults in rural areas. National Nutrition Monitoring Bureau, National Institute of Nutrition, Hyderabad.
35. O' DELL (1985). Bio-availability of and interaction among trace elements. In: *Trace Elements in Nutrition of Children*. Chandra RK (ed).. Nestle Nutrition Vevey/Raven Press, New York, pp. 41–62.
36. MORCK TA and COOK J (1981). Factors affecting the bio availability of dietary iron. *Cereal Foods World*, **26**, pp. 667–672.
37. MONSEN ER, HALLBERG L, LAYRISSE L, HEGSTED GM, COOK JD, MERTZ W, FINCH CA (1978). Estimation of available dietary iron. *Am J Clin Nutr*, **31**, pp. 134–141.

38. MONSEN ER (1988). Iron nutrition and absorption: Dietary factors which impact iron bio availability. *J Am Diet Assoc*, **88**, pp. 786–90.
39. COOK JD and MONSEN ER (1977). Vitamin c, the common cold and iron absorption. *Am J Clin Nutr*, **30**, pp. 235–241.
40. HALLBERG L and ROSSANDER L (1982). Absorption of iron from western type lunch and dinner meals. *Am J Clin Nutr*, **35** pp. 502–509.
41. SESHADRI S, SHAH A, BHADE S (1985). Hematologic response of pre school children to ascorbic acid supplementation. *J Human Nutrition Applied Nutrition*, **39A,** pp. 151–154.
42. NARASINGARAO BS (2007). . Bio availability of dietary iron and iron deficiency anemia. *NFI Bulletin*, **3,** pp. 1–6.
43. COOK JD and MONSEN ER (1976). Food iron absorption in human subjects. III. Comparison of the effect of animal proteins on non heme iron absorption. *Am J Clin Nutr*, **29,** pp. 859–67.
44. BJORN RASMUSSEN E and HALLBERG L (1970). Effect of animal proteins on the absorption of food iron in man. *Nutr Metb*, **23**, pp. 192–202.
45. NARASINGARAO BS, VIJAYASARATHY C, PRABHAVATHY TC (1983). Iron absorption from habitual diets of Indians studied by the extrinsic tag technique. *Ind J Med Res*, **77**, pp. 648–57.
46. HALLBERG L and TOSSANDER L (1982). Effect of different drinks on the absorption of non heme iron from composite meals. *J Human Nutr Appl Nutr*, **36A**, pp. 116–123.
47. HALBERG L and ROSSANDER L (1984). Improvement of iron nutrition in developing countries: Comparison of adding meat, soy protein, ascorbic acid, citric acid and ferrous sulphate on iron absorption from a simple Latin American type of meal. *Am J Clin Nutr*, **33**, pp. 577–83.
48. AUNG THAN BATU, THIEN–THAN, THANE-TOE (1974). Iron absorption from south East Asian rice based meals. *Am J Clin Nutr*, **29**, pp. 219–25.
49. LAYRISSE M, MARTINEZ-TORES C, GONSALEZ M (1974). Measurement of the total daily dietary iron absorption by the extrinsic tag model. *Am J Clin Nutr*, **27**, pp. 152–162.
50. ICMR (1998).Nutrient requirements and recommended dietary allowances for Indians. Indian Council of medical research, New Delhi, 1998.
51. PAWALOWSKI FS, SCHAD GA, SCOTT GJ (1991). Hook worm infection and anemia: Approaches to prevention and control. World Health Organization, Geneva.
52. GILLESPIE S and JHONSTON J (1998). Expert Consultation on anemia determinants and Interventions. *Micronutrient Initiative*, Ottawa.
53. ATUKORALA TMS, DE SILVA LDR, DE CHERING WHJC, DE C DASSENAEIKE TS, PERERA RS (1994). Evaluation of effectiveness of iron folate supplementation and anthelminthic therapy against anemia in pregnancy: a study in the plantation sector of Sri Lanka. *Am J clin Nutr*, **60**, pp. 286–292.
54. STOLTZFUS RJ, CHWAYA HM, MONTRESOR A, ALBONICO M, SAVIOLI L, TIELSCH JM (2000). Malaria, hook worms and recent fever are related to anemia and iron status indicators in 0-5y old Zanzibari children and these relationships change with age. *J Nutr*, **130**, pp. 1724–1733.
55. MENENDEZ C, KAHIGAWA E, HIRT R, VOUNATSOU P, APONTE JJ, FONT F (1997). Randomized placebo controlled trial of iron supplementation and malaria chemo prophylaxis for prevention of severe anemia and malaria in Tanzanian infants. *Lancet*, **350**, pp. 844–850.
56. BRABIN BJ (1983). An analysis of malaria in pregnancy in Africa. *Bulletin of World Health Organization*, **61,** pp. 1005–1016.

57. WHO (1991). Prevention and management of severe anemia in pregnancy. *World Health organization*, Geneva.
58. ZON LI, ARKIN C, GROOPMAN JE (1987). Hematologic manifestations of human immune deficiency virus (HIV). *Br J Hematology*, **66**, pp. 251–56.!!
59. SULLIVAN PS, HANSON DL, CHU SY, JONES JL, WARD JW (1998). Epidemiology of anemia in human immune deficiency virus (HIV) infected persons; results from multistage adult and adolescent spectrum of HIV disease surveillance project. *Blood*, **91**, pp. 301–308.
60. BAIN BJ (1999). Pathogenesis and patho physiology of anemia in HIV infection. *Current Opinions in Hematology* **6**, pp. 89–93.
61. FLEMING RE and BACON BR (2005). Orchestration of iron homeostasis. *N ENGL J Med*, **352**, pp. 1741–44.
62. EISENSTIN RS and BLEMINGS KP (1998). Iron regulatory proteins, iron responsive elements and iron homeostasis. *J Nutr*, **128**, pp. 2295–98.
63. INACG (1981). Iron deficiency in women. A report of the international nutritional anemia consultative group. New York and Washington.
64. VITERI FE (1997). Iron supplementation for the control of iron deficiency in populations at risk. *Nutr Rev*, **55**, pp. 195–209.
65. BEARD JL (2000). Iron requirements in adolescent females. *J Nutr*, **130**, pp. 440S-442S.
66. STEKEL A (1984). Iron requirements in infancy and child hood. In: *Iron Nutrition in Infancy and Childhood*. Stekel A. (ed). New York: Raven Press, pp. 1–10.
67. SIIMES MA (1984). Iron nutrition in low birth weight infants. In: Stekel A. ed. Iron nutrition in infancy and childhood. Raven press, New York, pp. 75–94.
68. WHO (2006). Optimal feeding of low birth weight infants. Technical Review. Karen E, Bahl R (eds). Geneva: World Health Organization.
69. HALLBERG L (1996). Iron requirements, iron balance and iron deficiency in menstruating and pregnant women. In: *Iron Nutrition in Health and Disease*. Hallberg L, Asp N.-G. (eds). London: John Libbey & Co, pp. 165–182.
70. ICMR (2009). Nutrient requirements and safe dietary allowances for Indians. A draft report of the expert group of the Indian Council of medical Research. National Institute of Nutrition, Hyderabad.
71. ICMR (1990). Nutrient requirements and recommended dietary allowances for Indians. A report of the expert group of the Indian Council of medical research. Indian Council of medical Research. National Institute of Nutrition, Hyderabad.
72. THANKACHAN P, WALCZYK T, MUTHAYYA S, KURUPAD A, HURRELL R (2008). Iron absorption in young Indian women: the interaction of iron status with the influence of tea and ascorbic acid. *Am J Clin Nutr*, **87**, pp. 881–886.
73. PATH (1996). Anemia detection in Health Services: Guidelines for program managers. 2n ed. Seattle, Washington: Program for appropriate technology in health (PATH).
74. INACG (1985). Measurement of iron status: A report of the international anemia consultative group (INACG). Washington D.C..
75. COOK JD, BAYNES RD, SKIKNE BS (1992). Iron deficiency and the measurement of iron status. *Nutrition Research Reviews*, **5**, pp. 189–202.
76. WHO/UNICEF/UNU (2001). Iron deficiency anemia: assessment, prevention, and control. Geneva, WHO/NHD/01.
77. GARDNER GW, EDGERTON VR, SENEWIRATNE B, BERNARD RJ, OHIRA Y (1977). Physical work capacity and metabolic stress in subjects with iron deficiency anemia. *Am J Clin Nutr*, **30**, pp. 910–917.
78. OHIRA Y, EDGERTON VR, GARDNER GW, SENEWIRARNE B, SIMPSON DR (1978). Non hemoglobin related effects on heart rate in iron deficiency anemia. *Nutr Rep Int*, **18**, pp. 647–651.

79. EDGERTON VR, OHIRA Y, HETTIARACHCHI J, SENEWIRATNE B, GARDNER GW, BERNARD RJ (1981). Elevation of hemoglobin and work tolerance in iron deficient subjects. *J Nutr Sci vitaminol*, **27**, pp. 77–86.
80. BASTA SS, SOEKIRMAN DS, KARYADI D, SCRIMSHAW NS (1979). Iron deficiency anemia and the productivity of adult males in Indonesia. *Am J Clin Nutr*, **32**, pp. 916–925.
81. EDGERTON VR, GARDNER GW, OHIRA Y, GUNAWARDENA KA, SENEWIRATNE B (1979). Iron deficiency anemia and its effect on worker productivity and activity patterns. *Br Med J*, **2**, pp. 1546–1549.
82. GOPALDAS T and GUJRAL S (2002). Empowering a tea plantation community to improve its micro nutrient health. *Food Nutrition Bulletin*, **23**, pp. 143–152.
83. HORTON S (2004). The economic impact of micronutrient deficiencies. In: Micronutrient deficiencies during the weaning period and the first years of life. Pettifor JM, Zlotkin S (eds).. Basel (Switzerland): Nestle Nutrition, Vevey/ Karger, pp. 187–202.
84. MALHOTRA S and SESHADRI S (1984). Effect of hematinics on the physical work capacity of anemics. *Ind Ped* **29**, pp. 529–533.
85. BHATIA D and SESHADRI S (1987). Anemia, undernutrition and physical work capacity of young boys. *Ind Ped*, **24**, pp. 133–139.
86. DAVIES KJA, DONOVAN CM, REFINO CM, BROOKS GA, PACKER L, DALLMAN PR (1984). Distinguishing the effects of anemia and muscle iron deficiency on exercise bio energetics in the rat. *Am J Physiol*, **246**, pp. E535–E543.
87. GERA T, SACHDEV HP, NESTEL P (2007). Effect of iron supplementation on physical performance in children and adolescents: systematic review of randomized controlled trials. *Indian Pediatrics*, **44**, pp. 15–24.
88. GOPALDAS T and GUJRAL S (2003). Multi nutrient package of iron, vitamin A and iodine to improve productivity and earnings of women tea pickers in south India. *Food Nutrition Bulletin*, **24**, pp. 218–223.
89. WEBB TE and OSKI FA (1973). Iron deficiency anemia and scholastic achievement in young adolescents. *J Pediatr*, **82**, pp. 827–833.
90. SESHADRI S, HIRODE K, NAIK P, MALHOTRA S (1983). Behavioral responses of young anemic Indian children to iron folic acid supplements. *Brit J Nutr*, **48**, pp. 233–240.
91. AGARWAL DK, UPADHYAYA SK, TRIPATHI AM, AGARWAL KN (1987). Nutritional status, physical work capacity and mental function in school children. New Delhi, Nutrition Foundation of India.
92. POLLITT E (2001). The developmental and probabilistic nature of the functional consequences of iron deficiency anemia in children. *J Nutr*, **131**, pp. 669S–675S.
93. SESHADRI S and GOPALDAS T (1989). Impact of iron supplementation on cognitive functions in pre school and school age children: the Indian experience. *Am J Clin Nutr*, **50**, pp. 675–686.
94. SACHDEV HPS, GERA T, NESTEL P (2005). Effect of iron supplementation on mental and motor development in children: Systematic review of randomized controlled trials. *Public Health Nutrition*, **8**, pp. 117–132.
95. ALLEN LH and GILLESPIE S (2001). What works? A review of the efficacy and effectiveness of nutrition interventions. Manila, ACC/SCN, Asian development Bank.
96. RASMUSSEN KM (2001). Is there a causal relationship between iron deficiency or iron deficiency anemia and weight at birth, length of gestation and perinatal mortality? *J Nutr* **131**, pp. 590S–603S.

97. AGARWAL KN, AGARWAL DK, MISHRA KP (1991). Impact of anemia prophylaxis in pregnancy on maternal hemoglobin, serum ferritin and birth weight. *Ind J Med Res* **94**, pp. 277–280.
98. COGSWELL ME, PARVANTA I, ICKES L, YIP R, BRITTENHAM GM (2003). Iron supplementation during pregnancy, anemia and birth weight: a randomized controlled trial. *Am J Clin Nutr*, **78**, pp. 773–781.
99. PREMA K, RAMALAKSHMI BA, NADHAVAPEDDI R, BABU S (1982). Immune status of anemic pregnant women. *Brit J Obst Gynecol*, **89**, pp. 222–225.
100. SRIKANTIA SG, BHASKARAM P, PRASAD JS, KRISHNAMACHARI K (1976). Anemia and immune response. *The Lancet*, **309**, pp. 1307–1309.
101. BHASKARAM P, SIVA PRASAD J, KRISHNAMACHARI K (1977). Anemia and immune response. *The Lancet*, **309**, p. 1000.
102. GERA T and SACHDEV HPS (2002). Effect of iron supplementation on incidence of infectitious illneses in children: systematic review. *Brit Med J*, **325**, p. 1142.
103. BRIGHAM D and BEARD J (1996). Iron and thermo regulation: A review. *Crit Rev Food Sci Nutr*, **36**, pp. 747–763.
104. AUKET MA, PARKYA SCOTT PH, WHARTON BA (1986). Treatment with iron increases weight gain and psychomotor development. *Arch Diseases Childhood*, **61**, pp. 847–849.
105. BHATIA D and SESHADRI S (1987). Growth performance in anemia and following iron supplementation. *Ind Ped* **30**, pp. 195–200.
106. SACHDEV HP, GERA T, NESTEL P (2006). Effect of iron supplementation on physical growth in children: systematic review of randomized controlled trials. *Public Health Nutrition*, **9**, pp. 904–920.
107. ALLEN L, BENOIST DE B, DARY Q, HURRELL R (2006). Guidelines on food fortification with micronutrients. Geneva, WHO/FAO.
108. NARASINGA TAO BS (1994). Fortification of salt with iron and iodine to control anemia and goiter: Development of a new formula with good stability and bio availability. *Food and Nutrition Bulletin*, **15**, pp. 32–39.
109. MADHAVAN NAIR K, BRAHMAM GNV, RANGANATHAN S, VIJAYARAGHAVAN K, SIVAKUMAR B, KRISHNASWAMI K (1998). Impact evaluation of iron and iodine fortified salt. *Ind J Med Res***108**, pp. 203–211.
110. NIN and ICMR (2005). Double fortified common salt (DFS) as a tool to control iodine deficiency disorders (IDD) and iron deficiency anemia (IDA). A Technical report. Hyderabad.
111. TAYLOR PG, MÉNDEZ-CASTELLANOS H, MARTÍNEZ-TORRES C, JAFFE W, BLANCO ML, JIMÉNEZ ML, LEETS I, TROPPER E, RAMÍREZ J, NIEVES ML, CASAL G, LAYRISSE M (1995). Iron bio availability from diets consumed by different socio economic strata of the Venezuelan population. *J Nutr*, **125**, pp. 1860–1868.
112. ACC/SCN (1991). Controlling iron deficiency. Nutrition policy discussion paper no 9. Administrative Committee on Co-ordination- Sub Committee on Nutrition, Geneva.
113. WHO (2009). Weekly iron–folic acid supplementation (WIFS) in women of reproductive age: its role in promoting optimal maternal and child health. Position statement. Geneva, World Health Organization, (http://www.who.int/nutrition/publications/micronutrients/weekly_iron_folicacid.pdf, accessed [date]).
114. DREYFUSS ML, STOLTZFUS RJ, SHRESTHA JB, PRADHAN EK, LECLERQ CL, KHATRY SK, SHRESTHA SR, KATZ J, ALBONICO M, WEST KP JR (2000). Hookworms, malaria and vitamin A deficiency contribute to anemia and iron deficiency among pregnant women in the plains of Nepal. *J Nutr*, **130**, pp. 2527–2536.

# 27

# Iron deficiency and iron deficiency anemia in adolescent girls

*Sheila C. Vir*

**Sheila C Vir,** MSc, PhD, is a senior nutrition consultant and Director of Public Health Nutrition and Development Centre, New Delhi. Following MSc (Food and Nutrition) from University of Delhi, Dr Vir was awarded PhD by the Queen's University of Belfast, United Kingdom. Dr. Vir, a past secretary of the Nutrition Society of India, is a recipient of the fellowship of the Department of Health and Social Services, UK, and Commonwealth Van den Bergh Nutrition Award. Dr Vir worked briefly with the Aga Khan Foundation (India) and later with UNICEF. As a Nutrition Programme Officer with UNICEF for twenty years, Dr. Vir provided strategic and technical leadership for policy formulation and implementation of nutrition programmes in India.

## 27.1 Prevalence of iron deficiency and anemia among adolescent girls

Adolescence, between the ages of 10–19 years [1], contributes to almost 20% population in developing countries. Adolescence is a stage of accelerated growth and development [2, 3, 4] when requirements for iron increases significantly. Iron deficiency and iron deficiency anemia (IDA) in adolescence is a major public health problem. As per the global estimates, 23% adolescent girls are anemic [5]. Incidence of anemia in school age children tends to increase with age and corresponds with acceleration in growth during adolescence (Figure 27.1). Studies indicate that the prevalence of anemia in school children increases from 10 years old upwards and remains high until 18 years of age during the growth period (Figure 27.1). The highest prevalence is between the ages of 12–15 years with over 50% girls reported to be anemic [6, 7]. This trend in prevalence of IDA with age is due to inability to meet the higher requirement for iron with increase in body mass which is correlated to variations in velocity of growth of adolescents [8, 9].

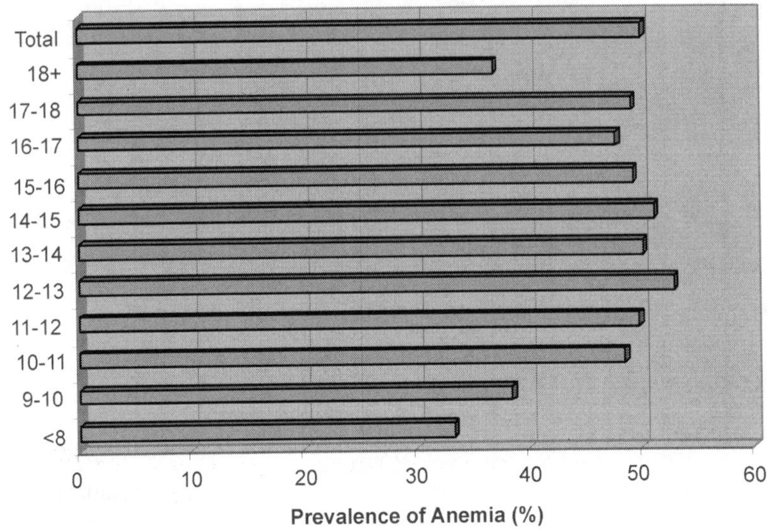


*27.1* Age-wise prevalence of anemia multi-centric study on adolescent girls [10]

In most South–East Asian countries almost half of the adolescent girls are anemic [11-21]. On the other hand, the prevalence of anemia in adolescent girls in USA and Norway is less than 6% (Figure 27.2).

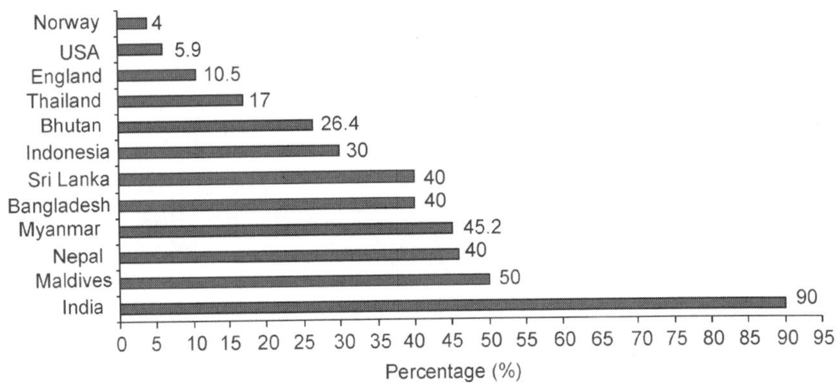


*27.2* Anemia prevalence in adolescent girls [11–21]

The high prevalence of anemia in adolescent girls in a region often corresponds with a high level of anemia during pregnancy. As indicated in Table 27.1, in all South Asian countries, except Thailand, one-third of adolescent girls were anemic while prevalence of anemia in pregnant mothers was over 40% (Table 27.1). Anemia is primarily due to iron deficiency and is in fact the long end stage of a relatively long process of deterioration in iron stores. Many more adolescents are in fact suffering from iron deficiency (ID) with its adverse effects on health and physical stamina, than are frankly anemic [22]. UNICEF/UNU/WHO/MI [23] indicate that there are approximately 2.5 cases of iron deficiency for each case of anemia. The functional consequences are known to occur prior to onset of clinical stage of iron deficiency.

*Table 27.1* Prevalence of anemia in adolescent population as compared to pregnant women in South East Asian Region countries

| *Country* | *Prevalence of anemia (percentage)* | |
|---|---|---|
| | *Adolescents girls* | *Pregnant women* |
| Bangladesh [10] | 40.0 | 75.0 |
| Bhutan [11] | 26.4 | 68.0 |
| India [12, 13] | 90.0 | 58.7[a] |
| Indonesia [14] | 30.0 | 51.0 |
| Maldives [15] | 50.0 | 68.0 |
| Myanmar [16] | 45.2 | 52.0 |
| Nepal [17] | 46.0 | 68.0 |
| Sri Lanka [18] | 40.0 | 40.0 |
| Thailand [19, 20] | 17.0 | 12.0 |

[a] Only India data specifies inclusion of adolescents.

## 27.2 Causes of iron deficiency and iron deficiency anemia in adolescent girls

Adolescent girls are at high risk of iron deficiency and anemia due to accelerated increase in requirements for iron, poor dietary intake of iron, high rate of infection and infestation as well as the social problem of adolescent pregnancy and conception.

(a) *Accelerated increase in requirement for iron during adolescence* – Iron deficiency anemia (IDA) occurs when iron stores in the body are depleted and supply to tissues is compromised resulting in fall of hemoglobin levels. Iron needs for the body increases sharply with accelerated growth spurt – adolescents on an average gain weight equivalent to 65% of their weight at the beginning of the period or 40% of their final weight, and a height gain equivalent to 15% of their adult height or 25% of an individual's attained height during adolescence [24, 25, 26]. The accelerated increase in lean body mass, blood volume and red cell mass results in increase in requirement for iron for the synthesis of myoglobin in muscles and hemoglobin in blood [27]. Figure 27.3 presents the continuous increase in the median requirements for absorbed iron for both boys and girls during adolescence [27]. The requirement peaks between the ages of 14–15 years. As shown in Table 27.2, the overall iron requirement increases two to three folds from a preadolescent level of approximately 0.6–0.9 mg iron per day to as much as 1.37–1.88 mg per day in adolescent

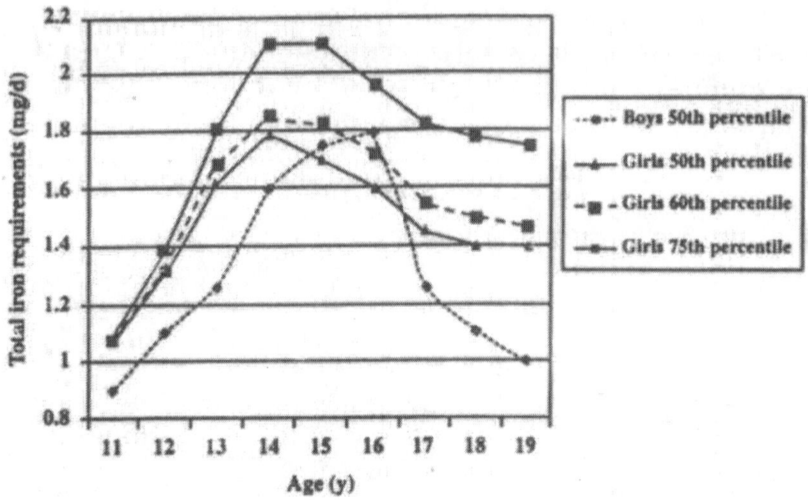


*27.3* Median requirements for absorbed iron (mg/day) during adolescence stage [27]

*Table 27.2* Iron intakes required for adolescent boys and girls, median basal iron losses, menstrual losses in women, and total absolute iron requirements as compared to children [22]

| *Group* | *Age* | *Body weight* | *Required Iron intakes for growth* | *Basal iron losses* | *Menstrual losses* | | *Total absolute requirements*[a] | |
|---|---|---|---|---|---|---|---|---|
| | | *Mean* | | *Median* | *Median* | *95th percentile* | *Median* | *95th percentile* |
| | *(Years)* | *(kg)* | *(mg/day)* | *(mg/day)* | *(mg/day)* | *(mg/day)* | *(mg/day)* | *(mg/day)* |
| Children | 0.5–1.0 | 9 | 0.55 | 0.17 | | | 0.72 | 0.93 |
| | 1–3 | 13.3 | 0.27 | 0.19 | | | 0.46 | 0.58 |
| | 4–6 | 19.2 | 0.23 | 0.27 | | | 0.50 | 0.63 |
| | 7–10 | 28.1 | 0.32 | 0.39 | | | 0.71 | 0.89 |
| Males | 11–14 | 45 | 0.55 | 0.62 | | | 1.17 | 1.46 |
| | 15–17 | 64.4 | 0.60 | 0.90 | | | 1.50 | 1.88 |
| | 18+ | 75 | | 1.05 | | | 1.05 | 1.37 |
| Females | 11–14[b] | 46.1 | 0.55 | 0.65 | | | 1.20 | 1.40 |
| | 11–14 | 46.1 | 0.55 | 0.65 | 0.48[b] | 1.90[c] | 1.68 | 3.27 |
| | 15–17 | 56.4 | 0.35 | 0.79 | 0.48[b] | 1.90[c] | 1.62 | 3.10 |
| | 18+ | 62 | | 0.87 | 0.48[b] | 1.90[c] | 1.46 | 2.94 |

[a] Total absolute requirements = Requirement for growth + basal losses + menstrual losses (females only)
[b] Non-menstruating
[c] Effect of the normal variation in hemoglobin concentration not included in this figure

boys and 1.40–3.27 in adolescent girls [22, 27]. Additional iron is therefore required by both adolescent boys and girls for the expanding red cell mass and growing body tissue.

The risk of iron deficiency increases significantly during the adolescent growth spurt for both boys and girls. In boys, following the phase of growth spurt, the need for iron decreases and there is a scope for overcoming deficiency of iron, However, in case of adolescent girls, the situation differs with requirements for iron continuing to remain high through the reproductive life to replace iron that is lost during menstruation – there is a regular loss of 12.5–15.0 mg iron per month or 0.4–0.5 mg iron per day in menstrual blood. Therefore in girls, following the growth spurt, the risk of iron deficiency continues to be of a public health concern through the entire reproductive age but this risk subsides for boys [28].

(b) *Low dietary intake and bio-availability of iron* – The primary cause of IDA in adolescence is lack of iron available to the body to meet the high requirements due to low dietary intake and poor bioavailability of iron consumed against the significant increase in requirements [29]. The data from India indicates that the diets of girls aged between 13 and 18 years provide much lower level of iron than the diets of boys in the same age group [30]. Low consumption of nutrients by adolescents reported from India indicates that over 50% adolescent girls consume less than 50% RDA for energy while over 70% girls consume less than 50% RDA of iron [31]. Similarly the Bangladesh study on adolescent girls attending school in Dhaka city [32] reveals that 31% of these girls consume less than 50% RDA of iron and 10% less than 50% energy. Similar findings of low intake of iron and energy are reported from other studies in adolescent girls in Bangladesh, Indonesia and India [33, 34, 35].

Besides low consumption of total dietary iron, the source of iron is important. Routine intake of monotonous diets based on cereals along with consumption of low quantities of meat, fish or fresh vegetables and fruits results in poor availability of iron. Such diet with high concentration of inhibitors and low concentration of enhancers lowers the bio-availability of dietary iron from cereal based diet. This is evident from data of India [36] where the prevalence of anemia is higher in Indian adolescents consuming a vegetarian diet (45.8%) as compared to those consuming a mixed diet, which includes animal food (30%).

Daily recommended intake of dietary iron varies widely when bioavailability of iron is taken into consideration (Table 27.4). Women in reproductive ages require only 19.6 mg daily of iron when diet is 15% bio-available compared to about 58.8 mg when diet is poor in vitamin C and animal protein and the bio-availability is only 5% [37]. Poor total intake of iron as well as low bio-availability of iron consumed results in iron deficiency and subsequently IDA.

In adolescents, there is also a tendency to frequently consume snacks prepared from cereals as well as a habit to consume carbonated drinks while there is a lower desire to eat fruits and vegetables. Moreover, habitual consumption of tea/coffee immediately after meals by adolescent girls also contributes to higher prevalence of anemia of 50% as compared to 34% in

*Table 27.3* Dietary intakes (energy, protein and iron) by adolescent girls in Bangladesh, Indonesia and India [33, 34, 35]

| | | *Bangladesh (Adolescent girls)* | *Indonesia (Adolescent girls 10–12 years)* | | *India* |
|---|---|---|---|---|---|
| | | | *Non-IDA* | *IDA* | |
| Energy (kcal) | Intake (RDA) | 1005<br>(1970 kcal (10–12 years)<br>2060 kcal (13–15 years)<br>2060 kcal (16–18 years)) | 1122<br>(1900) | 1126<br>(1900) | 1389 (10–12 yrs)<br>(1970)<br>1566 (13–15 yrs)<br>(2060)<br>1630 (16–17 yrs)<br>(2060) |
| Protein (g) | Intake (RDA) | 44<br>(-) | 43.8<br>(54) | 45.3<br>(54) | 37.8 (10–12 yrs)<br>(57)<br>42.0 (13–15 yrs)<br>(65)<br>43.9 (16–17 yrs)<br>(63) |
| Iron (mg) | Intake (RDA) | 18<br>(28) | 6.9<br>(14) | 8.3<br>(14) | 11.5 (10–12 yrs)<br>(19)<br>13.0 (13–15 yrs)<br>(28)<br>13.5 (16–17 yrs)<br>(30.0) |

* Figures in parenthesis indicate recommended dietery allowances (RDA)

*Table 27.4* Selected recommended daily intakes for iron by estimated dietary iron availability [37]

| *Dietary iron bioavailability (Percentage)* | *Children (1–3 years)* | *Children (4–6 years)* | *Women (19–50 years)* | *Women during pregnancy (2nd trimester)* | *Women during breast feeding (0–3 months lactation)* | *Men (19–50 years)* |
|---|---|---|---|---|---|---|
| | *(mg)* | *(mg)* | *(mg)* | *(mg)* | *(mg)* | *(mg)* |
| 15 | 3.9 | 4.2 | 19.6 | >50.0 | 10.0 | 9.1 |
| 10 | 5.8 | 6.3 | 29.4 | >50.0 | 15.0 | 13.7 |
| 51 | 11.6 | 12.6 | 58.8 | >50.0 | 30.0 | 27.4 |

Recommended daily intake for iron depends on the bio-availability of the diet: diet rich in vitamin C and animal protein = 15%; diet rich in cereals, low in animal protein, but rich in vitamin C = 10%, diet poor in vitamin C and animal protein = 5%.

those who do not consume tea/coffee after meals [33]. Although the iron density in the diets of both boys and girls is similar, the lower total food intake or energy intake by adolescent girls compared to boys, combined with menstrual losses cause adolescent girls to be at greater risk of iron deficiency and IDA [12]. In fact, in developing countries, 20% of women with normal menstruation have serious problems in meeting their iron requirements by food alone [34]. Social discrimination towards girl child as well as the frequent tendency of dieting play a crucial role in worsening the quality and quantity of diet and the dietary iron consumed by adolescents.

(c) *Frequent infectious disease and parasitic infections* – The frequent occurrence of infectious diseases and parasitic infestations in developing countries further increases requirements for iron and increases the chances of negative iron status and IDA. In a study in India, one-third of adolescents had a history of passing worms [38]. The prevalence of anemia was double in these girls (53.6%) compared to those who were not reported to be infested (25%). Infections and infestations interfere with food intake, assimilation and absorption, storage and use of many nutrients such as iron, vitamin $B_{12}$, folic acid, vitamin C, vitamin A etc which contribute to anemia. IDA during adolescence is primarily due to deficiency of iron resulting from low availability of dietary iron and less often due to deficiency of other nutrients and other conditions such as hookworm infestations, schistosomiasis and other infections [28]. However, the role of infestation and infection in contributing to iron deficiency and anemia cannot be ignored.

(d) *Adolescent pregnancy* – Added to the problem of poor dietary iron intake is the traditional practice of early marriage. Social pressure often results in most women conceiving within a year of marriage [39]. An onset of pregnancy during adolescence period of life further increases demands for iron and contributes to aggravating the iron deficiency and IDA. Table 27.5 indicates that in India, Bangladesh and Nepal [12, 35–37, 39, 40] over 50% girls are married by 18 years of age. In Indonesia, Thailand and Sri Lanka, 26, 22 and 12 per cent girls, respectively are married by 18 years of age. Studies on adolescent pregnant girls in Nepal and tribal India indicate risks and outcomes of pregnancy increases in such adolescent mothers with higher prevalence of anemia [41, 42].

*Table 27.5* Percentage of women aged 20–24 married by age 15 and 18 in selected countries of South East Asia Region

| *South East Asian Countries* | *Married by age 15 years (%)* | *Married by age 18 years (%)* |
|---|---|---|
| Bangladesh (1999–2000) [39] | 32.3 | 66.2 |
| India (2005–2006) [12] | 18.2 | 47.4 |
| Indonesia (2002–2003) [40] | 4.3 | 22.0 |
| Nepal (2005) [36] | 14.1 | 56.1 |
| Sri Lanka (2000) [35] | 1.5 | 10 |
| Thailand (1987) [37] | 2 | 20 |

Figure 27.4 presents an overview of the factors leading to higher iron requirements during adolescence and precipitation of anemia.

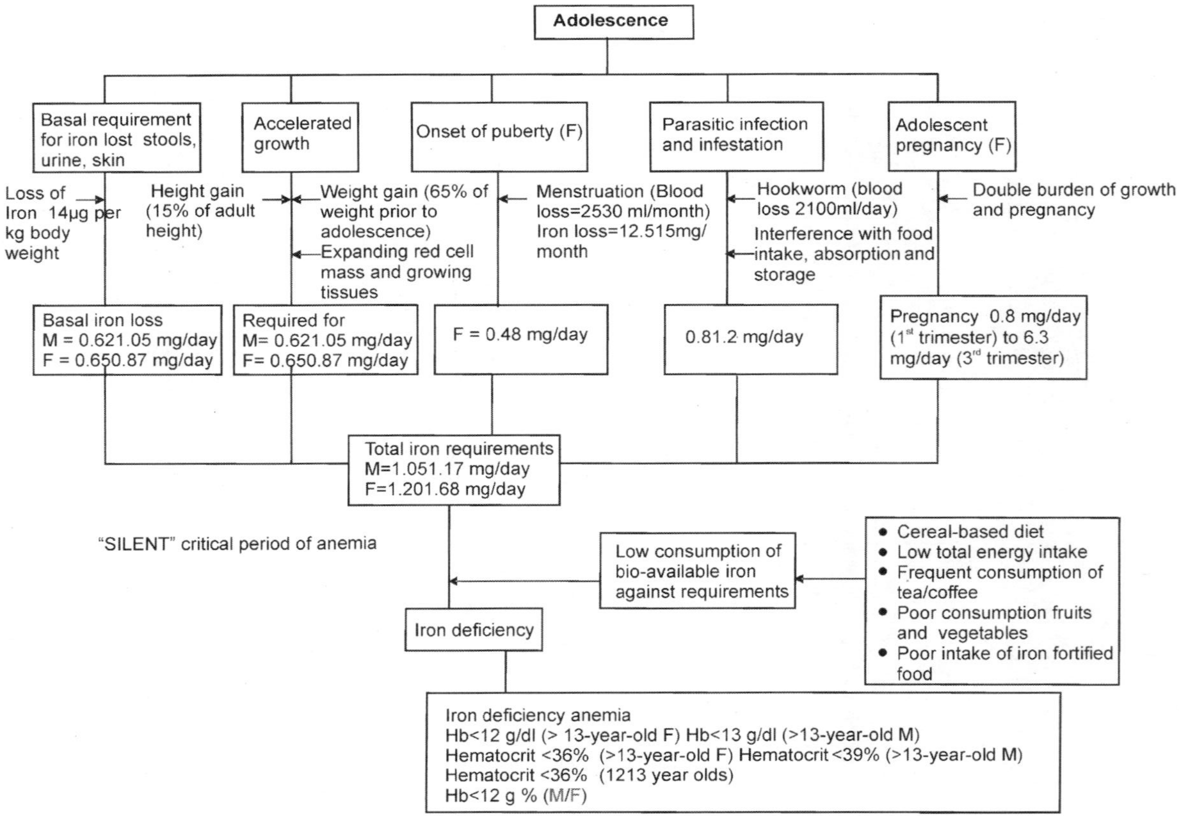


*27.4* Adolescence, a silent phase of iron deficiency and iron deficiency anemia – prevention is critical

## 27.3 Consequences of iron deficiency and iron deficiency anemia

Since 16th century, there are references to diseases commonly affecting adolescent girls which are characterized by pallor, fatigue, poor appetite and menstrual disturbances which seem to be related to iron deficiency [42]. In fact iron deficiency anemia during adolescence sets up a vicious cycle of anemia during pregnancy and childhood with serious consequences (Figure 27.5). Iron deficiency anemia adversely affects transportation of oxygen to tissues and accounts for the diminished work capacity and physical performance. IDA during adolescence has serious implications for a wide range of outcome: impaired physical growth, weakened cognitive development, reduced physical and work performance/capacity and diminished concentration in daily tasks and school performance, loss of appetite resulting in reduced food intake as well as irregular menstruation [12]. Iron deficiency adversely affects the immune system.

It has been estimated that each 1% decrease in hemoglobin results in a 1.5% decrease in work capacity and a 1–2% decrease in work output with economic consequences [23]. Anemic children exhibit poor attentiveness, poor memory and poor academic performance. It has been reported that anemia results in poor attention, concentration and scholastic performance [43, 44] and is associated with disturbances in attention and perception resulting in poor academic achievements [43]. Other clinical symptoms due to IDA include anorexia, flatulence, nausea, dimness of vision and headache which may ultimately affect school attendance, school retention and overall performance [28]. The serious implications of IDA needs to be seen with reference to its impact on lack of incentive to remain in schools, academic under achievements, poor school attendance and poor physical condition leading to poor economic productivity [45].

Iron deficiency in adolescent girls has serious implications on the future generation by adversely affecting the health of the fetus. Iron deficient adolescent girls have a higher risk of preterm delivery and having babies with low birth weight (LBW) [46, 47]. In fact anemia during adolescence limits growth and delays onset of menarche which may lead to cephalopelvic disproportion. IDA combined with early onset pregnancy results in increased maternal morbidity and mortality, increased risk of low birth weight, increased fetal morbidity and mortality as well as higher neonatal mortality [21, 48, 49]. These serious consequences are of special public health significance in developing countries where one third of adolescent girls are reported to be anemic [50] and 12 % of all women aged 15–19 years and 44% of married women aged 15–19 years are reported to have atleast one child [12]. In fact, severe anemia increases the risk of mortality of pregnant mothers with poor iron stores [51]. Investment in

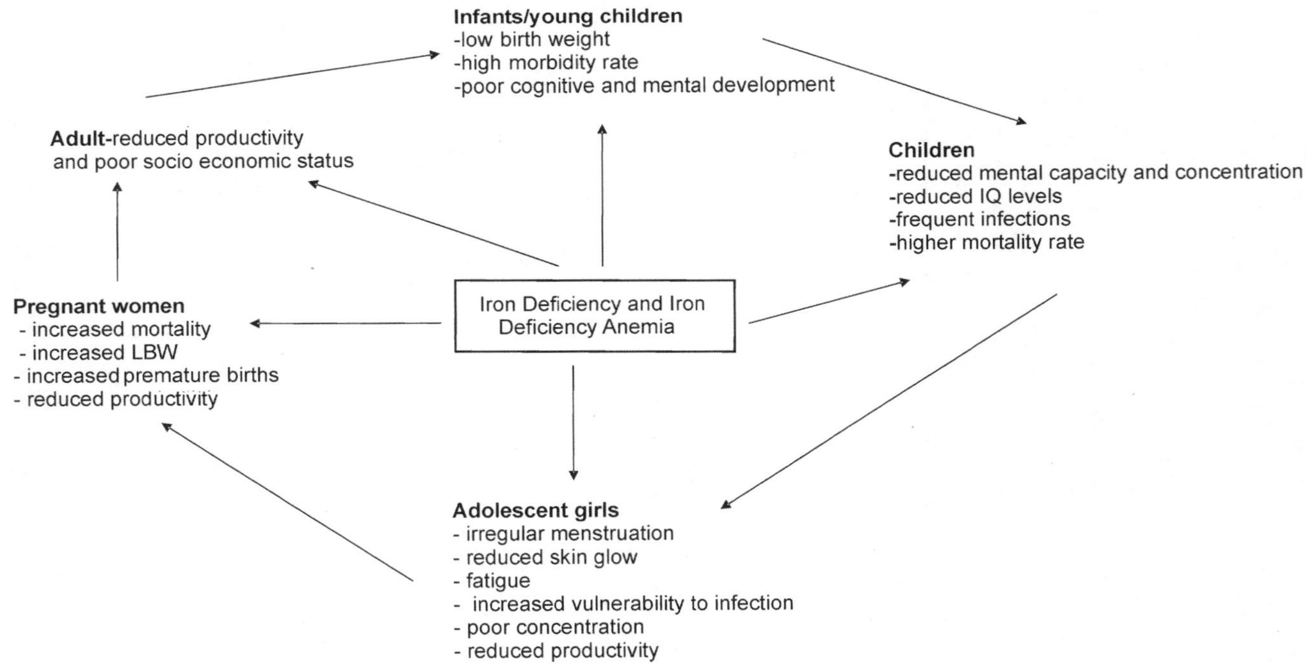


*27.5* Consequences of iron deficiency (ID) and iron deficiency anemia (IDA) during the life cycle [52].

building iron nutriture during adolescence is therefore critical not only for prevention of anemia and ill health during the adolescence phases of life itself but is crucial for mother's health and fetal development as well as child growth and development later in life (Figure 27.5).

With such serious adverse effect of iron deficiency and iron deficiency anemia, overcoming iron deficiency has significant impact on Millennium Development Goals (MDGs) as presented below in Box 27.1[52].

**Box 27.1 Iron deficiency and iron deficiency anemia (IDA) prevention in Women of Reproductive Age (WRA) help to achieve the MDGs [52]**

| *MDG goals* | *Impact of IDA prevention* |
|---|---|
| MDG # 1 Eradicate Extreme Poverty and Hunger | • Increases body's capacity to do work (for every 10% increase in HB – 15% increase in physical work)<br>• Reduces low birth weight<br>• Reduces undernutrition in under 5 year |
| MDG # 2 Achieve Universal Primary Education | • Reduces frequency and severity of infections/morbidity and mortality<br>• Improves School attendance, retention, learning capacity and school achievement |
| MDG # 3 Promote Gender Equality and Empower Women | • Anemia in girls – often more severe than in boys. Adversely influences school attendance and achievement.<br>• Reduces Gender disparity |
| MDG # 4 Reduce Child Mortality | • Reduces serious consequences on child health, including LBW, still birth<br>• Reduces Child mortality |
| MDG # 5 Improve Maternal Health | • Reduction of maternal anemia<br>• Reduces MMR (20% of maternal deaths are directly attributed to anemia) |

## 27.4 Prevention and control of iron deficiency and iron deficiency anemia

The most effective public health approach to prevent and control iron deficiency and iron deficiency anemia is a multiple integrated intervention comprising the following three main strategies – food-based approach, iron supplementation and public health interventions (Figure 27.6). The country strategy, however, needs to be based on analysis of the local situations. The most cost-effective means of determining whether iron deficiency is the cause of anemia is to measure changes in hemoglobin or hematocrit status in response to oral iron supplementation [53]. For addressing iron deficiency and IDA, participation of sectors other than health sector such as education, food industry and horticulture is important. Dietary diversification is the most sustainable approach, but is a difficult intervention to implement as a public health measure since both the actual quantity of iron intake and bioavailability of iron consumed is important. Foods with high bio-available iron (animal food) or foods that enhance the absorption of iron such as foods rich in vitamin C are expensive. Dietary measure such as iron fortification of basic food has been shown to be effective in reducing prevalence of iron deficiency anemia. Fortification aims to increase the intake of nutrient without bringing a change in customary diet. Many developing countries are in the process of introducing consumption of foods fortified with iron and other micronutrients. Wheat flour and maize meal are two major food vehicles that have been successfully used for fortification with iron in developed and developing countries. Standards for levels of iron used for fortification vary in different countries. For example fortification of wheat flour with Ferrous Sulphate used in Canada is 29–43 parts per million (ppm), Chile 30 ppm and Nigeria 35 ppm [54]. Regular use of cereal foods fortified with iron and salt fortified with iodine and iron as well as use of micronutrient mix as home or institutional fortificant is cost-effective and important to be promoted for addressing anemia in population including adolescent girls.

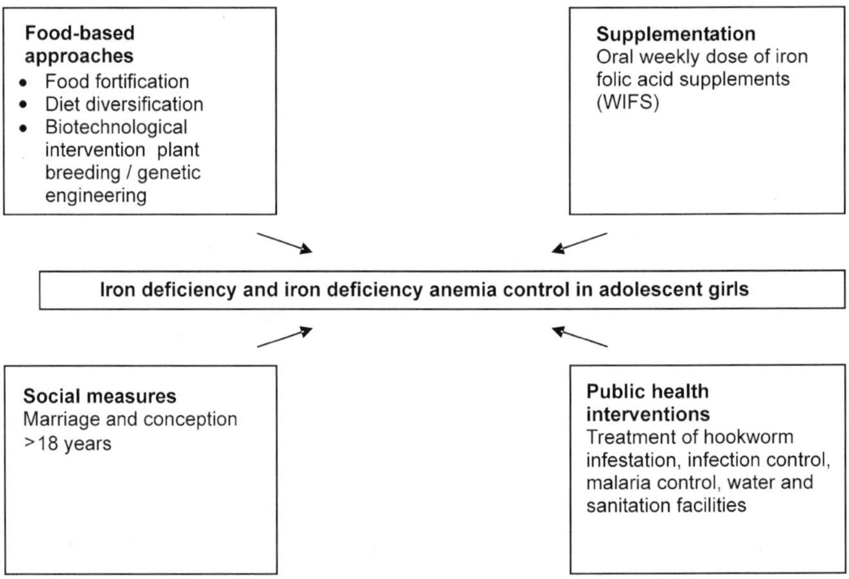


*27.6* Integrated strategy to address iron deficiency and iron deficiency anemia in adolescent girls

For improving iron status and prevention of iron deficiency anemia, regular use of iron-folic acid supplements is recommended as a public health approach. A joint consensus statement by UNICEF/UNU/WHO/MI emphasizes that in countries where anemia prevalence exceeds 40% in pregnant women or is above 20 percent among women in reproductive age group, universal iron supplements of adolescent girls (minimum those aged 12–16 years) and women of child bearing age is warranted [55]. In 1999, a meta-analysis was undertaken to study the efficacy of intermittent iron supplementation in the control of iron deficiency anemia in developing countries [56, 57]. The analysis was based on the results of a total of 22 completed trials of iron supplementation, including 9 studies with adolescent groups (Table 27.5). The results indicated a positive impact with weekly supplements in 5 of the 9 studies. The meta-analysis study concluded that "it appears under highly controlled conditions, supplementation can have an impact on anemia prevalence and that the daily and weekly approaches may have similar impact". Based on this conclusion, weekly supplementation with iron-folic acid was then recommended only in situations where there is a strong assurance of supervision and high compliance.

*Table 27.6* Efficacy of Daily and Weekly Iron Folic Acid Supplementation (WIFS) in various countries – meta-analysis study [55]

| *Countries* | | *% Prevalence of Anemia*** | | |
|---|---|---|---|---|
| | | *Weekly* | *Daily* | *Control* |
| East Jakarta | (B)* | 17.9 | 15.6 | 17.3 |
| | (E)* | 6.7 | 7.8 | 21.3 |
| India Baroda | (B) | 53.8 | 63.5 | 62.7 |
| | (E) | 66.2 | 44.4 | 60.1 |
| Delhi | (B) | 49.0 | 47.0 | 44.6 |
| | (E) | 48.2 | 30.9 | 57.8 |
| Mumbai | (B) | 65.0 | 61.6 | 64.8 |
| | (E) | 33.9 | 26.2 | 58.4 |
| Malawi | (B) | 11.1 | 12.8 | NA |
| | (E) | 12.0 | 11.9 | NA |
| Malaysia | (B) | 49.8 | NA* | 0 |
| | (E) | 9.0 | NA* | 10.1 |
| Mali | (B) | 29.6 | 37.1 | 28.9 |
| | (E) | 38.0 | 30.9 | 39.0 |
| Peru | (B) | 18.4 | 19.8 | 15.5 |
| | (E) | 17.3 | 10.9 | 22.7 |
| Sri Lanka | (B) | 25.0 | 18.5 | 19.8 |
| | (E) | 9.5 | 8.6 | 13.4 |

* (B) refers to Baseline and (E) refers to Endline
** Anemia criteria – Hb < 12 g/L

This global meta-analysis study was followed by a number of efficacy trials on use of weekly iron-folic acid (IFA) supplements for the adolescent girls population in Asia, Africa and South America [57–60]. Based on the results of these projects, weekly and not daily iron–folic acid supplement consumption is proposed as a preventive approach to improve iron status and for reducing the prevalence of anemia. The positive impact of weekly consumption of iron supplement is explained on the basis of the "mucosal block" hypothesis wherein administration of iron every seven days is assumed to allow time for shedding of cells loaded with iron from a previous dose, thereby increasing iron absorption [61, 62]. Additionally, weekly dosage instead of daily dosage is considered to result in avoiding a constant luminal and mucosal overload and thus preventing likely stimulation of gastro-intestinal symptoms [61–64]. Weekly dosage is expected to have fewer side effects with a positive impact on increasing compliance and reduction in anemia. The impact of weekly iron folic acid supplements (WIFS) in reducing prevalence of anemia is evident in a short period of 6–12 months from a study undertaken in non-school going adolescent girls in the state of Uttar Pradesh, India (Figure 27.7) [65].

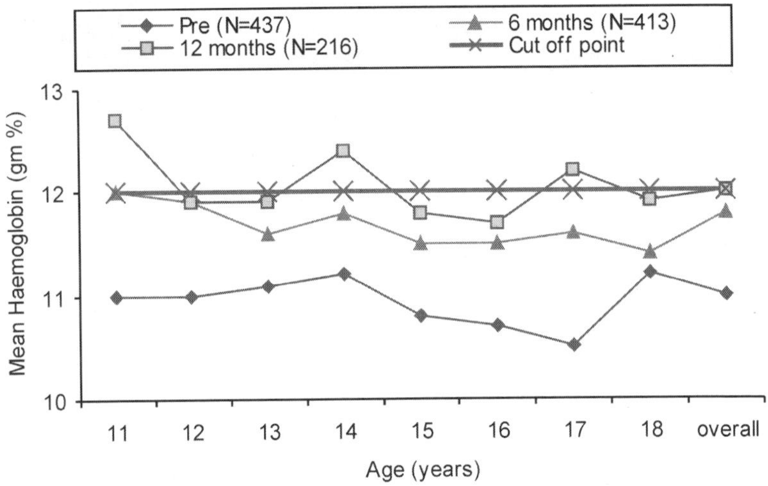


*27.7* Impact on hemoglobin levels following 6 and 12 months of weekly IFA consumption on adolescent girls [65]

Targeting adolescent girls with WIFS is critical for prevention of anemia since their high requirements, if not met, could lead to depleted iron stores even before the onset of pregnancy [66, 67]. WIFS is a low cost intervention and this is of advantage since consumption of supplements is recommended throughout the reproductive period. Menarche often sets in by 12 years of age and it is beneficial to ensure that adolescent girls regularly consume iron-folic acid tablets right from the onset of menarche. Intervention to address anemia at younger age of 10–14 years as compared to 15–18 years has been demonstrated to give a better response in weight gain and Body Mass Index (BMI) and in the regularization of menstrual cycle.

Regular consumption of IFA influences not only adolescent growth, physical output and educational performance but WIFS regime during adolescence is an investment for future and safe pregnancy [13]. Iron requirements during pregnancy are high and it is not always possible to absorb an adequate amount of supplementary iron, especially by those women who are iron deficient during pregnancy. Pregnancy itself is too short a period for addressing pre-existing anemia and in fact, it is noted that longer the pre-pregnancy preventive supplementation, the better its impact on iron nutrition during pregnancy [63]. Effort to improve iron status and anemia after the onset of pregnancy is therefore late and inadequate to meet the high requirements [65, 68]. Building pre-pregnancy iron stores contributes in lowering the risks of low birth weight, miscarriages and premature delivery since iron deficiency anemia as early as the first trimester itself increases the risks of premature delivery and low birth weight [36]. Building folic acid stores along with iron, prior to pregnancy, has the additional advantage of reducing the risks of neural tube defects (NTD) [69].

Regular consumption of WIFS during adolescence is envisaged to contribute to a set of behavior which is expected to have a beneficial effect in improving the acceptability as well as high compliance of IFA tablets during pregnancy. It is therefore obvious that actions for prevention of anemia need to be taken during adolescence itself and adequate iron status built up prior to the onset of pregnancy. Regular use of WIFS with the onset of menstruation is of special significance in developing countries where a very high percentage of girls enter pregnancy during the adolescence age itself. Along with WIFS, efforts to delay conception to over 18 years needs to be intensified for promotion of adolescent health and nutrition.

WIFS programme for adolescent girls implemented on a large scale in a few countries demonstrated a high compliance of supplement ranging from 42% to 94% and a reduction in anemia prevalence of 9.3% to 56.8% in a period of 6–12 months of intervention (Table 27.7) [65–68, 70–76]. In these programmes, the use of a fixed day approach (Iron day or WIFS day) facilitated in addressing the problem of forgetfulness which was noted to be the primary cause of poor compliance (Table 27.8).

*Table 27.7* Large scale WIFS programme from six countries [65–68, 70–76]

| Case study | Intervention period (months) | Compliance[c] (%) | (Baseline) anemia prevalence (%) | Reduction in anemia prevalence (%) |
|---|---|---|---|---|
| India[a] | 12 | 70–94 | 73.3–93.0 | 8.9–46.8% |
| Cambodia[b] | 6–12 | 98–100 | 58.0 | – |
| Egypt[b] | 6 | 92.2 | 30.0 | 20.0 |
| LAO PDR[b] | 6 | 74.5 | 43.0 | 53.4 |
| Philippines[b] | 12 | 64–99 | 33.3 | – |
| Vietnam[b] | 9–12 | 80–93 | 37.5–45.6 | 48.0–56.8 |

(a) WIFS composition – 100 mg elemental iron and 500 µg folic acid
(b) WIFS composition – 60 mg elemental iron and folic acid 0.3–3.5 mg
(c) All six countries – "Fixed" Day strategy used for WIFS Programme.

The programme issues considered important for effective implementation and outcome of the WIFS programme are political commitment to control anemia and resources allocated for procuring good quality supplements, regular supply of IFA tablets in attractive blister packs, effective logistic management, use of a fixed day in a week as "Iron Day" for effective programme management and promoting regular weekly consumption of tablet, appropriate communication and social mobilisation strategy for ensuring community support and improving compliance [70].

*Table 27.8* WIFS programme of India and Laos – percentage compliance [65, 70, 72]

| | *India (UP) (Adolescent girl – non-school)*[(a)] | *Lao PDR (WRAs)*[b] |
|---|---|---|
| WIFS routinely taken (%) | 86.0 | 74.5 |
| WIFS not taken (%) | 14.0 | 25.5 |
| • Forgetfulness | 52.4 | 50.0 |
| ▪ Side effects (vomiting, stomach ache, health problem) | 28.6([a]) | 5.8 |
| • Onset of pregnancy | – | 16.7 |
| • Others | 19.0 | 27.5 |

[(a)] Only 4% of total adolescent girls studied complained of adverse side effects
[(b)] Women in reproductive age (WRA).

A regular quality and quantity supply of IFA supplements along with a good delivery system and consistent efforts for creation of demand for supplements through social mobilisation and education activities is essential. Regular supply and linkage with suitable delivery systems, which involves not only health sector but other sector such as education and groups of adolescent girls ,youth and community groups is useful [70, 77, 78]. A social marketing strategy used in WIFS pilot project in India [79] and three large studies in Cambodia, Vietnam, the Philippines have demonstrated that a well planned communication strategy combined with attractive packaging has a substantial "value addition" effect [61–65, 80]. Blister packaging of 4 tablets/blister or 10 tablets/blister for meeting requirements of one–two months supply is practical for distribution and monitoring of WIFS.

Large scale unsupervised trials indicate that counseling of adolescent girls on positive attributes of WIFS and consuming tablets on a weekly designated day is effective in increasing compliance [68]. A study in Tanzania and India presents scientific evidence that a comprehensive communication strategy is effective for increasing acceptability and compliance even in the absence of supervision [65, 68]. Project findings demonstrate that adolescents who are reached through a well planned communication strategy view advantages for continuing WIFS to be much more important than discontinuing WIFS due to some minor side effects experienced. Communication strategy with a focus on the various benefits of WIFS such as improved learning, increase in concentration at school and work, higher level of energy, enhancement in skin glow or appearance as well as regularity of menstruation have been reported to be useful for mobilizing community and adolescent girls to regularly consume weekly dose of IFA tablets rather than information only on the side effects or emphasis on the future implications of WIFS on reproductive health. Monitoring distribution and consumption of IFA tablets through a special supplement record register as well as individual monitoring card has proved effective in improving compliance [68, 78]. In addition, periodic process and impact evaluation is recommended to be institutionalized to facilitate in programme adjustment and to check whether desired outcomes are being achieved.

WHO (2008) has recommended regular consumption of weekly iron-folic acid supplements for the women in reproductive age [81]. Box 27.2 presents details.

### Box 27.2 The WHO statement 2008 on WIFS for women in the reproductive age (WRA) group [81]

In 1998, a joint statement of UNICEF/UNU/WHO/MI emphasized universal regular iron-folic acid supplementation in regions where anemia prevalence is over 20% among women in reproductive age group or over 40% in pregnant mothers. In 2008, WHO issued a position statement on WIFS for women in the reproductive Age (WRA) Group [81]. The position statement is based on the consensus of a WHO Global Consultation on 'Weekly Iron and Folic Acid Supplementation (WIFS) for Preventing Anemia in Women of Reproductive Age' held in Manila, in April 2007 [82]. The WHO position statement is intended for a wide audience including implementing partners, scientists and governments involved in the design and implementation of public health interventions. Strategies to combat both iron deficiency and anemia, and to improve iron reserves and folate status of women of reproductive age (WRA) are emphasized to be integrated. In summary the statement highlights the following;

- In population where the prevalence of anemia in WRA is over 20% (or >40% in pregnant woman or children under 5 years) and mass fortification programme of staple foods with iron and folic acid are unlikely to be implemented within 1–2 years, WIFS should be considered a strategy.
- Recommended composition of WIFS being 60 mg elemental iron and 2800 µg folic acid (although evidence for the effective dose of folic acid for weekly supplementation is very limited). Upon confirmation of pregnancy, daily supplementation with 60 mg iron and 400 µg folic acid during pregnancy and first 3 months postpartum is recommended.
- WIFS programme must be integrated with other efforts to control iron deficiency and anemia and should be planned as long term self sustained interventions that woman of child bearing WRA will utilize during their child bearing years.

## 27.5 Anemia in adolescent girls in India and efforts launched at state level

Anemia prevalence rate in India is reported to vary between 48% and 90% [19, 83, 84]. A recent study on anemia prevalence in adolescent girls aged 10–19 years residing in eastern state of Assam, India [85] reported cent percent girls were anemic – 29.3% were mildly anemic (10–11 g%), while 58.5% girls had moderate anemia (7.0–9.9g%) and 12.3% had severe anemia (Hb <7g%). As per the national survey data [13] 55.8% adolescent age girls aged 15–19 years are anemic and of these 39% are reported to be mildly anemic. Prevalence of anemia is high across all socio-economic groups and 46.1% women in the highest economic group are anemic while in the lowest socio economic group, anemia prevalence is 64.3% [13].

Data from National family Health Survey [13] indicates 55.3% women in the reproductive age (WRA) are anemic and in only five states (Punjab, Manipur, Goa, Kerala and Mizoram) anemia prevalence is less than 40% while in 7 of the 28 states surveyed anemia prevalence is reported to be over 60% (Table 27.9). This India profile of anemia in WRA could be considered a proxy indicator of the situation of anemia in adolescent girls in various states of the country.

*Table 27.9* Anemia prevalence in women 15–49[(a)] years in India[(b)] – state-wise profile [13]

| *Percentage prevalence of anemia* | *States of India* |
|---|---|
| < 40% (5 states) | Punjab, Manipur, Mizoram, Goa, Kerala |
| > 40–60% (16 states) | Delhi, Haryana[(a)], Himachal pradesh, Jammu & Kashmir, Uttaranchal, Chhattisgarh[(a)], Madhya Pradesh[(a)], Uttar Pradesh, Arunachal Pradesh, Meghalaya, Sikkim, Gujarat, Maharashtra[(a)], Karnataka, Tamil Nadu |
| > 60% (7 states) | Bihar[(a)], Jharkhand[(a)], Orissa[(a)], West Bengal[(a)], Assam[(a)], Tripura[(a)], Andhra Pradesh[(a)] |

[(a)] Ten states have anemia prevalence over the national average of 55.3%.
[(b)] All India anemia prevalence is 55.3%.

A National Anemia Consultative Meeting of Government of India in 1997 recommended "adolescent girls on attaining menarche should continue one IFA tablet containing 100 mg elemental iron and 500 μg folic acid once a week. This should be accompanied by appropriate dietary counseling" [86]. The recommendations were based on the findings of the efficacy trails implemented in three regions of India with UNICEF support – Baroda, Delhi and Mumbai [83, 84, 87]. These trails compared the administration of daily iron folic acid (IFA) supplementation with weekly IFA. Additionally, the Consultation also reviewed the experience of social marketing of IFA tablets to adolescent girls, undertaken by a professional non government agency, *Parivar Seva Sansthan* for the State government of Delhi [79]. The Consultation highlighted the need for implementation of district level pilot projects for defining programme operational strategy. The Consultation recommended "The total duration for consumption of weekly dose of iron supplementation and its cost effectiveness and operational feasibility should be examined. These pilot projects should be carried out in 8–10 states in different regions of the country to facilitate in the formulation of the national policy for control of nutritional anemia among adolescents".

Following the National Consultation Meeting, WIFS programme was implemented in selected states of India [59]. The composition of the supplement used for WIFS was the same as that is supplied under the Reproductive Child Health (RCH) programme of the Government of India for the antenatal care (ANC) services, i.e. each tablet contains 100 mg elemental iron and 500 μg Folic Acid. The cost of annual supply of 100 tablets for a pregnant mother is estimated to be about 25 US cents while the cost for an adolescent girl consuming weekly iron supplement is estimated to be 12 US cents. The state programmes on anemia control in adolescent girls focus on weekly administration of IFA supplements to adolescent girls in school and out of school. The supplements are distributed free of cost. In some states biannual deworming is administered along with WIFS while in some states nutrition or family life education is also included in the package of services. For improving management and compliance, a "fixed WIFS day" approach is used [65, 66, 71, 84]. The health and education departments play a leading role in the WIFS programme for school going girls. The strategy for reaching girls out of school is noted to be more challenging and the system of Integrated Child Development Services (ICDS) is used along with the health sector for the distribution and monitoring of iron-folic acid supplement as well as for conducting education and community mobilisation activities. With one year's intervention, a substantial decrease in anemia prevalence has been reported – the decrease varies from 5% in the state of Jharkhand to 43% in state of Andhra Pradesh and 50% in the state of Uttar Pradesh [59]. These state level implementations demonstrated that routine consumption of weekly iron folic supplements is a cost-effective intervention to address anemia in adolescent girls and it is critical that WIFS programme for adolescent population is accorded a high priority in the public health programmes of the country. Box 27.3 presents experience of an adolescent anemia project implemented in one of northern states of India.

**Box 27.3 Uttar Pradesh – UMANG (Uplifting Marriage Age, Nutrition and Growth) Project [65]**

A 4-year project UMANG was launched in the state of UP in 2003 with the objective of preventing iron deficiency and reducing anemia in adolescent girls in school and out of school. The intervention included weekly iron–folic acid tablets, family life education, and deworming tablets every 6 months. A total of 150,700 adolescent school and non-school girls in a district (Lucknow) were reached. Girls in school were reached through teachers in the school system and both education and health departments played active roles. Girls out of school were reached through the ICDS Programme. IFA supplement were distributed directly to adolescent girls by ICDS workers (AWW) through formation of an adolescent girls group and a "girl to girl" approach. Consumption of iron–folic acid tablets was supervised for schoolgirls but not for non-school girls.

Hemoglobin levels were improved and anemia prevalence was reduced significantly at 6 months. No difference in the impact on hemoglobin levels or anemia prevalence was observed between supervised and unsupervised girls. Counseling on the positive effects of regular weekly iron–folic acid intake contributed to a high compliance rate of over 85%. Supervision in non-school system was not feasible but routine recording of distribution and consumption of IFA contributed to high compliance. The effect of supplementation on the prevalence of anemia and the compliance rate were assessed over a 4-year period. In 4 years, the overall prevalence of anemia was reduced from 73.3% to 25.4%. The cost of implementation was estimated to be US$0.36 per beneficiary per year. The results lead to the conclusion that weekly iron–folic acid supplementation combined with monthly education sessions and six monthly deworming is cost-effective in reducing the prevalence of anemia in adolescent girls. Appropriate counseling and effective monitoring system, irrespective of supervision, is critical for achieving positive *outcomes.* Following the success of UMANG project, the state government of Uttar Pradesh has included the weekly iron–folic acid supplementation programme for adolescent girls in schools as in the state implementation plan of the National Rural Health Mission (NRHM).

## References


1. UNICEF (2005). State of the World's Children. United Nations Press: New York.
2. WHO (2003). www.who.int/nut/ado.htm
3. HEALD FP and GONG EJ (1999). Diet, Nutrition, and Adolescence. In: Modern Nutrition in Health and Disease, 9th edn. Shils ME, Olson JA, Shike M and Ross AC (eds). Williams and Wilkins: Maryland, USA.
4. TRAVIS S (2003). Nutrition and Adolescent Development. Cornell Cooperative Extension. Division of Nutritional Sciences, Cornell University.
5. Micronutrient Initiative (MI) (2003). Iron improves life, MI Initiative.
6. VASANTHI G, FAWASHE AB, SUSIE H, SUJATHA T and RAMAN L (1994). Iron and nutritional status of adolescent girls from rural area and urban slum. *Indian Paediatrics*, **31**(2), p. 127.
7. AGARWAL DK, UPADHYAY SK, TRIPATHI AM and AGARWAL KN (1987). Nutritional status, physical capacity and mental work function in school children. *Nutrition Foundation of India (NFI)*. Scientific Report 6, p. 40.
8. VIR S (1991). Adolescent growth in girls – the Indian perspective. *Ind Paed.*, **27**(12), p. 1249.

9. EUROPEAN COMMUNITIES (1993). Nutrient and energy intakes for the European Community. EG-Report. Brussels Luxembourg: Commission of the European Communities.
10. SOEMANTRI AG, POLLITT E, KIM I (1985). Iron deficiency anaemia and educational achievements. *Am J Clin Nutr*, **42**, p. 1221.
11. MDG report (2005). BANGLADESH progress report 2005.
12. WHO Global database (1997). HFA country reports.
13. International Institute for Population Sciences (IIPS) and ORC Macro (2007). National Family Health Survey (NFHS) III, 2005-06, India, Mumbai: IIPS.
14. TOTEJA GS et al (2006). Prevalence of anaemia among pregnant women and adolescent girls in 16 districts of India. *Food and Nutrition Bulletin*, **27**(4).
15. Indonesia National Household Health Survey (2001).
16. WHO MDIS (2005).
17. National Hemoglobin and Nutritional Status Survey among Adolescents (2002).
18. SHAH BK and GUPTA P (2002). Anaemia in Adolescent Girls: A preliminary Report from Semi-urban Nepal. *Indian Paediatrics*, **39**, pp. 1126–1130.
19. HETTIARACHCHI et al (2006). Prevalence and severity of micronutrient deficiency: a cross-sectional study among adolescents in Sri Lanka. *Asia Pacific Journal of Clinical Nutrition*, **15**(1), pp. 56–63.
20. Thailand Health Profile (2001–2004).
21. ROSANNE A et al (2005). Only a small proportion of anemia in northeast Thai schoolchildren is associated with iron deficiency. *Am J Clin Nutr*, **82**, pp. 380–387.
22. DEMAEYER EM, DALLMAN P, GURNEY JM, HALLBERG L, SOOD SK, SRIKANTIA SG (1989). Preventing and controlling iron deficiency anaemia through primary health care: A guide for health administrators and programme managers. WHO. Geneva.
23. FAO/WHO (2002). Human vitamin and mineral requirements. Report of joint FAO/ WHO consultation, Bangkok, Thailand.
24. BRASEL J (1982). Changes in body composition during adolescence. In: *Adolescent Nutrition*. Myron W (ed.). . John Wiley & Sons, New York.
25. KURZ KM (1996). Adolescent nutritional status in developing countries. *Proc Nutr Soc*, **55**, pp. 321–231.
26. WHO (SEARO) (2006). Adolescent Nutrition: A Review of Situation in Selected South-East Asian Countries.
27. BEARD JL (2000). Iron requirements in adolescent females. *J. Nutr.*, **130**(25), p. 440S.
28. PASSI S and VIR S (2000). Functional consequences of nutritional anaemia in school age children. In: *Nutritional Anaemia*. Ramakrishnan U (ed), CRC Press.
29. ALLEN L and CASERLINA-SABEL (2000). Prevalence and causes of nutritional anaemia. In: *Nutritional Anaemia*, Ramakrishnan U (ed), CRC Press.
30. NATIONAL INSTITUTE OF NUTRITION (2006). National Nutrition Monitoring Bureau Report, Hyderabad, India.
31. NATIONAL NUTRITION MONITORING BUREAU (NNMB) (2002). Diet and nutritional status of rural population. Hyderabad, NIN, ICMR.
32. AHMED F, ZAREEN M, KHAN MR, BANU CP, HAQ N, JACKSON AA (1998). Dietary pattern, nutrient intake and growth of adolescent school girls in urban Bangladesh. *Public Health Nutr.*, **1**(2), pp. 83–92.
33. Guidelines for school health programs to promote lifelong healthy eating (1996). Centre for Disease Control and Prevention MMWR Recommendation Report, 45 (RR-9), pp. 1–41.

34. VITERI (2007). Global consultation on Weekly Iron-Folic Acid Supplementation for preventing Anemia in women of Reproductive Age Group.
35. Sri Lanka Demographic and health Survey (2000).
36. UNICEF (2005). Early marriage, a harmful traditional practice: A statistical exploration.
37. CHOI JW, PAI SH, IM MG, KIM SK (1999). Change in transferrin receptor concentration with age. *Lin Chem.*, **45**, p. 1562.
38. RAWAT CMS (2000). An epidemiological study of anaemia in adolescent girls in the rural areas of Meerut. MD thesis, Chaudhary Charan Singh University, Meerut, India.
39. Bangladesh Demographic and Health Survey (2007).
40. Indonesia Demographic and Health Survey (2007).
41. SHARMA AK, VERMA K, KHATRI S, KANNAN AT (2001). Pregnancy in adolescents: a study of risks and outcome in Eastern Nepal. *Ind Paed.*, **38**, pp. 1405–1409.
42. SHARMA V and SHARMA A (1992). Health profile of pregnant adolescents among selected tribal population of Rajasthan. *Ind J. Adol Health*, **13**(8), pp. 696–699.
43. LEVIN HM (1986). A benefit-cost analysis of nutrition program for anaemia reduction. *Res Observer*, **1**, p. 219.
44. WEBB TE and OSKI FA (1974). Behavioural status of young adolescents with iron deficiency anaemia. *J. Spec. Educ*, **8**, pp. 153–156.
45. DAMAYANTI D, SOEKARJO DD, SASKIA DE PEE, KUSIN JA, MARTIN W, BLOEM MW (2006). School-based supplementation: lessons learned in Indonesia. *SCN News*, **31**, pp. 14–18.
46. SCHOLL TO, HEDIGER ML, FISCHER RL, SHEARER JW (1992). Anaemia vs iron deficiency: Increased risk of preterm delivery in a perspective study. *Am J Clin Nutr*, Adolescent nutrition (5), pp. 985–988.
47. SCHOLL TO and HEDIGER ML (1994). Anaemia and iron deficiency anaemia: complications of data on pregnancy outcome. *Am J Clin Nutr*, **59**(2), pp. 492S-500S, discussions 500S–501S.
48. BRABIN L and BRABIN BJ (1992). The cost of successful adolescent growth and development in girls in relation to iron and vitamin A status. *Am J Clin Nutr*, **55**, p. 955.
49. VIR S (1998). Control of iron deficiency anaemia – a public health programme priority, Proceedings of XXXVI Nutrition society of India meeting, 26–27th Nov.
50. DEMAEYER E and ADIELS–TEGMAN M (1985). The prevalence of anaemia in the world. *World Health Statistics*, **38**, p. 302.
51. BRABIN BJ, HEKIMI M and PELLETIER D (2001). An analysis of anaemia and pregnancy related maternal mortality. *J. Nutr.*, **131**, pp. 604S–614S.
52. CAVALLI-SFORZA T, BERGER B, SMITASIRI S, VITERI F (2005). Weekly iron folic acid supplementation of women of reproductive age: impact overview, lessons learned, expansion plans, and contributions toward achievement of the millennium development goals. *Nutrition Reviews*, **63**(12), pp. S152–S158.
53. YIP R, STOLTZFUS R, SIMMONS W, (1996). Assessment of prevalence and nature of iron deficiency for population .The utility of comparing hemoglobin distribution. In: *Iron Nutrition in Health and Disease*. Hallberg L and Asp, N (eds).: John Libby and Co. Ltd, London, pp. 31–48.
54. LOTFI M et al, Fortification of Foods: Current Practice, Research and Opportunities. The Micronutrient Fortification of Foods: Current Practices, Research and Opportunities. The Micronutrient Initiative and International Agriculture Centre, Ottawa, Canada.

55. UNICEF/UNU/WHO/MI (1998). Technical workshop on preventing iron deficiency in women and children – technical consensus on key issues.
56. BEATON GH and MCCABE GP (1999). Efficacy of Intermittent Iron Supplementation in the Control of Iron Deficiency Anaemia in Developing Countries: An Analysis of Experience. Final report to the Micronutrient Initiative.
57. BERGER J, THANH HTK, TOMMASO CS, SUTTILAK S, KHAN NC, MILANI S, HOA PT, QUANG ND, VITERI F (2005). Community Mobilization and Social Marketing to Promote Weekly Iron-Folic Acid Supplementation in Women of Reproductive Age in Vietnam: Impact on Anemia and Iron Status. *Nutrition Reviews*, **63**(12), pp. S95–S108.
58. BOTHWELL TH (2000). Iron requirements in pregnancy and strategies to meet them. *Am J Clin Nutr*, **72**, pp. 257S–264S.
59. DWIVEDI A and SCHULTINK W (2006). Reducing anaemia among Indian adolescent girls through once-weekly supplementation with iron and folic acid. *SCN News*, **31**, pp. 19–23.
60. ANGELES-AGDEPPA I, SCHULTINK W, SASTROAMIDJOJO S, GROSS R, KARYADI D (1997). Weekly micronutrient supplementation to build iron stores in female Indonesian adolescents. *Am J Clin Nutr*, **66**, pp. 177–183.
61. WRIGHT AJ and SOUTHON S (1990). The effectiveness of various iron supplementation regimens in improving the Fe status of anaemic rats. *Br J Nutr.* **63**, pp. 579–585.
62. VITERI FE (1995). Iron deficiency in children: New possibilities for its control. *Int Child Health*, **6**, pp. 49–61.
63. SCHULTINK W (1997). Iron Supplementation Programme Compliance of target groups and frequency of tablet intake. *FNB*, **18**, pp. 64–70.
64. GROSS R et al (1997). Daily versus weekly iron supplementation: Programmatic and economic implications for Indonesia. *FNB*, **18**, pp. 64–70.
65. VIR SC, SINGH N, NIGAM A, JAIN R (2008). Weekly iron and folic acid supplementation with counseling reduces anaemia in adolescent girls: A large scale effectiveness study in Uttar radish, India. *Food and Nutrition Bulletin*, **29**(3), pp. 186–194.
66. KOTECHA PV, PATEL RZ, KARKAR PD, NIRUPAM S (2002). Impact evaluation of adolescent girl's anaemia reduction program, Vadodara district. Government of Gujarat and UNICEF.
67. SHARMA K and GANDHI H. A study on assessing the impact of adolescent anaemia control project among out of school adolescent girls, a midterm evaluation in Shivpuri district, Madhya Pradesh. Department of Women and Child Development, State Government of Madhya Pradesh, India and UNICEF.
68. Egypt's Adolescent Anemia Prevention Program (Ref – Ministry of Health and Population, Health Insurance Organization, 1999).
69. BOTTO LD et al (1999). Neural-tube defects. *New England Journal of Medicine*, **341**, pp. 1509–1519.
70. VIR SC (2009). Micronutrient and Child Health Workshop, 20–23rd October 2009, AIIMS, New Delhi.
71. SAIYED F (2008). UNICEF Patna field office report, India.
72. Preliminary report of operational trial of weekly iron folic acid supplementation (2007). Sekong province, Lao People's Democratic Republic. Ministry of Health and WHO.
73. PASRICHA SR, CARUANA SR, PHUC TQ, CASEY GJ, JOLLEY D, KINGSL S, TIEN NT, MACGREGOR L, MONTRESOR A, BIGGS BA (2008). Anemia, iron deficiency, meat consumption

and hookworm infection in women of reproductive age in Northwest Vietnam. *Am. J. Trop. Med. Hyg.*, **87** (3), pp. 375–381.

74. KANAL K, HALLEN JB, SFORZA TC, CRAPE B, SMITASIRI S and the Cambodian weekly iron folic acid program team (2005). Weekly iron folic acid supplements to prevent anemia among Cambodian women in three settings: process and outcomes of social marketing and community mobilisation. *Nutrition Reviews*. **63**(12), pp. S126–S133.
75. PAULINO LS, AGDEPPA IA, ETORMA UMM, RAMOS AC, SFORZA TC (2005). Weekly iron folic acid supplementation to improve iron status and prevent pregnancy anemia in Filipino women of reproductive age: The Philippine experience through government and private partnership. *Nutrition Reviews*. **63**(12), pp. S109–S115.
76. KHAN NC, THANH HTK, BERGER J, HOA PT, QUANG ND, SMITASIRI S, SFORZA TC (2005). Community mobilisation and social marketing to promote weekly iron folic acid supplementation: a new approach toward controlling anemia among women of reproductive age in Vietnam. *Nutrition Reviews*. **63**(12), pp. S87–S94.
77. NORSWORTHY B et al (2004). Effects of once-a-week or daily folic acid supplementation on red blood cell folate concentrations in women. *European Journal of Clinical Nutrition*, **58**, pp. 548–554.
78. GILLESPIE S (1998). Major issues in the control of iron deficiency. MI/UNICEF.
79. PARIVAR SEWA SANSTHAN, UNICEF (INDIA) (1997). Project on Social marketing of Iron Tablets, personal communication.
80. ADANK C, GREEN TJ, SKEAFF CM, BRIARS B (2003). Weekly high dose folic supplementation is effective in lowering serum homocysteine concentration in women. *Annals Nutr Metabol*, **4**, pp. 55–59.
81. WHO (2008). Weekly iron and folic acid supplementation (WIFS) in women of reproductive age: its role in promoting optimal maternal and child health.
82. WHO (2007). Global Consultation on weekly iron and folic acid supplementation (WIFS) for preventing anaemia in women of reproductive age, 25–27th April 2007, Manila, Philippines.
83. MEHTA MN (1998). Effectiveness of daily and weekly iron and folic acid supplementation in anaemic adolescent girls. Final report of the UNICEF research project, Bombay.
84. SESHADRI S (1998). Oral iron supplementation to control anaemia in adolescent girls. MS University of Baroda and UNICEF, India.
85. VIR SC (2008). Report on nutritional status of women and children in tea estate of Dibrugarh, Assam, UNICEF consultancy report.
86. Department of Family Welfare, Maternal Health Division, Ministry of Health and Family Welfare, Nirman Bhawan, New Delhi. National Consultation on control of nutritional anaemia in India 16–17th October 1997, GoI (1998).
87. AGARWAL KN (1998). Assessment of the prevalence of anaemia and iron stores in response to daily and weekly iron and folic acid supplementation in adolescent girls (10–18 years) from urban slums of northeast Delhi. UNICEF project report.

# 28

# Zinc – an essential micronutrient for health and development

*Sunil Sazawal* and *Pratibha Dhingra*

**Sunil Sazawal**, MD, MPH, PhD, is an Associate Professor, Johns Hopkins Bloomberg School of Public Health; Visiting Professor, Annamalai University, India; and the Director, Center for Micronutrient Research, New Delhi, India. Dr Sazawal is a physician by profession and has more than 20 years of research experience in conducting clinical and community-based trials of micronutrient interventions, especially in role of zinc and iron in reducing infectious diseases and mortality in children.

**Pratibha Dhingra**, PhD, is a Senior Research Scientist at the Center for Micronutrient Research, New Delhi, India. Dr Dhingra has more than 16 years of research experience in community-based health projects, with a special focus on role of micronutrients in preventing and improving the health, growth and development of children.

## 28.1 Introduction

Zinc is an essential micronutrient for all forms of life and plays a critical structural and functional role in multiple enzyme systems involved in gene expression, cell division and growth, immunologic and reproductive functions. Clinical zinc deficiency in humans was first described in Iran in 1961, when the consumption of diets with low zinc bioavailability due to high phytic acid content was associated with delayed sexual development and "adolescent nutritional dwarfism" [1] and later recognized in a group of patients from Egypt with hypogonadism, anemia and hepatosplenomegaly [2]. Since then, zinc insufficiency has been recognized as an important public health issue, especially in developing countries [3].

## 28.2 Biological functions of zinc

Zinc occurs in divalent state (Zn++) and is a bluish white metallic element (atomic number 30, atomic weight 65.4), which makes up about 0.002%

of the earth's crust and is the 23rd most abundant element. Zinc is associated with more than 200 distinct metalloenzymes, which have a diverse range of functions, including the synthesis of nucleic acids and specific proteins, such as hormones and their receptors [4]. Zinc also chelates with the amino acids cysteine and histidine, forming 'zinc fingers' that are important for protein transcription. Additional processes that are regulated by zinc include expression of the metallothionein gene, apoptosis and synaptic signaling. Zinc plays an important role in human metabolism and in the perpetuation of genetic material, including transcription of DNA, translation of RNA, and ultimately cellular division. Zinc deficiency at the gene regulatory level probably provides the common mechanism for many of the clinical signs of zinc deficiency such as growth failure, skin abnormalities and other signs that occur in various organs and organ systems. Of auxiliary interest is the absence of redox properties in zinc, which allows it to be transported in biological systems without inducing oxidant damage, as can occur with other trace elements, such as iron and copper.

## 28.3 Public health significance

Zinc Investigators' Collaborative Group, 2000 [5] has emphasized the significance of zinc in human nutrition and public health due to its role in normal growth/tissue repair; neural, cognitive and sexual development; immune function, resistance to disease and stress. Estimates indicate that approximately 20.5% of the world's population might be at risk of zinc deficiency [6]. Zinc affects health, mental/physical function, and survival of more than two billion people worldwide and ranks fifth in the leading risk factors for illness and disease in developing countries with high mortality [7]. Zinc deficiency is estimated to be responsible for 453,207 deaths globally [8]. Of these, 260,502 occur in Africa, 182,546 in Asia and 10,159 in Latin America. Zinc deficiency is considered responsible for 14.4% of diarrhea deaths, 10.4% of malaria deaths and 6.7% of pneumonia deaths among children between 6 months and 5 years of age [8]. A loss of nearly 16 million global disability-adjusted life years (DALYs) is attributed to zinc deficiency [9]. In India, estimated population at risk of inadequate zinc intake is as much as 25.9 % which is considered to be high risk category [7].

## 28.4 Zinc epidemiology

The epidemiological data on zinc deficiency has lagged behind that for other more well known vitamin and mineral deficiencies because of lack of scientific, practical, and accepted indicators for zinc deficiency. Population-based surveys have not been undertaken, marginal zinc deficiency is not characterized by a highly specific deficiency syndrome and severe clinical deficiency in humans is rare. Importance of mild zinc deficiency has been documented in the last decade in clinical trials of zinc supplementation.

Risk of zinc deficiency is highest among infants, young children, pregnant and lactating women, when there is an extra demand due to multiplicative cell growth. Risk factors include insufficient dietary intake due to poverty, food taboos, and special diets (i.e. vegetarian diets that are high in phytate and fiber). Dietary zinc intake of young children appears to be inadequate in many developing countries [10, 11]. Women of child-bearing age have inadequate dietary zinc intake in many populations [12, 13]. Eighty percent of women globally, and 100% women in developing countries, have inadequate zinc intake during pregnancy [14]. Individuals with malabsorption syndromes, diarrhea and parasitic diseases, acrodermatitis enteropathica, sickle cell disease, and cystic fibrosis are also at higher risk of zinc deficiency.

## 28.5 Clinical manifestations of zinc deficiency

Clinical manifestations of zinc deficiency are generally non-specific, vary widely, and depend on the severity of deficiency. The clinical manifestations in severe cases of zinc deficiency include bullous-pustular dermatitis, alopecia, diarrhea, emotional disorder, weight loss, intercurrent infections, hypogonadism in males and are fatal if unrecognized and untreated. Moderate zinc deficiency is characterized by growth retardation and delayed puberty in adolescents, hypogonadism in males, rough skin, poor appetite, mental lethargy, delayed wound healing, taste abnormalities, and abnormal dark adaptation. In mild cases of zinc deficiency in human subjects, the symptoms include oligospermia, slight weight loss, and hyperammonemia [15].

## 28.6 Dietary sources, intake, absorption and bioavailability

Zinc content in foods is closely related to their protein content. Richest sources of dietary zinc are animal products such as shellfish, poultry, beef, and other red meats. Nuts and legumes are relatively good plant sources of zinc. Foods from plant sources such as beans, lentils, chickpeas, and peas are relatively rich in zinc. Little zinc is found in white rice or wheat breads, as zinc is contained in the bran and germ portions of whole cereal grains, which are normally lost through milling. Dairy products contain only moderate amounts of zinc. Zinc content of some common foods is shown in Table 28.1. Zinc intake in developing countries is commonly sub-optimal due to usual consumption of foods with very poor sources of zinc.

*Table 28.1* Zinc content of some of the commonly consumed foods

| *Zinc category (mg/1000 kcal)* | *Foods* |
|---|---|
| Very poor (0-2) | Fats, oils, butter, cream, cheese, sweets, chocolates, soft drinks, alcoholic drinks, preserves |
| Poor (1-5) | Fish, fruits, refined cereal products, pastries, biscuits, cakes, puddings, tubers, plantains, sausages, chips |
| Rich (4-12) | Whole grains, pork, poultry, milk, low fat cheese, yoghurt, eggs, nuts |
| Very rich (12-882) | Lamb, leaf, and root vegetables, crustacea, beef, kidney, liver, heart, mollusks |

Zinc in flesh foods is more bioavailable than the zinc in plant foods because during their digestion certain L-amino acids and cysteine containing peptides are released, which form soluble ligands with zinc. Plant based diets often contain high levels of phytic acid (myoinositol hexaphosphate), dietary fiber, oxalate, tannin and lignin, the components known to inhibit absorption of dietary zinc. Of these, phytic acid, the major storage form of phosphorus in whole grains, legumes, oleaginous seeds and leafy vegetables, is the most potent inhibitor of zinc absorption as it forms insoluble chelates at alkaline pH [16]. However, lower inositol phosphates (i.e. tetra-, tri-, di-, and mono-inositol phosphates), formed by enzymatic or non-enzymatic hydrolysis of phytic acid, do not form insoluble complexes with zinc. The bioavailability of dietary zinc can be predicted from the ratio of phytic acid (Phy) to zinc (Zn) in the diets. The critical (Phy): (Zn) molar ratios associated with the risk of zinc deficiency are equivocal; ratios above 15 having been associated with biochemical, and in some cases, even the clinical signs of zinc deficiency in humans [17]. Soaking and fermentation of plant foods are among some strategies that can be used to reduce intake of phytic acid, as phytate is partially hydrolyzed to other analogous metabolites that have a lower capacity to bind zinc. The enzymatic action of yeast reduces the level of phytic acid in foods. Therefore, leavened whole grain breads have more bioavailable zinc than unleavened whole grain breads.

## 28.7 Physiology of zinc

### 28.7.1 Physiology and metabolism of zinc

The total body content of zinc is approximately 2 g and it is present in all the tissues/fluids of the body [18]. The skeletal muscle accounts for about 60%, bone for 30% and plasma 0.1% of the total body content of zinc. But plasma zinc has a rapid turnover rate, and its level appears to be under close homeostatic control. High concentration of zinc is found in the choroid of the eye as well as in prostatic fluids, semen ejaculates up to 1 mg and losses in menstruation are small (0.01 mg) [19, 20], other losses like normal daily zinc loss of hair are probably insignificant. Zinc is not stored in the conventional sense. Under conditions of bone resorption and tissue catabolism, it can be released and to some extent reutilized. Experimental studies in humans showed that in low zinc-containing diets (2.6–3.6 mg/day), plasma zinc and the activities of zinc-containing enzymes can be maintained within a normal range over several months indicating some zinc availability from tissues [21]. Zinc is lost from the body via kidneys, skin and the intestine; the endogenous intestinal losses can range between 0.5 and 3.0 mg/day depending on the zinc intake but exercise, diarrhea and fever could lead to large losses [22].

### 28.7.2 Zinc absorption

Zinc is absorbed mainly in the small intestine. Under normal circumstances the gastrointestinal tract adapts effectively to changes in zinc intake and/or nutriture with compensatory changes in the fractional absorption and excretion of endogenous zinc [23]. Pancreatic secretions deliver zinc into the duodenum equivalent to that provided by most meals. The intestine reabsorbs appropriate amounts of zinc from both dietary and endogenous sources to maintain favorable zinc balance. Zinc is absorbed both by passive diffusion and through a carrier-mediated process on the brush border of enterocytes. Zinc absorbed from the intestinal lumen is bound to many different molecules within the enterocytes, and metallothionein and cysteine-rich intestinal protein play a role in trans-mucosal transport.

### 28.7.3 Zinc homeostasis

Zinc homeostasis is affected by the liver and intestine at adequate and marginally adequate dietary zinc intakes [24]. When the body is at risk of zinc deprivation, intestinal absorption of exogenous zinc increases and there is a reduction in intestinal losses of endogenous zinc arising from intestinal conservation with an up regulation of carrier sites, and from a reduction in the pancreatico-biliary secretion of zinc, and to a lesser extent, increased renal conservation of the element [23]. These mechanisms are important because with the exception of the possible hepatic labile pool, there are no specific systemic stores of zinc and we are dependent on acquiring zinc from external sources [25].

Zinc transporters such as ZIP proteins (zinc importer proteins) and ZnT (zinc transporter proteins) have recently been recognized as two families of proteins involved in understanding the mechanisms of zinc-absorption and homeostasis. ZIP proteins transport zinc from the extracellular space and intracellular organelles into the cytoplasm [26]. ZnT proteins are primarily involved in the cellular efflux of zinc and in uptake of zinc by intracellular organelles. Thus, the net effect of these transporters is to decrease cytoplasmic zinc [27].

### 28.7.4 Zinc requirements

Varied estimates of zinc requirements have been proposed by several expert committees [28–32]. In 2004, the International Zinc Consultative Group (IZiNCG) Steering Committee [7] reviewed the methods used by the World Health Organization and Food and Nutrition Board/Institute of Medicine (FNB/IOM) committees to estimate zinc requirements, taking into consideration the methodology used to measure absorption, the types of diets and subjects from whom the data were derived, as well as the models used to summarize these data. Based on the review, this Committee followed the factorial approach used by the FNB/IOM but decided to base intestinal losses of endogenous zinc on the estimates derived by IZiNCG [7], and to use the NCHS/CDC/WHO reference body weights for laying down the zinc requirements. Using this approach for computing the estimated average requirement (EAR) of zinc [EAR *of zinc is the amount of zinc that must be absorbed to match the amount of endogenous zinc losses. Both intestinal and non-intestinal sources (urine, surface losses of skin/hair/nail/sweat) contribute to endogenous zinc losses*], the requirements for different ages and physiologic groups are laid down (Table 28.2).

*Table 28.2* Recommended dietary intake of zinc [31]

| *Children* | | | | *Adults* | | | |
|---|---|---|---|---|---|---|---|
| *Population group* | *Age* | *Males (mg/day)* | *Females (mg/day)* | *Population group* | *Age* | *Males (mg/ day)* | *Females (mg/day)* |
| Infants | 0-6 months | 2 (AI) | 2 (AI) | Adolescents | 14-18 years | 11 | 9 |
| Infants | 7-12 months | 3 | 3 | Adults | 19 years and older | 11 | 8 |
| Children | 1-3 years | 3 | 3 | Pregnancy | 18 years and younger | - | 12 |
| Children | 4-8 years | 5 | 5 | Pregnancy | 19 years and older | - | 11 |
| Children | 9-13 years | 8 | 8 | Lactation | 18 years and younger | - | 13 |
| - | - | - | - | Lactation | 19 years and older | - | 12 |

## 28.7.5 Interaction of zinc with other trace elements

A bi-directional interaction between copper and zinc has been postulated, one reducing the bioavailability of the other [33]. High levels of zinc (120–240 mg/kg) in the diets of rats have been reported to result in lower copper levels in the serum and liver. Dietary zinc deficiency has also been reported to cause mild increase in tissue copper levels. Conversely copper deficiency has been reported to result in mild increase in zinc absorption. Experimental zinc deficiency in guinea pigs caused significant reductions in plasma sodium (Na), potassium (K) and zinc (Zn) and increase in copper (Cu) and iron (Fe) content(s) of liver and kidney. Conversely, zinc supplementation improved the serum and tissue mineral levels whereas levels of hepatic Cu and Fe remained unchanged [11].

Zinc and vitamin A interact in several ways. Zinc is a component of retinol-binding protein, a protein necessary for transporting vitamin A in the blood. Zinc is also required for the enzyme that converts retinol (vitamin A) to retinal. This latter form of vitamin A is necessary for the synthesis of rhodopsin, a protein in the eye that absorbs light and thus is involved in dark adaptation. Zinc deficiency is associated with decreased release of vitamin A from the liver, which may contribute to symptoms of night blindness that are seen with vitamin A deficiency [34, 35].

In children with severe protein energy malnutrition, zinc supplementation improved serum retinol binding protein and retinol concentration [36]. Combined zinc and vitamin A synergistically reduced the prevalence of persistent diarrhea and dysentery. Zinc was associated with a significant increase in acute lower respiratory infection, but this adverse effect was reduced by the interaction between zinc and vitamin A [37].

The zinc to iron ratio in the diet may be of importance for the absorption of the individual trace elements [38]. In thirty-one adult subjects, simultaneous administration of zinc sulphate and ferrous sulphate in a ratio of Fe/Zn of 1:1 slightly inhibited zinc absorption while Fe/Zn ratio 2:1 and 3:1 inhibited zinc uptake [39]. High iron concentrations that are present in some supplements can reduce zinc absorption. The effect of iron on zinc will only occur when the iron to zinc ratio is very high (such as 25:1) and both are administered in solutions. Similarly, iron fortification of food has no adverse effect on zinc absorption and long term use of iron supplements does not impair zinc absorption or status. Thus, under most dietary conditions, Zn–Fe interaction is not likely to have a major influence on zinc requirement. But there is now evidence to suggest that iron supplementation with zinc may increase morbidity of infectious diseases [40] and the risk of adverse events especially in malarious areas [41], and may reduce linear growth in iron replete infants [42, 43].

There is also evidence that high calcium (2.0 g/d) reduced zinc absorption significantly whereas phosphorus (2.0 g/d) did not change the absorption. However, zinc balance was not significantly different with change in dietary calcium levels. Excess dietary calcium has been shown to decrease zinc absorption in animals, but such an effect is less conclusive in humans. While calcium phosphate decreases zinc absorption, calcium citrate-malate does not. The presence of phytate may also influence the effect of calcium on zinc absorption. Calcium may interact with zinc and phytate to form insoluble complexes, thus rendering zinc unavailable. Nonetheless, available data suggest that a calcium-rich diet has no significant inhibitory effect on zinc absorption, provided intake of zinc is adequate [44].

Studies on zinc-folate interaction have produced conflicting results. Some have shown low zinc intake decreases folate absorption, while others have not found such an adverse effect. Administration of 800 μg of folic acid daily for 2 weeks to a group of adults inhibited zinc absorption when the fractional rate of zinc absorption was higher than 30% [45]. This finding raises concern about pregnant women, who are often given supplemental folic acid to reduce the risk of birth defects. Otherwise, folate supplementation does not appear to have a deleterious effect on zinc status.

### 28.7.6 Zinc and immune response

Zinc is known to play a central role in the immune system, and zinc-deficient individuals experience increased susceptibility to a variety of pathogens. The immunologic mechanisms whereby zinc modulates increased susceptibility to infection have been studied for several decades. Zinc affects multiple aspects of the immune system, from the barrier of the skin to gene regulation within lymphocytes. Zinc is crucial for normal development and function of cells mediating nonspecific immunity such as neutrophils and natural killer cells. Zinc deficiency also affects development of acquired immunity by preventing both the outgrowth and certain functions of T lymphocytes such as activation, Th1 cytokine production, and B lymphocyte help. Likewise, B lymphocyte development and antibody production, particularly immunoglobulin G, is compromised. The macrophage, a pivotal cell in many immunologic functions, is adversely affected by zinc deficiency, which can dysregulate intracellular killing, cytokine production, and phagocytosis. The effects of zinc on these key immunologic mediators is rooted in the myriad roles for zinc in basic cellular functions such as DNA replication, RNA transcription, cell division, and cell activation. Apoptosis is potentiated by zinc deficiency. Zinc provides a biological basis for the altered host resistance to infections observed during zinc deficiency and supplementation [46–48].

## 28.8 Evidence from zinc supplementation studies on child health

### 28.8.1 Zinc supplementation and physical growth

Zinc-responsive growth stunting has been identified in many studies from several regions worldwide. A meta-analysis of growth data from zinc intervention trials recently confirmed the widespread occurrence of growth-limiting zinc deficiency in young children, especially in developing countries [49]. The meta-analysis showed a significant positive effect of zinc supplementation (ranging from 0.9 to 21.4 mg of zinc/day) on growth among prepubertal children [50]. Zinc supplementation produced a highly significant, positive impact on children's linear growth, with effect size of 0.170 (95% CI: 0.075 to 0.264, $p$ = 0.001) and weight gain, with a mean effect size of 0.119 (95% CI: 0.048 to 0.190; $p$ = 0.002). Although the exact mechanism for the growth-limiting effects of zinc deficiency is not known, research indicates that zinc availability affects cell-signaling systems that coordinate the response to the growth-regulating hormone, insulin-like growth factor-1 (IGF-1) [51].

### 28.8.2 Therapeutic effects of zinc supplementation and morbidity

*Effects of zinc on diarrhea*

Diarrhea is still the major cause of childhood mortality estimated to cause 2 million deaths and remains responsible for 18% of all child deaths [52, 53]. The adverse effects of zinc deficiency on immune system function are likely to increase the susceptibility of children to infectious diarrhea, and persistent diarrhea contributes to zinc deficiency and malnutrition. Zinc deficiency may also potentiate the effects of toxins produced by diarrhea-causing bacteria like E. coli [54]. Two measures of the effects of zinc supplementation on diarrhea have been reported in the literature. First, the 'therapeutic effect' which describes the effect of giving zinc supplementation to the child during an episode of diarrhea. Second, the 'preventive effect' which describes the effect of zinc supplementation given over a prolonged period on the occurrence and severity of diarrhea morbidity to all children in a population where there is some indication of zinc deficiency.

*Therapeutic effects of zinc supplementation on acute and persistent diarrhea*

The role of zinc supplement (5–45 mg/day) in acute diarrhea (<7 days duration) has been recently updated in a meta-analysis which included 14 randomized controlled trials (Figure 28.1) [55].

| Study or subcategory | N | Treatment Mean ± SD | N | Control Mean ± SD | WMD (random(22))* 95% CI | Weight % | WMD (random) 95% CI |
|---|---|---|---|---|---|---|---|
| 01 All age groups | | | | | | | |
| Al-Sonboli 2003 | 37 | 1.20 ± 0.80 | 37 | 2.50 ± 1.80 | | 6.94 | −1.30 (−1.93 to −0.67) |
| Bahl 2002 [13] | 402 | 1.60 ± 2.20 | 401 | 1.70 ± 2.50 | | 8.66 | −0.10 (−0.43 to 0.23) |
| Bhatnagar 2004 | 132 | 2.32 ± 1.54 | 134 | 2.69 ± 1.90 | | 8.21 | −0.37 (−0.79 to 0.05) |
| Boran 2006 | 150 | 3.02 ± 2.00 | 130 | 3.67 ± 3.20 | | 6.93 | −0.65 (−1.29 to −0.01) |
| Brooks 2005 | 86 | 5.00 ± 4.73 | 89 | 5.00 ± 4.81 | | 3.35 | 0.00 (−1.41 to 1.41) |
| Dutta 2000 | 44 | 2.93 ± 0.42 | 36 | 4.31 ± 0.71 | | 8.94 | −1.38 (−1.64 to −1.12) |
| Gregorio 2007 | 60 | 2.98 ± 0.92 | 57 | 3.67 ± 1.63 | | 7.83 | −0.69 (−1.17 to −0.21) |
| Hidayat 1998 | 739 | 3.50 ± 2.40 | 659 | 3.80 ± 2.60 | | 8.94 | −0.30 (−0.56 to −0.04) |
| Patel 2005'] | 102 | 4.34 ± 2.02 | 98 | 4.48 ± 1.98 | | 7.42 | −0.14 (−0.69 to 0.41) |
| Polat 2003 | 52 | 4.70 ± 1.40 | 54 | 5.20 ± 1.60 | | 7.31 | −0.50 (−1.07 to 0.07) |
| Roy 1997 | 37 | 5.10 ± 2.50 | 37 | 5.50 ± 2.70 | | 4.15 | −0.40 (−1.59 to 0.79) |
| Sachdev 1988 | 25 | 3.40 ± 1.80 | 25 | 3.80 ± 1.70 | | 5.10 | −0.40 (−1.37 to 0.57) |
| Sazawal 1995 | 456 | 4.50 ± 3.60 | 481 | 5.40 ± 3.40 | | 8.02 | −0.90 (−1.35 to −0.45) |
| Fischer Walker 2006 | 554 | 4.93 ± 3.90 | 556 | 4.49 ± 3.17 | | 8.19 | 0.44 (0.02 to 0.86) |
| Subtotal (95% CI) | 2,876 | | 2,794 | | | 100.00 | −0.50 (−0.82 to −0.18) |

Test for heterogeneity: $\chi^2 = 82.27$, df = 13 ($p < .00001$), $I^2 = 84.2\%$

Test for overall effect: $Z = 3.04$ ($p = .002$)

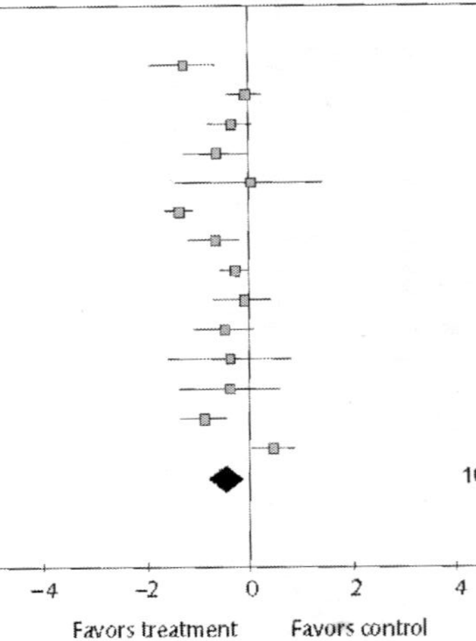


*28.1* Impact of zinc supplementation on mean duration of acute diarrhea, all age groups, WMD, weighted mean difference [55]

Current analysis of the adjunctive therapeutic benefit of zinc in acute diarrhea corroborates existing reviews [5] and provides evidence of reduction in duration of diarrhea by half a day. However, zinc supplementation was found to have no beneficial impact in infants under 6 months of age. Studies assessing the impact of zinc supplementation on the clinical outcome of the treated episode demonstrated 32% reduction in episodes of diarrhea lasting more than 7 days and a reduction in the frequency and/or volume of stools [56, 57]. Zinc supplementation given during a diarrheal episode and for a few days following the end of the episode (14 days) [58, 59] provides additional benefits, including decline in diarrheal incidence, and reduction in non-injury deaths. Boxes 28.1 and 28.2 present the experience with introduction of zinc supplementation in treating childhood diarrhea in India and other developing countries.

### Box 28.1 Experiences with introduction of zinc supplementation in treating childhood diarrhea in developing countries

In recent years, three large-scale effectiveness trials using zinc for the treatment of diarrhea have been completed in India, Pakistan, and Bangladesh through both tho public and the private sector health systems. Preliminary evidence suggests there was substantial reduction in diarrheal morbidity with zinc usage [60]. In these studies, the strategy was to give 20 mg elemental zinc daily in tablet/syrup form for 14 days along with ORS. In India [59], the study was conducted in rural Haryana and the strategy was to give 1 blister strip containing 14 dispersible zinc tablets (20 mg each) along with 2 ORS packets (to mix in 1 litre of water each) to all of the children aged 1 month to 4 years with diarrhea. Infants aged <6 months were to receive half a tablet in a teaspoonful of breast milk; older children were to receive 1 tablet dissolved in breast milk or clean water. The results demonstrated utilization of zinc supplements in 36.5% ($n = 1,571$) and 59.8% ($n = 1,649$) of diarrheal episodes occurring in the 4 weeks preceding interviews in the intervention areas [59]. The prevalence rates of diarrhea and pneumonia during the preceding 14 days were lower by 44% and 45% respectively in the intervention communities during the third quarterly survey. The numbers of hospitalizations for any cause, diarrhea, and pneumonia in the preceding 3 months were reduced in the intervention compared with the control areas (survey 3) (odds ratio for diarrhea hospitalizations, 0.69; 95% CI, 0.50 to 0.95; odds ratio for pneumonia hospitalizations, 0.29; 95% CI, 0.15 to 0.54). In a similar large-scale project in Matiari district in Pakistan, zinc supplements delivered by primary care government health workers to children with acute diarrhea produced a reduction in the subsequent incidence rates of diarrhea and mortality. These results have led to the incorporation of oral zinc sulfate for the treatment of diarrhea by the national primary health care programs and policies. In addition, the large effectiveness studies conducted in Bangladesh and in India [61, 62], have shown that when zinc and ORS are promoted together for the treatment of diarrhea, as part of a diarrhea control program, it led to increased ORS prescription rates, increased ORS use rates, decreased irrational antibiotic use rates, decreased anti-diarrheal use rates, and reduction in hospital rates.

**Box 28.2 Experiences with introduction of zinc supplementation in treating childhood diarrhea in Mali [63]**

Zinc for the treatment of childhood diarrhea was introduced in a pilot area in southern Mali to prepare for a cluster-randomized effectiveness study and to inform policies on how to best introduce and promote zinc at the community level. Dispersible zinc tablets in 14-tablet blister packs were provided through community health centres and drug kits managed by community health workers (CHWs) in two health zones in Bougouni district, Mali. Population-based household surveys with caretakers of children sick in the previous two weeks were carried out before and four months after the introduction of zinc supplementation. Household follow-up visits with children receiving zinc from the health centres and CHWs were conducted on days 3 and 14 after treatment for a subsample of children. A qualitative process evaluation also was conducted to investigate operational issues. Preliminary evidence from this study suggests that the introduction of zinc does not reduce the use of ORS and may reduce inappropriate antibiotic use for childhood diarrhea. Financial access to treatments, management of concurrent diarrhea and fever, and high use of unauthorized drug vendors were identified as factors affecting the effectiveness of the intervention in this setting.

In five studies that evaluated the effect of zinc supplementation on persistent diarrhea (episode that lasts 14 days or more) in children under 5 years of age, zinc-supplementation resulted in a significant reduction of duration of persistent diarrhea by 0.68 day and 21% lower probability of continuation of diarrhea on a given day. The meta-analysis showed a significant mean reduction of 42% (range, 10–63%) in the rate of treatment failure or death in children (<5 years of age) [55]. The benefit appeared to be more marked in children who were aged <12 months, were male, and had wasting or lowered baseline plasma zinc levels.

*Therapeutic effects of zinc supplementation on other illnesses*

Evidence of the benefit of zinc supplementation on pneumonia, malaria and tuberculosis in children under 5 years of age is insufficient and needs further evaluation [55].

## 28.8.3 Preventive effects of zinc supplementation

Brown et al [50] recently conducted a series of meta-analyses of the randomized controlled trials to quantify the impact of preventive zinc supplementation on morbidity, mortality and physical growth. A total of 55 individual trials i.e. 7 from Africa, 23 from Asia, 12 from South America, 11 from North America, 1 from Australia, and 1 from Europe were included in the analyses which enrolled 202,692 children.

*Preventive effects of zinc on diarrhea morbidity*

Zinc supplementation has been shown to reduce the incidence of diarrhea in several community and hospital based studies. The preventive effects of zinc supplementation on diarrhea have recently been updated by Brown et al [50] from 24 randomized controlled trials (Figure 28.2).

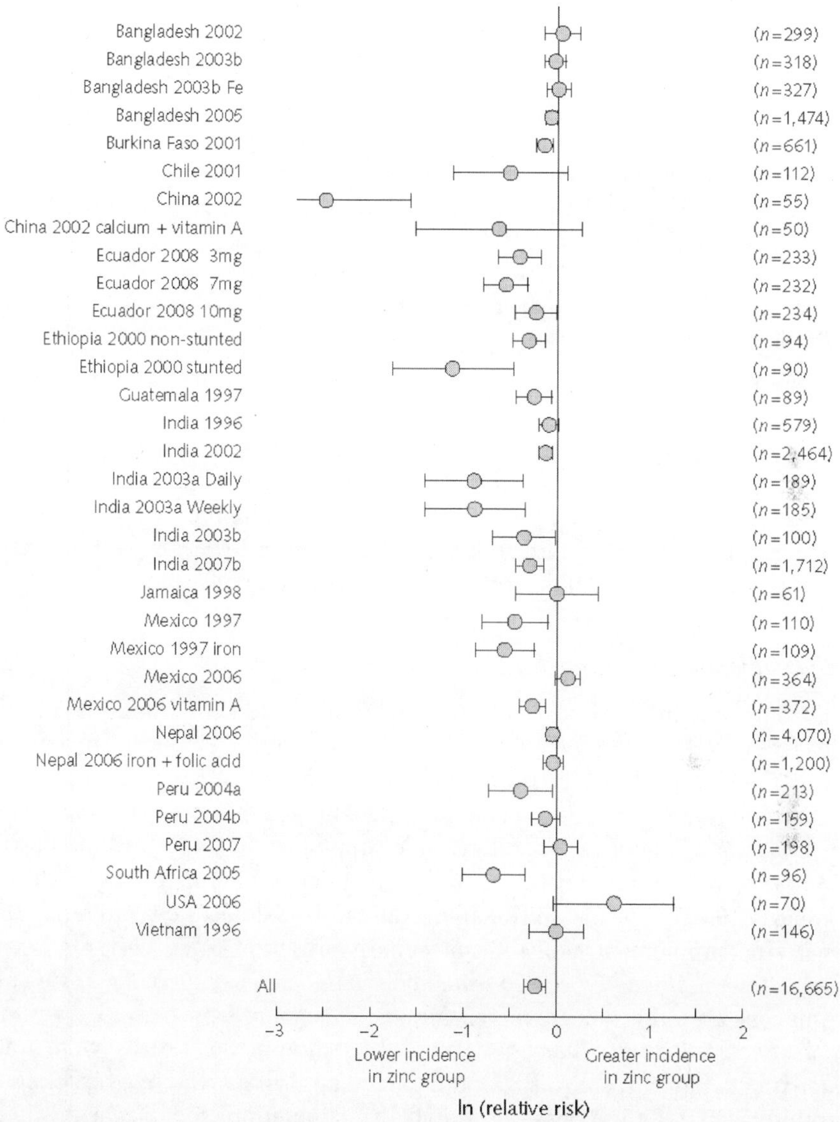


*28.2* Effect of zinc supplementation on diarrhea incidence from 24 intervention trials with 33 groupwise comparisons in which the supplements differed only bythe presence or absence of zinc [50].

Data from these studies which enrolled 16,339 children aged <4 years were pooled by using random-effect models with significant heterogeneity among children. The supplementation periods ranged from 2 weeks to 15 months and the dosage ranged from 1 to 70 mg per dose (median, 10 mg) mainly in the form of zinc sulfate. There was a significant 20% lower incidence of diarrhea among children who received zinc supplementation. The data indicated that the mean initial age of the study subjects was highly significantly associated with the magnitude of the effect of zinc supplementation. Among the subset of studies that enrolled children with the mean initial age greater than 12 months, the relative risk of diarrhea incidence was reduced by 27%. Data on duration of diarrhea from 9 studies which enrolled 1,692 children in the age group of 6 to 29 months indicated no significant effect of preventive zinc supplementation on duration of diarrhea.

*Preventive effects of zinc on pneumonia*

Zinc supplementation may also reduce the incidence of lower respiratory infections, such as pneumonia. Recently, Brown et al [50] have updated the meta-analysis, which included 12 randomized controlled trials with 16 group-wise comparisons, to evaluate the efficacy of zinc supplementation in respiratory illnesses among children between the mean initial ages of 0.9 and 49 months (Figure 28.3). Pooled data indicated that children who received a zinc supplement had significantly 15% reduction in lower respiratory tract infection or pneumonia than did those who received a placebo.

*Zinc supplementation and malarial morbidity*

In Gambia, using a twice-weekly 70 mg zinc supplementation, Bates et al [64] reported a 32% reduction in clinic visits due to malaria. In Papua New Guinea using daily 10 mg zinc supplementation, Shankar et al [65] reported a reduction of 38% in health center-based episodes of *Plasmodium falciparum*. Using a 12.5 mg daily zinc supplementation in Burkina Faso, Muller et al [66] found no effect in the incidence of *P. falciparum* malaria (relative risk of 0.98). Additionally, a randomized controlled trial reported that zinc supplementation did not benefit preschool-aged children with acute, uncomplicated *P. falciparum* malaria [67]. In a study in the Peruvian Amazon, children who received zinc or zinc plus iron had 15% fewer episodes of *Plasmodium vivax* infections though the results were not statistically significant [68]. A randomized controlled trial in over 42,000 children aged 1 to 48 months found that zinc supplementation did not significantly reduce mortality associated with malaria and other infections [69]. In a recently completed study in Burkina Faso, children who received zinc daily plus a single dose of vitamin A had 22% lower rate of fever and 30% reduction in malaria incidence [70].

In summary, there is still insufficient evidence to allow definitive conclusions to be drawn regarding the effect of zinc supplementation on

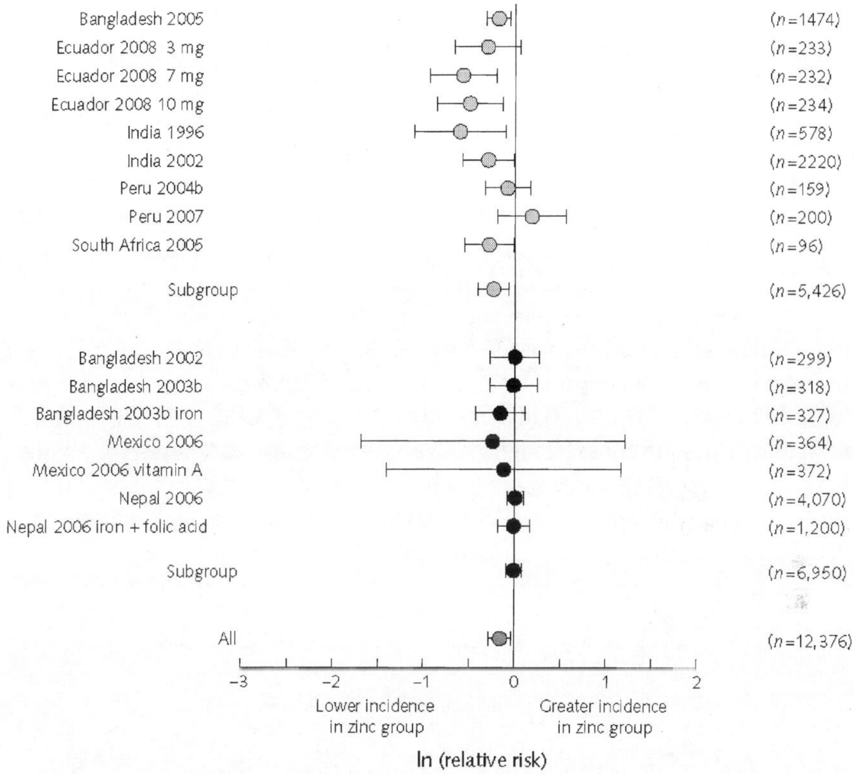


*28.3* Effect of zinc supplementation on the incidence of acute lower respiratory tract infection (ALRI)[a] from 12 intervention trials with 16 groupwise comparisons in which the supplements differed only by the presence or absence of zinc.

[(a)] Gray circles indicate studies in which ALRI was diagnosed by fieldworkers or physicians by using objective clinical signs: black circles indicate studies in which the diagnoise was based on caregiver reports of elevated respiratory rate or difficulty breathing [50].

the risk of malaria, although the weight of currently available information suggests that zinc may reduce the incidence of malaria, especially that of more severe cases that result in clinic attendance.

### *Zinc supplementation and mortality*

Given the effects of zinc supplementation on diarrhea and pneumonia morbidity, which are the main causes of mortality in preschool children, there is a strong case for the impact of zinc supplementation on mortality. To date there are ten studies with information on impact of zinc supplementation, given alone or with iron folic acid, on mortality. However, these studies are heterogeneous in terms of the study population. Seven studies measured the impact on unselected populations of young children (Burkina Faso,

Bangladesh, India, Nepal, Tanzania and Papua New Guinea) [65, 66, 69, 71–74]. Zinc supplementation had a marginal 6% impact on overall child mortality (Figure 28.4), there was an 18% reduction in deaths among zinc-supplemented children older than 12 months of age but it had no effect on younger children. Two studies which measured the impact of zinc supplementation on selected population, low birth weight (LBW) and small for gestational age (SGA) infants (Brazil, India) [75, 76], found 52–68% lower mortality rates among children who received zinc and showed a pooled RR for reducing mortality of 0.35. In these studies the children were followed up for <1 year, therefore the impact of zinc supplementation is not available beyond 1 year. These results are consistent with the analyses by birth weight in Nepal (2006), wherein they reported the relative risk of mortality was reduced by 44% [74]. One study carried out in Bangladesh enrolled ill children with diarrhea, with subsequent home based zinc supplementation for 14 days [61]. There was 51% lower rate of non-injury deaths in the group of children receiving zinc in addition to ORS as a part of diarrhea management than the group of children that was just receiving ORS.

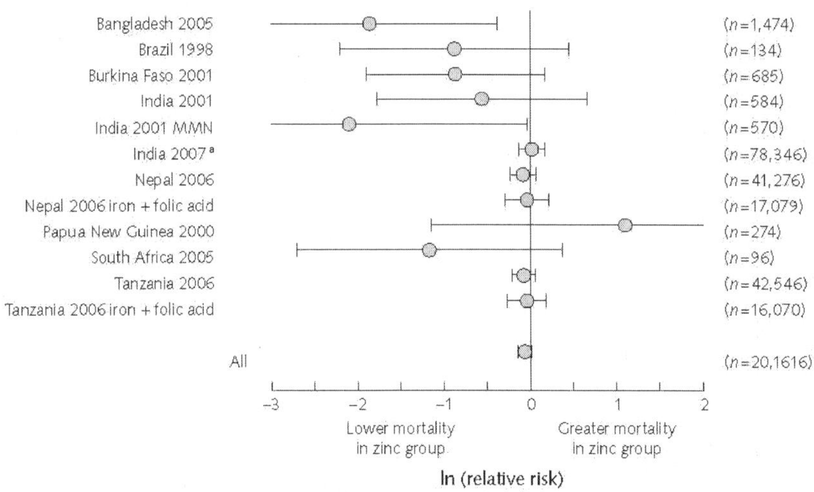


*28.4* Effect of zinc supplementation on childhood mortality from 10 intervention trials[(a)] is with 13 groupwise comparisons in which the supplements differed only by the presence or absence of zinc.

[(a)] The figure does not include the study by Bhandari et al. [73] (India, 2002; n = 2,482) because this study had no deaths in the zinc-supplemented group.

These combined sets of results indicate that providing preventive zinc supplementation in settings where there is an increased risk of zinc deficiency would reduce mortality among children greater than 1year of age and possibly among LBW infants. However, additional studies are needed to confirm the results.

### 28.8.4 Zinc supplementation and neurological/behavioral, mental and motor development of children

Low maternal zinc nutritional status has been associated with diminished attention in newborn infants and poorer motor function at six months of age. Zinc supplementation has been associated with improved motor development in very low-birth-weight infants, more vigorous activity in Indian infants and toddlers, and more functional activity in Guatemalan infants and toddlers [14, 77]. Additionally, zinc supplementation was associated with better neuropsychologic functioning (e.g. attention) in Chinese first grade students, but this was observed only when zinc was provided with other micronutrients [78]. Two other studies failed to find an association between zinc supplementation and measures of attention in children diagnosed with growth retardation.

Investigations of zinc supplementation on infants' development and behavior have yielded inconsistent findings [79]. There are 7 studies (provided nine groupwise comparisons) that reported on children's developmental outcomes in relation to zinc supplementation [50]. The study duration ranged from 1.9 to 12 months, and just two studies lasted more than 6 months. Two comparisons evaluated the impact of zinc supplementation versus placebo [80, 81], and the others provided additional micronutrients, such as iron [82, 84] or vitamin A [84, 85], to both groups. None of the studies found a significant positive effect of zinc on Mental Development Index (MDI). As with MDI, there was no significant overall impact of zinc supplementation on PDI (Psychomotor Development Index).

## 28.9 Zinc supplementation in pregnancy

Poor maternal zinc nutritional status has been associated with a number of adverse outcomes of pregnancy, including low birth weight, premature delivery, labor and delivery complications, fetal growth retardation, congenital anomalies and early postnatal infant immune dysfunction [86]. However, the results of maternal zinc supplementation trials in the U.S. and developing countries have been mixed [14]. Although some studies have found maternal zinc supplementation increases birth weight and decreases the likelihood of premature delivery, two placebo-controlled studies in Peruvian and Bangladeshi women found that zinc supplementation did not affect the incidence of low birth weight or premature delivery [87, 88]. Supplementation studies designed to examine the effect of zinc supplementation on labor and delivery complications have also generated mixed results, though few have been conducted in zinc-deficient populations [14]. A recent systematic review of 17 randomized controlled trials found that zinc supplementation during pregnancy was associated with a 14% reduction in premature deliveries; the lower incidence of preterm births was observed mainly in low-income women [89]. This analysis, however, did not find zinc supplementation to benefit other indicators of maternal or infant health. However, these results are quite limited, and more studies are needed to confirm these observations.

## 28.10 Effect of zinc on immune response in the elderly

Age-related declines in immune function are similar to those associated with zinc deficiency, and the elderly are vulnerable to mild zinc deficiency. However, the results of zinc supplementation trials on immune function in the elderly have been mixed. A randomized placebo-controlled study in men and women over 65 years of age found that a zinc supplement of 25 mg/day for three months increased levels of some circulating immune cells (i.e., CD4 T-cells and cytotoxic T-lymphocytes) compared to placebo [90]. However, other studies have reported zinc supplementation does not improve parameters of immune function, indicating that more research is required before any recommendations can be made regarding zinc and immune system response in the elderly.

## 28.11 Zinc toxicity

Zinc toxicity can occur in both acute and chronic forms. Acute adverse effects of high zinc intake include nausea, vomiting, loss of appetite, abdominal cramps, diarrhea, and headaches [31]. One case report cited severe nausea and vomiting within 30 minutes of ingesting 4 g of zinc gluconate (570 mg elemental zinc) [91]. Relatively speaking, zinc is non-toxic, non-accumulative compared to other trace elements such as lead, cadmium or arsenic and the proportion absorbed is inversely related to the amount ingested [92, 93]. Intakes of 150–450 mg of zinc per day have been associated with such chronic effects as low copper status, altered iron function, reduced immune function, and reduced levels of high-density lipoproteins [94]. Reductions in a copper-containing enzyme, a marker of copper status, have been reported with even moderately high zinc intakes of approximately 60 mg/day for up to 10 weeks [19]. The doses of zinc used in the Age-Related Eye Disease Study (80 mg per day of zinc in the form of zinc oxide for 6.3 years, on an average) have been associated with a significant increase in hospitalizations for genitourinary causes, raising the possibility that chronically high intakes of zinc adversely affect some aspects of urinary physiology [95].

## 28.12 Assessment of zinc status

The diagnosis of zinc deficiency is hampered by the lack of a single, sensitive, and specific low-cost indicator of zinc status. There are no generally accepted methods. Zinc status can be assessed by measurement of zinc in plasma, erythrocytes, leucocytes (lymphocytes/ neutrophils), platelets, urine, skin, sweat, saliva, and/or hair [96, 97].

### 28.12.1 Plasma/serum zinc concentrations

Plasma or serum zinc concentrations are the most widely used indicator for zinc status. In general, during zinc deficiency, plasma or serum zinc concentrations will decrease. The amount of zinc circulating in plasma is <0.2% of the total body zinc content, as most of the total body content of zinc is contained in muscle and liver. There are several confounding factors that may limit the use of plasma or serum zinc concentrations such as infection, inflammation, chronic disease, pregnancy and malnutrition. The cut off for plasma or serum zinc concentrations generally used to assess the risk of zinc deficiency is <10.71 μmol/L (<70 μg/dL) for pre-prandial samples and <9.95 μmol/L (<65 μg/dL) for post prandial samples.

Zinc plasma or serum concentrations can be measured by flame atomic absorption spectroscopy and most recent methods include flameless atomic absorption spectroscopy or inductively coupled plasma mass spectrometry. Plasma or serum should be separated as quickly as possible, as zinc concentrations may change if the plasma or serum has not separated from the blood within 1 hour. Hemolyzed samples should not be used, as zinc concentrations are higher in erythrocytes than in plasma. As zinc contamination may occur with use of regular blood-drawing equipments and supplies, trace element-free syringes, pipette tips and storage tubes should be used for the collection of plasma or serum for zinc determination.

### 28.12.2 Leucocyte and Erythrocyte Zinc Content

Leucocyte zinc content may be a useful indicator as leuocytes turnover is rapid but requires large quantity of blood sample (~10 ml), subject to contamination and is difficult to obtain from young children. Polymorphonuclear leucocytes can be collected relatively free from contamination with platelets but monocytes which are in themselves a very mixed population are difficult to collect free of contamination with platelets.

Leucocyte subsets have different zinc contents e.g. mean (SD): neutrophils 1.26 (0.27); monocytes 2.58 (0.65); lymphocytes 1.85 (0.32) μmol zinc/mg protein. Each has a different biological half-life (e.g. neutrophils 6 hours; monocytes 1–3 days; T lymphocytes 30 hours – 200 days). Pathophysiological changes in the relative proportions of the leucocyte subsets would lead to significant changes in the zinc content of the entire population. These phenomena could seriously limit the interpretation of mixed white cell analyses and the use of selected white cell subsets may seem to be more valuable. Analyses on selected separated subsets may prove to be more useful but are for the moment too impractical for routine or emergency use. In a systematic study of zinc supplemented children, leucocyte zinc concentrations were found to be a useful indicator of zinc deprivation [98].

Though, erythrocytes have a long shelf life (approximately 40 days), their zinc contents cannot be regarded as reliable indicators of recent or acute changes in zinc supply, unless zinc toxicity is suspected, but even so there are no adequate reference ranges to enable data to be evaluated.

### 28.12.3 Hair zinc concentrations

Although hair zinc has been used in literature due to ease of obtaining a sample, the limitations of determining hair zinc concentrations to detect severe zinc deprivation have been shown in animal models in which there is a paradoxical increase in zinc content of hair with severe zinc deprivation. This has been noted in malnourished children. A possible explanation for this is that as zinc supply becomes limiting, hair synthesis in the follicle is reduced such that despite the reduced supply of zinc, it accumulates in the hair root at a normal or increased rate.

### 28.12.4 Functional indices of zinc

Proxy indicators, such as activity of zinc metalloenzymes (alkaline phosphatase, carbonic anhydrase etc.), have been shown to be useful [99]. Serum alkaline phosphatase is low in severe zinc deficiency and returns to normal and a rise in serum alkaline phosphatase after zinc supplementation has been considered as a supportive indicator for the diagnosis of zinc deficiency. Increase in the plasma alkaline phosphatase following zinc supplementation to zinc deficient subjects has been frequently reported [100, 101]. Alkaline phosphatase level in serum responds to zinc depletion through a significant reduction in activity. Since the activity of this enzyme decreased before any sign of a lower food intake or reduced growth, it can be considered that the activity of serum alkaline phosphatase returns to the level of the control animals within 3 days of supplementation with zinc [100]. Improvement in serum alkaline phosphatase level was associated with corresponding improvement of clinical signs of zinc deficiency [99].

The metalloenzymes which responded with reduced activities in experimental zinc deficiency are alkaline phosphatase, pancreatic carboxy-peptidase, carbonic anhydrase, glutamic dehydrogenase, lactic and malic dehydrogenate, aldolase, NADH Diaphorase and pyridoxal phosphokinase. Metallothionein, a cytoplasmic metalloprotein, has been implicated in metabolism of zinc [102]. Experiments in rats indicated that metallothionein in hepatic and intestinal mucosal cells responded to altered dietary zinc content and serum zinc was directly related to metallothionein.

To assess an acute zinc deficiency state, measurement of zinc metalloenzymes or tissue, which has a rapid turnover rate, may be more practical. Labeled isotopes such as 69zn and 70zn have been used in absorption studies [103]. A good correlation between zinc status and the activity of the ribonuclease (RNase) has been observed.

## 28.12.5 Zinc pool – size and turnover rates

The exchangeable zinc pool (EZP) is the sum of the combined pools that exchange with zinc in the plasma within 48–72 hours and is thought to be critical for zinc dependent biological processes. The estimates of the size of the EZP have been found to be positively related to dietary zinc intake, especially the amount of absorbed zinc and fecal excretion of endogenous zinc. Once links to clinical, biochemical, or molecular effects of zinc deficiency have been achieved, the pool size and turnover measurements may be of value in evaluating the zinc status and zinc homeostasis [104, 105].

## 28.12.6 Growth faltering

Although growth faltering alone is not diagnostic of zinc deficiency, it is along with other factors a possible cause. A falling of height and weight measurements compared with normal standards or previous records of growth velocity may be one of the first clinical observations that suggest zinc deficiency. Growth faltering is a hall mark of severe zinc deficiency, and a rapid decline in growth velocity is the most striking clinical feature of mild zinc deficiency. Both linear and ponderal growth are negatively affected by inadequate zinc intake [106]. In populations where stunting is prevalent, growth of stunted children is most often significantly improved following zinc supplementation. Zinc supplementation had a positive impact on linear growth (effect size = 0.46) as well as, though small, but a highly significant impact on weight increments (effect size = 0.26 SD units) among those studies that enrolled stunted children (HAZ <-2SD). Thus the prevalence of growth stunting may be a useful indicator of poor zinc status in the population [107].

### 28.12.7 Dietary zinc estimates

Dietary zinc intake can be assessed quantitatively by a number of different methods, the simplest of which for population assessment is a modified interactive 24-hour dietary recall [108, 109]. Once the daily food intake is known, the total zinc intake can be estimated by multiplying the amount of each of the foods that are consumed by its zinc content, as recorded in local food composition tables or in databases available internationally, such as the US Department of Agriculture (USDA) food composition database [110]. For developing countries the World Food Dietary Assessment Program can be used [111]. The nutrient database associated with this system contains food composition values for 1800 foods from six countries (Egypt, Kenya, Mexico, Senegal, India, and Indonesia) and provides data for 53 nutrients and antinutritional factors that interfere with the absorption of nutrients including zinc, iron, dietary fiber, and phytate. Local databases are theoretically advantageous because the zinc content of foods can vary according to soil conditions, agronomic practices, and local food-processing techniques, although in many cases local food composition tables contain fewer food items and fewer replicate analyses per item. Moreover, these local tables frequently omit analyses of zinc and phytate. To estimate the amount of zinc available for absorption from the diet, the diet can be categorized according to its phytate–zinc molar ratio.

## 28.13 Scaling up programs to improve zinc nutrition

Despite the promising effects of zinc supplementation, public health programs have been slow to embrace zinc-related interventions. Reasons for the lack of large-scale programs to prevent zinc deficiency may include the limited information available on the prevalence of zinc deficiency and need for practical intervention strategies that could be incorporated into ongoing health programs. This section presents an abstracted overview of current public health programs and possible gaps in information needed to design large scale programs which has been reviewed in detail by Brown et al [112].

### 28.13.1 Assessment of population zinc status

Very few countries have systematically collected information on population zinc status, so the global prevalence of zinc deficiency remains unknown. To address this issue on an interim basis, IZiNCG has proposed using suggestive evidence of zinc deficiency, based on the rates of stunting of under-five children and information on the absorbable zinc content of the national food supply using FAO's food balance sheets [6].

National surveys of representative samples of the population are needed in high risk areas. Studies are also needed to validate the suggested cut-offs of zinc status indicators in relation to the functional effects of zinc deficiency. Additional field-applicable biomarkers of zinc status need to be developed. Finally, the suggestive evidence for classifying the population risk of zinc deficiency needs to be validated against objective biomarkers of zinc status.

### 28.13.2 Zinc intervention strategies

Three major nutrition-related strategies proposed to control zinc deficiency include supplementation, fortification, and dietary diversification/modification. The supplementation can further be divided into therapeutic and preventive supplementation.

*Therapeutic zinc supplementation for treatment of diarrhea*

This is by and large the most advanced component programmatically. Programs have begun in several countries, testing various approaches to training both health facility staff and community health workers, developing and delivering behavior change communication messages and consumer educational materials, and monitoring program progress. Private sector zinc programs are testing the feasibility of marketing zinc tablets and ORS as standalone products or packaging them together as a Diarrhea Treatment Kit (DTK).

Box 28.3 presents the WHO/UNICEF Zinc recommendations for treatment for diarrhea.

**Box 28.3 Zinc as a treatment for diarrhea – WHO/UNICEF recommendations**

Based on the updated meta-analyses of randomized, controlled intervention trials on children, the WHO/UNICEF recommended 20 mg zinc/day for 10–14 days for children with acute diarrhea and 10 mg/day for infants under 6 months of age in the form of sulfate, gluconate, or acetate. These updated recommendations take into account new research findings showing the beneficial effects of oral rehydration salts (ORS) containing lower concentrations of glucose and salts as well as of zinc supplementation. In combination with prevention and treatment of dehydration with appropriate fluids, breastfeeding, continued feeding and selective use of antibiotics, these two scientific advances – regarding ORS and zinc supplementation can drastically diminish the number of child deaths by reducing the duration and severity of diarrheal episodes and lowering their incidence [113, 114].

Subsequent to global recommendations upon review Indian Academy of Pediatrics (IAP) and Government of India also have revised guidelines for the use of zinc in diarrhea as given below (see Boxes 28.4 and 28.5):

**Box 28.4 Revised recommendations of the IAP National Task Force for use of zinc in diarrhea, May 2006**

1. All cases of diarrhea should receive zinc in addition to ORS. A uniform dose of 20 mg of elemental zinc should be given to all children older than 6 months and should be started as soon as diarrhea starts and continued for a total period of 14 days. Children aged 2 months to 6 months should be advised 10 mg per day of elemental zinc for a total period of 14 days.
2. Based on all the studies the group proposed that zinc salts e.g. sulphate, gluconate or acetate may be recommended.
3. The industry should be encouraged to prepare dispersible tablets that are reasonably priced, can be stored and transported easily. They can be dissolved in breast milk or water before use.

**Box 28.5 Recommendations by the Government of India, 2007**

Based on the WHO/UNICEF and the IAP recommendations and the data available on the evaluation of addition of zinc to current case management strategy in primary health setting [59] and personal communication of a larger study by Bhandari, *et al.* The Ministry of Health, Government of India has recommended that 20 mg of elemental zinc should be given to all children with diarrhea, older than 6 months, and should be started as soon as diarrhea starts and continued for a total period of 14 days. Children aged 2 months to 6 months should be advised 10 mg per day of elemental zinc for a total period of 14 days.

As part of global leadership mandate, USAID's Social Marketing Plus for Diarrheal Disease Control: Point-of-Use Water Disinfection and Zinc Treatment (POUZN) Project, has been implemented in 20 countries [115]. Box 28.6 presents the scaling up efforts of zinc supplementation programme in Nepal.

These efforts have focused on involving private companies to produce appropriate preparation for the diarrhea treatment and use social marketing approach to help scaling up its implementation. It is also recommended as part of standard case management in persistent diarrhea and in those with severe malnutrition.

### Box 28.6 Successful zinc supplementation scale-up in Nepal

In 2005, the Ministry of Health and Population requested assistance from the United States Agency for International Development (USAID) to support the integration of zinc into the government's diarrhea management programme.

In 2005, the Government of Nepal, through the Ministry of Health and Population's (MOHP) Child Health Division, is one of the first health ministries in the world to create a Zinc Task Force and prepare stakeholders for the introduction of zinc in line with the new World Health Organization (WHO)/UNICEF recommendations for standard management of childhood diarrhea, which includes ORS/ORT along with a 10–14 day regimen of pediatric zinc.

USAID's *Nepal Family Health Project* and UNICEF took the lead in providing commodities, training, and technical assistance to strengthen the skills of public sector health care providers in treating childhood diarrheas with both ORS/ ORT and zinc. At the same time, USAID/ Nepal funded the global *Social Marketing Plus for Diarrheal Disease Control: Point-of-Use Water Disinfection and Zinc Treatment (POUZN) Project*, implemented by Abt Associates in partnership with Population Services International, to introduce pediatric zinc in Nepal through the private sector as a companion piece to the introduction of zinc as the standard pediatric diarrhea treatment at public sector health facilities.

Both public and private sector programs have now been implemented in 30 targeted districts encompassing 65% of the population. The POUZN programme in Nepal, although active nationwide for only six months, has already successfully contributed to an increase in zinc use from 0.4% in 2005 to nearly 16% in 2008. Of users, 85% correctly took zinc and ORS together, and 67% correctly took zinc for the full 10 days, demonstrating the positive impact of the communications messages.

Box 28.7 presents the Scaling Up Zinc for Young Children (SUZY) project in Bangladesh.

### Box 28.7 Scaling Up Zinc for Young Children (SUZY) Project in Bangladesh

The Scaling Up of Zinc for Young Children (SUZY) Project was established in 2003 with the aim of setting Bangladesh on the path to covering all under-five children with zinc treatment of any diarrheal illness episode. ICDDR, B is the implementing and coordinating agency of the SUZY Project. Ministry of Health and Family Welfare (MoHFW) in collaboration with the SUZY team has developed two committees: (1) a National Advisory Committee, headed by the Health Secretary and (2) a Planning and Implementation Committee, headed by the Joint Secretary, Public Health and WHO. These two committees have been formed to have effective effort on policy decision. The National Advisory Committee of MoHFW approved the policy on using zinc in addition to ORS for under-five children suffering from diarrhea on 13 September 2006 and revised the National Diarrhea Treatment Guideline to incorporate zinc treatment in it.

A partnership was also created that included public, private, nongovernmental organization, and multinational sector agencies. Over a period of 3 years activities in support of preparing for the national scale up included formative and operational research, product registration and technology transfer, awareness building and orientation of health professionals, and preparation of mass media messages. In December, 2006 a national mass media campaign to promote a dispersible tablet zinc formulation, "Baby Zinc," for the treatment of childhood diarrhea was launched. All media messages linked zinc treatment to the continued use of oral rehydration salts (ORS). The scale-up of zinc treatment of childhood diarrhea rapidly attained widespread awareness, but actual use has lagged behind. Disparities in zinc coverage favoring higher income, urban households were identified, but these were gradually diminished over the two years of follow-up monitoring. The scale up campaign has not had any adverse effect on the use of ORS.

*Preventive zinc supplementation*

The evidence for preventive zinc supplementation on the functional outcomes of morbidity and mortality and physical growth, have been presented earlier. There has not been progress in scaling up preventive zinc supplementation. For scale up information is needed on the optimal safe and effective dose of preventive zinc supplements for children of different ages and the appropriate frequency and duration of supplementation, with and without other micronutrients. Information from effectiveness studies combining zinc supplementation with other routine health/nutrition contacts, such as growth monitoring, EPI, or periodic vitamin A supplementation activities is needed. Finally, the best way of integrating preventive and therapeutic supplementation programs would contribute a big step.

*Zinc fortification*

Several studies have evaluated the effects of fortifying different food products with multiple micronutrients, including zinc. Serum zinc concentrations of older infants did not respond to zinc-containing, multi-micronutrient fortified, cereal-based complementary foods in the four studies that measured this outcome [116–120]. Also there were no effects of the interventions on growth. In contrast serum zinc concentrations increased significantly among school children who received a multi-micronutrient fortified beverage between meals [121] or a multi-micronutrient fortified seasoning powder with meals [122]. Very little information is available from large-scale, programmatic interventions. Studies investigating the impact of home-based fortification using a mixture of vitamins and minerals packaged in small sachets containing a daily dose of micronutrients have focused mainly on the prevention of anemia and iron deficiency [123, 124]. Little is known about the impact of other micronutrients included in the multi-micronutrients mixture. In particular, there is limited information regarding their impact on zinc status. In general the health benefits of zinc included in "Sprinkles" have not yet been proven. Information is needed on the efficacy of zinc fortification programs (with and without other micronutrients), including their impact on biochemical indicators of zinc status and related functional outcomes. Similar information is needed for home fortification programs with zinc-containing micronutrient mixtures.

*Dietary diversification*

Diets in low income countries are predominantly plant-based and consumption of animal-source foods, such as meat, poultry, and fish, is often limited because of economic, cultural, and/or religious constraints. As a result, the zinc content of such diets is low and the efficiency of absorption is limited. Dietary inadequacy is probably the primary cause of zinc deficiency. To increase the zinc content in the diets, promotion of small-livestock husbandry, aquaculture, and production of other indigenous zinc-rich food has been proposed. At the household level, reduction of phytate content of the diet by using simple techniques to activate phytase, which is present naturally in cereals and legumes has been suggested. Such strategies have the added advantage of simultaneously improving the content and bioavailability of iron, vitamin B12, vitamin A, and calcium while enhancing protein quality and digestibility [125]. However there is little experience from large-scale programs to promote increased intake of zinc-rich foods. Practical information is needed on how best to identify locally available, low-cost, culturally acceptable zinc-rich foods and promote their consumption by those at risk of zinc deficiency. Information is also needed on best ways of implementing both large-scale and home-based food processing interventions to enhance zinc absorption from the usual diet [126, 127]. Agricultural interventions to increase dietary zinc content through improved agronomic practices and/or plant breeding need to be implemented and assessed.

## 28.14 Conclusion

Zinc is a crucial micronutrient because it affects few hundred enzyme systems, DNA replication and various immune mechanisms and modulates host resistance to several pathogens. Zinc nutrition is necessary for optimal child health, physical growth, and normal pregnancy outcomes. In recent years, global recognition of the importance of zinc nutrition in public health has been recognized and there is some understanding for the design and implementation of zinc intervention programs. Zinc supplementation reduces morbidity from diarrhea and pneumonia in high risk populations. A large body of evidence shows important therapeutic benefits with zinc administration during and after diarrhea and some studies also reported reduction in diarrhea morbidity in the subsequent 2–3 months without further supplementation. Zinc supplementation is also shown to have positive impact on growth in terms of height and weight gain in pre-pubertal children. In the interim, the present WHO strategy to focus on introduction of zinc for treatment of diarrhea is an important step forward. The administration of zinc with oral rehydration salts for diarrhea in the program settings resulted in increased use of these salts, decreased use of antimicrobials and harmful anti-diarrheal drugs, and also reduced hospital admissions. Further evidence is required for qualifying its use in treatment of other infectious diseases like pneumonia. In view of the available data on effect of zinc supplementation in reducing the diarrheal and pneumonia morbidity and child mortality, preventive zinc supplementation has a potential to contribute to achievement of the MDG 4 (reduction in child mortality) by 2015 [128]. In the long-term, measures to improve zinc intake of children, improvement of the overall diet, supplementation, food fortification, and sub-selection of crops with improved zinc content need to be explored and assessed. However, the challenges of delivery of zinc as a preventive intervention in a population like India where centralized food processing is not existent need to be sorted out before any program recommendation can be made. Effectiveness studies for novel ways to deliver zinc need to be undertaken to inform policy. More data and may be studies starting in pre-conception period are needed to make any firm conclusion about maternal supplementation during pregnancy.

## References

1. PRASAD AS, HALSTED JA, NADIMI M (1961). Syndrome of iron deficiency anemia, hepatosplenomegaly, hypogonadism, dwarfism, and geophagia. *Am J Med,* **31**, pp. 532–546.
2. PRASAD AS, MIALE A, FARID Z, SCHULER A, SANDSTEAD HH (1963). Zinc metabolism in patients with the syndrome of Iron deficiency anemia, hepatosplenomegaly, dwarfism and hypogonadism. *J Lab Clin Med*, **61**, pp. 573–549.
3. PRASAD AS (1988). Zinc in growth and development and spectrum of human zinc deficiency. *J Am Coll Nutr*, **7**(5), pp. 377–384.
4. HAMBIDGE M (2000). Human zinc deficiency. *J Nutr.*, **130**, pp. 1344S–1349S.
5. BHUTTA ZA, BIRD SM, BLACK RE, BROWN KH, GARDNER JM, HIDAYAT A, KHATUN F, MARTORELL R, NINH NX, PENNY ME, ROSADO JL, ROY SK, RUEL M, SAZAWAL S, SHANKAR A (2000). Zinc Investigators' Collaborative Group. Therapeutic effects of oral zinc in acute and persistent diarrhoea in children in developing countries: Pooled analysis of randomized controlled trials. *Am J Clin Nutr,* **72**, pp. 1516–1522.
6. WUEHLER SE, PEERSON JM, BROWN KH (2005). Estimation of the global prevalence of Zinc (Zn) deficiency using national food balance data. http://www zinc-health org/Health/Ab-s1p-ws cfm 2005.
7. International Zinc Nutrition Consultative Group (IZiNCG) Technical Document #1(2004). Assessment of the Risk of Zinc Deficiency in Populations and Options for Its Control. The United Nations University. *Food and Nutrition Bulletin*, **25**(1), pp. S94–S203.
8. FISCHER WALKER CL, EZZATI M, BLACK RE (2008). Global and regional child mortality and burden of disease attributable to zinc deficiency. *Eur J Clin Nutr.*, **63(5)**, pp. 591–597.
9. BLACK RE, ALLEN LH, BHUTTA ZA, CAULFIELD LE, DE ONIS M, EZZATI M, MATHERS C, RIVERA J (2008). For the Maternal and Child Undernutrition Study Group.

Maternal and child undernutrition: Global and regional exposures and health consequences. *Lancet*, **371**, pp. 243–260.

10. MURPHY SP, BEATON GH, CALLOWAY DH (1992). Estimated mineral intakes of toddlers: predicted prevalence of inadequacy in village populations in Egypt, Kenya, and Mexico. *Am J Clin Nutr.*, **56**(3), pp. 565–572.
11. GUPTA RP, VERMA PC, SADANA JR, GUPTA VK (1989). Effect of experimental zinc deficiency and repletion on sodium, potassium, copper and iron concentrations in guinea-pigs. *Br J Nutr*, **62**, pp. 407–414.
12. MUÑOZ EC, ROSADO JL, LÓPEZ P, FURR HC, ALLEN LH (2000). Iron and zinc supplementation improves indicators of vitamin A status of Mexican preschoolers. *Am. J Clin. Nutr*, **71(3)**, pp. 789–794.
13. TAMURA T and GOLDENBERG RL (1996). Zinc nutriture and pregnancy outcome. *Nutrition Research,* **16**, pp. 139–181.
14. CAULFIELD LE, ZAVALETA N, SHANKAR AH, MERIALDI M (1998). Potential contribution of maternal zinc supplementation during pregnancy to maternal and child survival. *Am J Clin Nutr.*, **68**(2), pp. 499S–508S.
15. PRASAD AS (1985). Clinical manifestations of zinc deficiency. *Annu Rev Nutr.*, **5**, pp. 341–363.
16. SANDSTROM B and LONNERDAL B (1989). *Promoters and Antagonists of Zinc Absorption.* C Mills (ed), Springer-Verlag, London.
17. FERGUSON EL, GIBSON RS, THOMPSON LU, OUNPUU S (1989). Dietary calcium, phytate and zinc intakes and the calcium, phytate, and zinc molar ratios of the diets of a selected group of East African children. *Am J Clin Nutr*, **50**, pp. 1450–1456.
18. JACKSON MJ (1984). Physiology of zinc: general aspects. *Zinc in human biology*, pp. 1–14.
19. BAER MT and KING JC (1984). Tissue zinc levels and zinc excretion during experimental zinc depletion in young men. *Am J Clin Nutr*, **39**, pp. 556–570.
20. HAMBIDGE KM and MERTZ W (1987). Trace elements in human and animal nutrition. In: *San Diego FL AP*, (ed). pp. 1–137.
21. LUKASKI HC, BOLONCHUK W, KLEVAY LM, MILNE DB, SANDSTEAD HH (1984). Changes in plasma zinc content after exercise in men fed a low-zinc diet. *Am J Physiol*, **247**, pp. E88–E93.
22. MILNE DB, CANFIELD WK, GALLAGHER SK, HUNT JR, KLEVAY LM (1987). Ethanol metabolism in postmenopausal women fed a diet marginal in zinc. *Am J Clin Nutr*, **46**, pp. 688–693.
23. LEE HH, PRASAD AS, BREWER GJ, OWYANG C (1989). Zinc absorption in human small intestine. *Am J Physiol*, **256**, pp. G87–G91.
24. TAYLOR CM, BACON JR, AGGETT PJ, BREMMER I (1991). Homeostatic regulation of zinc absorption and endogenous losses in zinc-deprived men. *Am J Clin Nutr*, **53**, pp. 755–763.
25. LOWE NN, BREMNER I, JACKSON NJ (1991). Plasma Zinc kinetics in the rat. *Br. Nutr.*, **65**, pp. 445–455.
26. EIDE DJ (2006). Zinc transporters and the cellular trafficking of zinc. *Biochim Biophys Acta*, **17**(63), pp. 711–722.
27. MCMAHON RJ and COUSINS RJ (1998). Regulation of the zinc transporter ZnT-1 by dietary zinc. *Proc Natl Acad Sci U S A* , **95**, pp. 4841–4846.
28. WORLD HEALTH ORGANIZATION (WHO) (1996). Trace elements in human health and nutrition. World Health Organization, Geneva.
29. NATIONAL RESEARCH COUNCIL (NRC) (2001). Institute of Medicine, Food and Nutrition Board. Dietary reference intakes for vitamin A, vitamin K, arsenic,

boron, chromium, copper, iodine, iron, manganese, molybdenum, nickel, silicon, zinc. Washington, DC: National Academy Press.

30. Panel on dietary reference values of the committee on medical aspects of food policy (1991). Dietary reference values for food energy and nutrients for the United Kingdom. Her Majesty's Stationery Office, London, p. 210.
31. INSTITUTE OF MEDICINE, FOOD AND NUTRITION BOARD (2001). Dietary Reference Intakes for Vitamin A, Vitamin K, Arsenic, Boron, Chromium, Copper, Iodine, Iron, Manganese, Molybdenum, Nickel, Silicon, Vanadium, and Zinc. Washington, DC: National Academy Press.
32. FAO/ WHO (2002). *Human Vitamin and Mineral Requirements*. Report of a joint FAO/WHO expert consultation. Rome.
33. OESTREICHER P and COUSINS RJ (1985). Copper and Zinc Absorption in the Rat: mechanism of Mutual Antagonism. *J Nutr*, **115**, pp. 159–166.
34. BORON B et al (1988). Effect of zinc deficiency on hepatic enzymes regulating vitamin A status. *J Nutr.*, **118**(8), pp. 995–1001.
35. CHRISTIAN P and WEST KP, JR (1998). Interactions between zinc and vitamin A: an update. *Am J Clin Nutr.*, **68**(2), pp. 435S–441S.
36. SHINGWEKAR AG, MOHANRAM M, REDDY V (1979). Effect of zinc supplementation on plasma levels of vitamin A and retinol-binding protein in malnourished children. *Clin Chim Acta.* **93**, pp. 97–100.
37. RAHMAN MM, VERMUND SH, WAHED MA, FUCHS GJ, BAQUI AH, ALVAREZ JO (2001). Simultaneous zinc and vitamin A supplementation in Bangladeshi children: randomised double blind controlled trial. *BMJ.* **323**(7308), pp. 314–318.
38. OLIVARES M, PIZARRO F, RUZ M (2007). New insights about iron bioavailability inhibition by zinc. *Nutrition* 2007, **23**(4), pp.292–295.
39. SOLOMONS NW and JACOB RA (1981). Studies on bioavailability of zinc in humans: effects of heme and nonheme iron on the absorption of zinc. *Am J Clin Nutr*, **34**, pp. 475–482.
40. OPPENHEIMER SJ (2001). Iron and its relation to immunity and infectious disease. *J Nutr*, **131**, pp. 616S–635S.
41. SAZAWAL S, BLACK RE, RAMSAN M, CHWAYA HM, STOLTZFUS RJ, DUTTA A, DHINGRA U, KABOLE I, DEB S, OTHMAN MK, KABOLE FM (2006). Effects of routine prophylactic supplementation with iron and folic acid on admission to hospital and mortality in preschool children in a high malaria transmission setting: Community-based, randomised, placebo-controlled trial. *Lancet*, **367**, pp. 133–143.
42. DEWEY KG, DOMELLOF M, COHEN RJ, LANDA RIVERA L, HERNELL O, LONNERDAL B (2002). Iron supplementation affects growth and morbidity of breast-fed infants: results of a randomized trial in Sweden and Honduras. *J Nut.*, **132**(3), pp.249–255.
43. LIND T, SESWANDHANA R, PERSSON LA, LÖNNERDAL B (2008). Iron supplementation of iron-replete Indonesian infants is associated with reduced weight-for-age. *Acta Paediatr.* **97**(6), pp. 770–775.
44. SPENCER H, KRAMER L, NORRIS C, OSIS D (1984). Effect of calcium and phosphorus on zinc metabolism in man. *Am J Clin Nutr*, **40**, pp. 1213–1218.
45. MILNE D B (1989). Effects of folic acid supplements on zinc-65 absorption and retention. *J. Trace Elements Exp. Med.*, **2**, pp. 297–304.
46. PRASAD AS (2008). Zinc in human health: effect of zinc on immune cells. *Mol Med.* **14**(5–6), pp. 353–357.
47. SHANKAR AH and PRASAD AS (1998). Zinc and immune function: the biological basis of altered resistance to infection. *Am J Clin Nutr.*, **68**(2), pp. 447S–463S.

48. SAZAWAL S, JALLA S, MAZUMDER S, SINHA A, BLACK RE, BHAN MK (1997). Effect of zinc supplementation on cell-mediated immunity and lymphocyte subsets in preschool children. *Indian Pediatr.*, **34**(7), pp. 589–597.
49. HAMBIDGE M and KREBS N (2000). Zinc and growth. In: *Roussel AM*, (ed.) Trace elements in man and animals 10: Proceedings of the tenth international symposium on trace elements in man and animals. New York: Plenum Press, pp. 977–980.
50. BROWN KH, PEERSON JM, BAKER SK, HESS SY (2009). Preventive zinc supplementation among infants, preschoolers, and older prepubertal children. Systematic Reviews of Zinc Intervention Strategies. International Zinc Nutrition Consultative Group Technical Document #2. *Food and Nutrition Bulletin*, **30** (1), pp. S12–S40.
51. MACDONALD RS (2000). The role of zinc in growth and cell proliferation. *J Nutr.*, **130**(5S), pp. 1500S–1508S.
52. BRYCE J, BOSCHI-PINTO C, SHIBUYA K, BLACK RE (2005). WHO Child Health Epidemiology Reference Group (2005) WHO estimates of the causes of death in children. *Lancet*, **365**, pp. 1147–1152.
53. MURRAY CJ, LAAKSO T, SHIBUYA K, HILL K, LOPEZ AD (2007). Can we achieve Millennium Development Goal 4? New analysis of country trends and forecasts of under-5 mortality to 2015. *Lancet*, **370**, pp. 1040–1054.
54. WAPNIR RA (2000). Zinc deficiency, malnutrition and the gastrointestinal tract. *J Nutr.* **130**(5S), pp. 1388S–1392S.
55. HAIDER BA and BHUTTA ZA (2009). The effect of therapeutic zinc supplementation among young children with selected infections: A review of the evidence. Systematic Reviews of Zinc Intervention Strategies. International Zinc Nutrition Consultative Group Technical Document #2. *Food and Nutrition Bulletin*, **30 (1)**, pp. S41–S59.
56. DUTTA P, MITRA U, DATTA A, NIYOGI SK, DUTTA S, MANNA B, BASAK M, MAHAPATRA TS, BHATTACHARYA SK (2000). Impact of zinc supplementation in malnourished children with acute watery diarrhoea. *J Trop Pediatr*, **46**, pp. 259–263.
57. AL-SONBOLI N, GURGEL RQ, SHENKIN A, HART CA, CUEVAS LE (2003). Zinc supplementation in Brazilian children with acute diarrhoea. *Ann Trop Paediatr*, **23**, pp. 3–8.
58. WINCH PJ, GILROY KE, DOUMBIA S, PATTERSON AE, DAOU Z, COULIBALY S, SWEDBERG E, BLACK RE, FONTAINE O (2006). Prescription and administration of a 14-day regimen of zinc treatment for childhood diarrhoea in Mali. *Am J Trop Med Hyg.*, **74**(5), pp. 880–883.
59. BHANDARI N, MAZUMDER S, TANEJA S, DUBE B, BLACK RE, FONTAINE O, MAHALANABIS D, BHAN MK (2005). A pilot test of the addition of zinc to the current case management package of diarrhoea in a primary health care setting. *J Pediatr Gastroenterol Nutr.* **41(5)**, pp. 685–687.
60. WHO/CAH and JHSPH (2008). Consultation to review the results of the large effectiveness studies examining the addition of zinc to the current case management of diarrhoea (India, Mali and Pakistan), New Delhi.
61. BAQUI AH, BLACK RE, EL ARIFEEN S, YUNUS M, CHAKRABORTY J, AHMED S, VAUGHAN JP (2002). Effect of zinc supplementation started during diarrhoea on morbidity and mortality in Bangladeshi children: community randomised trial. *BMJ.*, **325**(7372), p. 1059.
62. BHAN MK (2006). Personnel communication.
63. WINCH PJ, GILROY KE, DOUMBIA S, PATTERSON AE, DAOU Z, DIAWARA A, SWEDBERG E, BLACK RE, FONTAINE O (2008). Mali Zinc Pilot Intervention Study Group.

Operational issues and trends associated with the pilot introduction of zinc for childhood diarrhoea in Bougouni district, Mali. *J Health Popul Nutr.*, **26**(2), pp. 151–162.

64. BATES CJ et al (1993). A trial of zinc supplementation in young rural Gambian children. *Br J Nutr*, **69**, pp. 243–255.
65. SHANKAR AH et al (2000). The influence of zinc supplementation on morbidity due to Plasmodium falciparum: a randomized trial in preschool children in Papua New Guinea. *Am J Trop Med Hyg*, **62**, pp. 663–669.
66. MULLER O et al (2001). Effect of zinc supplementation on malaria and other causes of morbidity in West African children: randomized double blind placebo controlled trial. *BMJ*, **32**(2), p. 1567.
67. Zinc Against Plasmodium Study Group (2002). Effect of zinc on the treatment of Plasmodium falciparum malaria in children: a randomized controlled trial. *Am J Clin Nutr.*, **76**(4), pp. 805–812.
68. RICHARD SA, ZAVALETA N, CAULFIELD LE, BLACK RE, WITZIG RS, SHANKAR AH (2006). Zinc and iron supplementation and malaria, diarrhoea, and respiratory infections in children in the Peruvian Amazon. *Am J Trop Med Hyg*, **75**, pp. 126–132.
69. SAZAWAL S et al (2007). Effect of zinc supplementation on mortality in children aged 1-48 months: a community-based randomised placebo-controlled trial. *Lancet.* **369**(9565), pp. 927–934.
70. ZEBA AN, SORGHO H, ROUAMBA N, ZONGO I, ROUAMBA J, GUIGUEMDE RT, HAMER DH, MOKHTAR N, OUEDRAOGO JB (2008). Major reduction of malaria morbidity with combined vitamin A and zinc supplementation in young children in Burkina Faso: A randomized double blind trial. *Nutr J*, **7**, pp. 7–13.
71. BROOKS WA, SANTOSHAM M, NAHEED A, GOSWAMI D, WAHED MA, DIENER-WEST M, FARUQUE AS, BLACK RE (2005). Effect of weekly zinc supplements on incidence of pneumonia and diarrhoea in children younger than 2 years in an urban, low-income population in Bangladesh: randomised controlled trial. *Lancet.* **366**(9490), pp. 999–1004.
72. BHANDARI N, BAHL R, TANEJA S, STRAND T, MOLBAK K, ULVIK RJ, SOMMERFELT H, BHAN MK (2002). Effect of routine zinc supplementation on pneumonia in children aged 6 months to 3 years: Randomised controlled trial in an urban slum. *BMJ*, **32**(4), p. 1358.
73. BHANDARI N, TANEJA S, MAZUMDER S, BAHL R, FONTAINE O, BHAN MK (2007). Adding zinc to supplemental iron and folic acid does not affect mortality and severe morbidity in young children. *J Nutr*, **13**(7), pp. 112–117.
74. TIELSCH JM, KHATRY SK, STOLTZFUS RJ, KATZ J, LECLERQ SC, ADHIKARI R, MULLANY LC, BLACK R, SHRESTA S (2007). Effect of daily zinc supplementation on child mortality in southern Nepal: a community-based, cluster randomised, placebo-controlled trial. *Lancet.* **370**(9594), pp. 1230–1239.
75. SAZAWAL S, BLACK RE, MENON VP, DHINGRA P, CAULFIELD LE, DHINGRA U and BAGATI A (2001). Zinc supplementation in infants born small for gestational age reduces mortality: a prospective, randomized, controlled trial. *Pediatrics*, **10**(8), pp. 1280–1286.
76. LIRA P, ASHWORTH A, MORRIS S (1998). Effect of zinc supplementation on the morbidity, immune function, and growth of low-birth-weight, full-term infants in northeast Brazil. *Am J Clin Nutr.*, **68**(1), pp. 418S–424S.
77. SAZAWAL S, BENTLEY M, BLACK RE, DHINGRA P, GEORGE S, BHAN MK (1996). Effect of zinc supplementation on observed activity in low socioeconomic Indian preschool children. *Pediatrics.*, **98**(6), pp. 1132–1137.

78. SANDSTEAD HH et al (1998). Effects of repletion with zinc and other micronutrients on neuropsychologic performance and growth of Chinese children. *Am J Clin Nutr.*, **68**(2), pp. 470S–475S.
79. BLACK MM (1998). Zinc deficiency and child development. *Am J Clin Nutr.*, **68**(2), pp. 464S–469S.
80. ASHWORTH A, MORRIS SS, LIRA PI, GRANTHAM-MCGREGOR SM (1998). Zinc supplementation, mental development and behaviour in low birth weight term infants in northeast Brazil. *Eur J Clin Nutr*, **52**, pp. 223–227.
81. HAMADANI JD, FUCHS GJ, OSENDARP SJ, KHATUN F, HUDA SN, GRANTHAM-MCGREGOR SM (2001). Randomized controlled trial of the effect of zinc supplementation on the mental development of Bangladeshi infants. *Am J Clin Nutr*, **74**, pp. 381–386.
82. CASTILLO-DURAN C, PERALES CG, HERTRAMPF ED, MARIN VB, RIVERA FA, ICAZA G (2001). Effect of zinc supplementation on development and growth of Chilean infants. *J Pediatr*, **13**(8), pp. 229–235.
83. LIND T, LÖNNERDAL B, STENLUND H, GAMAYANTI IL, ISMAIL D, SESWANDHANA R, PERSSON LA (2004). A community-based randomized controlled trial of iron and zinc supplementation in Indonesian infants: Effects on growth and development. *Am J Clin Nutr*, **80**, pp. 729–736.
84. BLACK MM, BAQUI AH, ZAMAN K, AKE PERSSON L, EL ARIFEEN S, LE K, MCNARY SW, PARVEEN M, HAMADANI JD, BLACK RE (2004). Iron and zinc supplementation promote motor development and exploratory behaviour among Bangladeshi infants. *Am J Clin Nutr*, **80**, pp. 903–910.
85. TANEJA S, BHANDARI N, BAHL R, BHAN MK (2005). Impact of zinc supplementation on mental and psychomotor scores of children aged 12 to 18 months: A randomized, doubleblind trial. *J Pediatr*, **14**(6), pp. 506–511.
86. SHAH D and SACHDEV HP (2006). Zinc deficiency in pregnancy and fetal outcome. *Nutr Rev.*, **64**(1), pp. 15–30.
87. CAULFIELD LE, ZAVALETA N, FIGUEROA A, LEON Z (1999). Maternal zinc supplementation does not affect size at birth or pregnancy duration in Peru. *J Nutr.*, **129**(8), pp. 1563–1568.
88. OSENDARP SJ, VAN RAAIJ JM, ARIFEEN SE, WAHED M, BAQUI AH, FUCHS GJ (2000). A randomized, placebo-controlled trial of the effect of zinc supplementation during pregnancy on pregnancy outcome in Bangladeshi urban poor. *Am J Clin Nutr.*, **71**(1), pp. 114–119.
89. MAHOMED K, BHUTTA Z, MIDDLETON P (2007). Zinc supplementation for improving pregnancy and infant outcome. *Cochrane Database Syst Rev.*, **2**, CD000230.
90. FORTES C et al (1998). The effect of zinc and vitamin A supplementation on immune response in an older population. *J Am Geriatr Soc.*, **46**(1), pp. 19–26.
91. LEWIS MR and KOKAN L (1998). Zinc gluconate: acute ingestion. *J Toxicol Clin Toxicol*, **36**, pp. 99–101.
92. GALLERY EDM, BLOMFIELD J, DIXON SR (1972). Acute zinc toxicity in hemodialysis. *BMJ*, **4** (5836), pp. 331–333.
93. HELLER VG and BURKE AD (1972). TOXICITY OF ZINC. *J Biol Chem.*, **74**, pp. 85–91.
94. HOOPER PL, VISCONTI L, GARRY PJ, JOHNSON GE (1980). Zinc lowers high-density lipoprotein-cholesterol levels. *J Am Med Assoc*, **24**(4), pp. 1960–1961.
95. JOHNSON AR, MUNOZ A, GOTTLIEB JL, JARRARD DF (2007). High dose zinc increases hospital admissions due to genitourinary complications. *J Urol*, **17**(7), pp. 639–643.
96. HAMBIDGE KM, CASEY CE, KREBS NF (1986). *Trace Elements in Human and Animal Nutrition*. Academic, Orlando.

97. SANDSTEAD HH (1982). Nutritional role of zinc and effects of deficiency. *Curr Concepts Nutr*, **11**, pp. 97–124.
98. SIMMER K, KHANUM S, CARLSSON L, THOMPSON RP (1988). Nutritional rehabilitation in Bangladesh-the importance of zinc. *Am J Clin Nutr*, **47**, pp. 1036–1040.
99. ROTHBAUM RJ, MAUR PR, FARELL MK (1982). Serum alkaline phosphatase and zinc undernutrition in infants with chronic diarrhoea. *Am J Clin Nutr*, **35**, pp. 595–598.
100. PRASAD AS, MIALE A, FARID Z, SANDSTEAD H, SCHULER A, DARBY W (1963). Biochemical studies on dwarfism, hypogonadism, and anemia. *Arch Intern Med*, **11**(1), pp. 407–428.
101. PRASAD AS (1966). Metabolism of zinc and its deficiency in human subjects. Illinois.
102. RICHARD MP and COUSINS RJ (1976). Mammalian zinc homeostasis requirement for RNA and metallothionine synthesis. *J Nutr*, **106**(5), pp. 1591–1597.
103. AUGUST D, JANGHORBANI M, YOUNG VR (1989). Determination of zinc and copper absorption at three dietary zinc-copper ratios by using stable isotope methods in young adults and elderly subjects. *Am J Clin Nutr.*, **50**, pp. 1457–1463.
104. MILLER LV, KREBS NF, HAMBIDGE KM (2000). Development of a compartmental model of human zinc metabolism: identifiability and multiple studies analyses. *Am J Physiol Regul Integr Comp Physiol*, p. 279.
105. SIAN L, MINGYAN X, MILLER LV, NG LI, EBS NF, MBIDGE KM (1996). Zinc absorption and intestinal losses of endogenous zinc in young Chinese women with marginal zinc intakes. *Am J Clin Nutr*, **63**, pp. 348–353.
106. GIBSON R (1994). Zinc nutrition in developing countries. *Nutr Res Rev*, **7**, pp. 151–173.
107. BROWN KH, PEERSON JM, RIVERA J, ALLEN LH (2002). Effect of supplemental zinc on the growth and serum zinc concentrations of prepubertal children: a meta-analysis of randomized controlled trials. *Am J Clin Nutr*, **75**, pp. 1062–1071.
108. GIBSON RS (1990). *Principles of Nutritional Assessment*. Oxford University Press, New York.
109. GIBSON RS (1999). An interactive 24-hour recall for assessing the adequacy of iron and zinc intakes in developing countries. International Life Sciences Institute Press.
110. USDA WEBSITE (1999). <http://www.nal.usda.gov/fnic/cgi-bin/nut_search.pl>
111. BUNCH S and MURPHY SP (1994). User's guide to the operation of the world food dietary assessment program. *Office of Technology Licensing*. University of California, Berkeley, p. 21.
112. Brown KH information gaps for scaling-up programs to improve Zinc Nutrition 2007; 1-8 web site link: www a2z profect.org pdf Gap-Analysis-Zinc-Final.pdf. Accessed on 3rd September 2010.
113. FONTAINE O (2006). Zinc and treatment of diarrhoea. *Med Trop (Mars).*, **66**(3), pp. 306–309.
114. WHO/UNICEF (2004). Clinical management of acute diarrhoea. WHO/FCH/CAH/ 04.7. Geneva: WHO/UNICEF.
115. POUZN - AED PSP - One Private Sector partnerships for better health. Web site link: http:/www.psp - ones.com/section/task orders/pouzn/pouzn acd. Accessed on 3rd September 2010.
116. LARTEY A, MANU A, BROWN KH, PEERSON JM and DEWEY KG (1999). A randomized, community-based trial of the effects of improved, centrally processed

complementary foods on growth and micronutrient status of Ghanaian infants from 6 to 12 mo of age. *Am J Clin Nutr*, **70**, pp. 391–404.

117. OELOFSE A, VAN RAAIJ JM, BENADE AJ, DHANSAY MA, TOLBOOM JJ and HAUTVAST JG (2003). The effect of a micronutrient fortified complementary food on micronutrient status, growth and development of 6- to 12-month-old disadvantaged urban South African infants. *Internatl J Food Sci Nutr*, **54**, pp. 399–407.
118. FABER M, KVALSVIG JD, LOMBARD CJ and BENADE AJ (2005). Effect of a fortified maize-meal porridge on anemia, micronutrient status, and motor development of infants. *Am J Clin Nutr*, **82**, pp. 1032–1039.
119. LUTTER CK, SEMPERTEGUI F, RODRIGUEZ A, FUENMAYOR G, AVILA L and MADERO J (2006). Evaluacion e impacto del programa nacional de alimentacion nutricion PANN 2000. Washington DC: *Organizacion Panamericana de la Salud.*
120. BROWN KH, LÓPEZ DE ROMAÑA G, ARSENAULT JE, PEERSON JM and PENNY ME. Effect of mode of delivery of zinc (provided in a fortified food or as a liquid supplement) on the growth, morbidity and plasma zinc concentration of young Peruvian children. *Am J Clin Nutr*, in press.
121. ABRAMS SA, MUSHI A, HILMERS DC, GRIFFIN IJ, AVILA P and ALLEN L (2003). A multinutrient-fortified beverage enhances the nutritional status of children in Botswana. *J Nutr*, **13**(3), pp. 1834–1840.
122. WINICHAGOON P, MCKENZIE JE, CHAVASIT V, PONGCHAROEN T, GOWACHIRAPANT S, BOONPRADERM A, MANGER MS, BAILEY KB, WASANTWISUT E and GIBSON RS (2006). A multimicronutrient-fortified seasoning powder enhances the hemoglobin, zinc, and iodine status of primary school children in North East Thailand: a randomized controlled trial of efficacy. *J Nutr,* **13**(6), pp. 1617–1623.
123. ZLOTKIN S, ARTHUR P, SCHAUER C, ANTWI KY, YEUNG G and PIEKARZ A (2003). Home-fortification with iron and zinc sprinkles or iron sprinkles alone successfully treats anemia in infants and young children. *J Nutr*, **13**(3), pp. 1075–1080.
124. GIOVANNINI M, SALA D, USUELLI M, LIVIO L, FRANCESCATO G, BRAGA M, RADAELLI F and RIVA E (2006). Double-blind, placebo-controlled trial comparing effects of supplementation with two different combinations of micronutrients delivered as sprinkles on growth, anemia, and iron deficiency in Cambodian infants. *J Ped Gastroenterol Nutr*, **42**, pp. 306–312.
125. GIBSON RS, YEUDALL F, DROST N, MTITIMUNI BM and CULLINAN TR (2003). Experiences of a community-based dietary intervention to enhance micronutrient adequacy of diets low in animal source foods and high in phytate: a case study in rural Malawian children. *J Nutr*, **13**(3), pp. 3992S–3999S.
126. BROWN KH, ENGLE-STONE R, KREBS NF, PEERSON JM (2009). Dietary intervention strategies to enhance zinc nutrition: promotion and support of breastfeeding for infants and young children. *Food Nutr Bull.* **30**(1), pp. S144–171.
127. GIBSON RS and ANDERSON VP (2009). A review of interventions based on dietary diversification or modification strategies with the potential to enhance intakes of total and absorbable zinc. *Food Nutr Bull.* **30**(1), pp. S108–143.
128. BRYCE J and VICTORIA CG (2005). Child survival: countdown to 2015. *The Lancet*, **365** (9478), pp. 2153–2154.

# 29

# Vitamin A and zinc supplements for child survival – experiences and challenges ahead

*Anand Lakshman*

**Anand Lakshman,** a medical doctor with a Masters in Health Administration, has worked on tribal health issues in Karnataka and on the Revised National Tuberculosis Control Programme in West Bengal. Dr Lakshman, Coordinator Planning & Knowledge Management at the Micronutrient Initiative's (MI) Asia office, spearheaded MI's support to national programs in India, including vitamin A supplementation and therapeutic zinc supplementation.

## 29.1 Introduction

In 2008, a group of world-renowned economists in an exercise known as the Copenhagen Consensus [1], ranked micronutrient supplements as the top development priority out of more than 40 interventions, such as *The Doha Development Agenda*, Expanded Immunization Coverage for Children, Malaria Prevention and Treatment and Peace-keeping in post-conflict situations. The criteria used included the benefit–cost ratio, as well as feasibility and sustainability of the interventions. Specifically, it identified vitamin A supplementation for children (every 4–6 months, from age 6 months to 5 years) and therapeutic zinc supplementation along with oral rehydration therapy for diarrhea (10–14 days of supplementation, up to the age of 5) as interventions which can contribute significantly to reducing child mortality world wide with relatively modest investments. Global evidence summaries have suggested that vitamin A supplementation can reduce all-cause mortality for children 6–59 months by 23%, and several studies have indicated that therapeutic zinc supplements for diarrhea can reduce diarrheal mortality below the age of five by 50%.

## 29.2 Magnitude of the problem

Undernutrition remains a major issue in developing countries, being an underlying cause of 3.5 million deaths each year [2]. It is estimated that up to 219 million children are deficient in vitamin A [3] and over 1 billion people are susceptible to zinc deficiency [2]. Children with these deficiencies are significantly more likely to experience morbidity and mortality. Vitamin A deficiency in newborn babies, infants, and children accounts for about 6% of under-5 deaths, 5% of under-5 DALYs (disability-adjusted life years), and 1.7% of total DALYs lost. Zinc deficiency accounts for about 4% of under-5 deaths and DALYs and 1% of total DALYs lost. Vitamin A deficiency annually claims the lives of almost 670,000 children under five and zinc deficiency claims more than 450,000 lives [2].

*Table 29.1* Global deaths and DALYs in children under 5 years attributable to micronutrient deficiencies – 2004

| *Deficiency* | *Deaths* | *Percentage of deaths in children under 5 years* | *Disease Burden in 1000 Disability Adjusted Life Years* (DALYs) | *Percentage of DALYs in children under 5 years* |
|---|---|---|---|---|
| Vitamin A | 667771 | 6.5% | 22668 | 5.3% |
| Zinc | 453207 | 4.4% | 16342 | 3.8% |

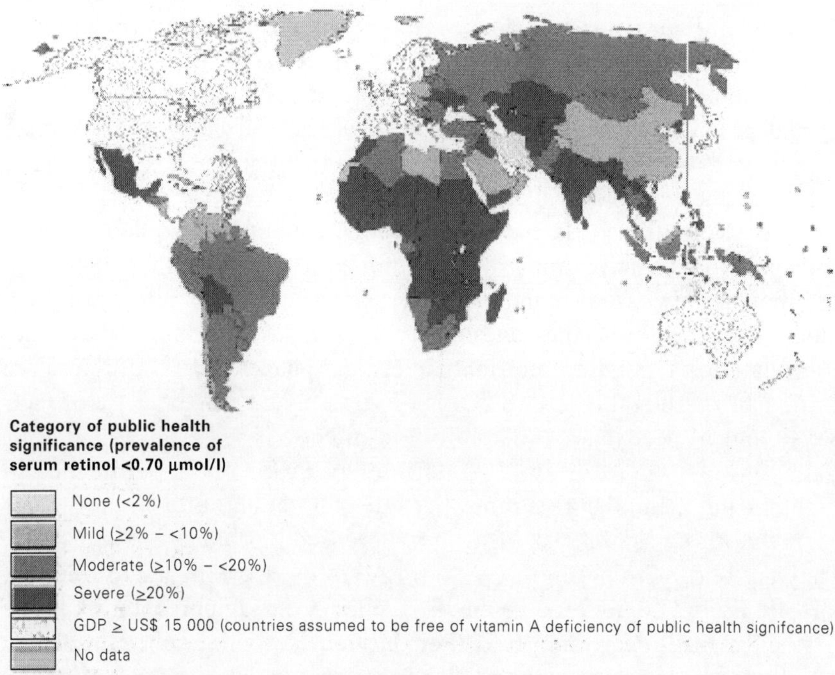


29.1 Global Prevalence of Vitamin A Deficiency (retinol) as a public health problem by country 1995–2005.

*Source*. WHO global prevalence of Vitamin A deficiency in population at risk 1995 2005. WHO global database on Vitamin A deficiency. Geneva, WHO, 2009.

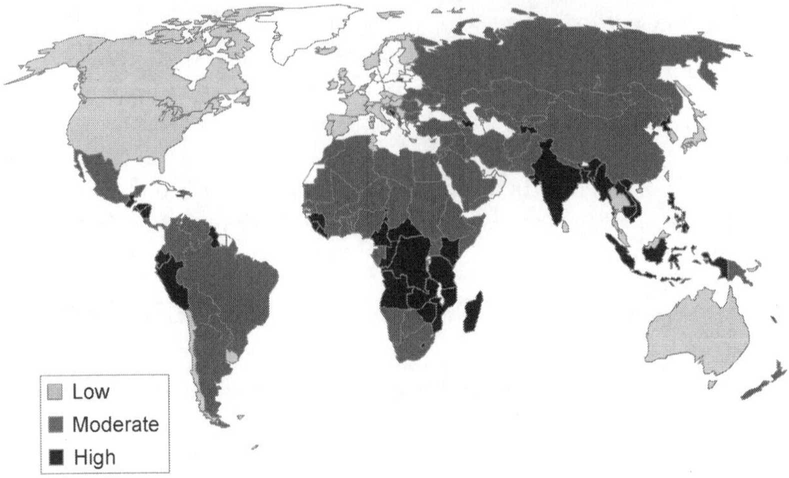


*29.2* National risk of zinc deficiency in children under 5 years [4]

## 29.3 The challenge

The diets of poor households in developing countries are lacking in many of the key vitamins and minerals, which are essential to keep people strong, healthy and productive. Dietary diversification, including consumption of animal products or more fruits and vegetables, can help satisfy human vitamin and mineral requirements. Though animal products are very good sources of the most bio-available forms of vitamin A, iron and of absorbable zinc; they are also costly food items which cannot be afforded by most poor people who have limited opportunities to diversify their meals. In addition, during periods of increased needs or acute vulnerability, everyday foods with high bulk and low density of vitamins and minerals do not contribute to the required nutrients in critical phases of life. Children are particularly vulnerable to deficiency of vitamin and zinc because of their physiological needs and vulnerability to infections.

In regions where vitamin A deficiency (VAD) is a public health problem and the under-five mortality rate is high, children under the age of five are at particular risk of further increased morbidity and mortality. They are born with negligible vitamin A stores, are exposed to frequent infections, and do not receive much vitamin A through breast milk in the first six months (particularly if their mother is malnourished). As they get older, even if some vitamin A rich foods are available in the household, young children cannot eat enough to prevent the effects of deficiency without being supplemented. To overcome deficiency in these children by eating fruits and vegetables alone, they would have to increase their intake many fold. Zinc deficiency may occur due to diets inadequate in bio-available zinc, certain diseases like diarrhea, loss of zinc in processing foods, and poor soil deprived of zinc with reduced zinc content in agricultural products. Zinc deficiency is also caused due to infections that decrease appetite and food intake (e.g. respiratory infections) and increase zinc loss.

The prevalence of zinc deficiency has not been adequately investigated, partly due to lack of suitable biomarkers. Based on the food balance data, it is estimated that a large section of the world population is at risk of developing zinc deficiency. The risk of deficiency is highest in populations, which consume predominantly cereal-based diets with little or no meat consumption.

Zinc occurs in a wide variety of food sources, but is found in highest concentrations in animal-source foods. Zinc content is also relatively high in nuts, seeds, legumes, and whole-grain cereals, and is lower in tubers, refined cereals, fruits, and vegetables. The absorption of zinc is inhibited by phytates and dietary calcium, and enhanced by protein. Thus predominantly plant-based diets with high phytate content and low consumption of animal-source foods contribute to low zinc consumption and limited absorption.

## 29.4 Vitamin A and zinc deficiencies – implications on child mortality

Both vitamin A and zinc have important roles in the immune system. The role of clinical vitamin A deficiency in measles mortality has been well understood for some decades, and a series of meta-analyses of the role of vitamin A in the early 1990s led to the consensus that vitamin A deficiency is associated with increased risk of mortality in children [5].

Evidence shows that in children 6–59 months, there is 47% higher chance of mortality due to diarrhea and a 35% higher chance of measles mortality associated with vitamin A deficiency in unsupplemented children.

The scientific evidence of the impact of zinc deficiency and those of zinc supplementation interventions are also quite recent and the meta-analyses mostly date after 2000. The increased risk of mortality associated with zinc deficiency is estimated to be 27% for diarrheal deaths, 18% for pneumonia related deaths, and 11% for malarial deaths. Similar effects of zinc deficiency on morbidity have been observed in trials of preventive zinc supplements in children aged 1–59 months [2]. Zinc deficiency is also associated with stunting, which has significant adverse effects on health and productivity. Studies suggest that therapeutic zinc for diarrhea can decrease mortality by 50%.

A series of large-scale trials of zinc supplementation among children suffering from diarrhea revealed that zinc-supplemented children had a significantly lower probability of continuing diarrhea (acute and persistent). In addition, zinc supplemented children had 26% faster recovery [6]. Zinc treatment also resulted in a 20% reduction in the chances of an episode lasting more than seven days. In a large trial in Bangladesh, mortality rates (excluding deaths from injury) were 51% lower in the cluster with therapeutic zinc supplementation for diarrhea, than the control [7]. Zinc-supplemented children had a 15% lower probability of continuing diarrhea on a given day in the acute-diarrhea trials and a 24% lower probability of continuing diarrhea and a 42% lower rate of treatment failure or death in the persistent diarrhea trials [6].

Appropriately, the Lancet journal series on child survival identified vitamin A supplementation and therapeutic zinc supplementation in childhood diarrhea as key proven interventions to reduce child mortality [8].

*Table 29.2* Under-5 deaths that could be prevented in 42 high-burden countries accounting for 90% of all child deaths if coverage of individual interventions were to be scaled up to 100% from estimated coverage in 2003 [8]

| | Mean estimated coverage of Target population (range among countries) |
|---|---|
| **Preventive Interventions** | |
| Breastfeeding (6–11 months) | 90% (42–100) |
| Measles vaccine | 68% (39–99) |
| Vitamin A | 55% (11–99) |
| Clean delivery (skilled attendant at birth) | 54% (6–89) |
| Tetanus toxoid | 49% (13–90) |
| Water, sanitation, hygiene | 47% (8–98) |
| Exclusive breastfeeding (<6 months) | 39% (1–84) |
| Newborn temperature management | 20% |
| Antibiotics for premature rupture of membranes | 10% |
| Antenatal steroids | 5% |
| Nevirapine and replacement feeding | 5% |
| Insecticide-treated materials | 2% (0–16) |
| Hib vaccine | 1% |
| Antimalarial intermittent preventive treatment in pregnancy | 1% |
| Zinc | 0% |
| Complementary feeding | † |
| **Treatment Interventions** | |
| Vitamin A | 55% (11–99) |
| Antibiotics for pneumonia | 40% |
| Antibiotics for dysentery | 30% |
| Antimalarials | 29% (3–65) |
| Oral rehydration therapy | 20% (4–50) |
| Antibiotics for sepsis | 10% |
| Newborn resuscitation | 3% |
| Zinc | 0% |

## 29.5 Approaches to address vitamin A deficiency

### 29.5.1 Food-based approaches

Ideally for children to be fully protected from VAD, they need to consume sufficient vitamin A to meet their physiological requirements. VAD can be controlled if dietary source and intake of vitamin A can be improved sufficiently and sustainably. Commercial marketing, community-based distribution, subsidized provision and/or social marketing of affordable vitamin A rich foods, and/or the development and increased cultivation of vitamin A rich foods, all can potentially help improving intake of vitamin A. However there is no comprehensive comparative assessment available of the extent and effectiveness of food-based approaches for VAD reduction vis-à-vis the health systems approach of providing periodic high dose vitamin A supplements (VAS).

Poverty is associated with poor quality diets which lack many micronutrients; poor diets lack protein and energy; diets low in animal products lack retinol. Improving diets could in principle tackle VAD and other issues simultaneously. This could involve increased production and consumption of micronutrient-rich foods, from commercial or home gardening sources, small livestock or aquaculture; nutrition education, mass media and programs aimed at changing food choices; steps to improve nutrient bioavailability by food processing or biotechnological measures. Increased intake of vitamin A from good plant sources such as red palm oil, orange flesh sweet potatoes etc, integrated with behaviour change support, can have a significant impact on nutritional status: giving red palm oil to children has been reported as having a small impact on reducing the prevalence of clinical VAD; providing it to mothers has been shown to increase maternal serum and breast milk retinol as well as infant serum retinol. However, much work remains to be done on resolving the logistics and costs of implementing such programs on wide scale.

Results from countries such as Nicaragua have shown that the widespread fortification of a commonly consumed food (sugar) in some settings can contribute to reducing VAD. Other countries are enriching other foods with vitamin A (South Africa: cereal flours; Bangladesh: edible oils); and World Food Program (WFP) policy requires international procured or donated vegetable oil to be fortified with vitamins A and D. However there is generally too little data to be able to assess the extent of the *effectiveness* of these approaches in reducing VAD in young children. The only evidence of large scale effectiveness relates to sugar fortification [9].

Prospects for achieving sustained improved widespread intake through food based approaches in the short term appear to be limited in countries with high child mortality rates and sub-optimal access to centrally processed foods. Such foods are often not accessible to the poorest and most deficient and this section of population may be the last to benefit from any enriched foods available other than through targeted feeding programs.

### 29.5.2 Health-systems-based provision of VAS

Where VAD is a public health problem, twice yearly provision of vitamin A supplements (VAS) to all children aged 6–59 months is accepted as a highly cost-effective way of improving intake. In addition, all cases needing therapeutic doses of vitamin A must be treated promptly in primary health care settings.

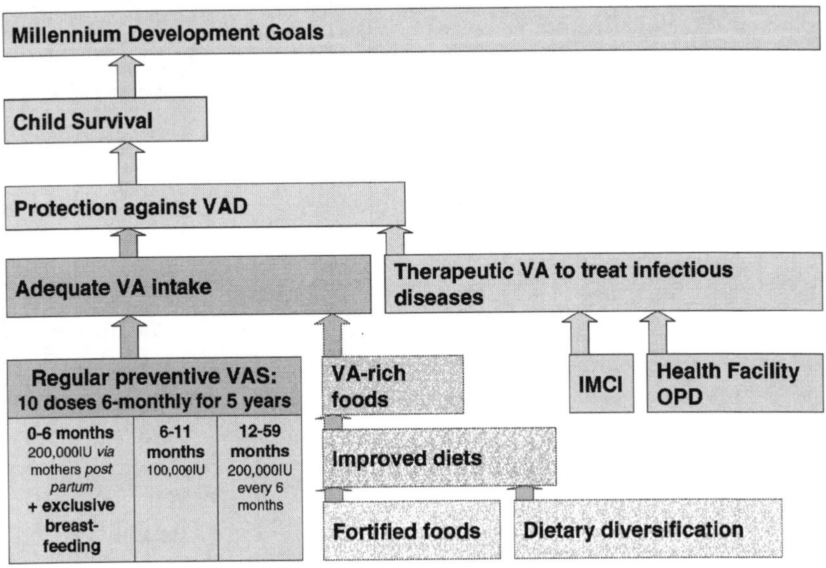


*29.3* The relationship between vitamin A and child survival

Thus, vitamin A is a critical nutrient which can promote child survival and help achieve the Millennium Development Goal No. 4.

### 29.5.3 Brief history of the VAS program for preschool children

India was one of the first countries in the world to launch a high dose vitamin A Supplementation program which was initiated in 1970 under the name "The National Prophylaxis Programme for Prevention of Blindness Due to Vitamin A Deficiency." Renewed focus on vitamin A supplementation at large scale began in the late 1990s when the World Health Organization (WHO), recognizing its impact on child survival recommended delivering VA supplements along with polio vaccination during immunization campaigns, called National Immunization Days (NIDs) and integrating its provision with other health services. As polio NIDs became widespread, increasing numbers of children under five received at least one high-dose of VAS each year. The scope of these immunization campaigns provided an opportunity for countries to achieve very high coverage of children under five every 6 months, however the strategy of linking vitamin A supplementation with polio NIDs was always recognized as being time-limited. As polio NIDs continue to be phased out, countries are faced with the challenge of maintaining the necessary high coverage twice a year, without the well-funded, vertical program of polio NIDs. Countries which achieved polio eradication or had only one NID in a year moved towards holding micronutrients days or integrated child health events to provide VAS and other complementary services to communities. This approach has been described as the 'REACH' (Regular Events to Advance Child Health). Many countries are now working to institutionalize twice yearly distribution using the existing health system infrastructure without the risk of drop in coverage. A series of assessments of supplementation programs in 20 countries with high under five mortality rates revealed that in many countries, vitamin A supplements are being distributed successfully through the routine, primary health care system when combined with regular, twice-yearly outreach of services targeting all children under five, such as Child Health Days [10]. Thus in many countries, national guidelines now define routine for vitamin A supplementation as a mix of facility-based, outreach and community-based interventions, though some countries continue to use polio NIDS for delivering at least one dose a year.

Until routine health services can reach all targeted children on a regular basis, outreach and biannual events such as Child Health Days will be critical to ensure full protection of children 6–59 months of age, not just with vitamin A supplements, but with other essential, preventive health services. Outreach entails not only extending the reach of the health services to all children who are live far from the health facility, but also to those older than 12 months who no longer receive regular immunizations.

For example, in Bangladesh, the strategy for vitamin A supplementation is two-fold: for children 6–11 months of age it is through the routine health services (Expanded Program of Immunization, 9 months of age measles booster) contact points, and to for children 12–59 months the twice-yearly Child Health Day approach is relied on, often called the National Vitamin A Plus Campaign. Conversely, in Kenya, twice-yearly coverage of children 6–59 months of age with vitamin A was over 80% when linked with immunization campaigns. However, in 2007 when the country decided to stop using campaigns and instead support increased delivery of routine services using fixed health facilities only (with no outreach), coverage for the full 6–59 month old age group dropped to approximately 20%. This drastic drop in coverage was not due as much to the 6–11 month old age group, whose coverage remained above 65% due to regular immunization contact points, but mainly due to the 12–59 month old age group whose coverage was less than 14% [11]. A similar problem is observed in India in those states that rely only on routine health services such as immunization contact points to deliver vitamin A supplementation, and which are only reaching children up to 18 months of age successfully. Child Health Days/Weeks or the Biannual Child Health & Nutrition promotion months as they are referred to in India, are a combination of fixed-site, outreach and community-based health days, offer the opportunity to strengthen the existing health system and deliver a package of essential child survival interventions. An example is in Ghana where their Child Health Days provide a package of services twice a year to over 80% of children 6–59 months, including vitamin A supplementation, immunization, deworming, re-treatment of insecticide-treated bed nets, issuing of child health cards and undertaking birth registration [10]. Another example is in Chattisgarh, India where a child protection month is celebrated twice a year (April and October) and delivers a package of services to over 85% of children. The services include vitamin A supplementation, deworming, growth monitoring, immunization focused on children never or partially vaccinated and salt testing for iodine content in households and community feeding centers.

In Indonesia, the months of February and August are designated "Vitamin A Months", where intensified communication and social mobilization encourages mothers to bring their children 6–59 months to their nearest health post for vitamin A supplementation, nutrition counseling, immunization and growth monitoring. In the Democratic Republic of Congo, the joint delivery of vitamin A and deworming is reported to boost the attendance of immunization and vitamin A supplementation programs [10]. Although such events require a significant amount of planning, strong logistical support and coordination among different departments of the Ministry of Health (EPI, Nutrition, Maternal Health for instance), the stakeholders and donors, they are very efficient in increasing coverage of several services at once.

The delivery two VA doses has became a key indicator of progress towards improved child health, and is reported annually in UNICEF's State of the World's Children report and has been adopted as an indicator of progress toward the MDG of reducing child mortality [11]. VAS provision is recognized as a key part of the 'arsenal of effective interventions against childhood killers.

**Box 29.1 Initiatives for VAS distribution in India**

In the late 1990s and early 2000s, States in India adopted various implementation strategies for VAS, as health falls under the State's mandate. Some States conducted vitamin A supplementation campaigns or distributed vitamin A along with pulse polio initiatives for achieving high coverage. However, these distribution mechanisms were halted by the Central Government in late 2001 due to reported side effects (vomiting and diarrhea) and 12 children dying after a vitamin A campaign in Assam (November 2001). Although a Government investigation found no evidence of a link between the vitamin A and the child deaths, the incidents were widely reported in Indian media and globally. The incident prompted the Government of India (GOI) to issue instructions to the States that they halt stand-alone vitamin A campaigns or vitamin A linked to polio National Immunization Days. This resulted in many States linking vitamin A with routine immunization, considerably lowering coverage.

Since 2004, VAS coverage has improved dramatically in most states. In part, this is because of increased advocacy for the program, increasing partner support, and movement toward a biannual approach. While most states include the first dose at the 9-month contact for measles, most also expand services to include older children during the biannual child health and nutrition promotion months.

The VAS program has been supported by a number of partners, including UNICEF, MI and A2Z, a USAID project and a variety of Indian NGOs including CARE and the Child in Need Institute (CINI) and the MI India trust (MII). These partners have helped in a variety of ways including help with procurement, training and capacity building, supervision and monitoring. The degree of support from partners varies considerably from state to state with most support focused on the states with higher child mortality.

## 29.5.4 Bottlenecks in achieving universal twice yearly VAS coverage

Assessments by MI and UNICEF in 2004, of the VAS programme in more than twenty countries, revealed several common findings with much still needed to be done to institutionalize ways of providing full and sustained protection against VAD to all children under five.

*Integration with routine health system efforts*

Many countries are working towards integrating VAS with routine immunization contacts at fixed sites and *via* outreach services. However the coverage currently achieved by these services is often sub-optimal. Second, this approach alone offers little scope to provide protection for children over a year old where immunization contacts focus on younger children. In a few cases, VAD control continues to be understood exclusively as a blindness prevention program; and the importance of VAS to child survival is not acknowledged.

*Resource commitments*

VAS in most countries is not included in government budgets; this weakens

VAS as a policy priority. Internationally, only a few donor agencies are actively funding vitamin A supplementation and investments in capacity and system strengthening approaches is inadequate and distribution costs are often not factored in adequately in donor contributions or in government budgets.

*Coordination issues*

Policy confusion and ineffective co-ordination at national level are exacerbated by mixed messages from the international community about primary health care (PHC) and child survival priorities and about the best strategies for controlling VAD. Insufficient collaboration and communication between many global initiatives makes it worse. VAD control programs end up fragmented between different units or departments, with gaps in policy and leadership, limited strategic choices, sub-optimal guidelines and poor co-ordination.

*Capacity issues*

Limited capacity and imperfect training in key operational areas, including supervision and monitoring, contribute to low rates of coverage.

*Monitoring performance*

Coverage estimation and denominators of children to be reached are not always reliable; and the emphasis placed on measuring percentage *(%) coverage* tends to obscure the importance of action at all levels to assure the provision of full and sustained protection for each child under five from VAD. Availability of sufficient supplies and other logistics and preparation of detailed micro-plans are not well monitored.

*Demand generation*

Following years of social mobilization alongside OPV, VAS does however seem reasonably well accepted by mothers and helps with their motivation to attend outreach or other contact points. However awareness of the benefits of VA is low with impact on night blindness being only consistent message that is known across communities.

*Supplies*

Supply chain, storage, inventory and logistics management are often weak with expiry of stocks and wastage being problems which are not effectively addressed.

In summary it appears from the analyses, that the factors critical to achieving universal coverage of twice yearly VA supplements among children under five are the existence and quality of policy guidelines, plans and strategies for delivering VAS; effectiveness of local championship and co-ordination of efforts to ensure that VAS is delivered to all children under five twice yearly; adequate state of the Primary Health Care infrastructure, availability of both financial, and appropriately trained human, resources; extent of advocacy about VAS and of public awareness about the benefits of VAS; quality and timeliness of monitoring, reporting and information exchange; availability and quality of operational support & training; and the efficiency of local supply chains & logistics.

## 29.5.5 Reaching the unreached children with VAS

In addition, well monitored programs are necessary to track progress, improve program delivery, and ensure that those intended to be reached are in fact being reached. Most countries will need complementary strategies to reach all children: the mainstream strategy to reach perhaps the first 80%, then the specialized, hard-to-reach strategy for the last 20%. The cost per child reached will vary between these two strategies, the "last 20%" expected to be the most costly to reach, but expected to yield a higher benefit.

Although there is a strong belief that children who are currently not reached by vitamin A supplementation program are the most vulnerable and those arguably most in need, there is yet no clear picture of who are the unreached.

Two studies from Indonesia suggest that children who are not supplemented come from lower socioeconomic status households, with lower immunization rates and lower parental education than children receiving supplements [12, 13]. Although it is assumed that the unreached live in geographically inaccessible areas, weak urban health infrastructure in poor urban areas makes health services such as vitamin A supplementation a challenge. Therefore in many cases, the unreached may also live in or around big cities such as Nairobi and Delhi. Ongoing operations research and pilot programs comparing alternative strategies to reach hard-to-reach populations will yield cost data and a better understanding of who are the unreached. Working with local and community-based organizations or using community extenders is one way to identify and reach the hard to reach.

**Box 29.2 Reaching the unreached – The Bangladesh experience**

A successful program in rural Bangladesh initiated in 2007 provides a good model for the rest of Asia, and the world, on how to reach the unreached. It was estimated that around 600,000 children in Bangladesh, primarily from socio-economically vulnerable households were not being reached with vitamin A supplementation. Building on an already successful two-district pilot project to reach hard-to reach children, local resource persons were trained and deployed as Vitamin A Extenders in more than 12 districts, who then coordinated with government health staff and trained special community volunteers. The volunteers collected data, conducted house-to-house visits, made follow-up visits and monitored distribution. Through this outreach, not only did 360,000 formerly unreached rural children receive vitamin A, but also essential information was collected about the needs of those children so they can receive additional health and social services. Key to this success was the use of active involvement of community groups and special volunteers, including women, active in the community in monitoring, collecting data and mobilizing families with previously unreached children. It cost about three times as much to reach this group of children as compared to those reached by regular distribution in 2007, although it is hoped that the differential could be reduced such that the "hard-to-reach" group would only cost 50% more than the regular distribution in future. [14]

## 29.5.6 Post-partum maternal and neonatal VAS

Post-partum vitamin A supplementation for breastfeeding mothers, which is recommended to ensure that all infants receive the immune-boosting protection of vitamin A in the first six months of life, lags behind supplementation for children 6–59 months of age. Programs exist in only two thirds of priority countries, and most are limited in scope. International recommendations also allow for low-dose supplementation of pregnant women with xerophthalmia, but coverage is not widespread.

### *Supplementing mothers – missed opportunities*

Opportunities exist to administer supplements to mothers at delivery in health facilities or more commonly at home. In Nepal, community health volunteers, many of them illiterate, administer vitamin A supplements to mothers soon after birth. Alternatively, mothers can receive their post-partum dose at the time of the newborn's first immunization contact for BCG. While BCG coverage is quite high in most countries (approximately 80%), not many countries actually use this opportunity to supplement new mothers with vitamin A, which clearly represents a missed opportunity.

### *Emerging research – neonatal high dose VA supplementation*

Review of recent evidence suggests that supplementing newborns with a single large dose (50,000 IU) within a couple of days of birth reduces neonatal mortality [15]. It appears that providing a vitamin A supplement to newborns in South Asia in the first 48 hours can reduce the risk of infant death by approximately 20% [15, 16]. As some other studies have not demonstrated similar benefits [17], the WHO is currently commissioning a set of studies to facilitate the generation of further scientific evidence in different geographical contexts. Further confusion exists as it has been shown in several studies that vitamin A supplementation of children 1–5 months of age has no effect on child morbidity or mortality rates.

## 29.6 Addressing zinc deficiency

It is clear from the results of numerous zinc supplementation trials that a wide range of health benefits can be realized by increasing the intake of zinc where intakes were previously insufficient [4]. The approaches to increase zinc intake can be classified under:

### 29.6.1 Food-based approaches

Strategies to diversify or modify the diet aim to enhance the access to, and utilization of, foods with a high content of absorbable zinc throughout the year. These strategies can involve changes in food production practices, food selection patterns, and traditional household methods for preparing and processing indigenous foods.

Agricultural strategies to increase total and/or absorbable zinc content in staple foods include the use of fertilizers and improved plant breeding and genetic modification while strategies to increase production and/or intake of zinc-rich foods include promoting small live stock production or aquaculture. Household processing methods such as soaking, germination and fermentation can help increase the absorbable zinc in the diet [4].

Fortification of both staples and snacks with zinc has been attempted but no evidence of impact is available at large scale.

### 29.6.2 Zinc supplementation

Research trials have indicated reduction of morbidities as well as impact on mortality with both preventive as well as therapeutic zinc supplementation. However the evidence for preventive zinc supplementation, especially with regards to reduction of mortality is not conclusive. Two large studies on the impact on zinc on mortality conducted in Nepal and in Tanzania [18, 19] reported a modest non-significant reduction in overall mortality in children under five years of age. When all of the prevention trials examining the impact on mortality of zinc supplementation in young children (excluding trials that only included selected specific groups such as low birth weight or malnourished children) are viewed together, a 9% reduction in mortality is observed [20].

There is however compelling evidence regarding the benefits of therapeutic zinc along oral rehydration therapy for childhood diarrhea which has built scientific consensus supporting low osmolarity oral rehydration salts and zinc for diarrhea management. This led to the joint WHO/UNICEF recommendation of administering 10–14 days of therapeutic zinc for children under 5 years of age along with oral rehydration. Zinc supplementation paired with low osmolarity oral rehydration solution (ORS) were recognized as important approaches to tackle childhood diarrhea which would be critical for achieving the Millennium Development Goal 4 on reduction of child mortality by two thirds of 1990 levels.

### 29.6.3 Global developments to introduce and scale up the new recommendations on use of zinc and change in guidelines for use of low osmolarity ORS

The new WHO/UNICEF recommendations on the clinical management of acute diarrhea, including the provision of zinc to all children with diarrhea treated in health facilities and at home, with ORS or recommended home fluids, were published in May 2004 [21]. Following this recommendation all WHO diarrhea management guidelines, including the Integrated Management of Childhood Illness (IMCI) treatment charts, were revised to incorporate these new recommendations. In March 2005, zinc was added to the WHO Model List of Essential Medicines [22].

New documents were developed by the WHO in collaboration with the Zinc Task Force to facilitate the adoption and implementation of the new diarrhea recommendations at country level, and to assist program managers and pharmaceutical manufacturers in choosing or producing zinc products adequate for use in the management of diarrhea.

### 29.6.4 Moving from efficacy to effectiveness to full scale programs: need for traction

In order to assist countries in including zinc supplementation in the management of diarrhea, three introduction studies were conducted in India, Mali and Pakistan. The aims were to assess potential constraints when implementing this new recommendation together with the administration of lower osmolarity ORS solution, as well as to determine the best possible delivery channels for zinc supplements. The preliminary results from these three large effectiveness studies clearly show that zinc encourages greater uptake of ORS and reduces inappropriate drug use. One study showed that an intervention that included caregiver education on the use of zinc and ORS during childhood diarrhea, and provision of both zinc and ORS by public and private health care providers to caregivers, was associated with reduction in the prevalence of diarrhea and pneumonia, and in all-cause, diarrhea, and pneumonia hospitalizations. The intervention also resulted in reduction in the use of unwarranted oral and injectable drugs during diarrhea, reduction in the out-of-pocket costs for care of diarrhea to the family, and substantial increase in the ORS use rates. [23]

Nevertheless, delays in moving from knowledge to action are being currently experienced. Policy initiatives, such as the joint WHO/UNICEF statement, have not yet acquired enough momentum to ensure widespread introduction of low osmolarity ORS and zinc across the world. Only about 53 countries have included therapeutic zinc in the diarrhea management policy, and fewer than 30 countries have initiated pilot programs so far [24]. Bangladesh is the only country to attempt a national scale-up, and Nepal is the first country to engage in large-scale social marketing, which now covers half its population [25]. Several other countries such as India, Guatemala and Bolivia have issued policy guidelines and are in the process of rolling out their programs.

The private sector is very critical in improving access to appropriate diarrhea treatment. The USAID supported POUZN (Point of Use Water Disinfection) project has supported the marketing of zinc products in India, Indonesia, and Tanzania by the private sector and raised awareness regarding the intervention and availability of product among health providers of both the formal and non-formal sectors. A diarrhea treatment kit (DTK), created by packaging together zinc tablets and ORS and delivered through both commercial retail outlets and NGOs, has been piloted successfully in Cambodia [25].

**Box 29.3 Steps in scaling up of the Zinc and ORS Program for childhood diarrhea**

- Awareness of the policy at all levels including states and districts.
- Defining roles and responsibilities of all stakeholders.
- Devising program strategy and its adaptation in different settings.
- Procuring supplies of zinc and ORS and logistics.
- Developing training material and program for training different cadres.
- Developing monitoring and evaluation systems that will include measurement of coverage and costs.
- Provide for mid-course corrections and continuing innovation.

**Box 29.4 The Bangladesh experiences of scale up Zinc and ORS Programme [26]**

Building upon the success of small-scale introduction through effectiveness trial activities in Matlab, the Gates-funded SUZY project was implemented in Bangladesh with the objective of nationally scaling up zinc. This is the first such example of efforts to nationally introduce zinc. Zinc, like ORS was listed as an over the counter (OTC) drug which was distributed through all possible channels, including the informal private sector.

The development of a local brand of zinc dispersible tablets was a key element of the strategy with an attractive tag line rhyming with a bicycle's ring "Cring... Cring... Baby Zinc" along with a logo of a playful boy and girl being used in all forms of advertising across the country.

Demand for this new product was created through two mechanisms:

- Provider promotion, and
- Mass media marketing once the product was well known from providers and the strategy was in place.

From what little has been reported it is known that while efforts to promote zinc through intensive provider engagement, mass media campaigns, and other strategies, corresponded to increased awareness, zinc coverage rates remained low with the Demographic Health Survey, 2007 reporting a 23% overall use rate with a 33% urban use rate and a 20% rural use rate.

### 29.6.5 Challenges of scale up of zinc use in childhood diarrhea in India

In India, the apex professional organization, the Indian Academy of Pediatrics (IAP) approved zinc as an adjunct therapy to ORS in the management of diarrhea in the year 2004 and the revised guidelines were endorsed in September 2007. The revised national policy for the treatment of childhood diarrhea announced by the Government of India in November 2006 include zinc as an adjunct to ORS in the management of acute diarrhea in the national program. The recommendation is that all cases of diarrhea receive a 20 mg zinc sulphate dispersible tablet; ½ tablet for infants aged 2 months to 6 months and 1 tablet for older children, for 14 days in addition to ORS. The policy emphasizes that (i) zinc tablets should be available in all parts of the country including at child care centres of ICDS or Anganwadi centres, (ii) that zinc be made an over-the-counter (OTC) formulation, (iii) an effective communication strategy be put in place and that (iv) health care providers are oriented and trained in the use of zinc along with ORS.

Zinc dispersible tablets are a part of the new treatment guidelines and the Government of India has already accepted zinc dispersible tablets (20 mg) as a part of supply kit A of the Reproductive Child Health Programme (RCH).

The following challenges are recognized to be critical for the successful scaling up the new diarrhea case management package in the Indian context:

*ORS use rates*

ORS use rates in India continue to remain low for the last 25 years. The strategy for scaling up zinc treatment should be a package along with ORS.

Recent programmatic trials have shown that when zinc is packaged with ORS, the ORS use rates go up dramatically. In addition to health facilities, community depot holders for zinc and ORS need to be created.

*Creating awareness in stakeholders*

All stakeholders including those at the state level need to be sensitized to the new diarrhea policy. This would include state and district level planners.

*Communications strategy*

A strong communications strategy with regional focus is essential for promotion of usage of ORS and Zinc. Although mass media would help boost the use rates the involvement of mass media should only occur once all the providers are sensitized and supplies are in place.

*Involvement of the private sector*

Data from various surveys show at large majority of diarrhea is treated by the private sector (formal and informal). Pediatricians and other formal providers will need to be sensitized through the provider associations. The new strategy should effectively reach networks of the informal private sector and sensitize them on the use of ORS and zinc as well.

*Formulations, pricing and supplies*

ORS and zinc are OTC products with a unique safety profile and therefore should be easily accessible and readily available to families close to their homes.

Dispersible tablets of zinc and ORS should be dispensed free of cost through the government system i.e. from the PHC and community based outreach workers such as Anganwadi workers and health community volunteers such as ASHA.

The private sector would have several options for dispersible tablets and syrups available in the market to choose from. However, keeping in mind the competition with antibiotics and anti-diarrheals, the pricing of these formulations should be such that the profit margin for the providers does not reduce substantially.

*Monitoring and evaluation systems*

Follow up action will need to be ensured at all levels and once the programs are in place, monitoring and evaluation systems need to be designed which are integrated with the existing systems and are able to guide decision making for improving the program reach and quality.

**Box 29.5 Zinc and ORS distribution in an emergency situation in Bihar**

In October 2008, large parts of the state of Bihar were ravaged by floods due to breach in the embankments of the river *Kosi* near the Indo-Nepal border, leading to a change in the course of the river which affected more than 4 million people living in 5 districts of the state (Araria, Purnea, Supaul, Madhepura and Saharsa) which are downstream from the breach in the river near the Nepal border.

The Government of Bihar as part of the flood relief measures planned to advance the biannual round of VAS distribution by 1 month in these 5 districts. They included the distribution of zinc and Low osmolarity ORS for children with diarrhea as part of the package of services.

The Government of Bihar with assistance from UNICEF and MI distributed 58,000 Diarrhea Treatment Kits (DTKs) (consisting of a 10 day course of zinc (in accordance with WHO guidelines) and 2 packets of low osmolarity ORS) to children suffering from diarrhea in five flood affected districts as part of a special child health package along with vitamin A supplementation (VAS) which is delivered twice a year, through a special biannual approach in Bihar.

The use of biannual VAS rounds to promote the use of zinc and ORS for the treatment of diarrhea was unique as it allowed multiple synergistic child health services to be provided at the same time. As part of the flood relief operations, it offered humanitarian aid in the time of crisis. Since zinc had not been distributed in the state along with ORS, the introduction of zinc during this period provided an opportunity to demonstrate positive attributes of zinc as a package of health services. It also provided an opportunity to check the effectiveness of the use of VAS biannual rounds as a means to promote the use and the knowledge of the use of zinc for treatment of diarrhea.

There were logistical difficulties in ensuring the availability of supplies at field level, given the nature of the emergency, with the process evaluation survey reporting that 14% of sites reporting not having received the DTKs and only 59% of sites reporting that the quantities supplied were adequate.

As it was a new intervention, the level of preparedness of frontline workers was not optimum, as only 74% of workers said that they recommended that zinc tablets be taken for 10–14 days.

## 29.7 Economic analysis of cost and benefit of vitamin A and zinc supplementation

The cost per child for achieving different levels of coverage of vitamin A supplementation and therapeutic zinc supplementation has been estimated for different parts of the world (see Table 29.3). It is generally accepted that it would cost more and be increasingly difficult to scale up coverage to reach the last 20% of the population who are likely to be the 'hard to reach'. These interventions are highly cost effective at these costs given the likely impact in terms of lives saved.

*Table 29.3* Estimates of total cost of supplementation per child per year, by region and level of coverage [27]

| Region(s) | Vitamin A, coverage 20–80% | Vitamin A, coverage 80–90% | Zinc, coverage 0–40% |
|---|---|---|---|
| South Asia, Sub-Saharan Africa, East Asia | $1.20 | $2.40 | $1.00 |
| Central Asia | $1.60 | $3.20 | $1.35 |
| Latin America and the Caribbean | $2.60 | $5.20 | $2.20 |

## 29.7.1 Vitamin A supplementation

VAS is relatively inexpensive on a per-child basis. Costs vary widely by region, tend to be lower in large-scale government programs than smaller non-government-organization programs, and are lower when vitamin A supplement delivery is combined with other health interventions. Reported costs are often substantially underestimated if personnel time is not included since the cost of capsule /VA syrup may be only 5–10% of costs. Other program costs include expenditure on training, logistics, promotional material etc.

Cost-effectiveness studies have estimated the per death-averted costs are less than US$ 500 as estimated in different contexts and regions, usually ranging from about US$228 through the Enhanced Outreach Strategy of using Child Health days in Ethiopia [28] to about US$ 327 in Nepal where community health workers are used for VA supplement distribution [29]. Costs per death averted vary depending on the number and proportion of the child population reached, number of doses received per child, and child mortality rates and the actual distribution costs involved [30]. This makes vitamin A supplementation among the most cost effective public health interventions in the world.

As there are no current zinc and ORS programs at significant scale, operational research is needed to develop and test varying delivery mechanisms in the public and private sectors (formal and informal), including comparative cost analysis. Estimates of cost-effectiveness by Robberstad et al [31] suggest that the incremental cost of zinc as part of case management is $0.47 per course of treatment, leading to an average cost of $73 per DALY gained, and $2,100 per death-averted. The cost of tablets range from $0.01 to 0.02 each, hence a course of the tablets costs about $0.10–0.19, with the additional costs representing distribution and administration. A broad cost analysis for a micronutrient investment plan for India estimated that it would cost US$0.35 per child per episode of diarrhea including programmatic costs such as training, communication material and monitoring, for a scale up of therapeutic zinc for childhood diarrhea [32].

Preliminary results from the economic evaluations performed in India and Pakistan based on the large-scale effectiveness trials have shown that zinc is cost effective in treating diarrhea in patients under 5 years as compared to ORS alone in this setting. The introduction of zinc led to a decrease in out of pocket payments for medicine/ consultation fees of over USD$1.00 per patient per episode.

## 29.8 Implications and conclusions

Vitamin A supplementation for young children and therapeutic zinc supplements for management of diarrhea in young children should be treated as priority interventions. Although, twice yearly vitamin A supplementation is now occurring in many countries as part of a minimum package of health services, the challenge is to ensure that the remaining 30% of children, who are not covered, are being reached to ensure and sustain universal supplementation for child survival. This requires additional resources to "do that last mile" and commitment from governments to mobilize and efficiently use supplementary resources. Countries which are lagging behind need to adopt best practices including twice yearly events like Child Health Days to extend the outreach of the primary health care system, identifying those who are regularly unreached, and using of vitamin A coverage as a health performance indicator.

Experience with zinc supplementation as an adjunct treatment for diarrhea is more recent. In spite of strong evidence of efficacy of zinc supplementation and more recently on effectiveness, very few countries have shown encouraging progress by revising their diarrhea management policy to include zinc, encouraging local production, ensuring sufficient supplies, and creating demand through social mobilization and marketing. It is essential that therapeutic zinc supplementation is integrated into the primary health care system at the community level. Such a strategy has been demonstrated to synergistically help boost ORS coverage as well. Twice yearly vitamin A supplementation through the REACH strategy and provision of ORS and zinc by community level providers to children with diarrhea will help achieve universal coverage with these essential child health interventions, which is a must for developing nations to reduce child mortality significantly and the world to achieve the Millennium Development Goals and move beyond.

## References

1. COPENHAGEN CONSENSUS (2008). Available at http://www.copenhagenconsensus.com/home.aspx (Accessed on 07.11.2009).
2. BLACK RE, ALLEN LH, BHUTTA ZA, CAULFIELD LE , DE ONIS M, EZZATI M, MATHERS C, RIVERA J (2008). The Maternal and Child Undernutrition Study Group, Maternal and Child Undernutrition: Global and Regional Exposures and Health Consequences, *The Lancet*, **371**(9608), p. 253.

3. MASON J, RIVERS J, HELWIG C (2005). Recent trends in malnutrition in developing regions: vitamin A deficiency, anemia, iodine deficiency and child underweight. *Food and Nutrition Bulletin*, **26**, pp. 57–162.
4. HOTZ C and BROWN KH (eds) (2004). IZINCG Technical Document No 1. Assessment of the risk of zinc deficiency in populations and options for its control. *Food Nutr Bull*, p. 25.
5. BEATON GH et al. (1993). Effectiveness of vitamin A supplementation in the control of young child morbidity and mortality in developing countries. Nutrition Policy Discussion Paper 13: Administrative Committee on Coordination—Subcommittee on Nutrition (ACC/SCN). Geneva, Switzerland: World Health Organization.
6. BHUTTA ZA, BIRD SM, BLACK RE, BROWN KH, GARDNER JM, HIDAYAT A, KHATUN F, MARTORELL R, NINH NX, PENNY ME, ROSADO JL, ROY SK, RUEL M, SAZAWAL S, SHANKAR A (2000). The Zinc Investigators' Collaborative Group. *Am J Clin Nutr*, **72**, pp. 1516–1522.
7. BAQUI AH, BLACK RE, ARIFEEN SE, YUNUS M, CHAKRABORTY J, AHMED S, VAUGHAN JP (2002). Effect of Zinc Supplementation Started During Diarrhoea on Morbidity and Mortality in Bangladeshi Children: Community Randomised Trial, *BMJ*, **32**(5), p. 1059. Downloaded from http://www.bmj.com on 25 September 2008.
8. JONES G, STEKETEE RW, BLACK RE, BHUTTA ZA, MORRIS SS and the Bellagio Child Survival Study Group (2003). How Many Child Deaths Can We Prevent This Year. *The Lancet*, p. 362, http://www.thelancet.com.
9. ARROYAVE G, MEJIA LA and AGUILAR JR (1981). The Effect of Vitamin A Fortification of Sugar on the Serum Vitamin A Levels of Preschool Guatemalan Children: A Longitudinal Evaluation. *Am. J. Clin. Nutr*, **34**, pp. 41–49.
10. AGUAYO VM, GARNIER D, BAKER SK (2007). Drops of Life: Vitamin A Supplementation for Child Survival. Progress and Lessons Learned in West and Central Africa. UNICEF Regional Office for West and Central Africa.
11. WAGSTAFF A and CLEASON M (2004). The Millennium Development Goals for Health: Rising to the Challenges. Washington DC: World Bank.
12. PANGARIBUAN R, ERHARDT JG, SCHERBAUM V, BIESALSKI HK (2003). Vitamin A Capsule Distribution to Control Vitamin A Deficiency in Indonesia: Effect of Supplementation in Pre-School Children and Compliance with the Programme. *Public Health Nutr*, **6**(2), pp. 209–216.
13. BERGER SG, DE PEE S, BLOEM MW, HALATI S, SEMBA RD (2008). Malnutrition and Morbidity are higher in children who are missed by periodic vitamin A capsule distribution for child survival in rural Indonesia, *Public Health*, **122**(4), pp. 371–378.
14. MICRONUTRIENT INITIATIVE. Annual Report 2008-09.
15. HAIDER BA and BHUTTA ZA (2008). Review of Vitamin A Supplementation in the Neonatal Period, Webappendix 11, Lancet Series on Maternal and Child Undernutrition, http://www.globalnutritionseries.org (accessed on June 18, 2008).
16. KLEMM RD, LABRIQUE AB, CHRISTIAN P, RASHID M, SHAMIM AA, KATZ J, SOMMER A, WEST KP, JR (2008). Newborn Vitamin A Supplementation Reduced Infant Mortality in Rural Bangladesh, *Pediatrics*, **122**(1), pp. E242–E250.
17. MALABA LC et al. (2005). Effect of postpartum maternal or neonatal vitamin A supplementation on infant mortality among infants born to HIV-negative mothers in Zimbabwe. *Am J Clin Nutr*, **81**, pp. 454–460.

18. SAZAWAL S, BLACK RE, RAMSAN M, CHWAYA HM, DUTTA A, DHINGRA U, STOLTZFUS RJ, OTHMAN MK, KABOLE FM (2007). Effect of Zinc Supplementation on Mortality in Children Aged 1–48 Months: A Community-Based Randomised Placebo Controlled Trial, p. 369.
19. TIELSCH JM, KHATRY SK, STOLZFUS RJ, KATZ J, LECLERQ SC, ADHIKARI R, MULLANY LC, BLACK R, SHRESTA S (2007). Effect of Daily Zinc Supplementation on Child Mortality in Southern Nepal: A Community-Based, Cluster Randomized Placebo-Controlled Trial, vol. 370, http://www.thelancet.com.
20. Report of Workshop to Review the Results of Studies Evaluating the Impact of Zinc Supplementation on Childhood Mortality and Severe Morbidity (Geneva, Switzerland, 15–16 September, 2006).
21. WHO/UNICEF (2004). Joint Statement on The Clinical Management of Acute Diarrhoea.
22. http://whqlibdoc.who.int/hq/2005/a87017eng.pdf (accessed on 09.02.2010).
23. BHANDARI N, MAZUMDAR S, TANEJA S, DUBE B, AGARWAL RC, MAHALANABIS D, FONTAINE O, BLACK RE, BHAN MK (2008). Effectiveness of Zinc Supplementation Plus Oral Rehydration Salts Compared with Oral Rehydration Salts Alone as a Treatment for Acute Diarrhoea in a Primary Care Setting: A Cluster Randomized Trial. *Pediatrics*, **12**(1), pp. E1279–E1285.
24. FISCHER CLW, FONTAINE O, YOUNG MW, BLACK RE. Zinc and Low-Osmolarity Ors for Diarrhoea: A Call to Action Four Years After the WHO/UNICEF Global Recommendation. Unpublished.
25. DARY O, HARVEY P, HOUSTON R, RAH J (2008). The Evidence on Micronutrient Programs: A Selected Review, *Micronutrient Forum.*
26. KOEHLMOOS T (2009). *Scaling Up Zinc For The Treatment Of Young Children With Diarrhoea. ICDDR*, B: Dhaka, Bangladesh.
27. HORTON S, BEGIN F, GREIG A, LAKSHMAN A (2008). Best Practice Paper, Micronutrient Supplements For Child Survival (Vitamin A And Zinc), Copenhagen Consensus Center, Working Paper.
28. FIEDLER JL and CHUKO T (2008). The Cost of Child Health Days: A Case Study of The Ethiopian EOS Program. *Health Policy and Planning*, **23**, pp. 222–233.
29. FIEDLER JL (2000). The Nepal National Vitamin A Program: Prototype to Emulate or Donor Enclave? *Health Policy and Planning*, **15**(2), pp. 145–156.
30. CHING P, BIRMINGHAM M, GOODMAN T, SUTTER R, LOEVINSOHN B (2000). Childhood Mortality Impact and Costs of Integrating Vitamin A Supplementation into Immunization Campaigns. *Am J Pub Health*, **90**(10), pp. 1526–1529.
31. ROBBERSTAD B, STRAND T, BLACK RE, SOMMERFELT H (2004). *Bulletin of the World Health Organization*, 82(7).
32. MICRONUTRIENT INITIATIVE (2007). India Micronutrient Investment Plan.

# 30

# Addressing micronutrient malnutrition through food fortification

*Saraswati Bulusu* and *Annie S. Wesley*

**Saraswati Bulusu**, PhD, in Biochemistry from Calcutta University, with specialization in Nutritional Toxicology, has undertaken special trainings in Program Monitoring and Evaluation at Tufts University, Boston, and Project & Financial Management at IIM Bangalore. Dr. Bulusu was a National Program Manager and the Managing Trustee of the Micronutrient Initiative, India, for more than 10 years and was responsible for developing various fortified low cost products and introduction of such products in the public and private systems. She is currently a nutrition specialist with UNICEF, Hyderabad office, India. She is a recipient of the Junior Scientist Award of the Indian Science Congress Association, Government of India.

**Annie S. Wesley** is a Senior Program Specialist at the Micronutrient Initiative, Ottawa, Canada since 1999. Dr. Wesley completed PhD in Food Science from the Central Food Technological Research Institute, Mysore, India and obtained post-doctoral experience in cereal chemistry and food technology from the Department of Grain Science and Industry, Kansas State University, USA and the Cereal Research Centre, Winnipeg, Canada. Currently she provides technical support in the area of food fortification to MI programs in Asia, Africa and the Middle East.

## 30.1 Introduction

Malnutrition is broadly categorized as macro malnutrition caused primarily due to deficiency of proteins and calories and micronutrient malnutrition caused due to deficiency of micronutrients such as vitamin A, vitamin $B_1$, vitamin $B_2$, vitamin $B_3$, folic acid, iodine, iron, calcium, zinc, selenium, etc. Data from developing country such as India show that percentage of children and adults with intake of major micronutrients below 50% recommended dietary allowances (RDA) is rather high (Table 30.1) [1]. Intake of iron is less than 50% of the RDA in all age groups, with the proportions varying from 70% to 80%. Similarly, vitamin A intake is less than 50% of the RDA in all age groups, with the proportions varying from

80% to 90%. There is increasing evidence to show that lack of micronutrients cause devastating damage to health and well being of the population [2].

*Table 30.1* Percentage of adults and children with nutrient intake below 50% of the RDA in rural areas of India in 2001

| Adults (% <50% RDA) | | | | | Children (% <50% RDA) | | | | |
|---|---|---|---|---|---|---|---|---|---|
| Age (year and sex) | Proteins | Calories | Iron | Vitamin A | Age (year and sex) | Proteins | Calories | Iron | Vitamin A |
| =18 F(L) | 13.9 | 1.3 | 71.1 | 86.7 | 1–3 | 17.4 | 38.0 | 72.1 | 87.5 |
| =18 F(P) | 15.4 | 1.6 | 68.1 | 82.4 | 4–6 | 6.3 | 24.1 | 70.7 | 87.3 |
| =18 F (NPL) | 4.7 | 1.4 | 67.9 | 85.7 | 7–9 | 11.2 | 19.0 | 76.2 | 90.0 |
| =18 M | 5.4 | 3.0 | 50.1 | 83.5 | 10–12 M | 19.2 | 16.8 | 80.7 | 87.8 |
| 16–17 F | 22.7 | 5.9 | 71.2 | 87.8 | 10–12 F | 23.8 | 8.5 | 77.5 | 87.8 |
| 16–17M | 24.7 | 6.6 | 73.3 | 87.8 | 13–15 M | 24.4 | 10.3 | 79.6 | 86.3 |
| | | | | | 13–15 F | 24.9 | 5.8 | 68.0 | 87.7 |

M – Male; F – female; L – lactating; P – pregnant; NPL – neither pregnant nor lactating.

Micronutrient malnutrition is commonly referred to as "hidden hunger", since micronutrient deficiencies often go unnoticed but cause individuals and families to suffer serious consequences including learning disabilities, impaired work capacity and illness, ultimately leading to death. Though micronutrients are required only in milligrams or micrograms, these nutrients are necessary for efficient metabolic activities and for functions such as growth, cognition, immune system and reproduction. It is therefore important to address micronutrient malnutrition right from the early childhood to reduce long-term effects on growth and development. The implications of micronutrient deficiencies on the millennium development goals are presented in Table 30.2 [3].

## 30.2 Micronutrient malnutrition – an overview

Nearly one-third of people, especially in the developing world, are affected by one or more micronutrient deficiencies, principally iron, iodine, vitamin A, folic acid or zinc [2]. The critical role of vitamins and minerals in the health and well being is demonstrated by the fact that iron, zinc and vitamin A deficiencies are among the first 15 of 26 major risk factors of the global burden of disease (Figure 30.1) [4].

A recent global progress report states that 35 percent of people in the world lack adequate iodine, 40 percent in the developing world suffer

*Table 30.2* Linkages between micronutrient deficiencies and Millennium Development Goals (MDGs) [3]

| Goal | Impact of vitamin A deficiency (VAD) | Impact of iron deficiency anemia (IDA) | Impact of iodine deficiency disorders(IDD) |
|---|---|---|---|
| | **On countries:** higher burden of death and disease to be managed | **On countries:** economic loss in affected countries = 1% of GDP | **On countries:** In iodine deficient population mean IQ lowered by 10–15% |
| **Poverty and hunger impact** (MDG1) | **On caregivers:** care for the sick/dying<br>**On families:** cost of funerals<br>**On families:** loss of future earnings | **On adults:** reduces productivity<br>**On caregivers:** care for the sick | **On adults:** negatively affects livelihoods<br>**On children:** impairs learning<br>**On caregivers:** care for the sick |
| **Education and literacy impact** (MDG2) | **On children:** decreased school attendance | **On children:** impaired mental development for 50% of 6–24 month-old children in developing world: hard to learn and keep jobs | **On children:** impaired mental development for 18 million children globally: 60,000 severely mentally retarded |
| **Gender equality impact** (MDG3) | **On women and girl children:** caring for sick young children affects earning a livelihood | **On adults:** impaired productivity increases risks to livelihood. Greater health impact on women. | **On women and girl children:** caring for sick young children affects earning a livelihood and school attendance |
| **Child mortality impact** (MDG4)<br>**Maternal health impact** (MDG5) | **On children:** Increased risk of death for >1 million young children yearly | **On children:** 15,000 infants at greater risk of death due to maternal anemia.<br>**On mothers:** Death of 50,000 women/year during pregnancy and childbirth | **On children:** increased risk of still births |
| **Major infectious disease impact** (MDG6) | **On children:** 40% of under-fives immuno-compromised by VAD with reduced protection against diarrhoea, measles, and other infections | **On people:** Impact of malaria exacerbated by iron deficiency<br>**On children:** anemia is linked to most malaria related deaths in young children | |

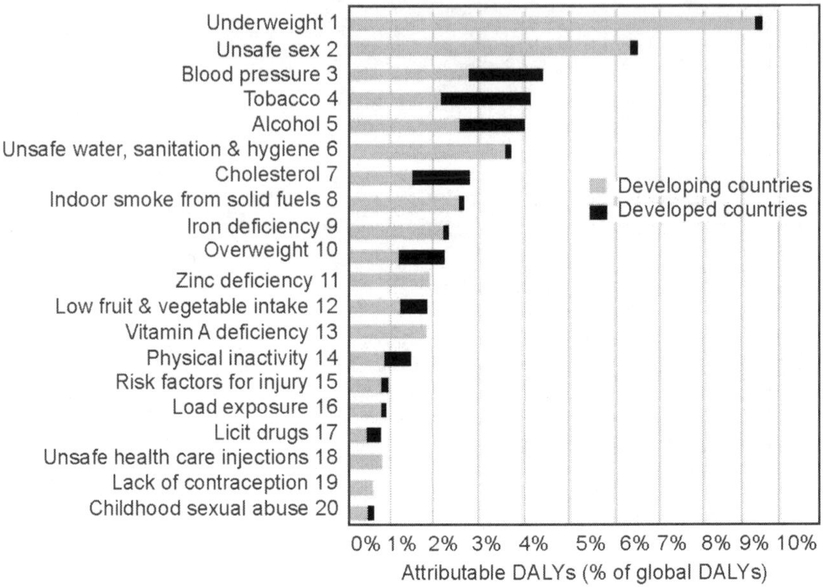


*30.1* Global disease burden.

from iron deficiency, and more than 40 percent of children are vitamin A deficient [2]. The situation in India is presented in Box 30.1.

## Box 30.1 Micronutrient Deficiency – Magnitude of Problem in India

According to the National Family Health Survey (NFHS)-3 India report [5], anemia prevalence is more than 79% in children 6–35 months of age, 56.2% in ever married women of 15–49 years, 57.9% in pregnant women 15–49 years and 24.3 % in men. In a study of pregnant women, anemia is reported to be over 80 percent in various regions of India [6]. As per National Nutrition Monitoring Bureau (NNMB) Report [1], the prevalence of conjunctival xerosis and Bitot spots, the signs of vitamin A deficiency was reported in 0.9% and 0.6% of pre-school children and 1.9% and 1.6% in school age children and 1.3% in adolescents. The prevalence of Bitot spots, the objective sign of vitamin A deficiency was more than the WHO cut-off level (0.5%) in several States. The prevalence of total goitre ranged between 3.3% and 13.7% in various states.

As discussed earlier (Table 30.1), data from National Nutrition Monitoring Bureau 2002 shows that in India, the intake of iron and vitamin A is less than 50% of the Recommended Dietary Allowance in all age groups. For iron, apart from a low dietary intake, there is also poor absorption due to a largely vegetarian diet. Such poor intakes are reflected in the nutritional status of the population in all age groups [7]. Added to these are other factors including lack of awareness, availability, accessibility, acceptability and affordability of micronutrient rich foods.

Though the extent of the micronutrient deficiencies are quite staggering these deficiencies can be prevented and even eliminated if populations consume small quantities of bio-available forms of required vitamins and minerals on a continuous and ongoing basis. According to a recent landmark document by the World Bank [8], the control of vitamin and mineral deficiencies is one of the most extraordinary development-related scientific advances of recent years. Probably no other technology available today offers as large an opportunity to improve lives and accelerate development at such a low cost and in such a short time [9].

The Government of India in 1993 adopted the National Nutrition Policy (NNP) and committed itself to achieve by 2000:

- Virtual elimination of iodine and vitamin A deficiency.
- Reduction of IDA in women by 1/3rd by the year 2000.
- Elimination of blindness due to VAD and reduction in prevalence of Bitot's Spots to less than 0.5%.
- Reduction in IDA among pregnant woman to 25% and
- Universal iodization of salt for reduction of IDD (Total Goitre Prevalence <10%).

India has come a long way in understanding the nature, magnitude and range of solutions to micronutrient malnutrition. Given the size and diversity of the nation, and the enormity and complexity of the problems of micronutrient deficiencies, the population's vitamin mineral requirements can be met only through a combination of strategies which have a synergistic effect as they can address multiple nutrient deficiencies simultaneously, foster the development of sustainable food production system, build partnerships among Government, consumer groups, food industry and other organizations and also promote self reliance and community participation. This concept is well reflected in the National Nutrition Policy, 1993. Fortification of foods with appropriate nutrients is recommended as one of the important priority actions.

## 30.3 Complementary strategies to overcome micronutrient malnutrition

Since neither the macro nor micro nutrient malnutrition occurs in isolation, there is a need to combine interventions for improving macro and micronutrients status in various development programs. As a consequence of the World Summit for Children, New York, 1990 [10], Ending Hidden Hunger Conference (1991) [11] and International Conference on Nutrition (Rome, 1992) [12], a number of developing countries intensified efforts to address the problem of micronutrient deficiencies.

The awareness on the micronutrient malnutrition has greatly increased in the past two to three decades. Most of the countries today are making efforts to approach the problem with real determination both at the national and community level [13]. For successful and sustainable micronutrient interventions, food fortification is recognised to be very essential.

Food fortification is a medium term approach to improve micronutrient intakes across the population on a consistent basis. Complementary to fortification, a short term approach during severe deficiency situations to ensure relief to vulnerable groups is being addressed through 'supplementation'. This involves administering high doses of the micronutrient in a concentrated supplement form to overcome the severe deficiency. An example is the six monthly high dose vitamin A supplementation being administered to children under 5 years of age in a number of developing countries. A longer term approach to ensure sustained outcome is through dietary diversification and involves ensuring access and encouraging population to consume foods rich in micronutrients including fruits and vegetables.

This chapter presents the various aspects of food fortification to meet the vitamin mineral needs of general population as well as specific target groups like women and children who are more susceptible to the deficiencies.

## 30.4 Food fortification

Food fortification can be described as a method of adding essential vitamins and minerals to foods to increase their nutritional value. According to *Codex Alimentarius*, fortification or enrichment is the addition of one or more essential nutrients to a food, whether or not it is normally contained in the food, for the purpose of preventing or correcting a demonstrated deficiency of one or more nutrients in the population or specific population groups [14]. The food to which the nutrients are added is called 'vehicle' for fortification and the added nutrients are called as 'fortificants'.

Fortification is the cheapest, most efficient and effective way to reach large populations with essential micronutrients. However, it is also important to recognize that food fortification is one part of a range of measures that influence the quality of food including improved agricultural practices, improved food processing and storage and consumer education to adopt good food preparation practices. Food fortification can be regarded as the best food based approach for solving the nutritional problems in developing countries.

## 30.5 History of food fortification

Food fortification is a public health initiative with a long history of being used effectively to remedy nutritional deficiencies that were causing widespread national public health problems. The earliest known nutrient supplementation of food was in 400 BC, when the physician Melanpus added iron filings to wine to increase Persian soldiers' strength. In 1833, the French agricultural chemist Jean Baptiste Boussingault urged his government to add iodine to salt to prevent goitre. It took until 1920 for his suggestion to be implemented. In the early 1920s, medical researchers announced that iodine could prevent goitre, which was widespread at that time. Fortification of salt with iodine proved to be an effective strategy in decreasing goitre incidence by 74–90% in the areas surveyed. It was so successful in reducing goitre and cretinism in affected populations that it prepared the way for future fortification of foods in the United States of America in 1922.

Between 1924 and 1944, iodine was added to salt, vitamins A and D to margarine, vitamin D to milk, and vitamins $B_1$, $B_2$, niacin and iron to flour and bread. The major impetus to fortification was World War II. Both the United Kingdom and the United States governments recommended voluntary fortification of flour and bread. By 1943, the US Army purchased only fortified flour or bread. In the UK, calcium, thiamine, niacin and iron were added to bread. These countries have added iron and vitamins to flour, bread and other foodstuffs with the intent of preventing or alleviating nutritional deficiencies in their population. Current efforts include enrichment of cereal grain-based foods with folate since such fortification has been demonstrated to reduce the annual incidence of neural tube birth defects by 25% [15].

## 30.6 Technical considerations

Food fortification has several advantages over other interventions as it does not necessitate a change in dietary patterns of the population, delivers a significant proportion of the recommended dietary allowances for a number of micronutrients on a continuous basis and does not call for individual compliance. It could often be dovetailed into the existing food production and distribution system, and therefore, can be sustained over a long period of time. The technical considerations in food fortification include selection of appropriate food vehicles that are consumed by a sizable proportion of the population and lend themselves to centralized processing on an economical scale. The product needs to be distributed through a wide network so that it reaches all parts of the country. When there is no single universally consumed vehicle in a country, fortification of a number of foods may be considered. The choice of food vehicle depends on local availability and consumption patterns.

A technical consultation by the Food and Agriculture Organization [14] agreed that, ideally, a fortified food should:

- *Be commonly consumed by the target population* – the food vehicle selected for fortification should be commonly consumed and needs to be identified as per the region. For example, in China soya sauce was identified as the choice for fortification because of the high consumption by the target population. Similarly, in India because of varied consumption patterns, wheat flour is regarded as the ideal food vehicle in North India, while rice is considered more suitable for the southern states of India.
- *Have a constant consumption pattern with a low risk of excess consumption* – salt is a good example here since its consumption is fairly constant, varying between 7 to 10 g per person per day.

Moreover, the unacceptable taste of additional salt prevents accidental excess consumption of the nutrients being carried through salt as the vehicle of fortification.

- *Have good stability during storage* – for example, vitamin A and D are the recommended nutrients for oil fortification because these two nutrients are fat soluble and have been demonstrated to have high stability during storage.
- *Be relatively low in cost* – commonly consumed foods like wheat flour and salt can be fortified at a very low additional cost. In India the additional cost of fortification of wheat flour with iron, folic acid and vitamin A in the state of West Bengal is approximately Rs. 1.50 (US$0.03) per beneficiary per year at a consumption profile of 100 grams per day.
- *Be centrally processed, with minimal stratification of the fortificant* – wheat that is centrally processed in large roller mills is being targeted for fortification in many developing countries. The particle size of the micronutrient premix used is close to that of wheat flour which minimizes separation or stratification of the nutrient in the flour.
- *Have no interaction between the fortificant and the food vehicle* – for double fortification of salt with iron and iodine, encapsulated form of iron is used to prevent interaction of the iron with salt as well as with iodine.
- *Be linked to energy intake* – while determining the levels of nutrients for fortification, the quantity of a specific food item consumed as well as the energy derived from the specific quantity is taken into consideration. This is essential since food intake, especially staple foods consumed by different age groups is generally proportional to their energy requirements. Taking into consideration both food and energy intakes helps in identifying the appropriate levels of micronutrients to be added to the food being fortified and ensuring that no single age group is getting either too low or too high levels of the micronutrients.

It is evident that selection of an appropriate vehicle is critical for a successful fortification programme. Staple foods and condiments are the obvious choice for fortification given their consistent consumption by large sections of the population. Commonly consumed foods used for fortification in different countries since early 1930s include wheat and corn flour, rice, oil, margarine, dairy products, salt, sugar and sauces (Table 30.3).

## 30.7 Technology for food fortification

The actual mechanics of adding the nutrients to the food is technically simple. It involves the use of a 'pre-mix' containing the required nutrients in a concentrated form and adding it to the selected food during processing and ensuring proper blending of the premix with the food. Depending on the food processing technologies, different addition methods have been developed [18]. Common examples include:

- **Dry mixing** for cereal flours and their products, powder milk, powder beverages
- **Dissolution in water** for liquid milk, drinks, fruit juices and in the water to be used for making bread, pastas, cookies etc.
- **Dissolution in oil** for adding lipid soluble vitamins to oily products like margarine.
- **Spraying technique** as for iodization of salt and some types of corn flakes – this process involves preparation of a solution containing the nutrients and spraying through a nozzle as the food to be fortified moves along the processing line.
- **Adhesion** as in sugar fortification where the vitamin A in powder form is adhered to the crystals surface by a vegetable oil.

*Table 30.3* Food fortification in developed countries [14, 16, 17]

| Year of initiation | Country | Nutrients/ Vehicles | Deficiency disorders to be controlled | Current status – current status- country policy |
|---|---|---|---|---|
| 19th to 20th century | France/ USA | Iodine in salt | Control of IDD (Cretinism, mental retardation) | Legislation in place to ensure that fortificant levels are defined and iodized and non-iodized salt are labeled |
| 1918 | Denmark | Vitamin A in margarine | Nutritional blindness | As per the current Danish food additive regulations, vitamin A is a permitted nutrient additive in margarine |
| 1930s | USA | Vitamin D in milk | Rickets | The U.S. Food and Drug Administration (FDA) standards are available for optional addition of vitamins A and D to milk. Evaporated milk must contain added vitamin D. Non-fat dry milk that is labeled "fortified with vitamins A and D" must be fortified with those vitamins. |
| 1940s | USA | Iron and B vitamins in wheat flour | Beri-beri, pellagra | FDA has set standards of identity for both wheat flour and enriched (fortified) wheat flour. Sale of non-fortified flour is not prohibited as |

| Year of initiation | Country | Nutrients/ Vehicles | Deficiency disorders to be controlled | Current status – current status-country policy |
|---|---|---|---|---|
| | | | | long as the product meets the labeling requirement. Nevertheless, given consumer interest in nutrition and value enhanced products most flour currently sold for household use is enriched with B vitamins, iron and folate. |
| 1980s | USA | Calcium in flour, dairy products and other foods | Osteoporosis (largely market driven) | Calcium fortification by the industry is allowed as an option. FDA permits a health claim regarding calcium and osteoporosis on foods that contain at least 20 percent of the reference daily intake (RDI) |
| 1998 | USA | Folic acid in wheat flour | Neural tube defects | FDA mandates that all enriched (fortified) wheat flour contains folic acid |

The technology of food fortification therefore involves careful consideration regarding selection of appropriate food vehicle and nutrients, levels of fortification, safety index, feasibility and sensory acceptability, bio-availability, storage and stability, methods of blending, efficacy and, last but not the least, the cost [19].

## 30.8 Fortificants

Clearer understanding of the interaction of fortificants with other dietary factors needs to be achieved if one is to optimize fortification programs. In cases where there is more than one demonstrated micronutrient deficiency in a target population, addition of more than one micronutrient to a single vehicle (multiple fortification) could be advantageous. With the expanding range of fortificant compounds available, and the need to use various food vehicles according to the designated target groups, it is important to consider the technologies best suited to achieve a fortified product with the desired properties.

In many cases identification of suitable vehicles is made difficult due to absence of reliable information on dietary habits of the target population. Fortificants must meet quality criteria specifications explicitly established for each application. Selection of an appropriate vehicle is a critical step in successful fortification to ensure stability, appearance, bioavailability and homogeneity. It is essential to undertake field testing of fortified food at several locations in the country in differing environmental conditions. This is important for understanding problems potentiated by scaling up production activities from pilot to industrial scale. The various fortificants and food vehicles which are commonly in use are presented below:

**(a) *Iodine*** – Salt is the most suitable vehicle for iodine fortification. Two chemical forms of iodine are currently used for iodization; these are iodates and iodides. The *Codex Alimentarius* standard for food grade salt [20] permits the use of both the sodium and potassium salts of iodides and iodates in the iodization of salt. According to international recommendations, the iodine concentration in salt at the point of production should be within the range of 20–40 mg of iodine per kg of salt (i.e. 20–40 ppm of iodine). Considering iodine losses from production site to households, adequately iodized salt at household level is recommended to contain 15 ppm of iodine [21]. The levels for iodization are, however, established by national authorities in light of the prevailing iodine deficiency. For example, Europe-wide uniform minimum and maximum levels (20 and 40 mg/kg salt) is adopted by all EU member states. The two forms of iodine also need to be harmonized in terms of equivalence to avoid trade barriers.

There are four major technologies that are used for addition of iodine to salt—dry mixing, drip feed addition, spray mixing and submersion. Program monitoring is important to ensure access to population of adequately iodised salt for elimination of iodine deficiency. Moreover, proper monitoring is critical for avoiding sporadic reports of thyrotoxicosis [22]. Prevalence of such side effect can be reduced by close monitoring of iodine levels in salt which can be adjusted based on monitoring of human urinary iodine excretion.

**(b) *Iron*** – Cereals are the most widely used vehicles for iron fortification although many others, such as milk products, sugar, curry powder, soya sauce, salt and cookies have been successfully used. Ferrous sulphate, Ferrous fumarate, elemental iron (particularly electrolytic form) and Sodium Iron Ethylene Diamine Tetra Acetate (NaFeEDTA) are examples of preferred iron fortificants. Selection of the iron fortificant is dependent on the food vehicle. The color of iron compounds is often a critical factor when fortifying lightly colored foods. The use of more soluble iron compounds (e.g. Ferrous sulphate) often leads to the development of off-colors and off-flavors due to reactions with other components of the food material, but they have the advantage of being highly bioavailable (Table 30.4). Vitamin C is known to increase the bioavailability of non-heme iron forms (iron from plant foods). In some countries bovine hemoglobin concentrate, which has an exceptionally high bioavailability, is being used as a heme-iron fortificant in local feeding programs.

The presence of phytates, polyphenols and calcium are known to adversely affect the bioavailability of non-heme iron fortificants. Increasing evidence indicates that in such cases sodium iron-EDTA may prove to be a better choice of fortificant in the future as iron from the EDTA-complex remains bioavailable even in the presence of iron absorption inhibitors. Given the wide variability of iron bioavailability, influenced by physical and chemical properties of the fortificant as well as the presence of substances which either inhibit or improve iron absorption, there is a need to develop convenient models for the evaluation of iron bioavailability. This is particularly important as an increasing range of iron fortificants with different physico-chemical properties, is being developed and marketed. It is also essential that surveillance data of iron status is interpreted with caution because of the known alteration of serum ferritin levels and other indicators of iron status in the presence of recent infection. Furthermore, it must be recognised that not all anemia is due to iron deficiency, although the latter is most common.

Several aspects of the interaction between iron and other nutrients, such as vitamin A, iodine, zinc and calcium, need to be investigated in relation to the possibility of multiple fortification. The stability and the cost of fortificant compounds as well as the bioavailability of the nutrients need to be considered.

**(c) *Vitamin A*** – Foods which have been successfully fortified with vitamin A include margarine, fats and oils, milk, sugar, breakfast cereals, and instant noodles with spice mix. Moisture contents in excess of about 7–8% in a food are known to adversely affect the stability of vitamin A. Beyond the critical moisture content there is a rapid increase in water activity which permits various deteriorative reactions to occur. Vitamin A is also shown to be very sensitive to light exposure and repeated heating, as may be experienced with vegetable oils used for frying, is known to significantly degrade vitamin A. Retinol palmitate (also called as vitamin A palmitate) is the frequently used form of vitamin A for fortification. Carotenoids can also be used as a source of vitamin A but its conversion and bioavailability is known to be affected by the vitamin A status of the individual and by dietary composition. A conversion factor of 6:1 (six milligrams of beta carotene equivalent to one milligram of retinol) is currently being applied in calculating intake [26], though a recent recommendation by US Institute of Medicine suggest a conversion of 12:1 [27]. The cost factor in using carotenoids as the source of vitamin A activity in fortification is generally considered prohibitive.

**(d) *Vitamin D*** – There are a limited number of food vehicles suitable for vitamin D fortification. These include margarine, vegetable oils and dairy products. Vitamin D metabolism is linked to calcium absorption and parathyroid hormone. Susceptible populations for marginal vitamin D status include children under three years of age, the elderly and any population where cultural practices or climatic conditions prevent exposure to sunlight. It is very important that a reliable, accurate, simple and rapid methodology

*Table 30.4* Characteristics of iron salts commonly used to fortify foods [23–25]

| Groups | Iron salts | Desirable characteristics | Undesirable characteristics | Uses | Average relative bioavailability (%) | |
|---|---|---|---|---|---|---|
| | | | | | Man | Vitamin C |
| | Freely water soluble<br>Ferrous Gluconate<br>Ferrous Ammonium citrate | Ferrous Sulphate<br>Water solubility | (a) Colour changes<br>(b) Fat oxidation<br>(c) Metallic taste<br>(d) Precipitation | cereal flours<br>Infant formulas | 100<br>89<br>– | Same<br>Same<br>12.9 times |
| Soluble in dilute acid | Ferrous fumarate<br>Ferrous succinate<br>Ferrous saccharate | | Slight risk of colour changes | Infant cereals, salt<br>Maize flour<br>Powdered drinks | 100<br>92<br>74 | Same<br>Same<br>Same |
| Water insoluble/ poorly soluble in dilute acid | Ferrous orthophosphate<br>Ferric ammonium orthophosphate<br>Ferric pyrophosphate<br>Elemental iron powders (Electrolytic carbonyl reduced and H-reduced) | No colour change<br>No flavour change | | Wheat flour<br>Infant cereals<br>Powdered drinks<br>Breakfast cereals | 25–32<br>45–58<br>21–74<br>–<br>5–100 | 4.0 times<br>Same<br>Same<br>–<br>– |
| Chelated iron compounds | NaFeEDTA | Fat oxidation<br>2–3 times better absorbed than FeSO4 from high phytate meals | Unwanted color reaction<br>Low absorption | High extraction flours<br>Infant cereals | more than 100 | No data available |

for the assessment of vitamin D status is carried out linked to the process of fortification. Without such assessment, it is difficult to make required adjustments to fortification practices based on feedback from comprehensive monitoring of the impact of fortification on vitamin D status.

**(e) *Vitamin E*** – Vitamin E, as tocopherol acetate, is added to fats and oils including margarine and fat spreads and breakfast cereals. Vitamin E intake is known to be related to the total dietary intake of fat and it has been shown to enhance absorption and bio-conversion of dietary carotenoids to vitamin A. Emerging evidence indicates that daily intake of vitamin E greater than 30 IU may afford protection against the development of degenerative diseases. Optimal levels of fortification of vitamin E should be reassessed based on such scientific evidence.

**(f) *Vitamin C*** – There are technologies available for vitamin C fortification of fruit juices, fruit juice drinks, other related beverages, dairy products and some breakfast cereals. High moisture content (greater than 7%) in the presence of oxygen is known to adversely affect the stability of vitamin C in cereals. There is a need to develop more stable vitamin C compounds and evaluate their use in the fortification of a range of vehicles. There is much ongoing investigation on the role of vitamin C in the prevention of anemia, chronic diseases such as cardiovascular disease, cancer and cataracts. Based on the outcome of such research it may be desirable to revise fortification practices for this vitamin.

**(g) *B-Complex vitamins*** – There are not many problems related to the technology of the addition of B vitamins to cereals and grains. The development of off-flavors due to the thermal instability of **thiamine** is easily circumvented by adding this vitamin following all heat treatments. The status of B complex vitamins is known to be marginal in populations with low consumption of animal foods (milk, meat, liver) and/or those which use low extraction (highly refined) products of cereals and grains such as flour as well as in populations in transition from rural to urban settlements [28]. Food fortification with B complex vitamins may be appropriate for such populations. The development of improved methodologies for the evaluation of B-vitamin status would be a valuable tool in establishing the need for fortification in target populations and in the monitoring of these programs. A confirmed association between dietary **folic acid** intake and neural tube defects has been reported. Based on this finding, addition of folic acid to wheat flour has been mandated in several countries [29]. Populations with marginal or low folic acid intake may therefore benefit from fortification of staples with folic acid. Furthermore, folic acid together with **vitamin $B_6$** and **vitamin $B_{12}$** has been reported to decrease plasma homocysteine levels; the latter is reported to be inversely associated with the development of ischemic heart disease [30]. Further investigation of these relationships is relevant to the evaluation of the adequacy of current fortification practices.

## 30.9 Planning food fortification intervention

Planning of food fortification begins by identifying the commonly eaten foods that can act as vehicles for one or more micronutrients. Food fortification aims to provide meaningful levels of the nutrient (usually 30% to 50% of the daily adult requirements) at normal consumption pattern of the selected food vehicle. The levels also need to take into account variations in food consumption by different age groups so that the safety of those at the higher end of the scale and impact for those at the lower end are ensured [31].

Ensuring an effective fortification program involves several components and stages that can be considered as part of a "food fortification cycle" (Figure 30.2). The sections of the cycle include:

(a) *Situation analysis* – Collect, review and analyze a range of information related to the problem of vitamin–mineral deficiencies and food vehicles with potential for fortification.

(b) *Determining feasibility* – Explore and confirm technical and economic feasibility of food fortification. The feasibility of any fortification program needs to be ascertained once its efficacy is established, as many a times an extremely efficacious program may not be feasible for implementation or scaling up. Similarly, identifying a feasible vehicle for fortification is equally important for the program to become successful.

(c) *Enabling partnerships* – Bring together a variety of sectors and organizations (most important the food industry and government) to pursue the common goal of reducing vitamin mineral deficiencies through food fortification. Success of partnership building in a fortification program has been depicted in details under wheat flour fortification.

(d) *Implementing program* – Developing an implementation plan with criteria and guidelines; identifying resource inputs; designing the support measures including advocacy and communications, ensuring that legislation is in place, steps to be followed towards formulating standards, ensuring regulation and assuring quality.

(e) *Monitoring and evaluation* – Collect, analyze and interpret data (quantitative and qualitative) and use of the information to identify problems for correction, or to help sustain successful activities. Monitoring and evaluation leads to re-assessment of the situation for further refinement of the program and so the cycle goes on. The cycle could be conceived as a sequential process where the development of one phase follows the previous stage. However, the different stages in the cycle are not necessarily sequential and often overlap. Also, it may not always be necessary to start at the beginning of the first phase and each phase may be of varying duration and timing.

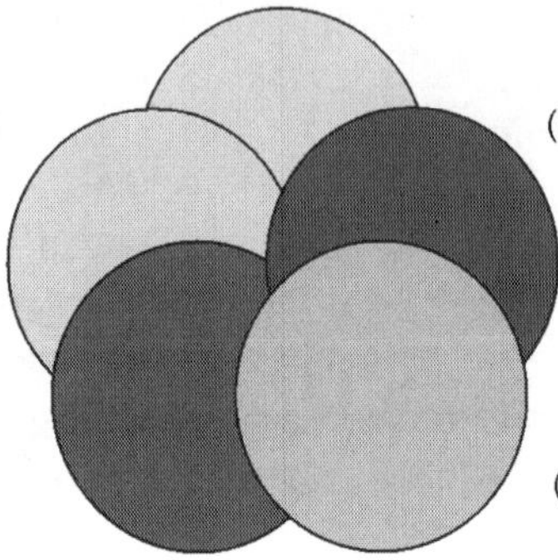


*30.2* The Food Fortification Cycle.

## 30.10 Global experiences with food fortification

Food fortification has played a major positive role in the health of the populations in several developed and developing countries over the last 70 years. As a result many nutritional deficiencies have been eliminated. More than 25 countries worldwide currently have mandatory fortification while several other countries practice voluntary food fortification.

Food fortification in the US was started with salt iodization in Michigan in 1922. In the 1930s and 1940s USA adopted fortification of flour and bread with niacin followed by multiple nutrients including iron. Flour fortification has been instrumental in reducing deaths attributed to pellagra, a condition caused due to niacin deficiency (Figure 30.3) [32]. The current low levels of iron deficiency in the USA are attributable to the wide consumption of fortified foods. Similarly, in Canada, flour fortification with B vitamins began in Newfoundland in 1944. Within four years, deficiencies reduced from 20% to negligible levels. The introduction of mandatory folic acid fortification of cereal-grain products after 1998 in the USA, Canada and Chile has resulted in 30 to 70% reduction of neural tube defects in newborns. It has been documented that even the voluntary fortification of foods, especially breakfast cereals, has contributed to the improvement in micronutrient intakes in many of the developed countries including France, Ireland, the United Kingdom and Spain [33]. The evidence from developed countries suggests that where the food industry is mature with effective quality assurance procedures and where commercially processed foods are widely consumed, fortification has played an important role in combating micronutrient malnutrition.

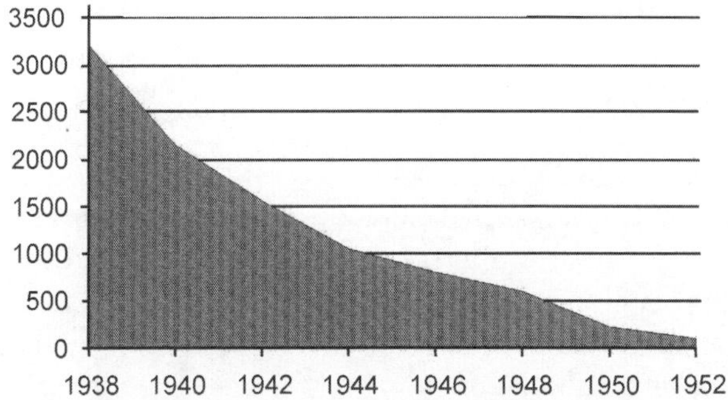


*30.3* Deaths from niacin deficiency in United States [32].

In the developing world also, there has been a rapid growth in fortifying a wide range of foods during the last two decades. The most successful global fortification experience is the fortification of salt with iodine. As of 2006 nearly two thirds of the salt consumed in the developing world is being iodized, protecting nearly 70 million newborns each year from the threat of mental impairment and other sub-clinical deficiency disorders [34].

Fortification of staple foods such as flour, oils, sugar, condiments, dairy products and a range of processed foods with micronutrients is also growing [35]. A successful program in Venezuela, started in 1993, enriched precooked corn flour with iron (50 mg), vitamin A (9500 IU), thiamine (3.1 mg), niacin (51 mg) and riboflavin (2.5 mg) per kilogram. The

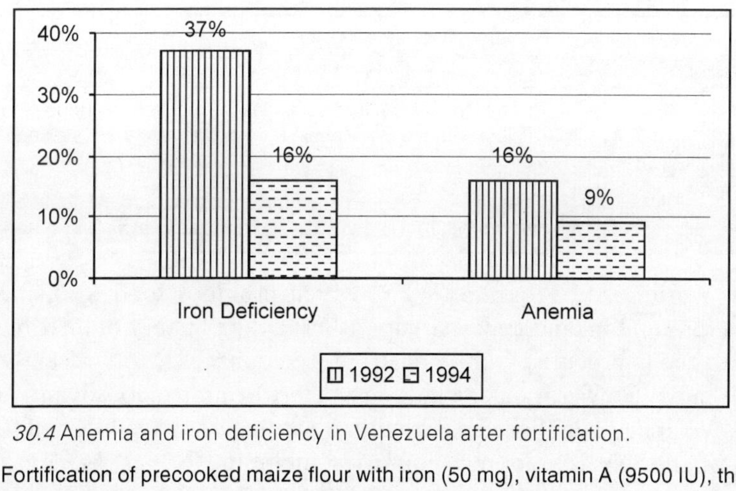


*30.4* Anemia and iron deficiency in Venezuela after fortification.

* Fortification of precooked maize flour with iron (50 mg), vitamin A (9500 IU), thiamine (3.1 mg), niacin (51 mg) and riboflavin (2.5 mg) per kilogram

prevalence of iron deficiency in school children dropped from 37 to 16% in just two years after the implementation of fortification program (Figure 30.4) [36]. Currently nineteen countries in Latin America and Caribbean have a national food fortification program in which iron and other micronutrients are added to at least one widely consumed food which is often wheat and/or corn flour.

In the Middle East and North Africa several countries introduced fortification with iron and folic acid to cereal flour. A program review by the Micronutrient Initiative (MI) in 2006 reported that while prior to 1998 only one country (Saudi Arabia) was fortifying flour, by 2005 a total of 13 countries in the region produced and consumed fortified flour containing at least iron and folic acid (in some instances vitamin A and other B complex vitamins also) on a national or sub-national scale - reaching more than 81 million consumers [37]. There is also growing interest and action on wheat flour fortification in Asia. Flour fortification at the national level is under implementation in Indonesia, Philippines, Pakistan and Nepal while several states in India have initiated or are planning to introduce it. The status of flour fortification in various countries across the world, along with the fortificants being used is presented in Table 30.5 [38].

It has also been demonstrated that choosing a food vehicle that is very specific to the country but consumed by large segments of the population could be effective. For example, soy and fish sauces fortified with iron are emerging as a major vehicle in China, Vietnam and Thailand because more than 80% of the population consumes these sauces regularly with a network of sauce factories operating under government supervision.

*Table 30.5* Fortification of staple food

| Staple cereal | No of countries | Primary micronutrients |
|---|---|---|
| Maize | 9 | Thiamin, riboflavin, folic acid, niacin, zinc, iron. At some places calcium, vitamin $B_{12}$, vitamin $B_6$ and vitamin a were also added |
| Rice | 2 | Thiamin, riboflavin, folic acid, niacin, zinc, iron |
| Wheat | 78 | Thiamin, riboflavin, folic acid, niacin, zinc, iron. At some places calcium, vitamin $B_{12}$, vitamin $B_6$ and vitamin a were also added |

The World Food Program (WFP) which provides food to displaced populations and in emergency situations has a long history of distributing fortified foods procured from industrialized countries. More recently the WFP is moving towards on-site milling and fortification of locally produced grains. WFP has established a capacity to produce fortified blended foods in 13 of the world's poorest countries including Nepal, Madagascar, Ethiopia and Malawi.

A national program to provide fortified milk to infants up to 18 months of age has helped reduce anemia in Chilean infants from 21% to around 1%. Fortified complementary foods provided through public feeding programs and commercial channels in Mexico, Ecuador and Chile had significant health and developmental impacts on children. In a number of situations where fortified foods are not accessible to children between 6 months to two years of age, multiple ways to deliver micronutrients to this age group has been experimented to enable mothers to either add them into the cooking pot or to mix them into the food they feed their infants. Such efforts have been successful in Bolivia, Guatemala, Sudan and Kenya as well as in several other countries. This approach is referred to as "Home Fortification" [39].

## 30.11 Food fortification in a developing country—experiences from India

To translate the National Nutrition Policy [40, 13] adopted by Government of India in 1993, into forceful, viable and sustained efforts, the National Plan of Action on Nutrition [ 41], was released by Government of India in 1995, which recommended a combination of interventions such as promotion of dietary diversification, nutrient supplementation, food fortification and public health measures to be implemented. The Department of Women and Child Development, Ministry of Human Resource Development, India along with the United Nations World Food Program in 2000, prepared a white paper on prevention of micronutrient malnutrition through the national programme of Integrated Child Development Services or ICDS [42]. The strategies for overcoming micronutrient malnutrition as mentioned in the white paper are as follows:

- Dietary diversification through behavior modification
- Fortification of foods with nutrients
- Horticulture interventions for adequate supply of nutrient rich foods
- Supplementation with specific micronutrients
- Sensitization of policy on issues related to prevention of micronutrient malnutrition

Government of India policy and the plan accepts food fortification as one of the most effective food based approach to address micronutrient deficiencies. The focus in planning a fortification program takes into consideration the fact that the prevention of malnutrition must address the problem at various stages of the life cycle. In developing countries like India, many of the staple foods are processed at the community level and they are often consumed in the areas where they are grown. However, the consumption of centrally processed foods is steadily increasing. Moreover, it is recognised that in situations like this where there is no single universally consumed and centrally processed food, fortification of a number of foods needs to be considered. The choice of the food vehicle depends on local availability and consumption patterns. In view of the diverse food consumption patterns and food processing situation in India, it is obvious that a single approach is not the answer. With the expanding range of fortificant compounds available and the need to use a combination of vehicles, it is essential to consider the technologies that are best suited to achieve a fortified product with the desired properties. In India food fortification has evolved over the past few decades through a number of trials which has resulted in the availability of several fortified foods and also led to increased interest in future potential for further expansion.

### 30.11.1 Initial efforts of food fortification in India

Initial efforts on food fortification in India were focused on improving the protein and energy levels of the diet and gradually progressed to fortification with vitamins and minerals. Fortification of tapioca flour with a high protein source like edible peanut flour and blending of 75 per cent edible peanut flour with 25 per cent of Bengal gram (Cicer arietinum) to produce Indian Multi-purpose Food (IMPF) were successfully tried at the Central Food Technological Research Institute (CFTRI) as early as 1950s [43, 44]. Though these products had significant nutritive value and established consumer acceptance, they were neither widely marketed through commercial channels nor promoted through government programs [45]. On the other hand, fortification of whole wheat flour *(atta)* with edible peanut flour introduced problems of consumer acceptability as confirmed by studies by the Protein Foods and Nutritional Development Association of India. Fortification of bread with lysine, vitamins and minerals tried by Modern Bakeries, a public sector organization of the Government of India showed significant improvement in the weight and height of children [46]. Elwood et al [47], using labeled iron in *chapati* , reported poor absorption of both iron in the wheat and from the iron salt used for fortification. Based on this finding, it was stressed that there was a need to discover or develop an iron salt that can be added to flour in relatively high concentration without adverse impact on the keeping quality or baking quality of wheat. Fortification of salt (with iron), consumed by all groups irrespective of age, economic status, and rural or urban setting was taken up by the Food and Nutrition Board of the Government of India in collaboration with the National Institute of Nutrition (NIN), wherein parameters like bio-availability, storage, and utilization of iron in Indian culinary practices were studied [48]. Fortification with iron of other foods like sugar [49] and tea [50] were also tried out.

## 30.11.2 Fortification of industrially processed foods

Many processed foods, infant foods and weaning foods (complementary feeding foods), manufactured by multinational companies are currently being fortified with vitamins, calcium, and iron, and in some cases with amino acids as per the specifications of the Indian Standards Institution (ISI) [51], with labels presenting specific amount of vitamins that a child of six months would derive from these foods in a normal day in comparison with his/her actual nutrient requirements. The micronutrient content in well known commercial baby foods shown in Table 30.6 indicates that all of the formulations are fortified with one or more essential vitamins and minerals. The level of micronutrients consumed through the baby foods is at least 100% of the child's actual requirement, many times more than the requirement (Table 30.7 and 30.8).

*Table 30.6* Micronutrient levels in samples of commercial baby foods (per 100 g)

| Nutrients | Amul | Glaxo spray | Lacto-gen | Sapan | Bal amul | Farex | Nestum |
|---|---|---|---|---|---|---|---|
| Calories | 450 | 574 | 474 | 454 | 391 | 375 | 366 |
| Calcium (mg) | 1.0 | – | – | 1.0 | 1.0 | 0.75 | 0.69 |
| Iron (mg) | 4.0 | 4.0 | 4.0 | 4.0 | 6.0 | 20 0 | 15.6 |
| Vitamin A (IU) | 1,500 | 1,500 | 1,500 | 1,500 | 1,500 | – | 1,875 |
| Vitamin D (IU) | 400 | 400 | 400 | 500 | 300 | 300 | 500 |
| Vitamin $B_1$ (mg) | 0.6 | – | 0.4 | 0.6 | 0.5 | – | 0.6 |
| Vitamin $B_2$ (mg) | 1.0 | – | 0.6 | 1.0 | 0.6 | – | 0.7 |
| Vitamin $B_6$ (mg) | 0.3 | – | 1.0 | 0.3 | – | – | 0.4 |
| Vitamin $B_{12}$ (ng) | – | – | 2.0 | 1.2 | – | – | – |
| Folic acid (ng) | – | – | – | – | – | – | 25 |
| Niacinamide (mg) | 6.0 | – | 6.0 | 6.0 | 5.0 | – | 6.0 |
| Calcium pantothenate (mg) | – | – | – | – | – | – | 4.6 |
| Vitamin E (ng) | – | – | – | – | – | – | 6.0 |
| Vitamin C (mg) | 30 | – | 40 | 40 | 50 | – | 45 |

Another industrially processed food which is being fortified is hydrogenated vegetable fat – referred as *vanaspati* in India. It is mandatory for *vanaspati* to be fortified with 25 International unit (IU) of vitamin A per gram (4% RDA). There has been substantial decrease in consumption of *vanaspati* in the pasty two decades and it is estimated that the consumption this type of fat is as low as 0.3 to 1.1 g/day/person. On the other hand, since 1993–94 the per capita consumption of edible oil has risen over a period of eleven years by as much as 30% in rural India and about 18% in urban India. In both rural and urban India, per capita consumption of oil other than groundnut oil, mustard oil, *vanaspati* and coconut oil has more than doubled. The oil varieties which have increased remarkably include sunflower oil, soyabean oil, other vegetable oil and rice bran oil. Fortification of oil, rather than any *vanaspati* is therefore considered important. There is however no mandatory fortification for any of these oils [52].

*Table 30.7* Vitamin and mineral intake of children—fortified commercial baby foods compared to actual requirements

| | Intake/day | Requirement | Percentage requirement |
|---|---|---|---|
| Vitamin A (IU) | 2,430 | 1,333 | 182. 3 |
| Vitamin D (IU) | 590 | 200 | 295. 0 |
| Vitamin $B_1$ (mg) | 0.91 | 0.6 | 151.7 |
| Vitamin $B_2$ (mg) | 1.39 | 0.8 | 173.8 |
| Vitamin $B_6$ (mg) | 0.62 | – | – |
| Niacinamide (mg) | 9.14 | 8.0 | 114.2 |
| Calcium (mg) | 1.62 | 0.4 | 405.0 |
| Iron (mg) | 7.64 | 7.0 | 109.0 |

*Table 30.8* Suggested fortification of commercial baby foods

| | Recommended dietary intake of a child of six months | Fortification of baby foods as at present per 100 g | Fortification on calorie basis (plus 10% extra) per 100 g | Percentage of excess fortification | ISI standards |
|---|---|---|---|---|---|
| Calories | 708 | 450 (as at present) | 450 | – | – |
| Vitamin A (IU) | 1,333 | 1,500 | 938 | 160 | 1,500 |
| Vitamin D (IU) | 200 | 400 | 140 | 286 | 200–300 |
| Vitamin C (mg) | 20 | 30 | 14 | 214 | 30 |
| Thiamine (mg) | 0.35 | 0.6 | 0.25 | 240 | 0.5 |
| Riboflavin (mg) | 0.43 | 1.0 | 0.30 | 334 | 1 0 |
| Niacinamide (mg) | 4.68 | 6.0 | 3.29 | 182 | 5.0 |
| Pyridoxine (mg) | 0.3 | 0.3 | 0.21 | 142 | 0.3 |
| Folic acid (ng) | 25.0 | – | 17.6 | – | 50.0 |
| Vitamin $B_{12}$ (ng) | 0.2 | – | 0.14 | – | 1.0 |
| Iron (mg) | 6.0 | 4.0 | 4.2 | – | 4.0 |

Other products like fortified breakfast cereals, noodles, milk, edible oils, fruit juices, breads, biscuits etc. are also flooding the Indian markets. However, most of these products are out of reach of the poor. The need for developing fortified products which are affordable, acceptable, scalable and sustainable is recognised. Moreover, it is also appreciated that a system needs to be introduced to ensure sustainability of these products to reach the entire population.

### 30.11.3 Fortification of food supplied under the government supported programmes

In India, several public programs such as the Integrated Child Development Services (ICDS), Mid Day Meal (MDM) and Targeted Public Distribution System (TPDS) provide supplementary food to various age groups.

ICDS has a life cycle approach of reaching children 6 months to 6 years of age, as well as adolescent girls and pregnant and lactating mothers. Too often they meet only the macro level requirements of energy and protein and do not address micronutrient deficiencies sufficiently. However, the *Ministry of Human Resource Development, Dept of Women and Child Development, Government of India wide their circular No. 5-17/2004-ND/Tech.FF dt. 12 July, 2005,* issued a notification to all the State Governments to fortify the supplementary nutrition component with multiple micronutrients providing 50% of RDA of selected nutrients to the children and women beneficiaries, as presented in Table 30.9 below.

*Table 30.9* Micronutrient levels in ICDS as per the Government of India guidelines

| Micronutrients | Per child per day |
|---|---|
| Iron | 15 mg |
| Vitamin A | 400 µg |
| Folic acid | 35 µg |
| Iodine | 100 µg |
| Zinc | 10 mg |
| Thiamin | 0.8 mg |
| Riboflavin | 0.8 mg |
| Ascorbic acid | 40 mg |
| Calcium | 400 mg |

Recently with efforts by Government of India and several State Governments and support from various international agencies, like WFP, CARE, MI and GAIN, fortified supplementary foods are being distributed through these public programs with encouraging results. Some of the success stories are highlighted below:

*(i) Point of use fortification of ICDS supplementary cooked food*

"Point of Use Fortification" is a term used to include both home fortification as well as fortification at the point of institutional or large cooking. In West Bengal, India, such point of use fortification is undertaken through the large Integrated Child Development Services (ICDS) programme. A local food item *Khichdi* (rice, lentils and oil mixture cooked to a soft semi-solid consistency), a supplementary food distributed through ICDS, is fortified with a multiple micronutrient premix "v*ita shakti*" which provides 500 IU of vitamin A, 14mg of microencapsulated iron (ferrous fumarate) and 0.05mg folic acid per day. Initially in 2006, fortified food reached 4.8 million beneficiaries .The strategy being cost-effective was scaled up by the State Government of West Bengal at their own cost (additional cost of fortification being Rs.9/- per annum) in the year 2006-07. This concept of addition of micronutrient mix such as "*vita shakti*" has been adopted in Africa where "*Rahama*" is added to food at home to overcome micronutrient deficiency problems among population.

The fortificant '*vita shakti*' is in the form of a powder and is recommended to be added to the prepared *khichdi* at the level of 0.25 mg at the ICDS village centre (referred as *Anganwadi* center or AWC ) using a measured spoon, calibrated to serve five beneficiaries. The addition of '*vita shakti*', the MI produced fortified premix, to the ICDS *khichdi* program is unique as it is community based with the micronutrient premix added at the child centre of ICDS *(AWC)* level. Fortification at the community level is advantageous as it instills ownership of the fortification program in the village community and demystifies the fortification process to local mothers, while ensuring that the fortified food is consumed at the proper levels by the targeted population. Community based programs also have the added benefit of using locally produced and consumed food vehicle which increases the acceptability, sustainability, and adherence to the fortification program.

The findings of the khichdi fortification programme revealed that the strategy was feasible and the product was acceptable as was indicated by the high program compliance by both ICDS workers who prepared the fortified *Khichdi* and by the enrolled children, who consumed it. Monitoring records showed no problems with the storage and preparation of the *Khichdi* at the Anganwadi center. In focus group discussions, ICDS workers reported no problems with the addition of the premix to the cooked *Khichdi*.

A study was undertaken on children in the Fortified Khichdi (FK) and Non Fortified Group(NFK) group .The study showed that *Khichdi* fortified with a microencapsulated ferrous fumarate and vitamin A premix was efficacious in improving iron status (Fig. 30.5 and reducing the prevalence of anemia, iron deficiency (ID) and iron deficiency Anemia (IDA) in pre-school aged children in West Bengal. The premix was also efficacious in increasing the serum retinol (SR) concentration of females in the targeted population [53].

The significant change in hemoglobin (Hb) concentration in children who received the fortified *Khichdi (FK)* was evident. (Fig. 30.6). Over a period of six months, the incidence of anemia was reduced from 19.1% in the FK at week 0 to 4.1% at week 24 against 32.6% in NFK at week 0 to 20.7% for week 24. Of the children in the FK who were still anemic after 24 weeks of intervention, 50% had hemoglobin concentration of 109.5g/L which further showed the ability of the fortified *Khichdi* to remove preschool aged children from an anemic state and maintain their nutrient stores at a sufficient level.

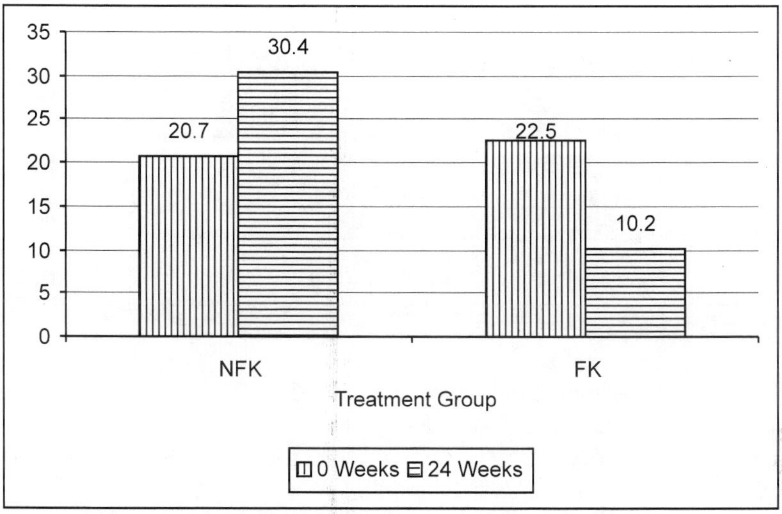


*30.5* Prevalence (%) iron deficiency for NFK and FK at 0 and 24 weeks.

Prevalence of iron deficiency Anemia was low in both FK and NFK at baseline, but the provision of fortified *Khichdi* almost eliminated IDA during the 6 month intervention (4.9% to 0.4%) while there was very little change in the prevalence of iron deficiency anemia (IDA) in children in NFK (9.6% to 9.3%). The fortified *Khichdi* was very effective in increasing ferritin level (Fig. 30.7) and in eliminating IDA in the target population during the relatively short intervention time.

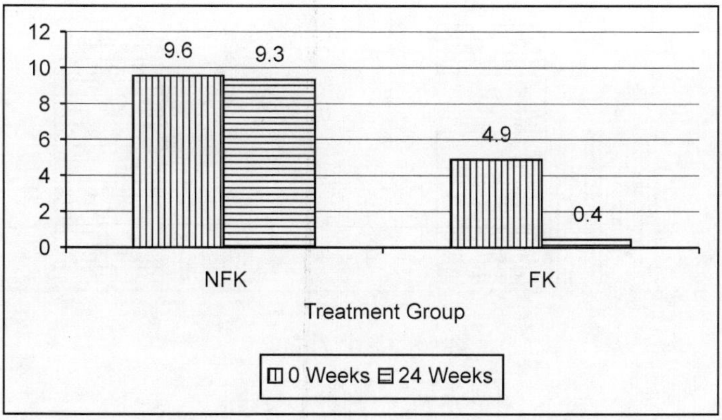


*30.6* Prevalence (%) iron deficiency anemia in children consuming for NFK and FK at 0 and 24 weeks.

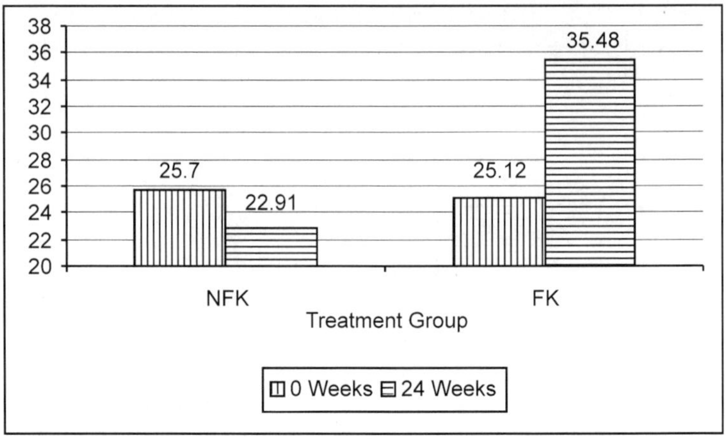


30.7 Serum ferritin concentration in anemic NFK and FK at 0 and 24 weeks .

Serum Retinol increased in both FK and NFK during the 6 month intervention (Fig. 30.8)

Serum retinol concentration was significantly different at baseline between the fortified (1.098 ±0.437) and NFK (1.226±0.505).

*(ii) Fortifification of factory produced Ready-to-Eat (RTE) foods*

Fortification of RTE food has been reported to be cost-effective strategy. RTE food , supplied as supplementary food in the ICDS programme, is produced at factory level using wheat and chick pea flour. RTE product which reached 0.35 million beneficiaries in four districts of Gujarat State was fortified with 50% of RDA levels of iron, vitamin A and folic acid.

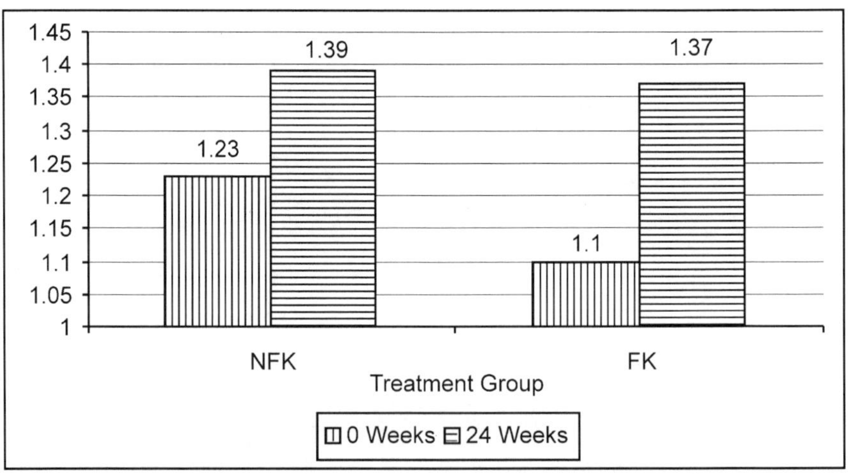


*30.8* Serum retinol concentration in NFK and FK at 0 and 24 weeks.

Unlike '*vita shakti*', the product was centrally fortified at production level. The impact assessment on the nutritional status of the beneficiaries consuming fortified ready-to-eat food showed a significant reduction in the prevalence of micronutrient deficiencies. In children the prevalence of vitamin A deficiency (serum retinol <0.7 μmol/1) decreased from 33% to 9% in the intervention district as compared to the control district. The prevalence of night blindness in children decreased from 2.0% to 0.1% in the intervention district (Panchmahal), and from 0.9% to 0.7% in the control district (Vadodra). There was no significant change in the anemia prevalence in children in intervention and control areas at endline—- anemia in women decreased from 83% to 73.5% in the intervention district, whereas the anemia prevalence in the control area remained more or less the same [54]. The reason for non-response in children was attributed to possible prevalence of worm infestation and other infections contributing to anemia which were not addressed. Following the initial trials, the project was scaled up to reach fortified complementary food distribution state wide in the state of Gujarat for under 3 year children.

*(iii) Fortification of food for the school feeding programme*

Improving the health and nutritional status of school-age children is important for improving school concentration, productivity and school performance. A good example of school feeding programme is the provision of supplementary food under the National Program of Nutritional Support for Primary Education, popularly called the Mid-Day Meal Scheme (MDM). *The National Advisory Council of India (28th August 2004) recommended that "From 1 July 2005, all mid-day meal schemes should include a component of "micronutrient supplementation", covering essential micronutrients such as Vitamin A, iron and iodine. Central assistance should be available for this component of the mid-day meal schemes and the necessary financial allocations should be made in the 2005-6 budget."* MDM program has recently begun to focus on a cooked food supplementation provided to school children five days a week, with a specified menu for each day of the week. Recipes prepared from rice / wheat, vegetable / dal are prepared for MDM and provide 450 calories and 12 grams of protein per day. The cooked food often lacked adequate micronutrient. In the State of Uttaranchal [55], a multiple micronutrient premix *"Sampoorna"* having 14 different micronutrients developed by WFP was used to fortify the mid day meal in all the schools in Tehri district. The premix was added at the rate of 0.25 g per child per day. Micronutrient levels provided per 0.25 g is presented below (Table 30.10).

*Table 30.10* Pre-mix (Sampoorna) composition per 0.25 g

| | |
|---|---|
| Vitamin A | 375 μg |
| Vitamin D | 3.75 μg |
| Vitamin E | 5.25 mg |
| Vitamin C | 26.25 mg |
| Vitamin $B_1$ | 0.68 mg |
| Vitamin $B_2$ | 0.68 mg |
| Vitamin $B_3$ | 9 mg |
| Vitamin $B_6$ | 0.75 mg |
| Vitamin $B_{12}$ | 1.35 μg |
| Folic Acid | 225 μg |
| Iron | 10 mg |
| Zinc | 4.2 mg |
| Copper | 0.45 mg |
| Iodine | 90 μg |

A cross-sectional randomized controlled study assessed the social acceptability of micronutrient fortified lunch meals cooked at schools. Subjects were randomly assigned to treatment and control groups. The treatment group consumed a weighed amount of cooked lunch meals fortified with locally produced multi-micronutrient premix and the control group consumed a weighed amount of the same meals but without added micronutrient premix. After having eaten, subjects were asked to rate, on a 3-point Likert scale using "smiley" faces, the pleasantness of smell, taste, and overall satisfaction with the food. The mean age of study children was 7.96 ± 1.64 y. The average amounts of food consumed by the treatment and control groups were 345 ± 114 and 360 ± 102.4 g, respectively. Addition of the multi-micronutrient premix to school meals did not significantly affect the mean amount of food consumed by the schoolchildren ($P > 0.05$; independent sample *t*-test). No significant differences were seen between treatment and control groups in terms of ratings for taste, smell, and the general acceptance of the micronutrient fortified or the unfortified school meals. In conclusion, the addition of a multiple micronutrient premix to school meals was well liked by schoolchildren and did not adversely affect their food consumption [56].

The study showed that, micronutrient fortification of cooked school meals by trained school authorities was effective in improving vitamin A, folate, iron and vitamin $B_{12}$ status of school children. The results are encouraging since such addition of micronutrient premix to meals at the school has advantages of being locally acceptable, sustainable and has low implementation cost since it is built on the already existing government school feeding program. However, for adoption of this fortification strategy in other regions may require adjustment to the micronutrient levels in the premix based on the micronutrient status and/

or consumption profile of the population in context, to avoid excessive intake of the vitamins and minerals. There is also the need for careful post fortification monitoring to ensure safety and potential effectiveness for the target populations.

*(iv) Fortification of wheat flour supplied through Targeted Public Distribution System (TPDS)*

The Planning Commission of India in its 10th Five Year Plan document has recommended *'food fortification'* as an important strategy for prevention and control of micronutrient deficiencies. Iron fortification of wheat flour (locally referred as *atta* ) is specifically referred in the Planning Commission document. A pilot project was implemented to test the operational effectiveness of fortified wheat flour in improving the iron and vitamin A status of the population in West Bengal (the Sadar sub-division of Darjeeling district) in India [54]. In this area, the government distributes high extraction wheat flour *(atta)*, 200 g/person/day to about 0.6 million beneficiaries below poverty line through the TPDS. Distribution of 200 g of wheat flour fortified with iron, folic acid and vitamin A, as per the composition of pre mix and wheat flour (Table 30.11) was undertaken through the public distribution system to four different target groups viz. pregnant and lactating women, pre school children, school age children and adolescent girls in the population. A *'Pre-post analysis'* with two cross-sectional surveys at baseline and 18 months after intervention was conducted . Kalimpong served as the control area for the same.

*Table 30.11* Composition of pre-mix and fortified wheat flour

| Micronutrient | Per 200 g of pre-mix | Per Kg of wheat flour | ICMR RDI | Per 200 g of wheat flour |
|---|---|---|---|---|
| Vit A | 3.33 IU | 3300 IU | 2000 IU | 660 IU |
| Folic Acid | 1.5 g | 1.5 mg | 100 µg | 300 µg |
| Iron | 60 g | 60 mg | 30 mg | 12 mg |

IEC (Information, education and communications) was undertaken to inform community of the benefits of the fortified product and for creating demand. Emphasis was on their benefits, consequences of deficiencies and significance of using the fortified atta. A workshop for the millers and PDS shop owners was organized. Additional teaching aids like wall writings, tableaux, posters, leaflets, danglers and street plays in the local language were also used for IEC activities. From the endline survey conducted after 24 months of intervention, a significant reduction in anemia prevalence was observed in all the target groups in the intervention area (Figure 30.9).

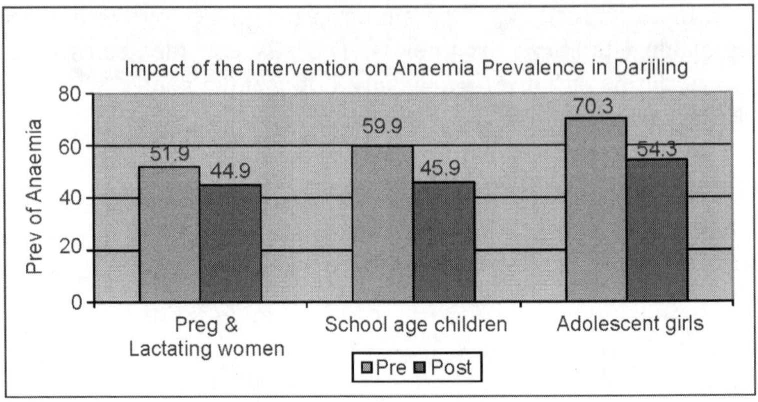


*30.9* Impact of fortified wheat flour* on prevalence of anemia.

* Wheat flour fortification details presented in Table 30.11

Though the quantity of flour distributed in the PDS is same for all age groups, the differences in the impact could be attributed to the consumption profile and needs in the respective physiological conditions. Process evaluation during the period of the study also revealed that there was no technical difficulty faced by the miller. Also, it was found that fortified wheat flour was acceptable to the population in terms of appearance, taste or storage quality of the flour. As the cost of fortification was nominal, (an additional 6 to 10 paise, one fifth of one US cent, per kg of fortified *atta*) which in fact is less than the seasonal fluctuation that occurs with wheat price, therefore it was not passed on to the consumer. However, the process did require one time investment by the miller towards installation and commissioning of a micro feeder to deliver the premix at a fixed flow rate, costing approximately INR 70,000/-(about US $ 1750), provided that the miller has all other infrastructure needed for wheat milling in place.

Based on the positive outcome, the fortification programme was scaled up in the entire state of West Bengal. By 2009, the fortified *atta* (called Enriched Atta) was being sold in the PDS outlets in 750 g poly pack bags at a cost of Rs 5/- which in fact is now being passed on to the consumer thereby demonstrating a sustainable, successful collaboration of the government and industry.

As a result of the success in one West Bengal, the supply of fortified wheat flour through the Public Distribution System has been introduced in many other states of the country such as Andhra Pradesh and Gujarat. The Roller Flour Millers Association of Gujarat has played an active role and have also launched a flour fortification program through the open market route [57]. Unlike in West Bengal, the premix formulation being used in Gujarat, as per the international recommendation, consists of two nutrients – ferrous sulphate 30ppm and folic acid 1.5 ppm i.e. (30mg of iron and 150µg of folic acid per kg of *atta*), [58]. The Government ensured political commitment at the highest level and also created an enabling environment to the millers by lending a logo, which helped in creating demand among the population.

Recognizing, wheat milling is commonly done at local village level using traditional hand milling technique or *chakkies*, a small scale *chakki* fortification programme was experimented in Sundernagar district of Gujarat. Small sachets containing 1.5 g of premix (equivalent to international recommendations of 30mg of iron and 150 µg of folic acid per kg of *atta)* have been developed with instructions of adding and mixing the contents to 10 kg of flour. Pioneering efforts in food fortification by the state government of Gujarat of about two years has resulted in overcoming the initial resistance and convincing the industry partners including roller flour millers, organized *chakki* operators and small *chakki* owners for fortifying flour. Encouraged by initial success, the state now extended the fortification program to include the distribution and utilization of fortified flour through the government feeding programmes such as the Public Distribution System, ICDS and the Mid Day Meal programs.

The flour fortification programme has been adopted in many states of India such as the Union Territory of Chandigarh, Governments of Tamilnadu, Kerala, Haryana, Punjab. The flour fortification programme is at different stages of implementation, with either a voluntary or a mandatory approach. The program is being implemented through the creation of an alliance among all stakeholders under the India Flour Fortification Network (IFFN). Government supports in monitoring the implementation of the fortification programme.

The main lesson learnt from India wheat fortification process is that the government support and commitment is an essential component for a sustainable fortification program. This support needs to be particularly in terms of a political will, lending a government logo, providing support for awareness generation and demand creation, and monitoring the program. Following ten years of implementation, the Ministry of Consumer Affairs, Food & Public Distribution of Government of India on January 24, 2008 issued a revised policy on the distribution of wheat flour to beneficaries of targeted public distribution system TPDS.

## 30.12 Fortification of selected food items

*(i) Fortification of salt*

Salt iodization has been in existence for over 70 years. In 1994 UNICEF and WHO recommended universal salt iodization (USI) as the prime approach to correcting iodine deficiency. Iodine is fortified with either potassium iodate ($KIO_3$) or Potassium iodide (KI). Compared to iodides, iodates are less soluble in water, more resistant to oxidation and evaporation, and do not require the co-addition of stabilizers being more stable under adverse climatic conditions. Potassium iodate ($KIO_3$) is thus preferred to potassium iodide (KI), especially in hot and humid climates, and is recommended for salt iodization. Most countries with tropical climates currently use potassium iodate though some countries are still using potassium iodide. Iodine is usually added to salt after the salt has been refined and dried. The common method is where a solution of $KIO_3$ is either dripped or sprayed at a uniform rate onto salt passing by on a conveyor belt. For the quality control purposes, the iodine content of salt can be determined quantitatively with the titration method, and qualitatively using rapid test kits [21].

The Government of India launched USI efforts in 1992. In India, the fortificant used is potassium iodate. The sustainability of the USI program is critical since IDD prevalence will raise if salt iodization effort weakens [59].

Building on the success of salt iodization, options for double fortifying salt with iron and iodine (commonly referred as Double fortified Salt or DFS) have been explored. Research on DFS over the decades have involved finding ways to prevent iron and iodine interactions through one of several ways including use of stabilizers , encapsulating/coating the iron or iodine with a non-reactive digestible material and identifying iron compounds with high degree of bio-availability but least reactivity with iodine.

Scientists at the National Institute of Nutrition (NIN) of India developed DFS by blending iodized refined common salt with ferrous sulphate as the iron source at 1000 ppm iron and sodium hexametaphosphate (SHMP) as a stabilizer at 1%. During the course of the past two decades, NIN successfully conducted production, sensory acceptability and efficacy trials of the product. The stability of the nutrients under laboratory conditions along with their bioavailability were found to be good but varied with the quality of salt used [60], therefore high quality dry refined salt is recommended to maintain the stability. A randomized double-blind study was carried out in 1996 for a period of two years among children belonging to backward communities attending four residential schools in and around Hyderabad, India. The study reported a generalized decrease in hemoglobin levels in both the groups. This decrease was attributed to an increase in physiological requirement for iron during the growth phase and the additional amount of iron supplemented through DFS (about 8±10 mg per day) perhaps being not adequate to increase the mean levels overall of hemoglobin [61]. However, in case of children with mild anemia (100–120 g/L Hb), a significantly greater increments in hemoglobin levels were noted in those receiving DFS (6.8 g/L) both at the end of 1 year and 2 years demonstrating significant association between improved hemoglobin and consumption of DFS. The studies confirmed that the DFS formulation by NIN is a viable option for salt which is refined and dry. The product has been field tested and commercialized to a limited extent.

The Micronutrient Initiative (MI) in collaboration with the University of Toronto identified ferrous fumarate as the iron compound suitable for DFS [62]. The process involves agglomeration of ferrous fumarate (to bring the particle size close to that of salt) and encapsulation or coating (to create a protective barrier around the iron particles). Use of small quantities of stabilizing and color masking compounds improved the product performance. The resulting 'iron premix' can be blended with iodized salt at the salt factory through a simple dry blending equipment. After a decade of research and pilot scale trials, the MI has transferred the technology to India in 2003 where the iron premix is being produced in Mumbai and blended with iodized salt at Tamil Nadu Salt Corporation (TNSC). The resulting double fortified salt containing iodine and iron is being used since then in the State Government sponsored mid day meal scheme in Tamil Nadu. Field studies confirmed iodine stability even under hot humid climates [63].

Micronized form of ferric pyrophosphate is another iron compound which has been tested by the research team at the Swiss Federal Institute, Zurich and has been shown to be an additional option for DFS [64].

In a controlled trial in rural areas around Bangalore, India in 2005, a double-blind, household-based intervention was conducted where 5–15 year old children receive iodized salt (IS) or two types of DFS with either encapsulated ferrous fumarate (EFF) or micronized ground ferric pyrophosphate (MGFePP), an alternate iron compound for comparison [65]. After 10 months the prevalence of anemia decreased from 16.8% to 7.7% in the MGFePP group and from 15.1% to 5.0% in the EFF group and the prevalence of iron deficiency dropped from 56.6% to 32.8% in the MGFePP group and from 52.4% to 34.6% in the EFF group demonstrating that both DFSs were efficacious in reducing the prevalence of anemia and iron deficiency in school-age children. In addition to improving the iron status, the EFF formulation showed better iodine stability relative to MGFePP in the presence of moisture confirming that the encapsulated ferrous fumarate is a useful option for producing DFS not only in refined dry salt but as well as lower grade salt with relatively higher moisture content since the encapsulation acts as a barrier preventing iodine losses. The light grey specs in DFS due to the iron premix were acceptable in most of the food preparations while consumer education was found to be important.

The DFS formulations by both NIN and MI target 1000 ppm of elemental iron (Table 30.12). At an average salt consumption of 10g/day these formulations provide 10 mg of iron per person per day meeting approximately 30% of the dietary requirements.

*Table 30.12* Characteristics of DFS formulations developed and tested by NIN and MI

| *Main Characteristics* | *NIN Formulation [60]* | *MI Formulation [65]* |
|---|---|---|
| Iodine (ppm), source | 30-40 as $KIO_3$ or KI | 30-40 as $KIO_3$ or KI |
| Iron (ppm), source | 1000 as Ferrous Sulphate | 1000 Ferrous Fumarate |
| Stabilization of iodine | SHMP and use of high quality dry salt | Encapsulation and stabilization by Soy Stearine and SHMP |

For quality control of DFS, it is recommended to check both iodine and iron levels at the production site. For field monitoring purposes, qualitative and semi-quantitative tests for DFS containing encapsulated iron has been developed by the University of Toronto [66].

(ii) *Fortification of sugar*

Sugar fortification with vitamin A in the form of retinyl palmitate at a concentration of 15 mg retinol per kg of sugar has been effective in reducing the prevalence of subclinical vitamin A deficiency in Central America [67].

**Box 30.2 Success of sugar fortification at the global level**

During the 1970s, the Institute of Nutrition of Central America and Panama (INCAP), which is associated with the Pan American Health Organization (PAHO), developed fortification technology and implemented sugar fortification programs in various Central American countries, with the first program launched in 1975 in Guatemala. The vitamin A compound in the form of beadlets is bound to the sugar crystal through a layer of vegetable oil to avoid segregation and stability was established to be 40–70% even after 9 months. Population based studies showed that the prevalence of vitamin A deficiency decreased from 22 to 5 percent over a one-year period, and retinol levels in breast milk and in hepatic reserves increased significantly. Mandatory sugar fortification has been established through a variety of legal instruments, with regulations prepared by the Ministries of Health.

In India, following review of Guatemala sugar fortification successful efforts, Vasantdada Sugar Research Institute (Pune) in collaboration with MI , National Federation of Cooperative Sugar Factories (New Delhi) and the Ministry of Food, Consumer Affairs and Public Distribution System developed a technology for fortifying large crystalline sugar available in India. A series of stability and segregation studies were also conducted with vitamin A in the form of retinyl palmitate at a concentration of 15 mg retinol per kg of sugar. With the financial support from the Government of India, MI installed and commissioned a pilot plant for fortifying sugar at

Shirpur, Maharashtra [68]. However, sugar fortification was not approved under the Prevention of Food Adulteration Act, 1955 by the government as sugar was not accepted as a very useful vehicle for fortification in India (neither with iron nor with vitamin A), as many of the lower economic groups were found to be using very little sugar.

(iii) *Fortification of edible oils*

Countries such as Nigeria, Morocco, Yemen, Bangladesh and Pakistan are implementing national programs to fortify cooking oils with vitamin A. Vitamin A is readily absorbed in the presence of oils and fats. The evidence for the biological effect of fortified oils and fats was reviewed in a report commissioned by SUSTAIN [69]. The review summarized studies before and after the fortification of margarine. In 1944, in Newfoundland it was reported that the percent of subjects with serum vitamin A below 20 µg/dl declined from 48% to 2% in a period of over four years. In Philippines, more recently, a shelf stable margarine was fortified with vitamin A. After consuming the margarine for six months, the percentage of children with serum retinol levels below 20 µg/dl fell from 25.6% to 10.1%. It was also demonstrated that soybean oil fortified with vitamin A in the form of retinol palmitate was well absorbed in humans who were fed fortified oil along with a rice-based diet. Significant increases in plasma retinol were reported. Differences in plasma retinol for subjects receiving uncooked versus cooked soybean oil were not statistically significant.

**Box 30.3 Success of oil fortification in India**

MI in collaboration with Central Food Technological Research Institute conducted studies on the stability of vitamin A in oils under different temperatures, varied cooking methods and for preparation of different products to suggest the levels of fortification under Indian culinary practices. In consultation with MI, Government of Gujarat was the first state to initiate edible oils fortification with vitamin A and D at the rate of 25 IU of vitamin A and 2 IU of vitamin D per gram of oil, and has also made it mandatory within the state [70]. All oil millers, packers and processors are fortifying the oil in the State. Fortified edible oils are also being procured and distributed under all government welfare programs like PDS, ICDS, MDM, at an additional cost of 3 paise per kilogram of oil. The quality control is being monitored through government approved laboratories under the Department of Food & Civil Supplies, Government of Gujarat.

(iv) *Fortification of rice*

For fortifying whole grain cereals like rice, a technology to produce simulated rice-shaped premix has been explored. Since rice grains are washed before cooking in many countries including India, rice fortification methods like addition of powder form of micronutrients or external coating methods practiced in North America were not considered suitable. During the past 10 years, extrusion methods were tried as a practical option where an iron compound with or without other micronutrients can be blended with rice flour and formed into rice shaped premix granules through the extrusion process. The target iron concentration of the premix is recommended to be set at 0.5 g or 1 g Fe/100 g of the premix so that when the premix (in shape of rice grains) is blended with natural rice grains at respective ratios of 1:100 or 1:200 the resulting fortified rice contains 5 mg iron per 100 g of rice. This fortification level would provide 15 mg of additional iron to a person consuming 300 g of rice per day. The premix composition and blending ratio can be adjusted based on rice consumption and targeted level of fortification.

Selection of an iron compound for fortification that is bioavailable but at the same time does not cause negative sensory characteristics has been a challenge. Color and sensory acceptability tests, using different iron compounds, conducted in Bangalore, India by St. John's National Academy of Health Sciences in collaboration with Rutgers University, USA and Institute of Food Science and Nutrition, Zurich, showed that extruded rice premix with excellent sensory characteristics and potential high bioavailability can be produced using micronized ferric pyrophosphate. The fortified rice produced using this premix closely resembled unfortified rice, showed less than 3% iron losses during rinsing and achieved a consistent texture when the fortified rice was cooked [71].

With support from the MI, an efficacy study was conducted in 2004 at St. John's National Academy of Health Sciences, Bangalore, India in schools located in urban slums around Bangalore where a Government subsidized lunch feeding program provided the students with a 200 to 300g meal of cooked rice daily. In a double-blind, 7 month school-based feeding trial, iron-depleted, 6 to 13 year old children were randomly assigned to receive either a rice-based lunch meal fortified with 20 mg Fe as Micronized Ground Ferric Pyrophosphate or an identical but unfortified control meal. Both the groups received deworming treatment. After 7months of feeding, there was a significant increase in body iron stores in both study groups, with a greater increase in the iron group than in the control group. Iron deficiency fell from 78% to 25% in the dewormed iron group and from 79% to 49% in the dewormed control group. Iron deficiency anemia decreased from 30% to 15% in the iron group but remained virtually unchanged in the control group (28% and 27%) [72].

In addition to the micro-nutrient iron, fortification of rice with vitamins A and B complex vitamins have also been tried by PATH. Efficacy studies on PATH technology, known as Ultra Rice, were conducted in India by the National Institute of Nutrition (NIN). The data from a recently concluded study [73] in school children revealed that consumption of rice fortified with iron Ultra Rice had positive impact on the iron stores as evidenced by significant increase in the serum Ferritin levels in the experimental group. It was also observed that the intervention led to a significant reduction in the incidence of morbidities among children in the experimental group as evidenced by a positive trend of lower proportion of children falling sick with increasing duration of intervention observed in the experimental group (31.7%) compared to control group (44.6%). Pilot testing indicated a price increase of 5 to 10% over the non-fortified rice depending on the nutrients included.

For rice fortification, premix production can be centralized at a large production facility as being done in China by DSM/Buhler collaboration or as a smaller scale production using pasta making equipment being established by PATH in India.

## 30.13 Innovative experiments with fortification

Innovative approaches to reach specific target groups with micronutrients have been explored in the past decaded (Table 30.13).

(i) *Hard-boiled sugar lozenges (nutri-candies)* are being increasingly used as a vehicle to provide essential micronutrients to young children through targeted programs along with food. The lozenges contain less than 3 g of sugar, center filled along with a number of micronutrients like, vitamin A, Iron, Folic Acid and vitamin C, at 50% of RDA levels for children. Vitamin C not only adds a citric flavor to make the candy more palatable but further enhance iron absorption.

A pilot project on distribution of nutri-candies in collaboration with the Government of West Bengal( Howrah district), was undertaken.The evaluation of the effectiveness of the fortified candies showed a 15% reduction in the prevalence of anemia among pre-school children over a span of 18 months (Figure 30.10a). However, no such change was observed in pregnant and lactating mothers as the level of fortification was only 25% of their RDA and not 50% as in the case of pre school children, and possibly not adequate to meet with the additional requirements of pregnancy. In case of adolescent girls, there was a reduction in anemia prevalence by 11% (Figure 30.10b) when paired samples were compared after a period of 18 months [74]. Efficacy trials conducted by the All India Institute of Medical Sciences showed a reduction by nearly 50% within a span of 12 weeks of candies administration [75]. The distribution of the nutri-candies at the ICDS Centre also had an impact on the percentage of children enrolled and attendance [76]. The principal advantages of supplying fortified candies through a programme like the ICDS was that the delivery could be targeted to a specific at-risk groups; distribution was simple and delivery of measured quantity of micronutrients could be ensured unlike in case

*Table 30.13* Compiled information on various fortified products developed and/or implemented by MI

| Product | Target group | Administration | Fortified Nutrients | Cost |
|---|---|---|---|---|
| Anuka/Sprinkles* | 6–24 mth old | Powder to be mixed with complementary food before consumption | Iron, Zinc, Vitamin A, Folic acid, Vitamin C – All 100% RDA except vit A) | 40 cents per child for 2 months intervention |
| Fortified Lozenges/ Candies | 2–6 years old, Adolescent girls, Pregnant and lactating woman | Consumed as such after food is consumed at the AWC | Vitamin A, Folic acid, Vitamin C and Iron 50% RDA for the children and 25% for pregnant and lactating women | $1.20 per beneficiary for a one year supply |
| Fortified Staples- Maize Meal and Wheat Flour | Entire Population | Consumed as such | Iron, Zinc, Vitamin A, Folic acid, B complex Vitamins – 25 to 50% RDA's for children & adults | $0.5 and $5 per metric ton |
| Double Fortified Salt | Entire Population | Recommended for use in cooking and as table salt | Iodine and Iron targeting about 100% RDA for iodine and 30% RDA for iron | 20 cents per person per year |
| Vita-Shakti/Rahma | Children 2-6 & Pregnant & Lactating Women in India & Entire Population in Africa | To be mixed to staple food after cooking | Iron, Vitamin A, Folic acid - 50% RDA for the children and 25% for pregnant and | 35–45 cents per person per year |

Sprinkles*—Two different formulations are available—one with 5 micronutrients as in case of Anuka, and the other with 15 micronutrients, covering all the B complex vitamins.

of fortification of staple food wherein, the variation in intake between individuals is large and difficult to control.

*(ii) Home fortificant–Anuka and Sprinkles*

A formulation for home fortification of complementary food, called *Anuka* developed in India with MI support, contains iron, vitamin A, folic acid, zinc and vitamin C (Table 30.13). *Anuka*, available in sachets, can be added to food just before feeding. It can therefore be regarded as complementary food supplement (CFS) for home fortification. The sachets are easy to use and provide the required dose of micronutrients to children regardless of the quantity of complementary food consumed. CFS provide 100% recommended daily allowances of nutrients in single-serve sachet form, which is added to and mixed with any semi-solid complementary food after it has been cooked and immediately prior to being fed to the child. The vitamin-C component provides a citric flavor and helps in the absorption of iron.

*Anuka* can be distributed to the mothers of target children (6–24 month olds), dispensed as dry powder in sachets. This product has undergone sensory trials, stability tests and acceptability studies. The tasteless dry powder has been tested at both room temperature and normal relative humidity as well as accelerated conditions and found to be stable for more than six months. When added to complementary foods, there is no appreciable change in taste or consistency of food and well accepted both by the service providers and receivers. An acceptability and feasibility study, supported by MI, was conducted in 14 blocks of Howrah District of West Bengal where sachets were distributed to mothers of children through the ICDS (Integrated Child Development Services) or Anganwadi Centers (AWCs) for 70,000 children. Positive results were

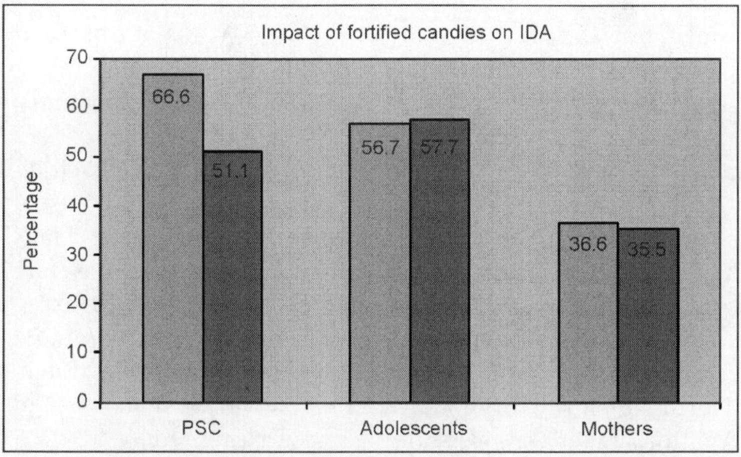


*30.10a* Effectiveness trials on anemia prevalence.

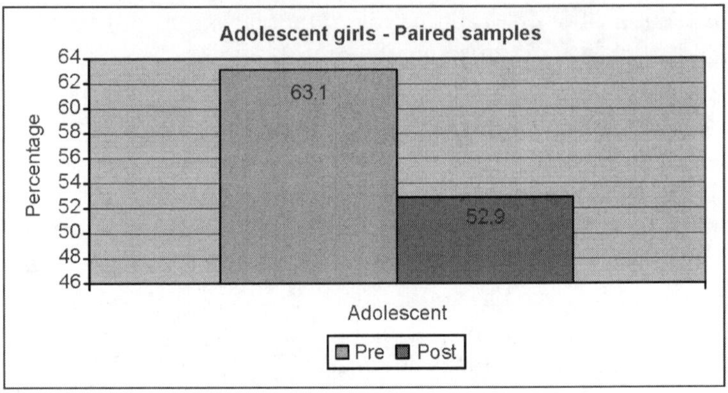


*30.10 b* Effectiveness trials on anemia prevalence.

noted with 80% to 85% compliance of usage by ICDS workers and mothers [77].

Another *Anuka* project was implemented by the state Government of Rajasthan. The impact on growth velocity of children (6–12 months), rate of weight and height increase, over a 6th month period demonstrated very positive results. There was an increase in compliance of the utilization of Anuka–multiple micronutrient sachets along with the complementary feeding, from 58% to 91% over a period of 6 months. The programme implementation involved technical consultations and standardization of recipes, partnerships and alliance building, developing state level master trainers, capacity building of functionaries as well as mothers. Weekly Distribution Day was designated wherein all children along with mothers/ caretakers assembled at the ICDS centre (AWC) and were distributed five sachets of *Anuka* along with complementary food mix. Presence of mothers at the AWC was ensured by the frontline ICDS worker or AWW. Demonstration of complementary food preparation was done by AWWs and grassroots health worker (ASHA) for mothers and caregivers on this day, along with enhancing capacities of mothers regarding usage of *Anuka* in complementary food. First dose of *Anuka* was given to each child by their mother, under supervision at the AWC during weekly distribution day. A total of 60 sachets were provided and consumed over a maximum period of 120 days. During home visit, the frontline workers (AWW and ASHA) were responsible to ensure the usage of *Anuka*. On the week following the distribution, AWW the empty sachets *of Anuka* were collected by these workers to confirm the compliance. Such close monitoring ensured high compliance. Over a span of 6 months intervention, under weight, stunting and wasting reduced by 3%, 21% and 1% respectively [78].

Sprinkles a multiple micronutrient premix developed by University of Toronto, Canada comprising iron, vitamin A, zinc, vitamin C and several other micronutrients and tested in several countries, when distributed to children in Mongolia [79] and China [80], reported high levels of feasibility, acceptability, compliance and efficacy, because of perceived benefits and ease of use. (*Details on sprinkles are presented in the chapter on Childhood Anemia*).

## 30.14 Public–private partnerships

Effective and sustainable fortification program is possible only if the public sector (which has the mandate and responsibility to improve the health of the population), the private sector (which has the experience and expertise in food production and marketing), and the social sector (which has grass-roots contact with the consumer) collaborate to develop, produce and promote micronutrient fortified foods [81]. The key players include (i) the Governments; (ii) Research and academic institutions; (iii) Food and premix manufacturing companies; (iv) Consumer organizations; (v) Development assistance agencies (vi) NGOs, and (vii) Media.

Food fortification serves the need of the public sector to reduce malnutrition and sustain economic growth. National governments play an equally important role by providing administrative support and prescribing the framework within which solutions are regulated and implemented. The private food industry contributes not only undertaking production of fortified foods but also in creating demand. Raising product quality through fortification stimulates demand for regional products, and intensifies competition and trade. The consumer once aware of the benefits of food fortification demands the product resulting in mobilizing industry to respond. International agencies provide technical, funding and advocacy support for development of intervention strategies.

The wheat flour fortification project in West Bengal, India summarizes the partnerships involved which played an important role in the success of the project (Figure 30.11). The role of each key player was as follows: implementation, monitoring and demand creation was done by the West Bengal Micronutrient Initiative Project (WBMIP) of unit office under the Department of Social Welfare (SW), Government of West Bengal; the Department of Food & Civil Supplies, Government of West Bengal issued the government notification about the policy/legislation of fortified *atta* and also increased the quota distributed through the PDS; the premix industry provided quality premix, the miller agreed to not only to install the micro-feeder at their own cost, along with the production of the quality product (fortified *atta*), but also imposed voluntary regulation at the factory; the local media viz. local newspapers, televisions etc assisted in increasing awareness and demand creation and last but not the least the well reputed non government organization, Child In Need Institute (CINI) conducted an impact assessment study, making it a successful pilot project.

Another good example of public–private partnership is IDD elimination through Universal Salt Iodization. The global experience of past years has demonstrated that coordinated action by all sectors of society is the key to eliminating iodine deficiency in any given country: the government authorities pursue policies that protect newborns from preventable brain damage by supporting and sustaining salt iodization as well as by monitoring progress; salt industry and vendors produce and sell adequately iodized salt at a fair price in cities and villages every day while civil society assists in public education regarding the dangers of iodine deficiency and ensuring that iodized salt is available.

The *Sangkap Pinoy Seal* program in the Philippines also is a good example of public–private collaboration. Since the program was launched in 1995, over thirty products from sixteen companies have attained the seal from the Department of Health. In Guatemala, the national program of sugar fortification with vitamin A is

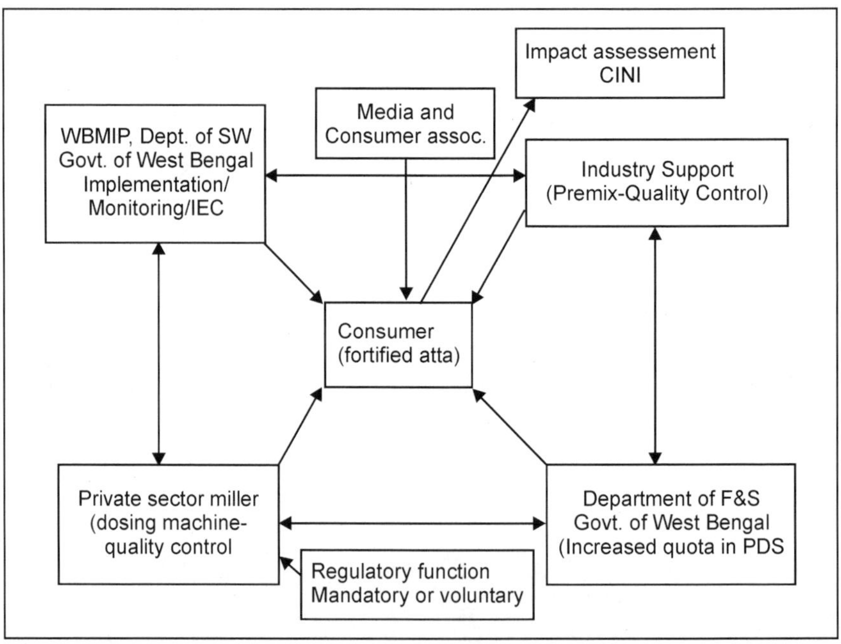


*30.11* Public–private partnership in food fortification–West Bengal case study.

implementedwith full cooperation of the sugar industry. In Vietnam, an alliance of private companies, research institutes, NGOs and donor organizations have jointly developed an iron-fortified fish sauce as well as vitamin-A fortified sugar. A private company provided the required technical expertise and developed a fortified drink called *Nutri-Delight*, and in partnerships with the governments, NGOs and universities who confirmed the efficacy of *the product*. The significance of such partnership is evident.

Table 30.14 defines the roles of each of the various partners in a Multi Sectoral Collaboration to build Public–Private Partnership model.

*Table 30.14* Multi-sectoral collaboration

| Sector | Role |
|---|---|
| Scientific Community | Identify problems and solutions, undertake efficacy trials |
| Government | Advocacy, resources and program support |
| Industry | Technical inputs, resources and marketing |
| Consumer Organizations | Consumer education to create demand |
| International/bilateral agencies | Advocacy, technical input, training, resources |

## 30.15 Monitoring and evaluation

Any fortification program needs to be accompanied with a good monitoring and evaluation system in place at production as well as at consumption level. Monitoring quality control at the production level is critical to ensure that the fortified food is produced according to the required procedures and contains adequate levels of the micronutrients. At consumption level, monitoring and evaluation comprises both product monitoring and its impact on the population.The latter includes anthropometric as well as clinical and biochemical measurements.

## 30.16 Regulations and standards

In order to undertake effective food fortification activities, it is important to ensure that laws and regulations provide legal authority and an adequate regulatory framework. Effective regulatory controls through established fortification standards protect consumers against the risk of purchasing and consuming nutritionally inadequate, deceptively mislabelled or misbranded, impure or unsafe foods. Regulations also create a 'level playing field' for food manufacturers and sellers. For example, the Prevention of Food Adulteration (PFA) of India defines standards for food items with micronutrients under the prevention of food adulteration rules of 1955 under appendix B. The standards of food items, as prescribed

*Table 30.15* Standards for food items as prescribed under the Prevention of Food Adulteration Rules, 1955 under Appendix B

| Name of the micronutrient | Name of the food | Prescribed level of added nutrients | | | Item no. in the appendix B | Other conditions, if any | Effective date |
|---|---|---|---|---|---|---|---|
| | | Minimum | maximum | Specific provisions | | | |
| Iodine | Iodized salt | 30ppm<br>15ppm | none | On dry weight basis | A.15.01 | Specific conditions of packing and labeling apply | 10/2/1988 |
| Iron | Iron fortified common salt | 850 ppm | 110ppm | As Fe | A. 15. 01 | Specific conditions of packing and labeling apply | 4/1/1985 |
| | Fortified atta | None | None | | A.18.01.01 | | 4/4/1960 |
| | Fortified maida | None | None | | A.18.02.01 | | 4/4/1960 |
| Vitamin A | Bakery shortening | 25 I.U | None | Synthetic vitamin A per gram at the time of packing and shall show positive test for vitamin A, when tested with Antimony trichloride(Carr price reagent as per I.S 886-1970 | A.19.01 | Specific conditions of packing and labeling apply | 10/10/1983 |
| | Bakery and industrial margarine | 30 I.U | None | Synthetic vitamin A per gram at the time of packing and shall show positive test for vitamin A, when tested with Antimony trichloride(Carr price reagent as per I.S 886-1970 | A.12.01 | | 14/8/97 |

under PFA, is presented in Table 30.15 and is being revised to be called "Integrated Food Laws".

## 30.17 Conclusion

Food fortification is a feasible and cost effective method to address the micronutrient deficiencies, along with other strategies like food diversification, supplementation as well as public health measures like immunization, deworming, safe water and sanitation. Experience gained in developed countries as well as developing countries clearly demonstrates that it is possible to select an appropriate fortification intervention based on the target population and suitable food vehicle. Partnership approach to end 'hidden hunger' between the governments, social sector organizations, private sector, academicians, civil societies and last but not the least the consumers need to play pivotal role in creating a demand for quality food and sharing the risks and rewards of combating micronutrient deficiencies.

## References


1. NATIONAL NUTRITION MONITORING BUREAU (NNMB) 2002 and 2006.
2. MASON J, RIVERS J, HELWIG C (2005). Recent trends in malnutrition in developing regions: Vitamin A deficiency, anemia, iodine deficiency, and child underweight. *Food and Nutrition Bulletin*, **26**(1), pp. 5–42.
3. MICRONUTRIENT INITIATIVE (2005). Controlling vitamin and mineral deficiencies in India—meeting the goal.
4. WHO (2002). The World Health Report 2002: Reducing risks, promoting healthy life. Geneva.
5. National Family Health Survey-III, (NFHS), Ministry of Health & Family Welfare, Government of India, 2005-06.
6. WHO BULLETIN (2006). Chapter V, p. 382.
7. RAJAGOPALAN S (2003). Nutrition challenges in the next decade, *Food and Nutrition Bulletin*, **24**(3), pp. 275–280.
8. WORLD BANK (2006). Repositioning Nutrition as Central to Development: A Strategy for Large Scale Action.
9. DEITCHLER M, MATHYS E, MASON J, WINICHAGOON P and TUAZON M (2004). Lessons from successful micronutrient programs Part II: Program implementation. *Food and Nutrition Bulletin*, **25**(1), pp. 30–52.
10. UNICEF (1990). World Declaration on the Survival, Protection and Development of Children. New York, USA.
11. Proceedings of "Ending hidden hunger"—A policy conference on micronutrient malnutrition. 10-12 October 1991, Montreal, Canada. Sponsored by WHO, UNICEF, World Bank, CIDA, USAID, FAO, UNDP.
12. World Declaration and Plan of Action for Nutrition (1992). International Conference on Nutrition. Rome, Italy.
13. DEPARTMENT OF WOMEN & CHILD DEVELOPMENT (1995). Ministry of Human Resource Development, GOI — Proceedings of the Workshop Held in Jaipur on "Strategy for Elimination of Micronutrient Malnutrition in India" November 1–2.

14. FOOD AND AGRICULTURE ORGANIZATION (1996). Food fortification: technology and quality control. Report of an FAO Technical Meeting held in Rome, 20–23 November 1995. FAO Food and Nutrition Paper. Rome: FAO.
15. RALOFF J (2004). Should Foods Be Fortified Even More. *Science News Online*, **166**(11). http://www.sciencenews.org/articles/20040911/food.asp (accessed October 23, 2006).
16. BISHAI D and NALUBOLA R (2002). The History of Food Fortification in the United States: Its Relevance for Current Fortification Efforts in Developing Countries; Economic Development and Cultural Change, University of Chicago Press, **51**(1), pp. 37–53.
17. PARK YK, CALVO MS, ROSS SA and YETLEY EA (1997). Sources of nutrients in the United States: food versus supplements. Presented at the 16th International Congress of Nutrition, Montreal, Canada, 27 July to 1 August 1997 (Abstr. PT14).
18. MANNAR MGV (2003). Food fortification. In: *Encyclopedia of Food Sciences and NutritionI*, 2nd ed. Cabellero B, Trugo LC and Finglas PM (eds.), pp. 2613–2621. Academic Press, Oxford.
19. ALLEN L, DE BENOIST B, DARY O and HURRELL R. (eds) (2006). Guidelines on Food Fortification with Micronutrients. Joint WHO and FAO publication, WHO Press, Geneva, Switzerland.
20. Codex Standard for Food Grade Salt; CX STAN 150-1985 Amend2-2001, Amend 3-2006.
21. WHO/ICCIDD/UNICEF (2001). *Assessment of Iodine Deficiency Disorders and Monitoring Their Elimination – A Guide for Program Managers*, 2nd edition, World Health Organization, Geneva.
22. CLARKE R (1995). Micronutrient Fortification of food: Technology and Quality control; working paper FAO Technical consultation on Food fortification. Rome, Italy, 20–23 Nov, 1995.
23. BOTHWELL TH and MACPHAIL P (1992). Prevention of iron deficiency by food fortification. In: *Nutritional Anemias*, Fomon SJ and Zlotkin S (eds). Nestlé Nutrition Workshop Series, **30.** Raven Press, New York, pp. 183–192.
24. HURRELL RF (1997). Preventing iron deficiency through food fortification. *Nutr. Rev.*, **55**, pp. 210–222.
25. INACG (INTERNATIONAL NUTRITIONAL ANEMIA CONSULTATIVE GROUP) (2002). Technical Brief on Iron Compounds for Fortification of Staple Foods. Life Sciences Institute-Nutrition Foundation. Washington, D.C.
26. MURPHY AP (1995). History of technology development of vitamin A fortification in developing countries, Working paper. FAO Technical consultation on Food Fortification. Rome, Italy, 20–23 Nov, 1995.
27. INSTITUTE OF MEDICINE (2004). Dietary Reference Intakes: guiding principles for nutrition labeling and fortification; Committee on Use of Dietary Reference Intakes in Nutrition Labeling. Food and Nutrition Board, Institute of Medicine (U.S.), National Academy Press, Washington, DC.
28. RUBIN SH, EMODI A, SCIALPI L (1977). Micronutrient additions to cereal grain products. *Cereal Chem.*, **54**(4), pp. 895–904.
29. MAHADEVAN B and BHAT VB (2005). Neural tube defects in Pondicherry. *Indian Journal of Pediatrics*, **72**.
30. RIDDELL LJ, CHISHOLM A, WILLIAMS S, MANN JI (2000). Dietary strategies for lowering homocysteine concentrations. *Am J Clin Nutr.*, **71**(6), pp. 1448–1454.

31. ORISS GD (1998). Food Fortification: Safety and Legislation. *Food and Nutrition Bulletin*, **19**(2), pp. 109–116.
32. MERTZ W (1997). Food fortification in the United States. *Nutrition Reviews*, **55**, pp. 44–49.
33. NESTLE and NALUBOLA (2003). Food Fortification is an effective public health intervention; Bureau for Global Health, U.S. Agency for International Development, Washington, DC.
34. UNICEF (2006). The State of the World's Children. New York: United Nations Children's Fund.
35. MANNAR MGV (2006). Successful food-based programs, supplementation and fortification. *Journal of Pediatric Gastroenterology and Nutrition*, **43,** pp. S47–S53.
36. LAYRISSE M, CHAVES JF, MENDEZ-CASTELLANO H, BOSCH V, TROPPER E, BASTARDO B and GONZALEZ E (1996). Early response to the effect of iron fortification in Venezuelean population. *Am J Clinical Nutrition*, **64**, pp. 903–907.
37. MANNAR MGV and WESLEY AS (2007). Food fortification. In: *Encyclopedia of Public Health*. Heggenhougen K (ed), Elsevier Inc., San Diego (in print).
38. JOHNSON Q, MANNAR V, RANUM P (2004). Fortification Handbook: Vitamin and Mineral Fortification of Wheat Flour and Maize Meal. In: *Micronutrient Initiative*. WESLEY A and RANUM P (eds).
39. ZLOTKIN SH, CHRISTOFIDES AL, ZIAUDDIN HYDER SM, SCHAUER CS, TONDEUR MC, SHARIEFF W (2004). Controlling iron deficiency anemia through the use of home-fortified complementary foods. *Indian J Pediatr*, **71**, pp. 1015–1019.
40. National Nutrition Policy (1993). Government of India Publication, Department of Women and Child Welfare, Ministry of Human Resource Development, New Delhi.
41. National Plan of Action on Nutrition (1995). Food and Nutrition Board; Department of Women and Child Development, Government of India.
42. Preventing Micronutrient Malnutrition Through ICDS; White Paper; Prepared by Department of Women & Child Development, Ministry of Human Resource Development, Government of India & United Nations World Food Product.
43. SUBRAHMANYAN V (1954). Investigation on rice substitutes. *Bulletin of the Central Food Technological Research Institute*, **3**(4), pp. 180–183.
44. SUBRAHMANYAN V, RAMA RAO G, KUPPUSWAMY S, NARAYANA RAO M, SWAMINATHAN M (1957). Indian multipurpose food. *Food Science*, **6**(4), pp. 76–80.
45. ORR E (1972). *The Use of Protein-rich Foods for the Relief of Malnutrition in Developing Countries, and Analysis of Experience*. Tropical Products Institute, London.
46. PRABHA S and BAGCHI K (1978). Effect of lysine-fortified wheat on the nutrition status of children. In: *Wheat in the Indian Diet.* Abrol YP and Pingle SV (eds).
47. ELWOOD PC, BENJAMIN IT, FRY FA, EAKINS JD, BROWN DA, DE KOCK PC, SHAH JU (1970). Absorption of iron from chapathi from wheat flour. *American Journal of Clinical Nutrition*, **23**, pp. 1267–1271.
48. NARASINGA RAO BS and VIJAYASARATHY C (1975). Fortification of Common Salt with Iron: Effect of Chemical Additives on Stability and Bio-availability. *American Journal of Clinical Nutrition*, **28,** pp. 1395–1401.
49. ZOLLER JM, WOLINSKY CA, PADEN CA, HOSKIN JC, LEWIS KC, LINEBACK DR, MCCARTHY RD (1980). Fortification of nonstaple food items with iron. *Food Technology*, **34**, pp. 38–47.

50. DISLER PB, LYNCH SR, CHARLTON RW, TORRANCE JD, BOTHWELL TH, WALKER RB, MAYET F (1975). The effect of tea on iron absorption. *Gut (British Medical Journal Publishing Group)*, **16**, pp. 193–200.
51. IS 14433 Part 1:1997-Infant Milk Substitutes, Specifications Part I.
52. PRESS INFORMATION BUREAU (1929). Government of India. Dated the 10 Vaisakha, 1929 Saka 30th April, 2007 PRESS NOTE Household Consumption of Various Goods and Services in India, 2004-05.
53. VARMA JL, DAS S, SANKAR R, MANNAR MGV, LEVINSON FL, HAMER DH (2007). Community-level micronutrient fortification of a food supplement in India: a controlled trial in preschool children aged 36-66 months. *American Journal of Clinical Nutrition*, **85**, pp. 1127–1133.
54. MANNAR MGV and BULUSU S (2007). Approaches to deliver micronutrients to young children and women through targeted public programs in India. *The Indian Journal of Nutrition and Dietetics*, **44**(1), pp. 50–51.
55. WFP-MI Joint Project Document (2007).
56. OSEI AK, HOUSER RF, BULUSU S and HAMER DH (2008). Acceptability of micronutrient fortification in school meals by school children in rural Himalayan villages of India. *Journal of Food Science*, **73**(7), pp. 354–357.
57. BULUSU S (2007). Strategies for Tackling Nutritional Deficiencies with Case Studies of Emerging Trends in Fortification in India and Abroad. *Food Fortification—A Gujarat Initiative*, pp. 115–124.
58. WHO/UNICEF/MI/ILSI (1998). Fortification of Flour to Control Micronutrient Deficiencies in Countries of the Eastern Mediterranean Middle East and North Africa, Report of a Joint WHO/UNICEF/MI/ILSI workshop, Lebanon (13-16 June 1998), WHO EMRO 1999.
59. VIR SC (2002). Current status of iodine deficiency disorders (IDD) and strategy for its control in India. *Indian Journal of Pediatrics*, **69**(7), pp. 589–596.
60. SIVAKUMAR B and NAIR KM (2002). Double fortified salt at cross roads. *Indian Journal of Pediatrics*, **69**(7), pp. 617–623.
61. NAIR KM, BRAHMAM GNV, RANGANATHAN S, VIJAYARAGHAVAN K (1998). Impact evaluation of iron & iodine fortified salt. *Indian Journal of Medical Research*, **108**, pp. 203–211.
62. DIOSADY LL, ALBERTI JO, RAMCHARAN K, MANNAR MGV (2002). Iodine stability in salt double fortified with iron and iodine. *Food and Nutrition Bulletin*, **23**(2), pp. 196–207.
63. OSHINOWO T, DIOSADY LL, YUSUFALI R, WESLEY A (2007). An investigation of the stability of double fortified salt during storage and distribution in Nigeria. *International Journal of Food Engineering*, **3**(4), pp. 1–20.
64. WEGMULLER R, CAMARA F, ZIMMERMANN MB, ADOU P, HURRELL RF (2006). Salt dual-fortified with iodine and micronized ground ferric pyrophosphate affects iron status but not hemoglobin in children in Cote d'Ivoire. *Journal of Nutrition*, **136**, pp. 1814–1820.
65. ANDERSSON M, THANKACHAN P, MUTHAYYA S, GOUD RB, KURPAD AV, HURRELL RF, ZIMMERMANN MB (2008). Dual fortification of salt with iodine and iron: a randomized, double blind, controlled trial of micronized ferric pyrophosphate and encapsulated ferrous fumarate in southern India. *American Journal of Clinical Nutrition*, **88**, pp. 1378–1387.
66. YUAN JS, LI YO, UE JW, WESLEY A, DIOSADY LL (2008). Development of field test kits for determination of microencapsulated iron in double-fortified salt. *Food and Nutrition Bulletin*, **29**(4), pp. 288–296.

67. MORA JO, DARY O, CHINCHILLA D, ARROYAVE G (2000). Vitamin A Sugar Fortification in Central America: Experiences and Lessons Learned; MOST, The USAID Micronutrient Program.
68. BULUSU S and SIROHI SS (1999). Pilot Plant Studies on Fortification of Sugar with Vitamin 'A' at Shirpur S.S.K. Ltd., Shirpur (Maharashtra). *Cooperative Sugar*, **31**(4), pp. 307–314.
69. BAGRIANSKY J and RANUM P (1998). Report on Vitamin A Fortification of PL 480 Vegetable Oil. *Sustain*, Washington DC.
70. NANDA SK (2007). Food Fortification in Gujarat Report, Government of Gujarat.
71. MORETTI D, LEE TC, ZIMMERMANN MB, NUESSLI J, HURRELL R (2005). Development and Evaluation of iron-fortified extruded rice grains. *Journal of Food Science*, **7**(5), pp. S330– S336.
72. MORETTI D, ZIMMERMANN, MB, MUTHAYYA S, THANKACHAN P, LEE TC, KURPAD AV, HURRELL RF (2006). Extruded rice fortified with micronized ground ferric pyrophosphate reduces iron deficiency in Indian schoolchildren: a double-blind randomized controlled trial. *Am J Clin Nutr*, **84,** pp. 822–829.
73. NIN (2009). Personal Communication.
74. BULUSU S and POPATIA Z (2006). Nutri-lozenges – An Innovation in Micronutrients. *Global Health Council Forum*, Washington, DC.
75. ANAND K, LAKSHMY R, JANAKARAJAN VN, RITVIK A, MISRA P, PANDEY RM, KAPOOR SK, SANKAR R, BULUSU S (2007). Effect of consumption of micronutrient fortified candies on the iron and vitamin A status of children aged 3-6 years in rural Haryana. *Indian Pediatrics*, **44**, pp. 823–829.
76. BULUSU S and JOSHI TP (2006). Fortified lozenges delivering multiple micronutrients to the communities in India – suck it and see. *Nutrition*, **3**, pp. 16–17.
77. BULUSU S, LAVIOLETTE L, MANNAR V, REDDY V (2006). Cereal fortification programs in developing countries. In: *Nestle Nutrition Workshop Series Pediatric Program—Issues in Complementary Feeding*. Agostoni C and Brunser O (eds). Nestle Nutrition Institute, **60**, pp. 91–105.
78. MI and UNICEF (2008). Home fortification of decentralized supplementary food with micronutrient sprinkle—Experience in ICDS, Tonk, Rajasthan by Directorate of ICDS, Government of Rajasthan, Department of Women and Child Development.
79. ZLOTKIN SH, SCHAUER C, CHRISTOFIDES A et al (2005). Micronutrient sprinkles to control childhood anemia. *PLoS Medicine*, **2**(1), pp. 24–28.
80. YEUNG DL, YAP J, CHENG C (2004). Consumer acceptance of a home food iron fortificant. [abstract]. In: International Nutritional Anemia Consultative Group [INACG] Symposium. Peru: ILSI Research Foundation, p. 18.
81. MANNAR MGV and VAN AMERINGEN M (2003). Role of public–private partnership in micronutrient food fortification. *Food and Nutrition Bulletin*, **24**(4), pp. S151–S154.

# 31

# Agriculture, food and nutrition security

*Deeksha Kapur*

**Deeksha Kapur** is Professor, Nutritional Sciences, School of Continuing Education, Indira Gandhi National Open University (IGNOU), New Delhi. She has been involved in designing and developing various professional and need-based programmes for distance learners since the past 20 years. She has extensive experience in imparting education and knowledge through various multimedia suited to open and distance education mode.

## 31.1 Introduction

The first Millennium Development Goal (MDG) is not simply about reducing poverty – there is a distinct focus on reducing hunger. Far from achieving the MDG goal of reducing hunger by half by 2015, some 75 million more persons were in fact added to the hunger trap during 2007, principally due to the rise in food prices [1]. The fact remains that 823 million people in developing countries are food insecure and undernourished. These chronically undernourished millions are caught in a vicious cycle – not getting adequate food regularly and therefore, not being able to lead a healthy and active life and without such a life, not being able to either produce or procure required food.

Undernutrition has significant economic consequences, leading to estimated individual productivity losses equivalent to 10 percent of lifetime earnings and gross domestic product (GDP) losses of 2–3 percent in the worst-affected countries [4]. Undernutrition is not merely a consequence of limited access to calories. Food must not only be available and accessible, but also be of the right quality and diversity (in terms of energy and micronutrients), be safely prepared, and be consumed by a healthy body, as disease hinders the body's ability to turn food consumption into adequate nutrition. Lack of dietary diversity and poor diet quality has led to micronutrient malnutrition or hidden hunger, even when energy intakes are sufficient. Hidden hunger can cause illness, blindness, and premature death as well as impair the cognitive development of survivors. Overcoming undernutrition requires effective and targeted attention to food (macro and micronutrients, clean drinking water) and non-food factors (such as agricultural production, trade, income, sanitation, governance and political stability). This chapter focuses on the concept of food and nutrition security, the global and the Indian perspective to food and nutrition security, the factors that influence food and nutrition security and finally a review on the policies and programmes for reducing food insecurity and vulnerability, particularly in the Indian context.

## 31.2 Food and nutrition security: understanding the basic concepts

Some key concepts related to food and nutrition security are defined in Box 31.1.

As highlighted in Box 31.1, the commonly accepted definition of food security is

> *"when all people, at all times, have physical, social and economic access to sufficient, safe and nutritious food to meet their dietary needs and food preferences for an active and healthy life".*

Food is here defined as any substance that people eat and drink to maintain life and growth. As a result, safe and clean water is an essential part of food commodities.

**Box 31.1 Food and nutrition security: some basic concepts [5]**

Hunger is a general concept to describe the sensation of not having enough to eat. FAO's indicator of hunger is 'undernourishment' – a measure of energy deficiency or food deprivation.
Vulnerability is defined as a function of 'exposure to risk and ability to cope'.
Food insecurity is defined as the lack of access to enough food for a healthy, active life style.
Food security is commonly defined as "when all people, at all times, have physical and economic access to sufficient, safe and nutritious food to meet their dietary needs and food preferences for an active and healthy life".
Nutrition security is defined as "physical, economic, environmental and social access to balanced diet and clean drinking water for every child, woman and man".
Food systems encompass activities related to production, processing, distribution, preparation and consumption of food; and the outcomes of these activities that contribute to food security, such as food availability, food access (including affordability, allocation and preferences) and food use (including nutritional value, social value and food safety).

It is interesting to note that food security as a concept evolved over time. Food security historically referred to the overall regional, national, or even global food supply and shortfalls in supply compared to requirements. But, with increased observation of insufficient food intake by certain groups (despite overall adequacy of food supply), the term has more recently been applied mostly at a community level, local, household or individual level [6].

## At the household level, food security is defined as

> *"access to food that is adequate in terms of quality, quantity, safety and cultural acceptability for all household members".*

A food-secure household is one in which all household members must be well nourished. In other terms they enjoy nutrition security. "Nutrition Security", therein, may be considered as adequate nutritional status in terms of protein, energy, vitamins, and minerals for all household members at all times [7] and thus in principle is more than food security as highlighted in Figure 31.1. Nutrition security is achieved for a household when secure access to food is coupled with a sanitary environment, adequate health services, and adequate care to ensure a healthy life for all household members. Nutrition security requires the following inputs:

- *Physical* – production and advocacy (communication and information).
- *Economic* – purchasing power — one must have the money to buy commodities for a balanced diet, for example, cereals, pulses, fruits and vegetables.
- *Environmental* – hygiene, sanitation and safe drinking water.
- *Social* – equity in gender terms, social factors including intra- and inter-family distribution of balanced diet.

The necessity to include nutrition into food security evolved over time (Figure 31.1). The nutrition focus includes the aspects of caring practices and health services and healthy environments to the definition and concept of food security (Figure 31.2).

Achieving food security therefore has the following three essential dimensions:

- Ensure a safe and nutritionally adequate food supply both at the national level and at the household level.
- A reasonable degree of stability in the supply of food, both from one year to the other and during the year.
- Ensure that each household has physical, social and economic access to enough food to meet its needs. This means that each household must have the knowledge and the ability to produce or resources to procure the food that it needs on a sustainable basis.

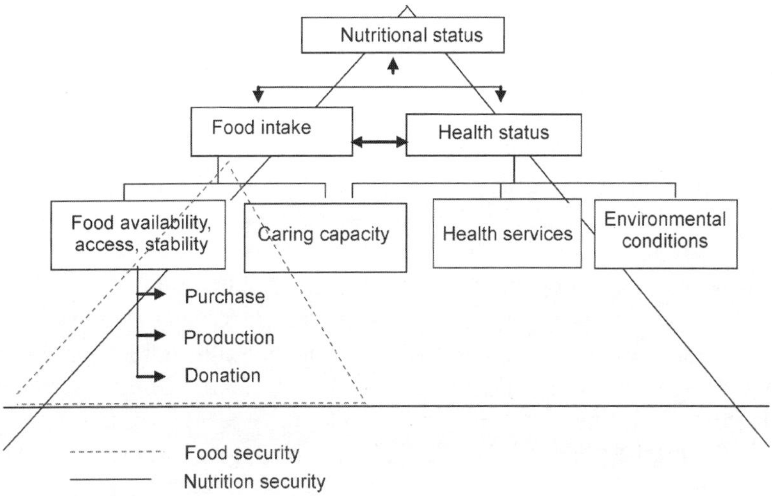


*31.1* Concept framework of the food and nutrition security and nutritional status at the household level [8].

As evident in Figure 31.2, the following four fundamental elements are essential: adequate food availability, adequate access to food, appropriate food utilization and its usage as well as food stability. More recently, the ethical and human rights dimension of food security has also come into focus.

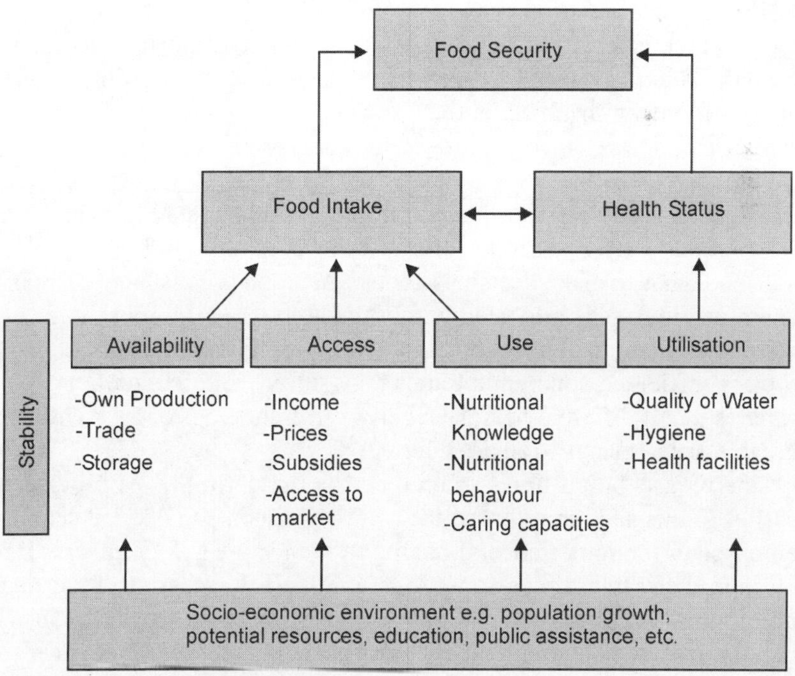


*31.2* Conceptual framework of food security [9].

Food availability is the amount of food that is physically present in a country or area through all forms of domestic production, stocks, commercial imports and food aid. Availability, in the context of food security, refers to the physical existence of food, be it from own production or the market trade. At the national level, food availability derives from the combination of domestic food stocks, commercial food imports, food aid and domestic food production, as well as the underlying determinants of each of these factors.

Food can be accessed through trade, barter, collection of wild foods and community support networks; it can also be received as a gift (or even through theft). Access is ensured when all households and all individuals within those households have sufficient resources to obtain appropriate foods for a nutritious diet. It is dependent on the household's ability to get food in the marketplace or from the other sources (gift, transfer etc.). Thus food access depends on household resources – labour, knowledge and purchasing power, which vary in relation to market integration, price policies and temporal market conditions. The primary determinants of food security for the majority of poor people are their income levels and the cost of food.

Utilization is commonly understood as the way the body makes the most of various nutrients in the food. This food security dimension is determined primarily by people's health status. Food use and utilization is determined by how much a person eats and how well a person converts food to energy, all of which affects proper biological use of food, nutritional status and growth. Adequate food utilization requires a diet providing sufficient energy along with all essential nutrients and potable water, adequate sanitation and access to health services and proper feeding practices and illness management.

Use and utilization thus have a socioeconomic and a biological aspect. If sufficient and nutritious food is both available and accessible, the household has to make decisions about what food is consumed (demanded) and how the food is allocated within the household. In households where distribution is unequal, even if the total quantity and nutritional value of food is sufficient, some individuals may suffer from food deficiency. The same is true if different persons receive different types of food which have greater or lesser nutritional value.

The phrase "at all times" mentioned in the definition of food security earlier in this section refers to the stability dimension of food security. It emphasizes the importance of having to reduce the risk of adverse effects on the other three dimensions: food availability, access to food or food utilization. Stability of food supplies refers to those situations in which populations are not vulnerable to losing access to resources and other forms of livelihoods due to extreme weather events, economic or market failure, civil conflict or environmental degradation and, increasingly, conflict over natural resources.

Food security must be determined and ensured at the macro (national), meso- (district, village etc.) and micro (household, family, individual) level by availability (agricultural, production and marketing), access (own income, transfer income) and use and utilization (nutrition behaviour, caring practices, as well as health status and its determinants) of food. Stability of availability, access and utilization is a further important aspect.

It is important to note that there has to be a paradigm shift from emphasis on food security at the macro level to nutrition security at the individual level. The overall outcome for food security is the nutritional status of the population. All three key elements (availability, access and utilization of food discussed above) are important for achieving a good nutritional status as highlighted in the Food Insecurity and Vulnerability Information and Mapping Systems (FIVIMS) framework (Figure 31.3). The framework suggests a hierarchical relationship where food security results from adequate food availability and access, as well as proper food utilization. Further the house-hold food access, care practices, health and sanitation coupled with adequate food consumption and utilization influence the nutritional status. Food use translates food security into nutrition security.

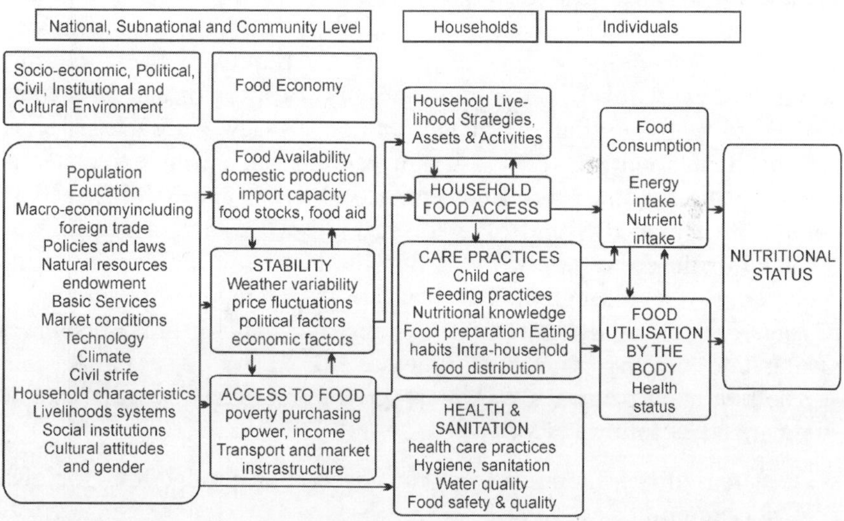


*31.3* The Food Security and Vulnerability Information and Mapping System (FIVIMS) framework [5].

Food security therefore depends on adequate and stable food availability, access to adequate and appropriate food, and proper use and good health to ensure that individual consumers enjoy the full nutritional benefits of available and accessible food. Availability is necessary but not enough to ensure access, which is necessary but not enough for effective use. But for most of the undernourished, the lack of access to food is a greater problem than food availability. Nobel Laureate Amartya Sen has famously written that "starvation is a matter of some people not having enough food to eat, and not a matter of there being not enough food to eat".

## 31.3 Agriculture: central to food and nutrition security

### 31.3.1 The global perspective

The world is generally food secure, producing enough food to meet the dietary needs of today's global population though future global food security should not be taken for granted because of uncertainties from growing resource scarcity and climate change.

Though, the world has more than enough food to feed everyone, yet 850 million are food insecure. Achieving food security requires adequate food availability, access, and use as already highlighted above. Agriculture, therein, plays a key role in (1) food availability globally (and nationally and locally in some agriculture-based countries); (2) income source to purchase food; and (3) foods with high nutritional value status.

Agriculture is central to poverty reduction and higher agricultural productivity is critical to the attainment of the MDGs. By increasing food availability, generating income for farmers, and improving the purchasing power and asset level of the poor, agricultural growth can contribute directly to MDG1 of halving hunger and poverty by 2015 and reducing childhood undernutrition [10]. Agriculture can also contribute to maternal and child health, nutrition and survival (MDG4 and MDG5) and to combating HIV/AIDS and other diseases (MDG6) by increasing the diversity of the food supply, increasing the micronutrient density of the staple crops (e.g. through biofortification), improving the overall quality of diets as well as by increasing income and making more resources available to prevent and manage illnesses [11, 12].

The five main pathways by which agriculture affects nutrition can be summarized as follows [13]:

- Increased consumption from increased food production (for own consumption),
- Increased income from sale of agricultural commodities (production for income),
- Empowerment for women agriculturalists and related gains in children's nutrition and welfare,
- Lower real food prices resulting from increased food production, and
- Macroeconomic growth arising from agricultural growth.

However, there is recent evidence that the global food production system is at an unprecedented level of risk from extreme supply deficits, particularly with respect to cereals. This trend could be amplified by climate change, which is expected to have significant impacts on agriculture and food production patterns world over through three major pathways: global warming, change in rainfall patterns and the increase in carbon dioxide concentration in the atmosphere. In a scenario of moderate climate change, it is projected that those most vulnerable to these changes would be the poor and landless in rural areas that are dependent on isolated rain-fed agricultural systems in semi-arid and arid regions. The future of global food supply is highlighted in Box 31.2.

**Box 31.2 Future of the global food scenario [10]**

Agriculture has been largely successful in meeting the world's effective demand for food. Yet more than 800 million people remain food insecure, and agriculture has left a huge environmental footprint. The future is increasingly uncertain. Models predict that food prices in global markets may reverse their long-term downward trend, creating rising uncertainties about global food security.

Climate change, environmental degradation, rising competition for land and water, higher energy prices, and doubts about adoption rates in future for new technologies present huge challenges and risks that make predictions difficult.

To meet the projected demand, cereal production will need to increase by nearly 50 percent and meat production by 85 percent from 2000 to 2030. Added to this is the burgeoning demand for agricultural feedstocks for biofuels, which have already pushed up world food prices.

## 31.3.2 The Indian perspective

Agriculture in India has contributed substantially to the national level food security through increased productivity and reduced dependence on imports. At the national level, a major achievement on the agricultural front in the post-Independence period has been the expansion of food grain production, enabling the country to acquire a degree of self-sufficiency in cereals production. The production of few important agricultural commodities in India is highlighted in Figure 31.4. International commodity prices are used to calculate the total value of each commodity produced and subsequently used in the ranking of the commodity. This is done to facilitate international comparative analysis of productivity at the national level.

Agriculture situation of India [15] is summarised below:

- With a production reaching ten times in past five years, India is today the second largest wheat producer in the whole world. India has the largest area in the world under wheat. India is also the second largest rice producer in the world. Pulses are sometimes called "poor man's meat". India's export of pulses has increased from Rs. 589.85 crores (USD million 131.46) in 2004–05 to Rs. 770.64 crores (USD Million 170.95) in 2006–07.

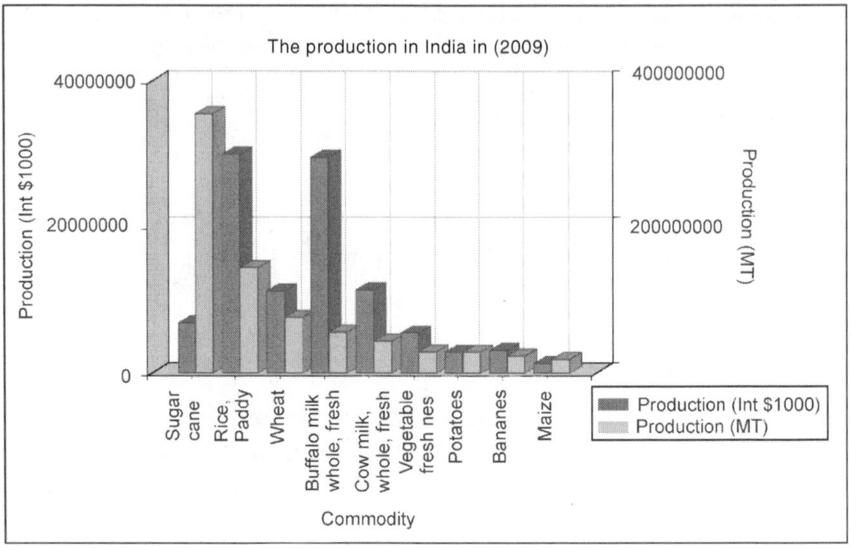


*31.4* The agricultural production in India [14].

- India is the fruit and vegetable basket of the world. India is the second largest producer of vegetables that account about 16 per cent of the world production. India ranks fifth in the world in cropped area under cultivation and production of potatoes. India is second largest onion growing country in the world. India produces 41% of world's mangoes, 23% bananas, 24% cashew nuts, 36% green peas and 10% onion.
- India is a world leader in the production of dairy and animal products.
- India retained its rank as the largest milk producer in the world with a total production of 100 million tonnes.

For operational purpose these statistics can be assumed to indicate that at the national level the aggregate production and supply of food is adequate to meet target consumption levels of our current population groups. However, despite the fact that India has attained near self-sufficiency in food grains, and the region as a whole was surplus in food grains, this food adequacy scenario did not translate into an increase in food grains consumption by the poor and improvement in the nutritional status of undernourished people in India. The limitation is not food supply, but food distribution. A detail review on food insecurity and vulnerability in India follows in Section 31.4.

## 31.4 Food insecurity and vulnerability

### 31.4.1 The global perspective

About 850 million people in the world are undernourished – a number that has hardly changed since the 1990–92 base period for the World Food

Summit and Millennium Development Goal commitments on reducing hunger by half by 2015. Of particular concern are hunger hotspots, marked by the widespread persistence and prevalence of food insecurity, especially in protracted crises. As of May 2006, 39 countries in the world were experiencing serious food emergencies and required external assistance for dealing with critical food insecurity: 25 in Africa, 11 in Asia and near East, 2 in Latin America and 1 in Europe [16]. A case study for food security in Cambodia is highlighted in Box 31.3.

**Box 31.3 Food security in Cambodia – a case study [9]**

Food security is a cross-cutting issue, and in a country such as Cambodia, rural poverty and food insecurity are strongly interlinked. In Cambodia most people depend, to an important extent, on their own capacity to produce food to meet their needs. They grow crops including their staple food (rice) as well as other annual and perennial crops, raise livestock, and harvest wild foods from fisheries and forests for food and income. Despite Cambodia being self-sufficient in rice at the national level, the country's rice balance varies significantly from area to area within the country, as well as from year to year. Crop agriculture is largely rice-based, with very limited diversification in many food-insecure areas of the lowland flood plains, while fish production (a main source of protein) is declining and increasingly under threat. Many rural households have insufficient land for crop production. Many rural people also depend on casual low-wage labour or informal-sector enterprises to make income with which to buy at least part of their food needs, and the food security of poor rural people can often depend mainly on income from such activities. Farmers seeking to sell their crops face a poorly developed road and market infrastructure, limited storage capacity, and high transaction costs. Net returns from rice production are very low, and the marketing strategies of households earn little profit. Purchasing power to buy food is generally very limited in rural areas due to the high incidence of poverty. Rice shortages (rice gaps for two months or more) at the household level are frequent and contribute to the indebtedness of rural households, which in turn leads to chronic food insecurity. High health expenditures erode the asset base and purchasing power of food-insecure and vulnerable households. Income and food from common-property resources (forests and fisheries) are particularly important for the poor, but concessions and environmental degradation have restricted their access to these resources.

Cambodia has some of the highest malnutrition rates in Asia, with 44% of children under five years of age stunted and 15% wasted. Micronutrient deficiencies such as Iodine Deficiency Disorder (IDD), Vitamin A Deficiency (VAD) and Iron Deficiency Anemia (IDA) are widespread and hamper the full use of human potential for development. There is limited access to safe water and proper sanitation. People's poor health status (resulting from limited access to quality health services and preventive health) impairs optimal utilisation of food, while poor quality diet and inadequate feeding and caring practices further exacerbate the problem.

In recent years, flooding and drought have become more frequent, but emergency response capacities remain insufficient. The current production system is very vulnerable to drought due to the lack of diversification and irrigation. Depletion of productive assets, as a result of indebtedness, leads to chronic food insecurity. The food needs of permanent vulnerable groups (female-headed households with children, elderly, disabled, people living with HIV/AIDS) are not sufficiently addressed as a result of disrupted rural social institutions and lack of social safety nets. While women in Cambodia play a major role in all components of food security, whether in food production, marketing, household income/budgeting or as care takers, their role is negatively impacted by issues such as high illiteracy rates among women, lack of education and knowledge, and poor health and nutritional status (e.g. very high maternal mortality rates and iron-deficiency anemia prevalence of 65% among pregnant women).

The elimination of food and nutritional insecurity in Cambodia, and the attainment of Cambodian Millennium Development Goal 1 to eradicate extreme poverty and hunger, demands a specific, comprehensive and integrated approach focusing on all three dimensions of food security: availability, access and use and utilization. Furthermore, food security and vulnerability need to be tackled at the national, household and individual level.

### 31.4.2 The Indian perspective

India is home to the world's largest food insecure population, with more than 200 million people who are hungry. On the 2008 Global Hunger Index (GHI), India ranks 66 out of 88 countries. Like the GHI, the 2008 India State Hunger Index (ISHI) has been calculated which shows that all Indian states have at least a "serious" level of hunger; there is not a single state with low or even moderate levels. India's poor performance on the GHI is primarily due to its relatively high levels of child malnutrition and undernourishment resulting from calorie deficient diets [17].

Though India has nearly attained self-sufficiency in food grains, and the region as a whole was surplus in food grains as mentioned earlier, this did not translate into an increase in food grains consumption by the poor. On the contrary, the calorie and protein intake of the poor in the country has declined over the years. Data from the National Sample Surveys [18–20] show a clear trend of decline in calorie intake. In rural India, the average calorie intake per capita per day fell from 2266 kcal in 1972–73 to 2183 in 1993–94, to 2149 in 1999–2000 and further to 2047 kcal in 2004–05. Between the same period, average per captia calorie intake in urban sector declined from 2089 to 2020 kcal. With reference to the names 2400 kcal for the rural sector and 2100 kcal for urban sector, the calorie deprivation extent increased from 69 to 85 percent in rural India and from 60 to 65 percent in urban India. The data also show a decline in cereal intake, a phenomenon clearly driven by distress rather than choice since it has occurred in a situation of declining overall calorie intake and persistence of high levels of malnutrition. Further, average daily intake of protein by the Indian population has also decreased from 60.2 to 57 grams in the rural area between 1993–94 and 2004–05 and remain stable around 57 grams in the urban area during the same period. However, a significant rise in per capita daily average intake of fat is observed during the decades (1993–94 to 2004–05) in both rural and urban areas. It has increased from 31.4 g to 35.5 g (13.1 percent) in rural areas and from 42 g to 47.5 g (13 percent) in urban areas. In spite of increasing oil and fat intake, the proportion of dietary energy from fat remains lower than 15 per cent.

In addition to energy deficiency, a lack of diversity in the diet is a key issue (e.g. cereals contribute a disturbingly high proportion of calorie intake, more than 80 percent, for the lowest decile, compared to approximately 50 percent for the highest decile). The Food Insecurity Atlas of Rural India, published by the Swaminathan Research Foundation 2001, gives a fairly complete picture of India's performance. In all the selected states for the study (Table 31.1), the average per capita consumption of cereal exceeds the norm of the Indian Council of Medical Research (ICMR) while that of other foods falls far short. Cereals seem to be the main dietary item and chief source of energy.

*Table 31.1* Food adequacy in India and in few selected Indian States relative to ICMR norms [21]

| *Food items* | *Unit consumption (state-wise)** | | | | | |
|---|---|---|---|---|---|---|
| | *Andhra Pradesh* | *Madhya Pradesh* | *Orissa* | *West Bengal* | *India* | *ICMR norm (grams/person per day* |
| Cereal | 1.05 | 1.13 | 1.26 | 1.19 | 1.04 | 420 |
| Cereal substitutes | 0.00 | 0.01 | 0.00 | 0.00 | 0.05 | 75 |
| Pulses | 0.58 | 0.81 | 0.38 | 0.35 | 0.58 | 40 |
| Vegetables | 0.53 | 0.45 | 0.47 | 0.51 | 0.48 | 125 |
| Fruit | 0.45 | 0.21 | 0.27 | 0.38 | 0.45 | 50 |
| Milk and milk products | 0.52 | 0.55 | 0.15 | 0.31 | 0.97 | 150 |
| Oils | 0.56 | 0.45 | 0.27 | 0.52 | 0.52 | 22 |
| Meat | 0.29 | 0.08 | 0.08 | 0.17 | 0.15 | 25 |
| Fish | 0.15 | 0.08 | 0.39 | 0.72 | 0.28 | 25 |

* ICMR norms equivalent to one unit.

The consumer expenditure survey of the NSSO during the 55th round covering the period from 1999 to 2000 [19] show that out of the total calorie intake of the average Indian, 68% in the rural areas and 55% in urban areas were derived from cereals alone. The contribution of cereals to the average intake of protein in the country was 67% in the rural sector and 57% in the urban sector. In rural areas, oils and fats accounted 7% of total calorie intake, milk and milk products accounted for 6%, pulses, nuts and oilseeds for 5% and sugar and honey for 5%. These contributions were somewhat higher in urban India – oils and fats 11%, milk and milk products 8%, pulses, nuts and oilseeds 7% and sugar and honey 6%.

Food security has come to be regarded principally as food grain security, mainly meeting the requirements of energy and proteins. However, for nutrition security, food production should ensure availability of diverse foods, which can ensure both macronutrients as well as micronutrient security. Food grains (cereals and millets) alone cannot meet the requirement of micronutrients like vitamins and minerals, and health promoting phyto-chemicals. It is not the case of "either/or" but "all". Nutrition security is a broader term and implies food grain security as well. In fact, diversification even within food grains to increase the production and availability of millets and legumes should be the demand.

Having reviewed the food and nutrition security scenario in India above, it is evident that currently we are in a paradoxical situation where somewhat food surpluses at the aggregate national level coexist with large undernourished and poor population. This scenario is well documented in the case study of food security in Orissa and Himachal Pradesh presented in Box 31.4. It is important to understand that the agriculture productivity and increased production can only ensure food security of the country and not that at individual or more precisely household level, which assumes a complex function of various socio-economic–environment factors as discussed in the next section.

### Box 31.4 Food security in Orissa – a case study [22]

Orissa is among the poorest of India's poor states. It depends largely on an undiversified agricultural economy. The poverty headcount rate is 47 percent. Poverty is an overwhelmingly rural phenomenon and is clearly linked to low land productivity, limited diversification of the agricultural economy (primarily paddy) and the lowest agricultural wages in the country. While the state, including some of the poorest districts, is virtually self sufficient in food grains, there is a significant portion of chronic food insecurity associated with particular areas and population groups. Inequalities are greater between the relatively better-off coastal areas and the more remote and inaccessible southern region. Regional differences are closely linked to differences among social groups, with poverty among castes and especially indigenous tribal people being strikingly higher than for other groups.

The pervasive and chronic food insecurity of poor communities in Orissa is captured by anthropometric measures as over half of the children between 1 and 5 are stunted. Almost half of all adult women and three quarters of all children under three in Orissa are undernourished. The infant mortality rate for Orissa is higher than any other state in India, while child malnutrition in Orissa is significantly higher than the national among the highest in India.

The proportion of labouring rural households with an average daily energy intake of less than 1800 kcal (less than 75 percent of the recommended minimum intake) was found to be 43 percent for the Coastal Plains, 57 percent for the Northern Plains and 69 percent for the Eastern Ghats. The vulnerable group category with the greatest prevalence of extreme food insecurity (defined as calorie intake per capita per day below 1800 kcal for people who are 40 percent below a poverty line income) was rural artisan households (73 percent), while more than half of all marginal farming households and labouring rural households (52 to 58 percent) were also considered extremely food insecure. Children of labouring rural households and marginal farming households emerged as the most affected by extreme undernourishment (hunger), particularly in the districts of Gajapati and Nuapada where between 56 and 80 percent were found to be consuming less than 1800 kcal per day.

Findings contributing the poor scenario of Orissa include (a) *Human capital* – Alarmingly poor education levels and awareness of basic health and sanitation issues among poor communities. (b) *Social capital* – Traditional extended family and community and civil society support systems have been significantly undermined as a result of entrenched poverty and shocks such as natural disasters. (c) *Natural capital* – Unsustainable farming practices and declining soil fertility are key factors causing slow growth in the agricultural sector and worsening rural livelihood conditions. (d) *Physical capital* – Poor rural connectivity is a major factor underlying limited market development. In addition, the low capital value of the dwellings of vulnerable households has negative implications for access to formal credit services. (e) *Financial capital* – More than 75 percent of all poor rural households are found to be indebted (mostly through informal and often exploitative arrangements). The majority of loans are taken to meet basic consumption requirements. In most households more than 50 percent of income is regularly used for repayments.

The central challenge facing policy makers in Orissa involves managing a transition away from an underdeveloped agricultural economy, while ensuring basic levels of human welfare and equitable access to resources. Central to this achievement is an increase of labour productivity within agriculture and, simultaneously, expansion of non-agricultural employment opportunities in both rural and urban areas. Eleven specific priority areas of intervention for reduced vulnerability and enhanced food security following a twin-track approach addressing both rural/agricultural development while addressing also immediate food needs of the most vulnerable in Orissa have been suggested:

| *TRACK 1*<br>*Rural development* | *TRACK 2*<br>*Addressing immediate food needs* |
|---|---|
| • greater investment in dryland/ agricultural technology<br>• adaptive agricultural research<br>• watershed development<br>• irrigation and water management<br>• pro-poor land policy reform<br>• joint forest management and Non Timber Forest Products (NTFP) promotion<br>• developing financial services<br>• diversification e.g. through horti-culture, animal husbandry and fish production<br>• improved agro-processing<br>• promotion of small scale industries and micro-enterprises<br>• developing tourism and mining sectors | • strengthening of disaster management capacities<br>• strengthening anti-poverty programmes for enhanced social protection<br>• food storage |

**Food security in Himachal Pradesh: a case study [5, 22]**

Whilst Himachal Pradesh is comparably less food insecure, the state does face a range of challenges related to undernourishment and malnutrition. Anthropometric measures show that close to every second child under five in HP are underweight and 41 percent of adult women are anaemic, only slightly lower than the national figure. The main causes of food insecurity and vulnerability include increased fragmentation of land, limited or no access to welfare provisions and public services related to migration, weak infrastructure and lack of accessible credit institutions.

Key interventions to address the causes of food insecurity and vulnerability in Himachal Pradesh have been identified. These include increased investment in irrigation; improved extension services; ensuring social service provision and basic human welfare; and continued assurance of high levels of investment in constructing and maintaining rural infrastructure as a prerequisite for sustainable and broad-based economic growth.

## 31.5 Factors underlying the current state of food and nutrition security

As will be discussed in this section, many factors have contributed to the current food insecurity situation prevailing worldwide, though it is difficult to quantify their contributions. Among the most important factors it is possible to list environmental factors such as climatic changes, stock levels, increasing food prices, biofuel and agricultural commodities, food supply etc. A briefly review of these factors follows.

### 31.5.1 Global perspective

*(i) Food pricing and food security*

Agricultural commodity prices rose sharply in 2006 and 2007 and continued to rise even more sharply in the first three months of 2008. The continuing surge in prices is led by vegetable oils, which on an average increased by more than 97 percent during the same period, followed by grains with 87 percent, dairy products with 58 percent and rice with 46 percent. This is a very large increase for poor people who depend on a single staple food (particularly cereals) for the bulk of their caloric intake, and typically spend 20–40 percent of their income on this one commodity alone.

A critical trigger for the price hikes has been the decline in the production of cereals in major exporting countries, which beginning in 2005 and continuing in 2006, declined annually by 4 and 7 percent, respectively. The gradual reduction in the level of stocks, mainly of cereals, since the mid-1990s, is another supply side factor that has had a significant impact on markets recently.

However, in spite of the soaring prices in global commodity markets, in particular of tradable cereals such as wheat, rice and maize, the most recent data on the food use of these key cereals have not shown much of a decline on a per capita basis. These trends however, must be interpreted cautiously. Even if cereal consumption of the poor does not change, this does not imply that there are no important welfare effects. The poor may defend their intake of cereals, but only at the expense of reduced consumption of more nutritious foods such as meat and dairy products, and reduced expenditures on education and health. As one example, Block et al (2004) [23] found that when rice prices increased in Indonesia in the late 1990s, purchases of more nutritious foods were reduced in order to afford the more expensive rice. This led to a measurable decline in blood haemoglobin levels in young children (and in their mothers), increasing the probability of developmental damage. A negative correlation between rice prices and nutritional status has also been observed in Bangladesh [24]. Reductions in expenditures on education and health care can also obviously have adverse long-term consequences on their efforts to escape poverty. Households under distress may liquidate assets (distress sales) and deplete savings with uncertain prospects for re-building them.

### *(ii) Climate, agriculture and food security*

Climate change is expected to have significant impacts on agriculture and food production patterns through three major pathways: global warming, change in rainfall patterns and the increase in carbon dioxide concentration in the atmosphere [25]. The present crisis of food insecurity world over is a combination of rising demand for agricultural products, due to population growth and economic development in emerging countries; the rapid expansion of biofuels; insufficient supply as production is negatively affected by climate change, in particular drought and floods, and water availability.

Developing countries are particularly vulnerable because their economies are closely linked to agriculture, and a large proportion of their populations depend directly on agriculture and natural ecosystems for their livelihoods. The Asian countries most vulnerable to climate change are Afghanistan, Bangladesh, Cambodia, India, Lao PDR, Myanmar and Nepal. Afghanistan, Bangladesh, India and Nepal are particularly vulnerable to declining crop yields due to glacial melting, floods, droughts, and erratic rainfall, among other factors.

Several studies have looked at the sensitivity of specific crops to projected changes in the climate, to assess vulnerability of systems based on these crops. These are highlighted in Box 31.5.

#### Box 31.5 Assessing and mapping vulnerability [26]

*Wheat in the Indo-Gangetic Plains.* Wheat is a crop of temperate climate, and rising temperatures may make many currently important wheat areas too hot for the crop. A study from the International Maize and Wheat Improvement Center (CIMMYT) details possible climate shifts in the Indo-Gangetic Plains of South Asia, a region of 13 million hectares that extends from Pakistan across northern India, Nepal and Bangladesh, and which grows 15% of the world's wheat. According to the study, by 2050 more than half of its area may become heat-stressed for wheat, with a significantly shorter season for the crop.

*Rice in the mega-deltas of Asia.* The Mekong and Red River Deltas in Vietnam, the Irrawaddy Delta in Myanmar and the Ganges–Brahmaputra Delta in Bangladesh and India are vital for world rice production. But the impacts of climate change – increased flooding and salinity – pose a major threat.

*Maize in sub-Saharan Africa and Latin America.* Scientists at the International Center for Tropical Agriculture (CIAT) and the International Livestock Research Institute (ILRI) have taken outputs from climate simulation models and data from various sources to simulate the growth, development and yield of maize crops over sub-Saharan Africa and Central and South America. The results showed an aggregate yield decline by 2055 for smallholder rain-fed maize production of 10%, representing an annual economic loss of the order of US$2 billion.

It is important to understand that climate change has the potential to act as a 'risk multiplier' in some of the poorest parts of the world, where agricultural and other natural resource-based systems are already failing to keep pace with the demands on them. Some of the anticipated costs of climate change are highlighted in Box 31.6.

**Box 31.6 The costs of climate change [26]**

A recent study by the International Food Policy Research Institute (IFPRI), highlights some of the anticipated costs of climate change, which include:

- 25 million more children will be malnourished in 2050 due to climate change without serious mitigation efforts or adaptation expenditures
- Irrigated wheat yields in 2050 will be reduced by around 30% and irrigated rice yields by 15% in developing countries
- Climate change will increase prices in 2050 by 90% for wheat, 12% for rice and 35% for maize, on top of already higher prices.
- At least US$7 billion a year are necessary to improve agricultural productivity to prevent adverse effects on children.

It is estimated (Figure 31.5) that, twenty five million more children will be malnourished in 2050 due to effects of climate change (Figure 31.5). Further, with climate change, average calorie availability in Asia in 2050 is expected to be about 15 percent lower and cereal consumption is projected to decline by as much as 24 percent compared to a no climate change scenario. To counteract the effects of climate change on nutrition, additional annual investments of 7 billion USD per year is estimated (Figure 31.5).

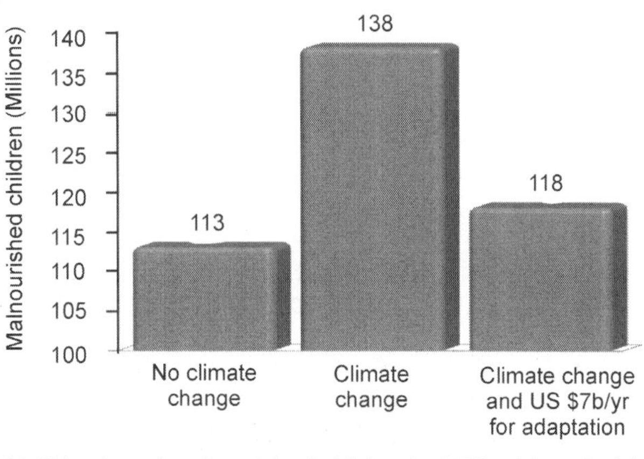


*31.5* Number of malnourished children in 2050 with and without climate change [27].

### *(iii) Biofuels and agricultural commodities*

There is a growing international consensus that the rapid increase in demand for biofuel feedstocks has contributed significantly to the current rise in food prices. The emerging biofuels market is a new and significant source of demand for some agricultural commodities such as sugar, maize, cassava, oilseeds and palm oil. The increase in demand for these commodities has been one of the leading factors behind the increase in their prices in world markets which, in turn, has led to higher food prices.

The most important biofuels today are ethanol and biodiesel. Ethanol is produced predominantly from sugar cane and maize and, to a far lesser degree, from wheat, sugar beet and cassava. Biodiesel mostly uses rapeseed but also palm oil, soybean oil and jatropha. Sugar from Brazil and maize from the United States of America (USA) dominate global ethanol production. Together they comprise around 80 percent of global production. China, the European Union (EU) and India are other significant ethanol producers. In 2007, approximately 23 percent of USA coarse grain production was used to produce ethanol, as was about 54 percent of Brazil's sugar-cane crop. In the EU, about 47 percent of vegetable oil production was used in the production of biodiesel causing higher imports of vegetable oil to meet domestic consumption needs.

These commodities, which have predominantly been used as food and/or feed, are now being grown as raw material (feedstock) for producing biofuels. Significant increases in the price of crude oil allow them to become viable substitutes in certain important countries that have the capacity to use them.

Availability of food can be threatened to the extent that land, water and other productive resources are diverted from food production to biofuel production. This competition for natural resources occurs whether edible or non-edible crops are cultivated for bioenergy purposes. The degree of competition among food, feed and fuel uses of biomass hinges on a variety of factors, including crop selection, farming practices, agricultural yields and the pace at which next-generation biofuel technologies develop.

Utilization of food, as discussed earlier refers to peoples' ability to utilize, i.e. absorb, nutrients. This is closely linked to health and nutrition factors, such as access to clean water, sanitation and medical services. When biofuel feedstock production competes for water supply, it could make water less readily available for household use, threatening the health status and, thus, the food security status of affected individuals.

Further growth in biofuels could exert additional pressure on the stability of food supplies. The use of food crops (or crops which compete with them for land resources) for biofuels may establish an effective floor price for these commodities, and price volatility from the petroleum sector will be more strongly transmitted to the agricultural sector, increasing the risk of food insecurity. This impact will be enhanced as import dependence is expected to grow for most low income food deficit developing countries, and as price transmission increases between global and national markets with greater market liberalization and the forces of globalization.

## 31.5.2 Indian perspective

*(i) Impact of Green Revolution on food security*

As a result of the Green Revolution[(1)], India's total food grain production increased from 50 million tons in 1950–51 to over 200 million tons in the year 2000–01 – a four-fold increase. The population during the same period increased from 300 millions to 1000 millions (1 billion) [28]. Thus, the increase in food grain production surpassed population growth and India turned from a 'nation' with a 'begging bowl', to a country with food grain reserves to provide some degree of national food security. This impressive achievement, however, has some worrisome aspects.

- The Green Revolution concentrated primarily on cereals like rice and wheat, which responded to innovations in agriculture technologies leading to development of high yielding varieties. However, these crops are water guzzling – particularly paddy and have had adverse environmental impact. Production of millets (referred as coarse cereal), legumes/pulses and oil seeds, which are less water demanding and nutritionally better endowed, has remained almost static.
- Apart from scientific and technological reasons, the pricing policy of the government in terms of minimum support price and procurement price as well as PDS has favoured production of rice and wheat, leading to the neglect of millets and legumes.

Higher support price for fine cereals is responsible for the accumulation of cereal stocks, which reached 60 million tons in mid 2002; but has come down since.

Farmers, who traditionally raised millets, have shifted to growing and eating fine cereals with adverse impact on nutrition, environment, and threat to biodiversity with regard to some of the local minor millets.

---

[(1)] A significant increase in agricultural productivity resulting from the introduction of high-yield varieties of grains, the use of pesticides, and improved management techniques.

### Box 31.7 Green Revolution in India

The term "Green Revolution" is a general one that is applied to successful agricultural experiments in many Third World countries. It is not specific to India. But it was most successful in India.

The world's worst recorded food disaster happened in 1943 in British-ruled India known as the, Bengal Famine, an estimated *four million* people *died* of hunger that year alone in eastern India that included today's Bangladesh. The initial theory put forward to 'explain' that catastrophe was that there was an acute shortfall in food production in the area. While food shortage was a contributor to the problem, a more potent factor was the result of hysteria related to World War II which made food supplies a low priority for the British rulers. The hysteria was further exploited by Indian traders who hoarded food in order to sell at higher prices.

Nevertheless, when the British left India in 1947, food security was a paramount item on free India's agenda. This awareness led to the Green Revolution in India and also framing legislative measures to ensure that businessmen would never again be able to hoard food for reasons of profit.

The term "Green Revolution" in India is specifically applied to the period from 1967 to 1978. The Green Revolution changed India from a starving nation to one of the world's leading agricultural nation.

There were three basic elements in the method of the Green Revolution in India:

(1) Continued expansion of farming areas;
(2) Double-cropping existing farmland;
(3) Using seeds with improved genetics. The most noteworthy high-yield value (HYV) seed was the K68 variety for wheat.

The Green Revolution resulted in a record grain output of 131 million tons in 1978–79. This established India as one of the world's biggest agricultural producers. No other country in the world which attempted the Green Revolution recorded such level of success. India also became an exporter of food grains around that time.

Yield per unit of farmland improved by more than 30 per cent between 1947 (when India gained political independence) and 1979 when the Green Revolution was considered to have delivered its goods.

The crop area under HYV varieties grew from 7 per cent to 22 per cent of the total cultivated area during the 10 years of the Green Revolution. More than 70 per cent of the wheat crop area, 35 per cent of the rice crop area and 20 per cent of the millet and corn crop area, used the HYV seeds.

### *(ii) Food supply – situation in India*

The decline in per capita net availability of cereals and pulses over the last 15 years (from 510 g per capita a day in 1991 to 463 g in 2004) in India has been unprecedented. While a few years ago, it appeared that there was no threat to self-sufficiency in food grain production, the situation is of concern.

The estimates for the requirement of cereals in 2020 range from 224 to 296 million tonnes. The High Level Committee on Long Term Grain policy (Abhijit Sen Committee) arrived at an intermediate projection of 260 million tonnes. To achieve this, starting from the production level of 191 million tonnes of cereals in 2004–05, in the next 15 years, production will have to increase by 69 million tonnes to meet the demand of 2020. In the last 15 years, cereal production increased by only about 29 million tonnes. In the next 15 years, the achievement needs to be doubled to meet the projected requirement. The present rate of growth of cereal and food grain production will not be adequate to meet these demands. Major changes are needed in terms of agricultural strategy, as spelt out in the Reports of the National Commission on Farmers [29].

*(iii) Land fragmentation*

One clear cause of food insecurity and vulnerability in some parts of the Indian region is the increased fragmentation of land. The fragmentation has made farming households more vulnerable to weather-induced or market-based shocks and many farming households have difficulty maintaining sufficient food production with only a marginal piece of land. However, households with access to proper irrigation seem to be better off in terms of coping with marginal land areas. The fragmentation has also led to an increase in both agricultural and non-farm labourers putting a downward pressure on wages and thereby increasing the vulnerability of these livelihoods.

*(iv) Poverty, purchasing power and food security*

In India, availability of foodgrains is not the real problem since the country has achieved self-sufficiency in the matter of foodgrains. This implies that there is no longer a requirement to import foodgrains. In fact, the country is in a position to export same food items. However, the problem of suppressed demand, due to poverty, is of concern since the prevailing poverty amongst a large number of household essentially those living below poverty line (BPL) is the major constraint for achieving household's food security. In 2004–2005, the Planning Commission based on National Sample Survey (NSS) estimated that 27.5% of the population was living below the poverty [30]. The criterion used by 61st round of the National Sample Survey (NSS) was monthly per capita consumption expenditure below Rs. 356.35 for rural areas and Rs. 538.60 for urban areas. It is estimated that 75% of the poor are in rural areas, most of them are daily wagers, self-employed householders and landless labourers. More recently, an expert group constituted by the Planning Commission, Government of India, to review the methodology for estimation of poverty line recommended that actual private expenditure per capita on food, education and health consistent with optimal nutrition, educational and health outcomes should be used to define poverty line. It has been estimated that if these revised criteria are applied, poverty at all India level in 1993-94 was 51% in rural areas, 31.8 in urban areas and 45.3% in the country as a whole compared to the 1993-94 official estimation of 37.2% rural, 32.6% urban and 36% combined. A 2007 report by the state-run National Commission for Enterprises in the Unorganised Sector (NCEUS) reported that 25% of Indians, or 236 million people, lived on less than 20 rupees per day with most working in "informal labour sector with no job or social security, living in abject poverty".

In India, large scale unemployment is a great aggravating factor and in conjunction with rapidly growing population, severely impairs the purchasing power of a large number of households or forces the families to acquire purchasing power at a certain social cost like child labour.

To ensure food security, we have to ensure adequate supply (also called availability) as well as intake. Intake by individuals depends on many factors, most importantly on purchasing power and availability of food of appropriate quantity and quality at affordable prices. The contributions that agriculture makes to food security need to be complemented by medium-term programs to raise incomes of the poor, as well as insurance and safety nets, including food aid, to protect the chronic and transitory poor. The Government of India (GoI) has, since independence, implemented multiple initiatives – policies, programmes. In the next section we focus on such initiatives and strategies.

## 31.6 Policies and programmes for reducing food insecurity and vulnerability in the Indian context

To address widespread poverty, food insecurity and vulnerability, the Government of India (GoI) has, since independence, implemented multiple initiatives such as the Integrated Child Development Services (ICDS) Programme, the Mid Day Meal (MDM) Programme, the Mahatma Gandhi National Rural Employment Guarantee Act (MGNREGA), social protection initiatives (Anti-poverty programmes, Public Distribution System or PDS), community-based food and nutrition programmes, and, in recent years, the National Plan of Action on Nutrition and the National Rural Health Mission. Though macro-level food self-sufficiency has been achieved, partly through the establishment of national systems for public grain procurement and distribution, this has proved insufficient to ensure micro-level food security for the poor. A brief description of the programmes and initiatives taken by the government to address the food insecurity and vulnerability issue are highlighted herewith.

### 31.6.1 Social protection initiatives

It is now well recognized that the availability of food grains is not a sufficient condition to ensure food security to the poor. It is also necessary that the poor have sufficient means to purchase food. The capacity of the poor to obtain food can be ensured in two ways – by raising the incomes or supplying food grains at subsidized prices. While employment generation programmes attempt the first solution, the Public Distribution System (PDS) is the mechanism for the second option. Our government has made consistent efforts to improve availability of food for the poor. Besides the PDS, other programmes such as, the Antyodaya Anna Yojana (AAY), the Annapurna Scheme, National Food for Work Programme (NFFW) have also been launched. Few of these central government sponsored social protection initiatives are presented below:

*(i) The Public Distribution System (PDS) and the Targeted Public Distribution System (TPDS)*

PDS continues to be a major instrument of Government's economic policy for ensuring food security to the poor. 'Rationing', as it was originally called, has a long history in India, dating from the Second World War. Introduced by the British government, the PDS was retained after independence as a deliberate social policy. Over time, the PDS, evolved into a national social safety system. In 1984, Government of India created the Ministry of Food and Supplies with the Department of Civil Supplies in charge of the PDS. With a network of more than 4.62 lakh Fair Price Shops (FPS) distributing commodities worth more than Rs 30,000 crores annually to about 160 million families, the PDS in India is perhaps the largest distribution network of its kind in the world. The Central government, through Food Corporation of India (FCI), has assumed the responsibility for procurement, storage, transportation and bulk allocation of food grains to the State Governments. The operational responsibility, including identification of families below the poverty line, issue of Ration Cards and supervision of the functioning of Fair Price Shops (FPS), rest with the State Governments. Under the PDS, presently the commodities, namely wheat, rice, sugar and kerosene, are being allocated to the States/UTs for distribution. Some States/UTs also distribute additional items of mass consumption through the PDS outlets such as cloth, exercise books, pulses, iodized salt and tea, etc.

The PDS gave way to the Revamped PDS (RPDS) in 1992 with focus on disadvantageous area. The PDS as it was being implemented, was widely criticized for its failure to serve the population Below the Poverty Line (BPL), its urban bias, limited coverage in the States with high concentration of the rural poor and lack of transparent and accountable arrangements for delivery. Therefore, in June 1997, the Government of India modified the PDS into a two-tiered structure known as The Targeted Public Distribution System (TPDS) with focus on the poor. This was the new beginning of targeting the PDS.

**TDPS beneficiaries**

The beneficiaries of the TPDS were identified on the basis of a specific poverty line:

(i) Households existing below the poverty line (BPL households), whose entitlements were subsidized, and
(ii) Above-the-poverty-line households (APL) who were allocated food grain at cost price.

The BPL households were determined on the basis of population projections of the Registrar General of India for 1995 and the state-wise poverty estimates of the Planning commission for 1993–94.

At present the Government provides 35 kg of food grains, including wheat and rice to 65.2 million families classified as living below the poverty line (BPL). These subsidized rations are made available at a price of Rs. 4.15 per kg for wheat and Rs. 6.65 per kg for rice. To focus the TPDS further, Antyodaya Anna Yojana (AAY) was launched. The TPDS is often considered a key initiative in promoting food security. However, a number of implementation challenges are evident such as non-availability of rationed foodstuffs, problems faced by the poor in accessing BPL entitlement cards, corruption etc. Critics of India's long standing grain procurement and distribution systems have also raised concerns regarding poor cost efficiency and long-term market distortion resulting from such a system.

*(ii) Antyodaya Anna Yojana (AAY)*

Antyodaya means "*uplift of the last*". The Antyodaya Anna Yojana scheme, launched in 2000, is to provide special food-based assistance to destitute households. The scheme reflects the commitment of the Government to ensure food security for all and improve the PDS so as to serve the poorest in the rural and urban areas. It is estimated that 5% of the population are unable to get two square meals a day on a sustained basis through out the year. Their purchasing power is so low that they are not in a position to buy food grains round the year even at BPL rates. It is this 5% of the population (ten million of the poorest BPL families) which constitutes the target group of AAY. The scheme provides food grains at the rate of 35 kg per family per month. The food grains are issued by the Government of India @ Rs.2/- (US cents 4.25) per kg for wheat and Rs. 3/- (US cents 6.5) per kg for rice. After the identification of Antyodaya families, distinctive ration cards known as 'Antyodaya Ration Cards' are issued to the families based on which the ration is provided.

*(iii) Sampoorna Gramin Rozgar Yojana (SGRY)*

The Prime Minister in his Independence Day speech in 2001 announced the introduction of a Food for Work Programme to be called "Sampoorna Gramin Rozgar Yojana" (meaning Complete Rural Village Scheme) in all the States/UTs for organizing various employment generation programmes. The main objective of the scheme is to give security to the rural poor. Generation of supplementary employment for the unemployed poor in the rural area is the focus of the scheme. Under the Scheme, food grains are given as part of wages to the rural poor at the rate of 5 kg per man-day. Fifty lakh tonnes of foodgrains are distributed to the labourers as a part of wages at the BPL rate under this programme. Special component of Sampoorna Gramin Rozgar Yojana is also initiated with a view to extending support to the people affected by natural calamities in States/UTs.

*(iv) National Food for Work Programme (NFFWP)*

The National Food for Work Programme has been conceived with the objective to provide additional resources apart from the resources available under the Sampoorna Grameen Rozgar Yojana (SGRY) to 150 most backward districts of the country so that generation of supplementary wage employment and providing of food-security through creation of need based economic, social and community assets in these districts is further intensified. Distribution of foodgrains as part of wages under the NFFWP is the focus of the programme and based on the principle of protecting the real wages of the workers besides improving the nutritional standards of the families of the rural poor. Under the scheme, foodgrains are given as part of wages to the rural poor at the rate of 5 kg per man-day. More than 5 kg foodgrains can be given to the labourers under this programme in exceptional cases subject to a minimum of 25% of wages to be paid in cash. The State Governments also takes into account the cost of foodgrains paid as part of wages, at a uniform BPL rate. The workers are paid the balance of wages in cash, such that they are assured of the notified minimum wages.

*(v) Mahatma Gandhi National Rural Employment Guarantee Act (NREGA)*

The scheme known as the National Rural Employment Guarantee Act (NREGA) was launched in February 2006 in 200 districts, and was expanded to cover additional 130 districts in 2007–08 and eventually covered all the 593 districts in India by 2008. On October 2, 2009, the scheme has been renamed as Mahatma Gandhi National Rural Employment Guarantee Act or NREGA. The scheme is a landmark in the history of social security legislation in India and promises to be a major tool in the struggle to secure the right to food.

The scheme provides for the enhancement of the livelihood security of the households in rural areas of the country by providing at least one hundred days of guaranteed wage employment in every financial year to every household whose adult members volunteer to do unskilled manual work at the statutory minimum wage of Rs. 100/day. The scheme has been introduced with the aim of improving the purchasing power of the rural people, primarily semi or un-skilled work to people living in the rural India, whether or not they are below the poverty line. About one-third of the stipulated work force is women. The Central Government outlay for the scheme is Rs. 39,100 crores (US$ 50 m) in the financial year 2009–10.

*(vi) The Right to Food Act*

The President of India in August 2009 announced that India would soon pass a Food Security Act which will ensure at least 25 kg of grain (wheat/ rice) at Rs. 3/kg to every household below the poverty line. Aside from an overarching obligation to protect everyone from hunger, as well as to promote sustainable and equitable food production, essential provisions of the proposed Right to Food Act include:

- a universal Public Distribution System (providing at least 35 kgs of grain per family); special food entitlements for destitute households (including an expanded Antyodaya programme);
- consolidation of all entitlements created by recent Supreme Court orders (e.g. cooked mid-day meals in primary schools and universalization of ICDS);
- support for effective breastfeeding (including maternity entitlements and crèches); safeguards against the invasion of corporate interests in food policy; and
- elimination of all social discrimination in food–related matters.

## 31.6.2 Programmes/assistance targeted toward specific needy sections of the population

In addition, following programmes targeting specific sections of the society, often at individual level to address intra-household inequities or to address the issue of meeting the gap in nutritional requirements and other social needs have been launched.

*(i)* National Social Assistance Programme (NSAP)

The National Social Assistance Programme (NSAP) came into effect from

15th August, 1995. It introduces a National Policy for Social Assistance benefit to poor households in the case of old age, National old Age Pension Scheme (NAOPS), death of primary bread-winner National Family Benefit Scheme (NFBS) and maternity National Maternity Benefit Scheme (NMBS). Under the maternity scheme, benefit is provided in the form of a lump sum cash assistance (Rs. 500) to pregnant women of households below the poverty line. The benefit is restricted to pregnant women for upto the first two live births provided they are of 19 years of age and above.

The Schemes under NSAP are implemented through the State/UT Governments with assistance from the Panchayat and Municipal functionaries.

*(ii) Annapurna Scheme*

Annapurna is yet another scheme started in 2000, addressing the food security of senior citizens, who though eligible have remained uncovered under the National Old Pension Scheme. Under the Annapurna Scheme, 10 kg of food grains per month are to be provided 'free of cost' to the beneficiary. The gram panchayat is required to identify, prepare and display list of persons eligible to receive benefits under the Annapurna Scheme. The Department of Public Distribution, Ministry of Consumer Affairs and Public Distribution ensure the supply of the required food grains.

*(iii) Village Grain Bank Scheme*

Village or Community Grain Bank Scheme was launched during 1996–97 by the Ministry of Tribal Affairs with a focus on remote tribal-dominated areas for the prevention of starvation deaths. A revised Village Grain Bank Scheme for establishment of Grain Banks in chronically food scarce areas was approved by Ministry of Finance in February 2006 for the period 2005–07 subject to its evaluation in the 11th Five Year Plan. The main objective of the scheme is to provide safeguard against starvation during the period of natural calamity or during lean seasons. The grain banks are set up in food scarce area like the drought prone areas, the hot and cold desert areas, tribal areas and the inaccessible hilly areas. An evaluation of the Grain Bank Scheme implemented in Andhra Pradesh is presented in Box 31.8.

*(iv) Nutritional Programme for Adolescent Girls (NPAG)*

A Pilot Project – "Nutritional Programme for Adolescent Girls"(NPAG) – was launched by the Planning Commission initially for a period of two years (2002–04) in 51 identified districts on a pilot project basis to provide free food grains to undernourished (weight < 35 kg.)

## Box 31.8 Evaluation of Grain Bank Scheme in tribal areas of Andhra Pradesh [31]

The community managed grain banks have been established in the tribal areas of Andhra Pradesh during 1990s under externally aided Andhra Pradesh Tribal Development Project (APTDP) and Andhra Pradesh Participatory Tribal Development Project (APPTDP), funded by IFAD, Rome. Besides, Government of India have also formulated the scheme of grain bank in the year 1996–97 to arrest the starvation deaths in the vulnerable areas of 12 States identified by the Central Planning Committee which included the Chenchu areas of Andhra Pradesh. The main objectives in establishing the grain bank are

- to combat the problem of food grains scarcity during the lean season.
- to avoid or reduce dependency on local money lenders or traders for borrowing grains during the lean season at exorbitant rates of interest.
- to promote the habit of self-help among the tribals.

The Tribal Cultural Research and Training Institute (TCR & TI) has conducted Evaluation of Grain Banks in the year 2001 established under APTDP in Tribal Sub Plan areas of East Godavari District and also in Sundipenta ITDA area where the Government of India Scheme of Grain Banks has been under implementation. The specific objectives underlying the study were as follows:

- Community mobilization strategies adopted in the formation of grain banks.
- Modus operandi of grain banks.
- Physical and financial targets and achievements under different schemes.
- Impact on already existing local lending system operated by money lenders and traders.
- Identifying the factors contributing to the success/failure of grain banks.
- Lacunae in the implementation of the scheme.
- Perceptions of the beneficiaries and functionaries for effective functioning of the scheme.

**Observations and recommendations**

- There was no follow-up after establishing grain banks which led to closure of most of the grain banks. Hence, it was suggested to ensure sustainability of all grain banks by way of motivation, training of beneficiaries and regular monitoring.
- Constitution of mandal-level community mobilization committees by involving local functionaries to ensure timely motivation especially during harvesting season and also prompt recoveries.
- There are no permanent storage structures in most of the areas and the collected grain are stored in private houses which are not in good condition. It is essential to ensure construction of storage structures with a part of beneficiary contribution and the beneficiaries should be trained in safe storage methods.
- Under Government of India scheme, rice was distributed at the rate of 1 quintal per family without educating the beneficiaries regarding the modalities of the scheme and repayment procedures. Hence they are under the impression that it was a free supply of rice and need not be paid back. It is required to educate all the beneficiaries regarding the modalities of the scheme before distributing rice for the sustainability of the scheme.
- The functionaries of grain banks should be imparted proper training for ensuring transparency in recording the details of loan transactions. If necessary, one of the educated local functionaries should be attached to them for maintenance of the accounts.

adolescent girls (11–19 years) and expectant and nursing mothers. This scheme was restarted in 2005–06, with the coverage confined to only adolescent girls. As per the revised guidelines of the programme, undernourished adolescent girls as identified by weight would be beneficiaries under the programme, irrespective of financial status of the family which they belong. Free foodgrains, 6 kg per beneficiary per month, is provided to the adolescent girls initially for a period of three months. Those beneficiaries, who cross the cut off point for weight, are discontinued from the programme. Those who in spite of receiving food grains for three consequent months do not show improvement in nutritional status, are investigated by ICDS workers and, if necessary referred to doctor for investigation and treatment, but continue to receive free foodgrains for the next three months. Besides the free food grains, beneficiaries are given regular health check ups and referral services and are imparted appropriate nutrition education.

*(v) National Programme of Nutritional Support to Primary education (Mid-Day Meal Programme)*

The National Programme for Nutritional Support to Primary Education, (popularly known as the MDM) was launched as a centrally sponsored scheme on 15th August 1995. Its objective was to boost "universalization of primary education, by increasing enrolment, retention and attendance and simultaneously impact on nutrition of the students in primary classes". It was implemented in 2408 blocks in the first year, and covered the whole country in a phased manner in the year 1997–98. The programme originally covered the children of primary stages (classes I to V) in Government, local-body and Govt.-aided schools and was extended in October 2002 to cover children studying in Education Guarantee Scheme (EGC) and Alternative and Innovative Education Centres. The revised MDM scheme is entitled "National Programme of Nutritional Support to Primary Education (NP–NSPE), 2004 and covers over 100 million school children. The central Government provides the following assistance to the States under the MDM programme (a) Free supply of food grains through Food Corporation of India (FCI) @ 100 g of wheat/rice per student per day, and (b) Subsidy for the transport of the food grain from the nearest FCI depot to the primary school – subject to a maximum of Rs. 50 per quintal.

MDM provides either cooked lunches or foodgrains to assure food security without caste or gender bias. Its goal is to eliminate classroom hunger and promote balanced socialization along with free and compulsory education to all children. As per provision mentioned in the programme, the meal is to be provided for 200 working days in a year and the rate of mid day meal is Rs. 2 (US 4 cents) per child per day. The meal/food supplement distributed as part of the programme provides roughly 350–450 kcal and 20–30 g protein per child per day, which is expected to meet one-third of the energy and half of the protein Recommended Dietary Intakes of the children.

The MDM has been successful in significantly increasing school enrolment, improving attendance and keeping students in school. It has been especially beneficial to girls who were earlier discriminated into leaving school prematurely. Conjunctively, the choice of cooks (preferably women) from the lower caste (Dalit) and the construction of cooking sheds have helped to further increase employment and income among the specially targeted socially weaker castes and gender.

### *(vi) Integrated Child Development Services (ICDS) Scheme*

Started in 1975, the Integrated Child Development Services Programme (ICDS) is one of the most unique, community-based outreach programmes in the world.

ICDS is the only major national programme that addresses the health and nutrition needs of children under the age of six. It seeks to provide young children with an integrated package of services, including supplementary nutrition, health care and pre-school education. Since the needs of a young child cannot be addressed in isolation from those of his or her mother, the programme also extends to adolescent girls, pregnant women and nursing mothers.

ICDS provides a package of services that consists of supplementary nutrition, immunization, health check-up, referral services, non-formal pre-school education, and nutrition and health education. The nutrition norms for the programme are highlighted in Table 31.2. The programme provides an integrated approach for delivering basic services through community-based Anganwadi workers and helpers, supportive community structures and women groups through the ICDS centres, better known as "Anganwadis". Besides this, the ICDS Centre is a meeting place where women and mothers' groups can come together to promote awareness and joint action for child development and women empowerment. The programme is estimated to cover over 4.8 million expectant and nursing mothers and over 23 million children under the age of six. Of these children, more than half participate in early learning activities.

*Table 31.2* Nutritional norms

| *S. no.* | *Category* | *Revised (per beneficiary per day)* | |
|---|---|---|---|
| | | *Calories (kcal)* | *Protein (g)* |
| 1. | Children (6–72 months) | 500 | 12–15 |
| 2. | Severely malnourished children (6–72 months) | 800 | 20–25 |
| 3. | Pregnant women and nursing mothers | 600 | 18–20 |

## 31.6.3 Poverty programs and the evolution of public works

The 'Rural Works Programme', first initiated in 1970/1, was later re-designated as the 'Drought Prone Areas Programme' (DPAP). The 'Food-For-Work Programme' was started in 1977 with the aim of utilizing the surplus food stocks of the times. The 'National Rural Employment Programme' (NREP) evolved in 1980. The 'Rural Landless Employment Guarantee Programme' (RLEGP) was instituted in 1983 to address the plight of the core rural poor. In 1989 NREP and RLEGP were merged to form the Jawahar Rozgar Yojana (JRY) programme that prioritized backward, schedule caste and schedule tribe classes (SC/ST), women and bonded labour. Central and state governments shared the expenses, and wages were paid partly in cash and partly in food. Labour-intensive projects were preferred and operationalized by stipulating a desired wage-to-material cost ratio. In 1993 the JRY was again modified, and two of the programme components were dropped and made as independent programmes i.e. – the 'million wells' and Indira Awaas Yojana for rural housing – JRY programme, redesigned again in 2001, and renamed as Jawahar Gram Samridhi Yojana.

In November 2004 the 'Food-For-Work' (FFW) was launched which is planned to be managed with NREGA.

## 31.6.4 Agriculture initiatives to improve food security

Many new initiatives have been undertaken by the governments world over to ensure that the synergies between agriculture and nutrition are successfully exploited and lead to food security and better overall development outcomes. Programmes such as the National Food Security Mission, the Horticulture Mission, the Rashtriya Krishi Vikas Yojana in India and the Conditional Cash Transfer Programmes developed in Mexico in late nineties are reviewed in this section.

*The National Food Security Mission (NFSM)*

The objective of the National Food Security Mission is to increase production and productivity of wheat, rice and pulses on a sustainable basis so as to ensure food security of the country. The approach is to bridge the yield gap in respect of these crops through dissemination of improved technologies and farm management practices. The programme has three missions – one each for rice, wheat and pulse.

The implementation of the NFSM is expected to result in increasing the production of rice by 10 million tones, wheat by 8 million tones and pulses by 2 million tones by 2011–12.

*National Horticulture Mission*

National Horticulture Mission was launched by the Government of India during the year 2005–06 (Tenth Five Year Plan) with the objective to promote holistic growth of the horticulture sector in India and to enhance horticulture production.

To achieve the above objectives, the mission has adopted the following strategies:

1. Ensure an end-to-end holistic approach covering production, post harvest management, processing and marketing to assure appropriate returns to growers/producers.
2. Promote R&D technologies for production, post-harvest management and processing.
3. Enhance acreage, coverage, and productivity through.
   - Diversification from traditional crops to plantations, orchards, vineyards, flower and vegetable gardens.
   - Extension of appropriate technology to the farmers for high-tech horticulture cultivation and precision farming.
4. Assist setting up post harvest facilities such as pack house, ripening chamber, cold storages, Controlled Atmosphere (CA) storages etc, processing units for value addition and marketing infrastructure.
5. Adopt a coordinated approach and promotion of partnership, convergence and synergy among R&D, processing and marketing agencies in public as well as private sectors, at the national, regional, state and sub-state levels.
6. Promote National Dairy Development Board (NDDB) model of cooperatives which are appropriate and feasible to ensure support and adequate returns to farmers.
7. Promote capacity-building and human resource development at all levels.

*Rashtriya Krishi Vikas Yojana*

The Rashtriya Krishi Vikas Yojana was launched as a central and state sponsored scheme by Government of India in August 2007 with the aim of achieving 4% annual growth in the agricultural sector during the XI Five Year Plan period by ensuring a holistic development of agriculture and allied sectors. The beneficiaries to the programme include individual, families, communities, women and children. The objectives of the scheme, in general, are (i) to provide incentives to the State for increasing public investment in agriculture and allied sectors, and in particular, to ensure that agriculture for the State and districts are prepared based on agro-climatic conditions, availability of technology and natural resources; (ii) local needs/crops/priorities are better reflected in the agricultural plan of the State; (iii) reduce yield gaps in important crops through focused interventions; (iv) maximum returns is obtained by farmers in agriculture and allied sectors; (v) increase in production and productivity of various components of agriculture and allied sectors by addressing them in a holistic manner.

*Conditional Cash Transfer Programme (CCT)*

Conditional Cash Transfer Programme is a novel approach to social safety net developed in Mexico in the late nineties. CCT programme involves the direct transfer of cash to poor households, with the condition that the household undertake specific actions such as enrolling and maintaining their children in schools, and complying with a schedule of health visits for mothers, young children and other household members. CCT programmes are usually targeted to the poor households or other vulnerable population groups, and benefits are often specifically targeted to the women in the household [32]. The overarching goal of CCTs is to reduce poverty and food insecurity in the short term while providing an incentive for poor families to invest in their children and hence alleviate poverty in the long term. The CCT programme is expected to influence nutrition through a combination of several pathways; one potential pathway is through increasing income and access to food, thereby increasing household food consumption, another pathway may be through improved water and sanitation and/or greater use of health services and the resulting prevention and better control of infectious diseases. The CCT programme of Mexico is being critically reviewed for adoption in India policy.

Global and the Indian perspective of food and nutrition security, presented in the chapter, highlights the fact that access to food and good nutrition is largely governed by socio-economic, environmental factors. An integrated approach to address poverty, unemployment, targeting alternate and sustainable livelihood and economic empowerment is essential. Social protection initiatives, rural development schemes and policies, micro-enterprises, employment generation schemes etc., are all vital links to ensure food security at household level, particularly in rural areas. An integrated approach together with economical agricultural productivity is critical to mitigate food security challenges, to a great extent, in developing countries.

## References

1. SWAMINATHAN MS, Oct 2, 2008, Hindu.
2. India at a Glance. http://devdata.worldbank.org/AAG/ind_aag.pdf. Accessed on 11/7/08.

3. FAO Statistical Year Book. www.fao.org/statistics/yearbook/vol_1_2/pdf/India.pdf. Accessed on 11/7/08.
4. Agriculture for Development, World Development Report, 2008. The World Bank, Washington DC. Accessed on 14 December 2009.
5. Understanding the Dynamics of Food Insecurity and Vulnerability in Himachal Pradesh, India. ESA Working Paper No 07-22. FAO, May 2007.
6. FOSTER P. (1992). The world food problem: Tackling the causes of undernutrition in the Third World. Boulder.
7. QUISUMBING AR et al. (1995). Women: The key to food security. IFPRI Food Policy Report. Washington.
8. GROSS, R. et al. (1998). Community nutrition: definition and approaches. Encyclopedia of Human Nutrition. M. Sadler, S. Strain and B. Caballero (eds).
9. Food Security and Nutrition. Cambodian Food Security and Nutrition website. http://www.foodsecurity.gov.kh/CamSituation.aspx
10. ROSEGRANT MW, MSANGI S, SULSER T and RINGLER C (2007). "Future Scenarios for Agriculture: Plausible Futures to 2030 and Key Trends in Agricultural Growth." Background paper prepared for the World Development Report 2008.
11. BOUIS H (2002). Plant breeding: A new tool for fighting micronutrient malnutrition. Journal of Nutrition. 132(3):491S.
12. VON BRAUN J, SWAMINATHAN MS, ROSEGRANT MW (2004). Agriculture, Food Security, Nutrition and the Millennium Development Goals. 2003–2004. Annual Report Essay. IFPRI: Washington DC.
13. World Bank and International Food Policy Research Institute (2007). From agriculture to nutrition, Pathways, Synergies and Outcomes. Report No. 40196-GLW. Washington DC.
14. The Agricultural Production in India. http://faostat.fao.org, Accessed 15 December 2009.
15. Agricultural and Processed Food Products Export Development Authority. http://www.apeda.com/apedawebsite/six_head_product/FFV.htm. (Accessed on 27/8/08).
16. Food Security, Policy Brief. Issue 2, FAO, June 2006.
17. 2008 India State Hunger index: Key Findings and Facts. *http://www.ifpri.org/publication/2008-india-state-hunger-index-key-findings-facts.* Accessed 30th January 2010.
18. Nutritional Intake in India, 2004-2005, NSS 61st Round. July 2004 – June 2005. National Sample Survey Organisation. Report No. 513 61/1.0/6). Ministry of Statistics & Programme Implementation. Government of India, May 2007.
19. Nutritional Intake in India 1999-2000. NSS 55th Round. July 1999 to June 2000. Report No. 471(55/1.0/9). National Sample Survey Organisation. Ministry of Statistics & Programme Implementation. Government of India. August 2001.
20. Reported Adequacy of Food Intake In India: 1993–94, Fifth Quinquennial Survey of Consumer Expenditure, Nss 50th Round July 1993 – June 1994, Report No.415; National Sample Survey Organisation, Department of Statistics, Government of India. http://mospi.nic.in/rept%20_%20pubn ftest.asp?rept_id=415&type=NSSO. Accessed on 11/7/08.
21. The Food Insecurity Atlas of Rural India, Swaminathan Research Foundation (2001).
22. Understanding the Dynamics of Food Insecurity and Vulnerability in Orissa, India. ESA Working Paper No 07-28. FAO, October 2007 (22).

23. BLOCK S, KIESS L, WEBB P, KOSEN S, MOENCH-PFANNER R, BLOEM MW and TIMMER CP (2004). Macro shocks and micro outcomes: child nutrition during Indonesia's Crisis. Economics and Human Biology, 2(1): 21–44.
24. TORLESSE H, KIESS L and BLOEM MW (2003). Association of household rice expenditure with child nutritional status indicates a role for macroeconomic food policy in combating malnutrition. J Nutr, 133(5): 1320–1325.
25. Climate Change, Water and Food Security. Technical Background Document From the Expert Consultation Held on 26 to 28 February 2008, FAO, Rome. ftp://ftp.fao.org/docrep/fao/meeting/013/ai783e.pdf. Accessed on 24-7-08.
26. Climate Change: Impact on Agriculture and Costs of Adaptation, International Food Policy Research Institute (IFPRI), 2009 (26).
27. Projections by the International Food Policy Research Institute. http://www.ifpri.org/pressroom/briefing/impact-climate-change-agriculture. Accessed 15th January 2010.
28. Government of India. Planning Commission, Report of the Steering Committee on Nutrition for the Tenth Plan (2002–2007), September 2002.
29. National Commission on Farmers. http://kisanayog.gov.in/. Accessed on 28-8-08.
30. Poverty Estimates for 2004–05, Planning Commission, Government of India, March 2007, http://www.planningcommission.gov.in/news/prmar07.pdf. Accessed 21 July 2008.
31. Evaluation of the Grain Bank Scheme in Andhra Pradesh. Tribal Cultural Research and Training Institute. www.aptribes.gov.in. Accessed 15-12-09 (31)
32. ADATO AND HODDINOTT (2007). Conditional Cash Transfer programme. A magic bullet for reducing poverty? 2020 Focus Brief on Worlds poor and hungry people IFPRI : Washington DC.

# 32

# Food and nutrition situation in India

*K. Vijayaraghavan*

**K. Vijayaraghavan,** formerly Head of Department of the Division of Community Studies at the National Institute of Nutrition, India, is a medical graduate with Masters in Community Health and Nutrition from the University of London. During his forty years of research experience, Dr. Vijayaraghavan was involved with the National Nutrition Monitoring Bureau (NNMB) and is recognized for his research contributions in the areas of prevention of vitamin A deficiency, household food security studies, micronutrients deficiencies of iron and iodine, and development and implementation of behavioural change communication.

## 32.1 Introduction

India, though has made substantial progress in improving life expectancy at birth and reducing infant and maternal mortality since independence, still it shelters a large proportion of population suffering from ill-health and preventable undernutrition. Undernutrition contributes to 35% of all deaths due to all major causes like diarrhea, pneumonia, malaria, measles etc [1]. Despite an unequivocal commitment in the Constitution of India that *"State shall regard the raising of the level of the nutrition and the standard of living of its people and the improvement of public health among its primary duties"*, malnutrition continues to be an important public health problem in India even after about 60 years of independence, with a major share of undernourished people in the world.

The UN General Assembly, in the year 2000, adopted the Millennium Development Declaration [2] with nutrition related goals: to halve the proportion of the world's people who suffer from hunger by the year 2015; to reduce maternal mortality by three quarters; and under five year child mortality by two thirds, of their current rates. India is signatory to the Millennium Development Goals. Adequate food and good nutrition being the basic human need, is recognized in the Millennium Development Goals (MDGs), which emphasize eradication of extreme poverty and hunger and promote the empowerment of women as effective ways to combat poverty, hunger and disease and to stimulate sustainable development.

### 32.1.1 Hunger in India

The International Food Policy Research Institute (IFPRI) developed the Global Hunger Index (GHI) [3] as an approach to measuring and tracking progress on hunger, and seeking solutions to preventing hunger and improving nutrition (See Box 32.1).

**Box 32.1 Global Hunger Index (GHI)**

- The GHI has been developed by the International Food Policy Research Institute (IFPRI) as a tool for calculating hunger and malnutrition. It supports the measurement of progress of the global fight against hunger and thus helps in monitoring of the UN Millennium Development Goals.
- The GHI was established in 2008 for 120 developing countries and newly industrialized countries.
- It combines three equally weighted indicators: (a) the percentage of the population undernourished (reflecting the share of the population with insufficient dietary intake); (b) the prevalence of underweight children among under-fives (indicating the proportion of children suffering from weight loss and/or reduced growth); and (c) the mortality rate of children under the age of five (partially reflecting the mortality as a result of synergy between dietary intake and unhealthy environments).
- The GHI contributes to a comprehensive understanding of hunger; provides for a quick overview; makes visible factors characterizing the specific food security situation in a country and facilitates making apparent the progress and failures in the fight against poverty and hunger.
- The GHI is, of course, limited by the collection of accurate data by various governments and international agencies.

India's GHI score is 23.7, which ranks it 66th out of 88 countries. The GHI of some of the developing and third world countries for the year 1990 and 2008 is presented in Table 32.1 which shows that as compared to the year 1990, there is an improvement in the over all situation of global hunger in 2008. The GHI of India is worse than all its neighbouring countries, except Bangladesh.

*Table 32.1* Global Hunger Index of some developing countries

| | *2008* | | *1990* |
|---|---|---|---|
| *Country* | *GHI* | *Rank* | *GHI* |
| Mauritius | 5.0 | 1 | 6.1 |
| Malaysia | 6.5 | 10 | 9.5 |
| China | 7.1 | 15 | 11.6 |
| Thailand | 9.9 | 23 | 18.4 |
| Sri Lanka | 15.0 | 39 | 19.1 |
| Nepal | 20.6 | 57 | 27.6 |
| Pakistan | 21.7 | 61 | 25.3 |
| **India** | **23.7** | **66** | **32.5** |
| Bangladesh | 25.2 | 70 | 32.3 |

## 32.1.2 Indian State Hunger Index (ISHI)

It was calculated on the same lines as Global Huger Index for 17 states in 2008 (See Box 32.2).

**Box 32.2 India State Hunger Index (ISHI)**

- The ISHI is a tool to calculate hunger and malnutrition at the regional level in India.
- It is constructed in the same fashion as the Global Hunger Index (GHI) 2008 for 17 states in India, covering more than 95 percent of the population.
- The India State Hunger Index (ISHI) represents the index calculated using a calorie undernourishment cut-off of 1,632 kcal per person per day to allow for comparison of the India State Hunger Index with the Global Hunger Index 2008. The ISHI score for India using this cut-off is 23.3 and corresponds more closely with the GHI 2008 score for India of 23.7 than any other calorie cutoff.
- The ISHI ranges between 13.6 in Punjab and 30.9 in Madhya Pradesh.
- Punjab is ranked 34 in the 2008 country rankings while MP is ranked 82.
- Twelve of the 17 states fall into the "alarming" category, and Madhya Pradesh into the "extremely alarming" category.
- ISHI scores though are closely aligned with poverty, there is little association with state level economic growth.
- High levels of hunger are seen even in states that are performing well from an economic perspective.
- Inclusive economic growth and targeted strategies to ensure food sufficiency, reduce child mortality and improve child nutrition are urgent priorities for all states in India.

All the 17 states had Inter State Hunger Index (ISHI) scores well above the "low" and "moderate" hunger categories and 12 states fall into the "alarming" category, with Madhya Pradesh in the "extremely alarming" category (Figure 32.1).

While the ISHI scores are closely aligned with poverty, there is little association with economic growth at the state level. Therefore, high levels of hunger are seen even in states that are performing economically well. Inclusive economic growth and targeted strategies to ensure food sufficiency, reduction in child mortality and improvement in child nutrition are urgent priorities for all the states in India. It is particularly essential to improve the food security among the socio-economically vulnerable sections of the society through out all the seasons but especially during the times of stress and disasters such as drought.

## 32.2 Food security

The FAO (1992) [4] reported that at least one fifth of the world's population – about 800 million people of the developing countries – suffer from chronic

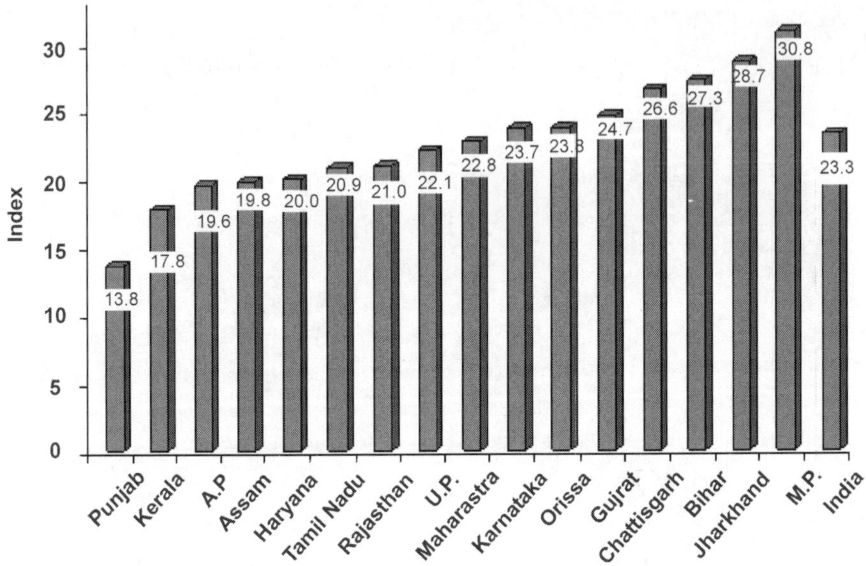


*32.1* Interstate Hunger Index – India (IFPRI, 2009).

undernutrition. These undernourished millions are trapped in a vicious cycle of not getting adequate food regularly, unable to lead a healthy and active life and inability to either produce or procure required food. In India, the results of the National Sample Survey Organization (NSSO) indicate that self-reported hunger at the national level is about 2%; in the rural areas it is 2.4% while in the urban areas it is only 0.5% (5). In other words, the household food security, in the opinion of the community, is satisfactory. Access to adequate food, which is one of the fore-most basic needs of life, is the fundamental right of every single human being on this earth. There can be food security in the population only when every one at all the times has both physical and economic access to sufficient food to meet their dietary needs for a productive and healthy life (USAID, 1992) [6].

The FAO Committee on World Food Security (1983) [7] incorporated the following specific goals for food security (i) ensuring adequacy of food supplies and (ii) maximizing stability, emphasizing thus that availability, access, affordability and adequacy are essential for food security. Food security, thus, should include physical, economic and social access to a balanced diet, safe drinking water, environmental hygiene and primary health care. This requires concurrent attention to the availability of food, the ability to buy needed food and the capability to absorb and utilise the food in the body. Thus, food as well as non-food factors, such as drinking water, environmental hygiene and primary health care are involved in food security.

### 32.2.1 Production and availability of foods in India

The food security in India, at the national level, is reportedly improving with the estimated overall production of food grains at 217.3 MT in 2006–07 as compared to about 108 MT in 1970–71. In India, though apparently food security at the national level may have been achieved, household and/or individual food security continues to be an important problem particularly among the low socioeconomic groups of population.

The productions of food grains, between 1950–51 and 2006–07, increased at an average annual rate of 2.5 per cent, marginally higher than the average annual population growth rate of 2.1% during the corresponding period. As a result, India almost became self-sufficient in food grains with hardly any imports during 1976–77 to 2005–06. However, the production of pulses shows no increase in the fifteen years in the period 1990–2005 (Figure 32.2). Consequently, the consumption of pulses has declined from 42 g per capita per day (72 g in 1956–57) to 33 g per capita per day during the same period.

*Table 32.2* Production of food grains – time trends [8]

| | *Year* | | | | |
|---|---|---|---|---|---|
| *Crop* | *2003–04* | *2004–05* | *2005–06* | *2006–07* | *2007–08** |
| Rice | 88.5 | 83.1 | 91.8 | 93.4 | 94.1 |
| Wheat | 72.2 | 68.6 | 69.4 | 75.8 | 74.8 |
| Coarse cereals | 37.6 | 33.5 | 34.1 | 33.9 | 36.1 |
| Pulses | 14.9 | 13.1 | 13.4 | 14.2 | 14.3 |
| Total foodgrains | 213.2 | 198.4 | 208.6 | 217.3 | 219.3 |

*Estimates

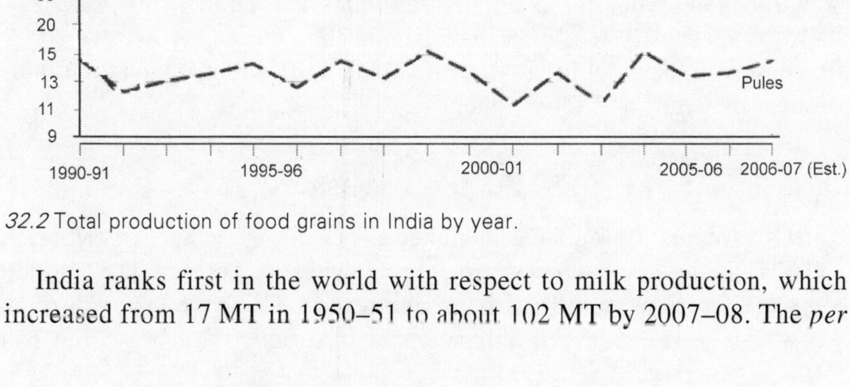


*32.2* Total production of food grains in India by year.

India ranks first in the world with respect to milk production, which increased from 17 MT in 1950–51 to about 102 MT by 2007–08. The *per capita* availability of milk has also increased from 112 g in 1968–69 to 246 g per day during 2006–07. Though it is still low compared to the world average of 265 g per day, it is more than the recommended intakes per consumption unit (sedentary adult male) (Figure 32.3) [9]. The efforts of the governments in the dairy sector are currently concentrated on the promotion of dairy activities in non-Operation Flood area with emphasis on building up cooperative infrastructure, revitalization of sick dairy cooperatives and federations and creation of infrastructure at state level for production of quality milk and milk products.

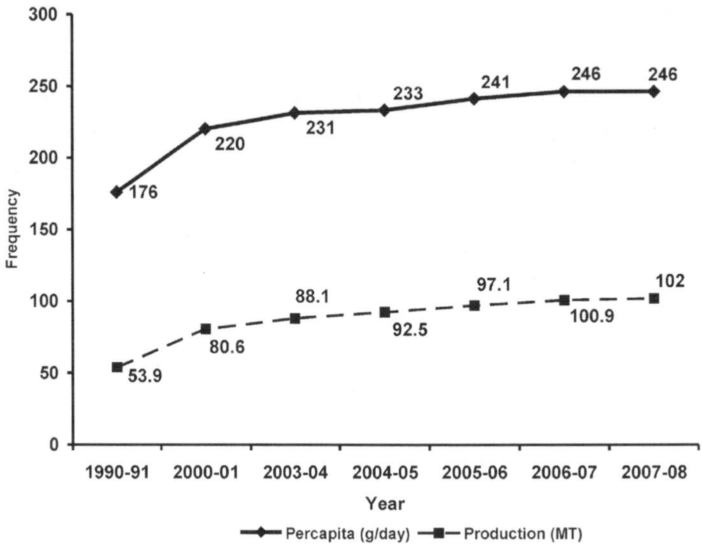


*32.3* Production and availability (per capita) of milk in India – Time Trends.

While there are debates and concerns about food security, it is important to recognize that we are yet to achieve nutrition security, meaning that the diets do not yet provide all the nutrients in proper amounts. Though the production of cereals appears adequate, the *per capita* availability of pulses, the only rich source of protein for the poor, actually shows a decline as compared to that in 1960–61. Unfortunately, the food insecurity is observed all round the year for protective foods like pulses, milk and milk products, making it difficult for the individuals to meet their nutrient requirements.

### *32*.2.2 National Food Security Mission

The Government of India has launched a National Food Security Mission (NFSM) to increase the production of rice, wheat and pulses. The Mission aims at increasing food grains production of the above crops through expansion in the area and enhancement in productivity; restoring soil fertility and its productivity; creating employment opportunities; and enhancing farm level economy to restore confidence of farmers of 305 targeted districts. The districts are selected in different states with emphasis on specific food crops and are referred as (1) Rice districts, (2) Wheat districts, and (3) Pulse districts [10].

Besides the NFSM, the government launched the National Horticulture Mission (NHM), which was initiated during 2005–06 for holistic development of the sector with the objectives to enhance horticulture production through area-based regionally differentiated strategies; improve nutritional security and income support to farm households; establish convergence and synergy among ongoing programmes for horticulture development; and, promote, develop and disseminate technologies. The area and production of horticultural crops is presented in Table 32.3. Following the launch of the NHM, an increase in area and production is evident. In 2006–2007, of the total horticulture production, vegetables contributed to 59.8% and fruits to 30.9%.

*Table 32.3* Area production of vegetables, roots and tubers and fruits [9]

| *2004–05* | | *2005–06* | | *2006–07* | |
|---|---|---|---|---|---|
| *Area ('000 ha)* | *Production ('tonnes)* | *Area* | *Production* | *Area* | *Production* |
| 6744 | 101246 | 7131 | 110106 | 7211 | 111770 |

## 32.3 Dietary consumption pattern in India

Indian population, by and large, depends, on foods of plant origin with cereals – rice and wheat – forming the bulk of the dietaries. NNMB surveys [11, 12] reveal that the consumption of protective foods like pulses, vegetables, milk and milk products is woefully inadequate and much below the ICMR recommended dietary allowances (Table 32.4).

*Table 32.4* Consumption of foods (g/day) among rural communities – NNMB

| *Food* | *Cereals* | *Millets* | *Pulses* | *GLV* | *Other vegetables* | *Roots and tubers* | *Milk* | *Oils* | *Sugar and jaggery* |
|---|---|---|---|---|---|---|---|---|---|
| *Consumption* unit* | 344 | 52 | 28 | 16 | 49 | 60 | 82 | 14 | 14 |
| RDI (ICMR) | | 460 | 40 | 40 | 60 | 50 | 150 | 20 | 300 |

* For consumption unit, see Box 32.3.

Over the years, the practice of consumption of qualitatively superior diet consisting of mixed cereals, containing particularly coarse grains

**Box 32.3 Consumption unit**

Diet surveys involve assessment of diet and nutrient intakes of different individuals belonging to different ages and physiological groups. In such cases, the usual practice is to assess the requirements of different groups in terms of those of the average man by applying calorie coefficients, which are referred to as consumption units. The energy consumption of an average male doing sedentary work is taken as one consumption unit, which corresponds to energy requirements of 2400 kcal/day. The other coefficients are worked on the basis of their calorie requirements as a proportion of the above. For more information on the consumption units for different age and physiological groups details are available in a document on nutritive value of foods [13].

like millets, is showing a significant decline. The surveys conducted by the NNMB [11] indicate that the intake of coarse grains like millets is confined mostly to the States of Gujarat (maize, *bajra*), Maharashtra (*Jowar*), Karnataka (*ragi*) and Madhya Pradesh. Even the NSSO surveys indicate that there has been a significant decline in the consumption of coarse cereals like millets during 1972–73 and 1999–2000 (Table 32.5).

*Table 32.5* Time trends in consumption of coarse cereals in India [14]

| *Group* | *Rice and Wheat (kg/month)* | | *Coarse cereals (kg/month)* | |
|---|---|---|---|---|
| | *1972–73* | *1999–2000* | *1972–73* | *1999–2000* |
| Lowest income | 3.4 | 8.3 | 2.4 | 1.4 |
| Pooled | 10.5 | 11.3 | 4.8 | 1.4 |

Though a large majority of the population is non-vegetarian, the contribution of animal foods is very small and infrequent, mainly due to economic reasons. The diets, thus, are poor in micronutrients. High levels of poly-phenols and phytates in the Indian diets further interfere with the absorption of nutrients leading to inadequacy of micronutrients.

The National Nutrition Monitoring Bureau (NNMB) under the auspices of the Indian Council of Medical Research (Box 32.4) has been presenting annual data on diet and nutritional status for the past 40 years.

## 32.4 Trends in nutrient intake

The nutrients intakes for the age group 1–3 years and 4–6 years against the RDA are presented in Tables 32.6 and 32.7, respectively. The data is based on the 2002 and 2006 NNMB report for the rural region in 9 states (Andhra Pradesh, Gujarat, Karnataka, Kerala, Madhya Pradesh, Maharashtra, Orissa, Tamil Nadu and West Bengal) of the country [11, 12].

**Box 32.4 National Nutrition Monitoring Bureau** (www.nnmbindia.org)

- The Indian Council of Medical Research (ICMR) established the National Nutrition Monitoring Bureau (NNMB) in 1972 – with Head quarters in National Institute of Nutrition, Hyderabad – in the States of Kerala, Tamil Nadu, Karnataka, Andhra Pradesh, Maharashtra, Gujarat, Madhya Pradesh, Orissa, West Bengal and Uttar Pradesh.
- The main objectives of the NNMB are to collect data on a continuous basis on dietary and nutritional status of the population in each of the States, and to evaluate the on-going National Nutrition Programmes, identify their strengths and weaknesses and recommend mid-course corrections to improve their effectiveness.
- Initially, the Bureau carried out annual surveys in four randomly selected districts from four strata formed on the basis of certain developmental criteria at the district level, from each State. From the year 1982, the NMMB has been adopting the sample frame of National Sample Survey Organization (NSSO) developed for its Consumer Expenditure Surveys covering a sub-sample of villages, which enabled sufficient spatial representation of the sample. The NSSO adopts a two stage stratified random sampling method in which the villages formed the first stage units (FSU), while the households (HHs) formed the second stage units (SSU). For the purpose, each State is divided into different agro-economic regions. Each region within a State consists of groups of contiguous districts having similar cropping pattern and population density. A district or part of the district with rural population of less than 1.8 millions forms one stratum. Districts with rural population of more than 1.8 million are divided into two or more strata by grouping contiguous *talukas/tehsils* having similar cropping pattern and population density.
- Such an approach helped in calculating, in future, unbiased estimates of the diet and nutrition situation of the community by applying design-based multipliers obtained from the NSSO.
- The unique feature of NNMB is conducting two repeat surveys in rural areas in the same villages which were surveyed in the years 1975–79. The results of the repeat surveys helped in assessing the changes in diet and nutritional status of rural communities.
- The results of all the annual surveys are published in the form of technical reports – to date 25 technical reports have been published. The results of the surveys carried out till the year 1995 were compiled as a publication entitled "25 years of National Nutrition Monitoring Bureau" (1997).
- The National Nutrition Monitoring Bureau (NNMB) also carried out special studies on micronutrient deficiency (MND) survey in 10 states including biochemical estimations of serum vitamin A, hemoglobin and urinary iodine.
- The bureau also conducted a cross-sectional survey of assessment of hypertension and diabetes mellitus in the rural areas.

*Source*: www.nnmbindia.org

About 70% of the children in the age group of 1–3 years and 4–6 years consume inadequate amounts of energy (Tables 32.6 and 32.7). The protein intake is inadequate (<70 percent RDA) in 40 percent of 1–3 year old children, while less than 10 percent of the 4–6 year old children consume inadequate protein daily. Thus, it is clear that the primary limiting factor in the Indian dietaries, among the poorest segments of rural India, is 'food

*Table 32.6* Trends in intakes of nutrients for preschool children (1–3years) [11, 12]

| *Nutrient* | *RDA* | *2002* | | | | *2006* | | | |
|---|---|---|---|---|---|---|---|---|---|
| | | *Intake* | *% RDA* | *%consuming % RDA* | | *Intake* | *%RDA* | *%consuming %RDA* | |
| | | | | > 70 | < 50 | | | > 70 | < 50 |
| Energy (kcal) | 719 | 729 | 101.3 | 29.5 | 38.0 | 719 | 100.0 | 28.9 | 41.7 |
| Protein (g) | 22 | 19.5 | 88.6 | 62.3 | 17.4 | 20.2 | 91.8 | 63.3 | 18.9 |
| Fat (g) | – | 12.1 | – | 22.7 | 63.1 | 10.7 | – | – | – |
| Calcium (mg) | 400 | 221 | 55.2 | 18.5 | 69.7 | 245 | 61.2 | 29.6 | 58.3 |
| Iron (mg) | 12 | 5.3 | 44.1 | 15.1 | 72.1 | 5.7 | 47.5 | 19 | 66.8 |
| Vitamin A (μg) | 400 | 106 | 26.5 | 8.0 | 87.5 | 129 | 32.2 | 9.4 | 85.8 |
| Thiamin (mg) | 0.6 | 0.4 | 66.6 | 39.1 | 43.7 | 0.5 | 83.3 | 42.5 | 42.9 |
| Riboflavin (mg) | 0.7 | 0.3 | 42.8 | 18.7 | 69.8 | 0.3 | 42.8 | 21.6 | 66.4 |
| Niacin (mg) | 8 | 5.1 | 63.7 | 36.2 | 41.8 | 5.2 | 65.0 | 38.7 | 40.7 |
| Vitamin C (mg) | 30 | 17 | 56.6 | 23.0 | 66.1 | 17 | 56.6 | 14.8 | 76.5 |
| Free Folic Acid (μg) | 30 | 20.4 | 68.0 | 40.0 | 37.5 | 20.3 | 67.6 | 38.8 | 41.1 |

*Table 32.7* Trends in mean dietary intakes of nutrients for preschool children (4–6 years) [11, 12]

| *Free Folic Nutrient* | *RDA* | *2002* | | | | *2006* | | | |
|---|---|---|---|---|---|---|---|---|---|
| | | *Intake* | *% RDA* | *% consuming %RDA* | | | *%RDA* | *% consuming %RDA* | |
| | | | | >70% | <50% | Intake | | >70% | 50% |
| Energy (kcal) | 1690 | 1066 | 63.0 | 30.6 | 24.1 | 1020 | 60.3 | 25.9 | 31.3 |
| Protein (g) | 30 | 28.2 | 94.0 | 73.4 | 6.5 | 28.7 | 95.6 | 72.9 | 8.6 |
| Fat (g) | – | 15 | – | 29.7 | 51.2 | 12.7 | – | – | – |
| Calcium (mg) | 400 | 239 | 59.7 | 28.1 | 55.3 | 272 | 68.0 | 34.0 | 49.5 |
| Iron (mg) | 18 | 8.1 | 45.0 | 15.3 | 70.7 | 8.6 | 47.7 | 18.3 | 66.4 |
| Vitamin A (μg) | 400 | 127 | 31.7 | 9.6 | 87.3 | 166 | 41.5 | 10.9 | 84.0 |
| Thiamin (mg) | 0.9 | 0.7 | 77.7 | 44.6 | 26.3 | 0.7 | 77.7 | 45.0 | 28.6 |
| Riboflavin (mg) | 1 | 0.4 | 40.0 | 5.6 | 83.0 | 0.4 | 40.0 | 6.4 | 82.5 |
| Niacin (mg) | 11 | 8.1 | 73.6 | 49.1 | 23.4 | 7.9 | 71.8 | 45.8 | 27.9 |
| Vitamin C (mg) | 40 | 24 | 60.0 | 25.3 | 60.7 | 25 | 62.5 | 25.8 | 63.1 |
| Free Folic Acid (μg) | 40 | 30.2 | 75.5 | 49.0 | 24.9 | 28.8 | 72.0 | 44.7 | 31.7 |

gap' and not protein deficiency as was, hitherto, believed. However, decreasing trend in consumption of pulse is of concern since it would adversely influence the quantity and quality of protein. More than two-thirds of the households and individuals consume less than 70% of RDA of other vital nutrients like vitamin A, iron and vitamins B-complex. In the case of younger children in the age group of 1–3 years, over 80 percent children consume less than 70 percent RDA of vitamin A, while almost 70 percent consume less than 50% RDA of iron.

The nutrient intakes of adolescent girls in the age group of 10–12 years are presented in Table 32.8. The proportion of the adolescent girls consuming less than 50 percent RDA of energy seems to increase between the years 2002 to 2006. The intake of iron, calcium and vitamin A is rather low.

*Table 32.8* Trends in mean dietary intakes of nutrients for adolescent girls (10–12 years) [11, 12]

| | | 2002 | | | 2006 | | |
|---|---|---|---|---|---|---|---|
| *Nutrient* | *RDA* | *Intake* | *% consuming (% RDA)* | | *Intake* | *%consuming (% RDA)* | |
| | | | *>70 %* | *< 50 %* | | *>70 %* | *<50%* |
| Energy (kcal) | 1970 | 1500 | 56.6 | 8.5 | 1389 | 46.7 | 16.6 |
| Protein (g) | 22 | 39.4 | 41.1 | 23.8 | 37.8 | 35.5 | 27.5 |
| Fat (g) | 57 | 18.9 | 51.3 | 30.5 | 14.8 | – | – |
| Calcium (mg) | 600 | 304 | 22/0 | 63.2 | 307 | 21.8 | 65.2 |
| Iron (mg) | 19 | 12.1 | 11.2 | 77.5 | 11.5 | 27.5 | 51.9 |
| Vitamin A (μg) | 600 | 174 | 9.2 | 87.8 | 205 | 9.2 | 87.4 |
| Thiamin (mg) | 1.0 | 1.0 | 65.6 | 19.0 | 0.9 | 59.7 | 21.7 |
| Riboflavin (mg) | 1.2 | 0.5 | 10.5 | 74.0 | 0.5 | 8.2 | 78.7 |
| Niacin (mg) | 13 | 11.7 | 70.4 | 8.5 | 11.1 | 63.0 | 16.2 |
| Vitamin C (mg) | 40 | 32 | 35.0 | 51.9 | 33 | 36.8 | 50.5 |
| Free Folic Acid (μg) | 70 | 42.4 | 29.0 | 42.0 | 39.3 | 25.4 | 46.9 |

The average energy nutrient intake among adult women seems to decrease in all these groups of adult women such as non-pregnant-non-lactating as well as pregnant and lactating women (Tables 32.9, 32.10 and 32.11). In the case of pregnant women, almost a third have energy intake of less than 70 percent RDA. In the case of micronutrients, a very high percentage of women consume less than 50 percent of RDA.

*Table 32.9* Trends in mean dietary intakes of nutrients for adult women [11, 12]

| | | 2002 | | | 2006 | | |
|---|---|---|---|---|---|---|---|
| *Nutrient* | *RDA* | *Intake* | *% consuming (% RDA)* | | *Intake* | *% consuming (% RDA)* | |
| | | | >70% | <50% | | >70% | <50% |
| Energy (kcal) | 1875 | 1878 | 89.1 | 1.4 | 1738 | 81.0 | 4.2 |
| Protein (g) | 50 | 48.2 | 78.3 | 4.7 | 46.5 | 76.3 | 5.9 |
| Fat (g) | – | 27.6 | 77.0 | 10.9 | 21.8 | – | – |
| Calcium (mg) | 400 | 445 | 60.9 | 24.5 | 443 | 60.5 | 23.2 |
| Iron (mg) | 30 | 14.1 | 14.7 | 67.9 | 13.8 | 15.3 | 68.6 |
| Vitamin A (μg) | 600 | 219.8 | 11.2 | 85.7 | 254 | 11.8 | 84.3 |
| Thiamin (mg) | 0.9 | 1.2 | 86.1 | 4.5 | 1.1 | 83.2 | 5.6 |
| Riboflavin (mg) | 1.1 | 0.6 | 26.7 | 47.9 | 0.6 | 24.4 | 50.8 |
| Niacin (mg) | 12 | 14.9 | 91.1 | 1.9 | 14.2 | 86.6 | 4.3 |
| Vitamin C (mg) | 40 | 44.7 | 51.4 | 14.4 | 47 | 51.2 | 33.3 |
| Free Folic Acid (μg) | 100 | 51.6 | 17.0 | 55.3 | 50.6 | 16.1 | 55.9 |

## 32.4.1 Intrafamily distribution of nutrients

An analysis of intra-family distribution of dietary energy in the households was carried out by comparing the adequacy of energy intakes, as per the RDI, of those of preschool children in each household with those of their parents and other elders. The intra-family distribution of dietary energy was assessed from 24-hour dietary recall data collected by the NNMB in seven states in India during 1996 97. The energy consumption, expressed

*Table 32.10* Trends in mean dietary intakes of nutrients for pregnant women [11, 12]

| *Nutrient* | *RDA* | *2002* | | | *2006* | | |
|---|---|---|---|---|---|---|---|
| | | *Intake* | *% consuming (% RDA)* | | *Intake* | *% consuming (% RDA)* | |
| | | | *< 50* | *> 70* | | *< 50* | *> 70* |
| Energy (kcal) | 2175 | 1933 | 1.6 | 75.5 | 1726 | 7.5 | 63.6 |
| Protein (g) | 65 | 49.7 | 15.4 | 48.4 | 46.8 | 18.2 | 46.5 |
| Fat (g) | – | 25.9 | 12.8 | 75.0 | 22.5 | – | – |
| Calcium (mg) | 1000 | 463 | 24.5 | 61.2 | 456 | 67.4 | 17.1 |
| Iron (mg) | 38 | 14.0 | 68.1 | 15.4 | 14.0 | 80.2 | 5.3 |
| Vitamin A (μg) | 600 | 227 | 82.4 | 13.3 | 261 | 83.4 | 12.3 |
| Thiamin (mg) | 1.1 | 1.2 | 8.5 | 82.4 | 1.1 | 15.0 | 73.8 |
| Riboflavin (mg) | 1.3 | 0.7 | 54.8 | 16.0 | 0.6 | 62.6 | 15.5 |
| Niacin (mg) | 14 | 15.1 | 3.2 | 87.8 | 13.7 | 8.6 | 73.8 |
| Vitamin C (mg) | 40 | 45 | 36.2 | 50.5 | 42 | 36.9 | 45.5 |
| Free Folic Acid (μg) | 400 | 53.1 | 55.3 | 21.8 | 50.3 | 100.0 | 0.0 |

*Table 32.11* Trends in mean dietary intakes of nutrients for lactating women [11, 12]

| *Nutrient* | *RDA* | *2002* | | | *2006* | | |
|---|---|---|---|---|---|---|---|
| | | *Intake* | *% consuming (% RDA)* | | *Intake* | *% consuming (% RDA)* | |
| | | | *> 70* | *< 50* | | *> 70* | *< 50* |
| Energy (kcal) | 2425 | 2028 | 82.3 | 1.3 | 1878 | 71.6 | 3.7 |
| Protein (g) | 75 | 50.3 | 46.9 | 13.9 | 49.6 | 47.1 | 13.4 |
| Fat (g) | – | 25.9 | 74.9 | 13.2 | 22.1 | – | – |
| Calcium (mg) | 1000 | 408 | 54.9 | 27.4 | 447 | 17.6 | 72.0 |
| Iron (mg) | 30 | 14.6 | 15.3 | 71.1 | 14.7 | 17.6 | 66.5 |
| Vitamin A (μg) | 950 | 212 | 9.3 | 86.7 | 249 | 7.9 | 89.9 |
| Thiamin (mg) | 1.2 | 1.3 | 83.8 | 7.8 | 1.2 | 84.4 | 6.6 |
| Riboflavin (mg) | 1.4 | 0.6 | 15.1 | 64.1 | 0.6 | 15.2 | 63.7 |
| Niacin (mg) | 16 | 16.3 | 83.8 | 3.0 | 15.5 | 81.9 | 4.2 |
| Vitamin C (mg) | 80 | 48 | 53.9 | 32.3 | 46 | 24.2 | 64.3 |
| Free Folic Acid (μg) | 150 | 57.6 | 23.4 | 45.4 | 55.2 | 3.5 | 83.5 |

as percentage of recommended dietary intake (%RDI) for preschool children, schoolchildren, and adolescents was compared with that of adult men and women in the same households. The data on energy consumption of adult males and females and children from +1 to +4 years is presented in Table 32.12, which presents the comparison of the percentage of preschool children consuming adequate energy according to different ages with that of adults when their diets were either adequate or inadequate. The results revealed that about one third of the preschool children had inadequate intakes of energy even when their adult counterparts had an adequate intake [15]. There were no difference between sexes in any of the age groups, with respect to intra-family food distribution.

The time trends in the intra-family distribution of dietary energy were assessed by comparing the data with those collected in 1975–80 using the

*Table 32.12* Adequacy (%) of energy consumption by age – preschool children and adults

| *Energy consumption category* | | *% of children age-wise (years) in specific energy consumption category* | | | |
|---|---|---|---|---|---|
| *Adult male (M) and female (F)* | *Child* | *1+* | *2+* | *3+* | *4+* |
| Both M and F adequate | Adequate | 13.0 | 33.9 | 42.5 | 32.0 |
| Both M and F adequate | Inadequate | 57.7 | 41.1 | 33.1 | 42.1 |
| Either M or F inadequate | Adequate | 1.8 | 4.6 | 6.6 | 4.0 |
| Either M or F inadequate | Inadequate | 17.6 | 12.9 | 10.2 | 14.0 |
| Both M and F inadequate | Adequate | 1.0 | 1.2 | 1.3 | 0.5 |
| Both M and F inadequate | Inadequate | 8.9 | 6.3 | 6.3 | 7.4 |

same procedures in the same villages. The analysis revealed a significant increase in the proportion of preschool children consuming inadequate energy, although both adult men and women were consuming energy-adequate diets during 1996–97 as compared to those surveyed in 1975–80. These results reflect the inappropriate child feeding and caring practices prevailing in the community, perhaps, due to mothers' ignorance about the child's energy requirements indicating the need for effective nutrition education for parents regarding appropriate feeding of their children for meeting the nutritional needs.

## 32.4.2 Socioeconomic status and diet

The socioeconomic status of the households plays an important role in the dietary pattern of the families. The dietary consumption among the landless agriculture labor and the socially backward scheduled castes and scheduled tribes, particularly, is not satisfactory. Poverty and ignorance are the major determinants of dietary consumption in these households. Even if all their income is spent on food, the poor families will not be able to meet the nutrient requirements. The average per capita consumption expenditure for rural and urban population as per 61st Round of NSSO (2004–05) is Rs. 558.78 and Rs. 1,052.36, respectively. In the rural households, on an average the consumption expenditure on food is about 55 per cent and remaining 45 per cent on non-food items. Rural population divided on the basis of their monthly per capita expenditures (MPCEs) exhibit consumption patterns as presented in Table 32.12. Rural poor (below poverty line/BPL) are spending about 31–35 per cent of their total consumption expenditure on non-food items and remaining on food items (Table 32.13).

NSSO consumption expenditure surveys indicate that expenditure on food has declined without any apparent increase in the cereal consumption, except in the lowest income group. It might be because cereal requirements, perhaps considered to be important by the community, are being met.

*Table 32.13* Expenditure on food and nonfood items according to MPCE**

| *MPCE Classes of Rural Population (Rs)* | *Expenditure %* | |
|---|---|---|
| | *Food* | *Non-food* |
| 0–235 | 68.45 | 31.55 |
| 235–270 | 67.16 | 32.84 |
| 270–320 | 66.35 | 33.65 |
| 320–365 | 64.78 | 35.22 |
| 365–410 | 63.99 | 36.01 |
| 410–455 | 62.93 | 37.06 |
| 455–510 | 61.61 | 38.39 |
| 510–580 | 60.11 | 39.88 |
| 580–690 | 58.02 | 41.98 |
| 690–890 | 53.92 | 46.08 |
| 890–1155 | 49.80 | 50.20 |

*BPL – Below Poverty Line
**MPCE – Monthly Per Capita Expenditure of BPL is Rs. 356.30
(Source: NSSO, 2004–05)

Unfortunately, the pulse consumption among all the segments showed a decline due to the continuous escalation of prices. Consequently dietary diversification is observed mainly in middle and high-income groups in urban and rural areas. There has been only a small increase in energy consumption among the poor despite widespread distribution of subsidized foods through Public Distribution System (PDS) to the BPL families. On the other hand, the energy consumption of the urban high-income group is achieved through increased quantities of sugar, oil, milk and milk products and lowering quantities of cereals. Such changes in the energy density of the diet and sedentary lifestyles are likely to lead to steep increase in over weight and obesity among this group.

## 32.5 Nutritional status – trends in children and adults

NNMB surveys indicate that Indians of lower socio-economic group, in general, are shorter and lighter as compared to the international standards. In fact, the median heights and weights of Indian preschool children of rural areas are comparable to the 5th percentile of the international standards. In other words, only the upper 5% of Indians have measurements comparable to an average well fed normal child. Until recently, for comparison purposes and to assess the extent of undernutrition, the heights and weights of National Centre for Health Statistics (NCHS) of USA were being used as international standards. The earlier NNMB data was based on the NCHS standards. The analysis of data by the NNMB using the NCHS standards and the recently developed WHO Multicentre Growth Reference Study (MGRS) revealed that the overall prevalence of underweight and stunting is less when the MGRS standards are used on the same children, as compared to the figures arrived by using NCHS reference standards, while the prevalence of wasting is higher [12].

The data for the national survey, National Family and Health Survey, 2006, are calculated on the basis of the WHO–MGRS Standards [17].

Trends in the nutritional status of children 1–5 years are presented in Figs. 32.4, 32.5 and 32.6. This is based on the surveys conducted by the NNMB [16] at different points of time for the 10 states covered by the NNMB between 1975 and 2006. It should be recognized that while in the repeat surveys, the same villages were surveyed in 1975–79 and 1996–97, the sample covered in the routine annual surveys during the years 2002 and 2006 is an independent sample selected using NSSO sample frame [11, 12]. They are presented based on Mean-2SD classification using NCHS standards for reference. The anthropometric values below Mean-3SD represent severe underweight, stunting or wasting. It should be noted that Mean-2SD values in the Figs. 32.4, 32.5 and 32.6 also include Mean-3SD. The values between <Mean-2SD and Mean-3SD represent moderate undernutrition. The data reveals that there has been a gradual reduction in the prevalence of underweight and stunting among the Indian preschool children during the last 3 decades. However, with respect to wasting in preschool children during the same period, the prevalence of wasting did not show any appreciable change, except for a small increase in 2002. This is not surprising since there have been changes in both height and weight. The samples in 2002 and 2006, as already indicated are independent samples based on NSSO sample frame.

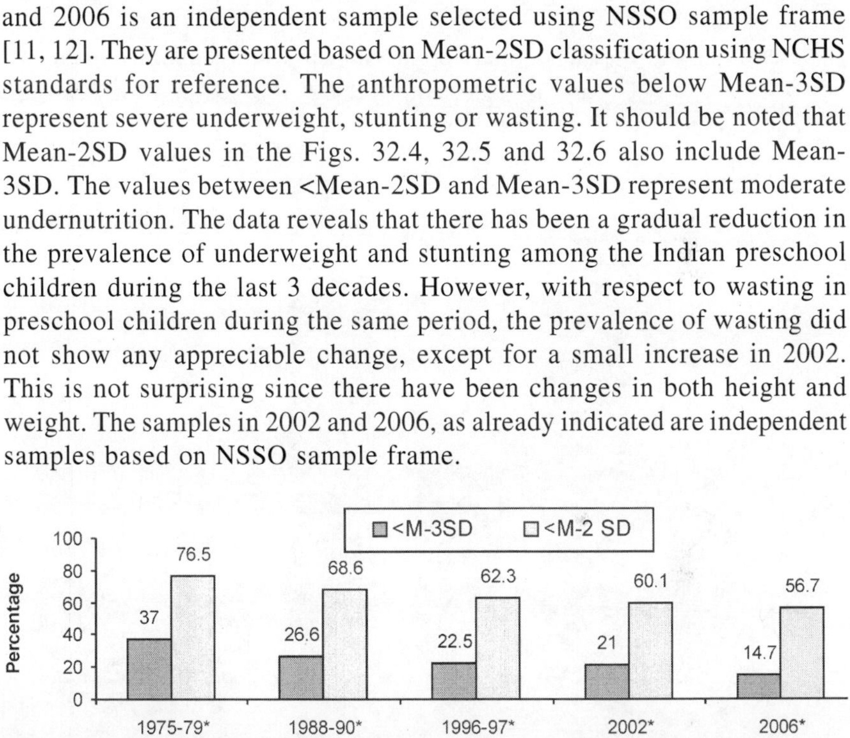


*32.4* Trends in underweight (weight for age) for preschool (1-5 years) children.

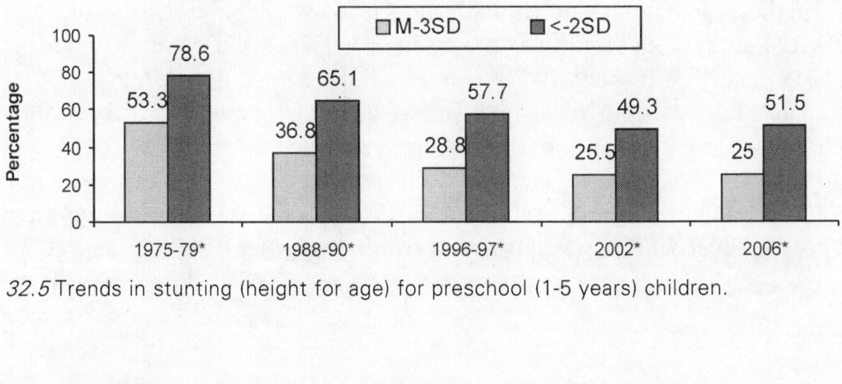


*32.5* Trends in stunting (height for age) for preschool (1-5 years) children.

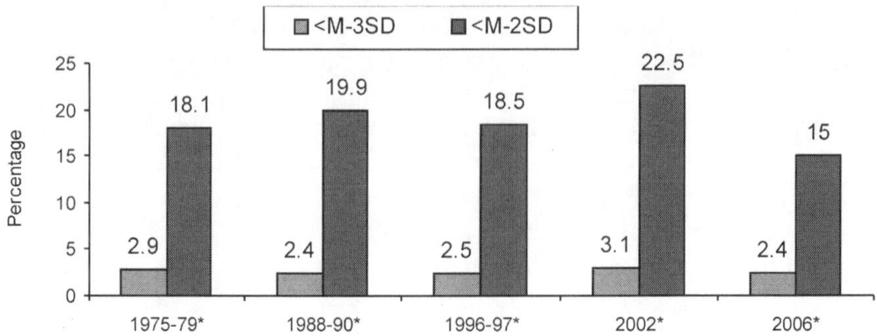


*32.6* Trends in wasting (weight for height) for preschool (1–5 years) children.

A comparison data on underweight, stunting and wasting in under 5 years children between NNMB-2006 and NFHS-3 using WHO-MGRS standards are presented in Fig. 32.7.

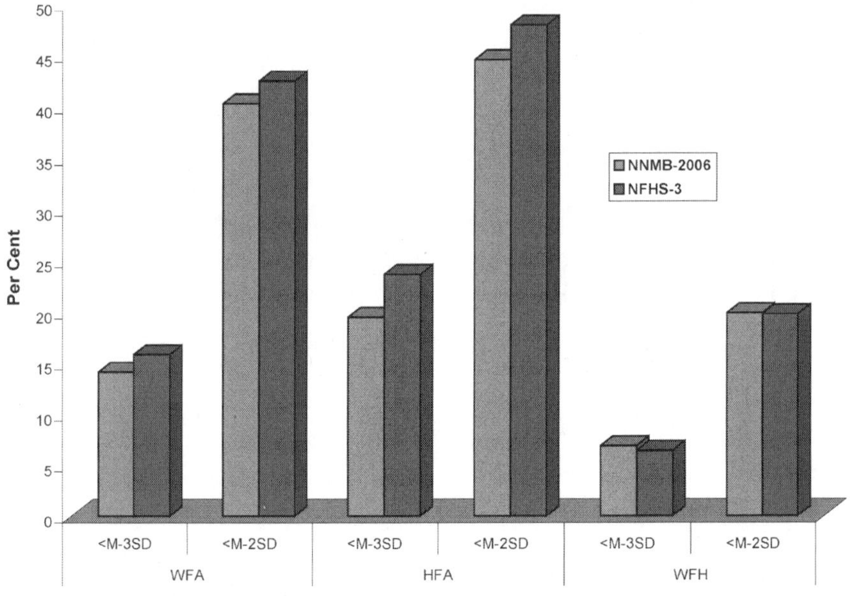


*32.7* Nutritional status of under five year children - NNMB - 2006 and NFHS - 3.

In the case of adults, nutritional status is assessed by body mass index or BMI (weight in kg divided by height in $m^2$). The classification of James et al [18] using BMI index is presented in Table 32.14.

The adults with BMI less than 18.5 in general are considered as chronic energy deficient, while those with values between 20 and 25 are treated as normal. The values 25+ and <30 indicate overweight (pre-obese), while >30 is considered to indicate obesity. Based on the BMI, overweight and obesity have been classified into various categories of I, II and III as

*Table 32.14* Classification of nutritional status by BMI

| *Classification* | *BMI (kg/m²)* |
|---|---|
| Underweight | <18.5 |
| Normal range | 18.5–24.9 |
| Pre-obese (Overweight) | 25.0–29.9 |
| Obese class I | 30.0–34.9 |
| Obese class II | 35.0–39.9 |
| Obese class III | ≥ 40.0 |

shown in Table 32.14. The BMI provides a reliable estimate of body fat in a great majority of individuals and has been recommended by the WHO. In view of the relative ease and accuracy of the basic measurements required for assessment, the BMI is widely used as an indicator of the risk of underweight as well as for classification of overweight.

The major limitations of BMI are that it does not distinguish between weight associated with either muscle or fat. Heavily muscled athletes will have a higher BMI but a relatively low fat content and conversely with increasing age, the lean tissue of the body decreases, so elderly subjects may have a normal BMI but excessive amount of fat. Also, BMI does not assess the fat distribution in the body.

NNMB surveys [12] indicate that about 37% of the males and 39% of the females have chronic energy deficiency (CED: <18.5), while 57% of the males and 52 % of females have normal BMI. The prevalence of central obesity was about 33% in men (Waist–Hip Ratio >0.95) and 77% in women (Waist–Hip Ratio >0.80). Figures 32.8 and 32.9 present the national data on nutritional status of adult men and women.

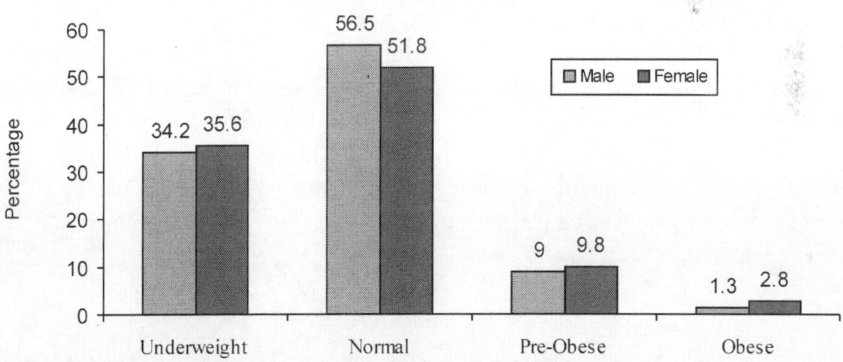


*32.8* Nutritional status (BMI) of adult men and women [17].

The classification of BMI in children and adolescent is complex as they are still growing and their stature and body composition is changing at different rates and times in different populations. The International Obesity Task Force (IOTF) based on the data obtained of BMI of more than 10,000 children in the age group of 6–18 years from each of the six countries –

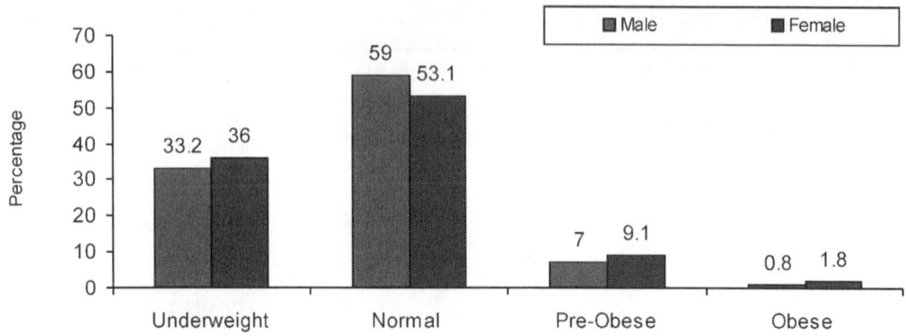


*32.9* Trends in nutritional status (MBI) of adult men and women.

Hong Kong, the Netherlands, Singapore, Brazil, Great Britain and the United States suggested the IOTF classification. According to this classification, children with BMI value between 85th and 95th percentile are considered as overweight and those with BMI value above 95th percentile for specific age and sex as obese [19].

## 32.6 Conclusion

Despite large investments by the governments, the extent of undernutrition remains high mainly due to unsatisfactory implementation of the programmes. This is evident from the reports that only a third of the eligible persons are reported to be using any services under the Integrated Child Development Services (ICDS) while only a quarter are availing supplementary feeding [17]. Inappropriate child feeding practices, poor food availability in the family, unsafe drinking water and lack of sanitation lead to high child undernutrition and mortality. With the threat of double burden of undernutrition and diet related non-communicable diseases glaring at the country, it is critical to ensure that there is intensive effort to reduce undernutrition through proper implementation of the existing programmes and working with the community to address the problem of child feeding, maternal care, large family size, poverty and ignorance.

## References

1. JONES G, STEKETEE RW, BLACK RE, BHUTTA ZA, MORRIS SS and the Bellagio Child Survival Study Group (2003). How many child deaths can we prevent this year? *Lancet*, **362**, pp. 65–71.
2. United Nations (2001). General Assembly, 56th session. Road map towards the implementation of the United Nations Millennium Declaration: report of the Secretary-General. New York: United Nations.
3. MENON P, DEOLALIKAR A and BHASKAR A (2009). Inter State Hunger Index-Comparisons of Hunger Across States, Washington, DC: IFPRI.

4. Food and Agriculture Organization (1992). Malnutrition in the World. Nutrition the Global Challenge. International Conferences on Nutrition, p. 3. Rome: FAO.
5. SAXENA NC (2008). Hunger, Under-nutrition and Food Security in India, UNDP workshop, Delhi, December.
6. USAID (1992). Policy Determination PD-19, Definition of Food Security, USAID, New York
7. FAO (1983). World Food Security: A Reappraisal of the concepts and approaches, Rome: FAO.
8. Ministry of Agriculture (2009). Agriculture statistics at a glance, Department of Agriculture and cooperation, Government of India.
9. Ministry of Finance, Govt. of India, Economic Survey 2007–08, (http://indiabudget.nic.in/ub2007-08/ubmain.htm
10. Ministry of Agriculture (2007). National Food Security Mission-Operational Guidelines, New Delhi: Department of Agriculture and Cooperation, Government of India.
11. National Nutrition Monitoring Bureau (2001). Diet and Nutritional Status of Rural Population, NNMB Technical Report No. 21, NNMB, NIN, Hyderabad.
12. National Nutrition Monitoring Bureau (2006). Diet and Nutritional Status of Rural Population and Prevalence of Hypertension among adults in Rural Areas, NNMB Technical Report No. 24, NNMB, NIN, Hyderabad.
13. GOPALAN, C et al. (1995). *Nutritive Value of Indian Foods*, Hyderabad: National Institute of Nutrition.
14. National Sample Survey Organization (2001). Department of Statistics, Government of India.
15. VIJAYARAGHAVAN K, SURYA PRAKASAM B and LAXMAIAH A (2002). Time Trends in the intrafamily distribution of dietary energy in rural India, *Food & Nutrition Bulletin*, **23,** pp. 390–394.
16. National Nutrition Monitoring Bureau, Report of Second Repeat Surveys 1996–97– Rural (1999), Technical Report No.18, National Nutrition Monitoring Bureau, National Institute of Nutrition, Hyderabad.
17. International Institute for Population Sciences (IIPS) and ORC Macro, 2007. National Family Health Survey (NFHS) III, 2005-06, India, Mumbai: IIPS.
18. JAMES WPT, FERRO-LUZZI A and WATERLOW JC (1988). Definition of chronic energy deficiency in adults. Report of Working Party of IDECG. *Eur J. Clin. Nutr* **42**, pp. 969–981.
19. COLE JC, MARY CB, KATHERINE MF, WILLIAM HD (2000). Establishing a standard definition for child overweight and obesity worldwide: international survey. *Br Med Journal*, **320**, pp. 1240–1243.

# 33

# Food and nutrition in natural and manmade disasters

*Deepti Gulati*

**Deepti Gulati**, MSc (Food and Nutrition), is currently a Senior Programme Associate with Global Alliance for Improved Nutrition (GAIN). Prior to GAIN, she was a Senior Nutritionist with UN World Food programme. She has extensive experience of working with the government as Deputy Director, National Institute of Public Cooperation and Child Development, Government of India. Deepti is Masters in Foods and Nutrition from MS University, Baroda, India. The author has received fellowships from the International Agriculture Centre, Netherlands and from the United Nations University in 'Management of Community Nutrition Programmes'.

## 33.1 Natural and manmade disasters

There are various definitions of disaster. WHO defines disaster as "an occurrence disrupting the normal conditions of existence and causing a level of suffering that exceeds the capacity of adjustment of the affected community" [1].

The definition by UN/ISDR is "a serious disruption of the functioning of a community or a society causing widespread human, material, economic, or environmental losses which exceed the ability of the affected community or society to cope using its own resources" [2].

Disasters whether natural or man-made, cause immense stress and instability. High profile disasters, like earthquakes, cyclones, floods, tsunamis, landslides, avalanches, conflicts etc., take heavy toll of life, while silent disasters like drought, starvation, epidemics, chronic malnutrition etc., take an even heavier toll of life. The disasters may be brief or protracted. All disasters – silent or otherwise – result in emergencies.

In the unstable aftermath of disasters, there are periods in which conditions become more or less acute, and the sequence and duration of these periods are unpredictable. The acuity of conditions may build to a peak (as in a drought or floods) or start at a pinnacle and then taper down and start mending (as in an earthquake). Transition from disasters to normality takes time and people affected by disasters usually need external support to cope and to return to normalcy.

Disasters can be categorized broadly into three categories:

- *Sudden disasters* – natural disasters, which affect food access and / or cause population displacements (floods, cyclones, earthquakes etc.).
- *Slow-onset disasters* – these are usually droughts and crop failures.
- *Complex emergencies* – these can involve conflict, widespread social and economic disruption and large population displacements, within the country or outside.

Whatever be the type of disaster, availability of food and its access to people affected by disaster, always gets highly compromised. The nature of food and nutrition problems depends on the type of disaster, its duration and size of the area affected, and the nutritional status of population prior to disaster. Disasters demonstrate their serious adverse impact on the nutritional status. Both protein energy malnutrition (PEM) and micronutrient malnutrition can occur. Malnutrition contributes to mortality amongst those affected by the disasters. Such mortality is often more pronounced in disasters such as internal political conflicts and wars, which result in large scale displacements of population groups within and outside the country, forcing people to stay in the refugee camps. In such situations, water and sanitation facilities are poor or non-existent and people's access to food is minimal. This results in high levels of malnutrition. Ethiopia, Somalia and Sudan have been affected by war/conflict over a very long period. In the worst phase of conflict in these countries, malnutrition incidence was reported to be as high as 80% in Somalia in 1992 and Southern Sudan in 1993. Micronutrient deficiencies – vitamin A, vitamin C, iron deficiency anemia and niacin are also commonly observed in refugee camps [3].

*Thus, human nutrition is nowhere more critically grave than in the situations where the normal channels of food access have been disrupted or cut off because of natural or man-made disasters. Nothing is more important than providing food when people find themselves suddenly, and often critically, in need, following a storm, earthquake, flood or other disaster emergency.*

Besides just the food and nutrition scenario, the environment itself gets greatly affected and contributes to the multiplier effect of the disaster. In fact, disasters trigger on a cycle of malnutrition, infection and ill health: disease burden increases and the malnourished individuals are many times more likely to succumb to infectious diseases resulting from environmental degradation perpetuated by the disaster. Hunger, poor performance of health and social service systems, low immunization coverage, and poor provision of primary care, render people more susceptible to disease and death.

### 33.1.1 Nutritional emergencies in natural or manmade disasters

Emergencies resulting from natural or man-made disasters are characterized by abnormal conditions of stress and instability (Box 33.1 and 33.2). Even though every emergency is unique and challenging, certain departures from normal, characterize nutritional emergencies. These include:

- *Changes in livelihood strategies*. Normal strategies for earning income and obtaining essential goods and services are interrupted or become less efficient. Less desirable (begging/selling off jewellery or household goods) and less-efficient strategies (eating lesser amounts of food or working on compromised wages) are referred to as coping strategies and these are adopted or expanded (Box 33.3).
- *Expansion of poverty, both in prevalence and intensity*. Incomes drop and possessions, necessary to households' short- or long-term viability, are lost.
- *Reduced availability of and/or access to staple foods*. Food and productive resources are destroyed, production fails, trade is interrupted and/or access to markets is blocked.
- *Changes in household and community structures and functions*. Death, disability, migration or conscription to armed forces removes people from households and communities. Those who remain must compensate, assuming new roles. Political rifts, armed conflict or competition for diminishing resources increases intra- and intercommunity tensions, disrupting normal operations.
- *Increased susceptibility to death and disability*. Several new threats, such as malnutrition, increased disease transmission, interruption of or blocked access to health services, inadequate water and sanitation and loss of protective infrastructure, goods and services, increase the susceptibility to death and disability (Box 33.2).

Disasters are major challenges to nutrition, health and food security. People in the areas with recurrent disasters face the problem of "transitory food insecurity" due to displacement or damage to household stocks. Inadequacy and uncertainty of food supply makes them food insecure and undernourished. Populations that are chronically undernourished are less likely to survive these crises. Disasters reduce a community's ability to effectively mobilize resources for the crisis management, making it difficult for people to cope up with the situation.

**Box 33.1 India's vulnerability to natural disasters**

India has been traditionally vulnerable to natural disasters on account of its unique geo-climatic conditions. Floods, droughts, cyclones, earthquakes and landslides have been a recurrent phenomena. About 60% of the landmass is prone to earthquakes of various intensities; over 40 million hectares is prone to floods; about 8% of the total area is prone to cyclones and 68% of the area is susceptible to drought. In the decade 1990–2000, an average of about 4344 people lost their lives and about 30 million people were affected by disasters every year. The loss in terms of private, community and public assets has been astronomical. [4]

People are thus caught in a hunger trap. Within these population groups, women and children are the worst affected. Familiar images of mothers with their children, standing amidst the wreckage of floods, cyclones, earthquakes, and other major disasters, reinforce the correct scenario that women and children are the first and foremost victims; they are vulnerable, poor, marginalized, and lack socio-political influence. *Worldwide, women and children are 14 times more likely to die in a disaster than men are.* [6]

In the critical situations arising from disasters, the humanitarian aid agencies step in to provide various types of assistance. Food assistance is of paramount importance as without enough food, any other humanitarian assistance intervention is likely to be less effective. Health interventions alone will not be enough to prevent illnesses that are compounded by lack of adequate nutritional intake, and even if there are adequate hygiene facilities, people will continue to be susceptible to risk of disease because of weakened immune systems and diminished bodily reserves.

**Box 33.2 Global scenario**

Earthquakes, floods, drought, and other natural hazards continue to cause tens of thousands of deaths, hundreds of thousands of injuries, and billions of dollars in economic losses each year around the world. According to the EM-DAT global disaster database maintained by the Centre for Research on the Epidemiology of Disasters (CRED) in Brussels, 354 natural disasters were recorded in 2008. Asia remained the most affected continent. Nine of the top 10 countries with the highest number of disaster-related deaths were in Asia. The human and economic losses caused by natural disasters in 2008 were devastating. More than 235,000 people were killed, 214 million people were affected and economic costs were over 190 billion US$ [5].

Disasters represent a major source of risk for the poor and wipe out development gains and accumulated wealth in developing countries.

*Purpose of food aid*

Very often during the disasters like floods/cyclones/earthquakes, there is widespread destruction, resulting in reduced access to food due to diminished household food stocks, crop destruction, easy access to markets etc. In such situations, food aid may perhaps be the only way of restoring people's access to food.

**Box 33.3 How people respond in disasters?**

Recurrent natural disasters undermine people's livelihoods, force poor households to resort to unsustainable practices in order to meet basic food needs:

- Reduce food – fewer meals – low cost food
- Work as labour/service-job
- Seasonally migrate for employment
- Sell animals – jewellery, land, self
- Permanent out-migration

When people are unable to gain access to enough food, they are more likely to engage in short-term survival strategies like excessive disposal of household assets, leading to destitution, ill health and other long-term negative consequences. Food aid can thus act as one of the most crucial interventions and an important mechanism to sustain life, protect or restore people's self-reliance, reduce the need for them to adopt potentially damaging coping strategies and help to re-establish their capacity to respond to future shocks.

The purpose of food aid is to:

(a) Sustain life by ensuring adequate availability and access to food by people affected by disaster.
(b) Provide sufficient food resources to eliminate the need for survival strategies, which may result in long-term negative consequences to human dignity, household viability, livelihood security and the environment.
(c) Provide a short-term income transfer or substitution to people to allow household resources to be invested for recovery.

Hence whenever situational analysis demands that food aid is an appropriate response, it should be undertaken in a manner that not only meets short-term needs but also, as far as possible, contributes to restoring long-term food security.

## 33.1.2 Planning for an effective food aid

Measures to prevent malnutrition following a disaster include assuring that food supplies are nutritionally complete, that food is distributed equitably among affected population, safe drinking water is available and there is adequate sanitation. In the absence of both, adequate nutrition and proper sanitation, it is difficult to prevent the onset of malnutrition.

Following steps are to be followed in order to ensure effective food aid programme:

- Estimate the quantity of food available.
- Calculate the dietary needs of the affected population.

- Determine the food rations in accordance with the characteristics of the population and estimated duration of the effects of disaster.

Food aid and feeding interventions have demonstrated that these play a vital role in disaster management and have made a difference. However, these need to be coupled with a development approach. The transition from receiving relief aid to community development can be difficult. Agencies may withdraw their personnel and resources, leaving the community with some of the immediate needs met but little reserves to cope long term. On the other hand, the community may become over-dependent on outside help if the agencies remain for too long. Neither approach enables the underlying vulnerability to be addressed, nor capacity and preparedness to develop.

Local data highlighting rising rates of malnutrition (refer to section 33.5 for details) can lead to increased efforts directed at prevention or if necessary, application for food intervention. Building capacity of vulnerable community should be the focus with emphasis on multidisciplinary involvement for addressing nutrition concerns during disasters.

## 33.2 Understanding concepts of vulnerability, disaster-preparedness and building capacities

During the last 30 years, there has been a manifold increase in the number of disasters and complex humanitarian emergencies and food insecurity of the community has been the core issue. Individuals, communities, and countries face various challenges in different ways; some seem well able to cope with adverse situations and overcome them, and others are completely overwhelmed.

**Box 33.4 Disaster and malnutrition**

Malnutrition is commonly associated with food insecurity and poverty. In most developing countries, the malnutrition is high amongst all population groups and amongst these, women and children have much higher levels of malnutrition. Disasters perpetuate environment degradation. So in any disaster situation, when the access and availability to adequate food and safe water is highly compromised, reduced food intake and lack of varied diet during a disaster predisposes people to protein-energy malnutrition and micronutrient deficiencies.

Malnutrition, lack of safe water supply and any sanitation services, displacement due to loss of property, etc. make people highly vulnerable and they have an increased risk of infectious diseases such as cholera, typhoid fever, diarrhea, acute respiratory infections and measles. Malnourished individuals are many times more likely to succumb to infectious diseases that result from environmental degradation perpetuated by the disasters.

It is important to prepare the communities to deal with the disasters and build their coping capacity so that their vulnerability is reduced (Box 33.4).

Hence it is essential to understand the concepts of vulnerability, disaster preparedness and capacity building. It is also essential to understand the importance of the interaction between vulnerability, and disaster-preparedness as these are inextricably linked. Therefore, the agencies providing aid to the disaster-affected populations also need to direct their efforts at enabling populations to build their own capacity and decrease their vulnerability – communities need to be enabled to mobilize as much of their own strengths as possible, so that their preparedness for any future disaster is enhanced.

### *Vulnerability*

In the disaster reduction context, vulnerability has been defined as "the conditions determined by physical, social, economic, and environmental factors or processes, which increase the susceptibility of a community to the impact of hazards" [1]. WHO defines vulnerability as "the predisposition to suffer damage due to external events" [2].

For example, those people living near the coastal areas are vulnerable to cyclones and tsunamis; those near the rivers are vulnerable to annual floods; those people who are living in the arid zones, are highly vulnerable to hunger as these areas are drought-prone, and those living in the seismic zones are vulnerable to earthquakes. These people suffer colossal damages whenever there are external events like droughts/cyclones/floods/earthquakes, etc. Unless the capacity of these people is built and they are supported to cope with these hazards, they would always be at the receiving end of the calamity or such external events.

In a disaster, vulnerability of communities will be influenced not only by the nature, extent, and time-scale of the disaster but also by community's capacity to cope with it, which means "the ability of the community to use available resources and abilities to face adverse consequences". This capacity to cope is influenced by factors such as prior experience, access to information, and cultural norms. In fact, the following formula has been proposed which indicates the relationship of vulnerability, hazards and coping capacity: V = H – C, where V is *vulnerability*, H is *hazards/disasters* and C is the *coping capacity*. Addressing vulnerability and capacity to cope aims to increase disaster preparedness i.e. the measures taken in advance to help ensure effective response to the impact of hazards [2].

To illustrate this, let us take an example of Orissa. Orissa has a very big coastline (over 430 km) and is visited by cyclones almost annually, making the people in the coastal areas very vulnerable to the cyclone fury. In October 1999 when the super cyclone hit Orissa, there were only 23 cyclone shelters of the Red Cross operating under the Orissa Disaster Mitigation Programme (ODMP) where people could seek rescue. About 2,000 persons occupied each shelter, which was designed only for about 1,500 people. Nevertheless, according to the Orissa Government's Relief Commissioner, these Red Cross shelters saved around 40,000 lives. Equipment of the shelters such as megaphones, generators, first aid kits, water containers etc. ensured that at least no one staying in these shelters died.

In this case, the vulnerability is the exposure of people to recurrent cyclones (which is the hazard) and the coping capacity is the availability of shelters. Hence, if the coping capacity to meet with the hazards/disasters is enhanced, the vulnerability due to hazards/disasters is reduced.

Since the super cyclone, Government of Orissa has constructed many such cyclone shelters across the cyclone-prone areas so that the vulnerability of the people to hazards of cyclones is greatly reduced.

Recognizing and understanding vulnerability in the context of disaster preparedness is fundamental in designing programmes for appropriate capacity building of the community and aiding in their quick recovery from the aftermath of the disasters.

However, in order to help the communities to build their coping capacity for facing the challenges of disasters, it is critical to interact with and listen to the local community. This will help to understand what factors onset the disasters and make these communities vulnerable. For example, activities like indiscriminate digging of deep bore-wells for water without any mechanism of water harvesting/re-charging, depletes water table leading to severe water crises, and arbitrary tree-felling leads to low rain falls. Many similar activities exploit and degrade the environment, which results in making the area become arid and drought prone.

Displacement, loss of buying power and erosion of coping and caring capacities, limit people's access to health services and often contribute to an overall increase in morbidity and mortality.

Discussions with community members help in identifying key issues that explain why a community is not able to cope with the disasters. Once the dynamics of vulnerability and inability of community to cope is understood, it becomes easier to partner with the community to develop mechanisms for reducing their vulnerability.

### *Disaster preparedness*

Disaster preparedness refers to "activities and measures taken in advance to ensure effective response to the impact of hazards" [2]. This includes the use of early warnings and measures to evacuate people from areas that might be affected.

The WHO definition of preparedness is "the measures that ensure the organized mobilization of personnel, funds, equipment and supplies within a safe environment for effective relief" [1].

However, the extent to which vulnerability is addressed by building a community's capacity is a key factor in determining its disaster preparedness (Box 33.5). When preparedness is directed towards the threat of a specific phenomenon like an earthquake, flood, or famine, knowledge gained from experience of comparable situations should be of value.

A key issue in nutrition and disaster preparedness is that development of capacity in vulnerable populations and disaster management must go hand in hand. Food aid and feeding interventions from outside have been vital in disaster management and have made a difference, but these need to be coupled with a development approach.

**Box 33.5 ASHRAYA project**

Due to the Super Cyclone, around 800,000 homes were demolished and 1.9 million badly damaged. CARE initiated ASHRAYA project to build better, stronger homes that could withstand future punishing storms, in the worst affected villages of Astarang, Balikuda, Mahakalpara and Rajnagar. The project was undertaken in partnership with local people. Rather than adopt a small number of villages, CARE spread the intervention over a larger area by building only 10 to 15 'core houses' in each village usually having a population of about 100 people and handed it over to the community for use during emergencies.

The core house is designed to withstand cyclones, has a flat roof so that people can shelter from floods, and is not vulnerable to fire and can therefore also act as a safe storage place for grain.

In addition, local people were encouraged to build their own core houses – and to learn new building methods as a result.

*Capacity building*

According to UN/ISDR, capacity to address disaster is "a combination of all the strengths and resources available within a community, society or organization that can reduce the level of risk, or the effects of a disaster" [2]. This includes physical and human resources as well as leadership and management.

**Box 33.6 The National Disaster Management Authority, India**

The National Disaster Management Authority (NDMA) with Prime Minister of India as its chairperson is the lead agency in India, which is authorized to deal with all types of natural and man-made disasters. It deals with prevention, mitigation and preparedness in pre-disaster phase, and response, rehabilitation and reconstruction in post-disaster phase. NDMA has a "National Disaster Management Operations Centre" with the state-of-the-art multi-faceted communication systems, to carry out the tasks of capacity development, training and knowledge management.

WHO indicates that capacity for emergency management consists of timely sharing of all the relevant information with people in authority and with the community so that the resources and procedures can be activated instantly to minimize the impact of disasters [1]. This can happen only if there is a systematic approach and well-laid out advance plans, which people in authority have been trained to understand and execute efficiently and effectively; and there is a receptive and responsive community that has been readied before hand to meet with such exigencies.

Hence, a country's ability to deal and manage a disaster in an urgent, organized and effective manner depends upon its advanced planning and effective systems that have been put in place, which can be activated as and when the need arises.

Capacity building for disaster prevention and mitigation also implies that there is a clear line of command authorizing the trained personnel at different levels to take quick decisions and implement the set of actions without the tardy processes of sanctions and approvals.

Therefore, for the areas prone to disaster, we must develop an early warning system, which provides accurate "information" about the impending disaster. Then, there must be specifically designated people/officers who receive this information, interpret it and are authorized to initiate action *without delay.* Each country must have its own specified agency/department/partner institution(s) that have the responsibility to put into action the mechanism to deal with any kind of disaster or any eventuality that may take place.

Enabling communities for disaster preparedness and building their capacity to cope with the disasters and enhancing the ability for disaster management at the country/state/district level must be addressed together if we wish to reduce the vulnerability from future eventualities. Unless the underlying vulnerability and its relation to disaster preparedness are addressed, the damage from the disasters cannot be minimized.

### 33.2.1 Role of humanitarian aid organization

In the immediate response to disaster, the affected community uses its own knowledge about local needs and capabilities and this helps in the speedy recovery and development processes. The role of humanitarian aid organisations is not to take over the affected communities unnecessarily, but to enable these communities to take control over the decisions. The humanitarian aid organisations must take account of potential expertise and contribution from within the affected populations and offer help and support that is culturally appropriate and acceptable. Otherwise their support / programmes may be limited in time and effectiveness.

### 33.2.2 Early warning systems (EWSs)

Early warning is "provision of timely and effective information, through identified institutions, that allows individuals exposed to a hazard (impending risk/danger) to take action to avoid or reduce their risk and prepare for effective response" [1]. Effective EWSs can predict a specific sequence of events that may result in disasters. This EWS helps in the identification and understanding of the hazard, the related impending risk and the extent of damage that can result. Hence, by using an EWS, the impending events are forecast and monitored, and understandable warnings disseminated to the population and those in authority, leading to an appropriate and timely action in response. This can thus minimize the havoc and reduce the loss of life, property and livestock.

Using preliminary indicators of natural disasters, EWSs can predict most of the disasters. However, EWSs have been mostly used in the area of drought prediction, possibly due to its slower onset and the large numbers of people potentially affected. Also, EWSs related to 'food security' use indicators like information on rainfall, state of crops, market prices, migration of workers, population movement, changes in nutritional status, and mortality rates, etc., which are easier to predict [7].

Based on the EWSs, impending crisis can be assessed and its management is planned accordingly. EWSs can be a very useful tool in helping the humanitarian aid organisations to estimate the seriousness of the impending disaster and help the organisations to decide when best to intervene for maximum effectiveness and prepare plans. These plans should be used as intervention strategies ready for immediate implementation if required. It is advisable that planned interventions, based on the EWSs *are implemented before any population displacement begins.* The commencement of migration often reflects that the situation is already serious.

## 33.3 Food insecurity and malnutrition – identification and measurement

Nutrition and health are inextricably linked and the factors that influence nutrition, ultimately affect health. Dietary inadequacies are a major contributing factors resulting in malnutrition, which influences and compromises resistance to diseases. It is well understood that poor nutritional status leads to lowered immunity and thus to increased morbidity from infectious diseases such as measles, malaria, or tuberculosis. The disease/nutrition cycle affects infants and young children in particular.

The nutritional status in children under 5 years responds rapidly to acute food shortages and high levels of malnutrition in this age group are used as proxy indicator of acute malnutrition in the overall population. Hence, in populations affected by disasters and complex emergencies, ascertaining the level of malnutrition should be given priority.

Marasmus (severe wasting), kwashiorkor (where oedema is a key feature), or a combination (marasmic kwashiorkor) are often present in children affected by disasters. Besides "protein energy malnutrition" (PEM), there may be micronutrient deficiencies in the population. The body also requires adequate stores of micronutrients to prevent deficiency in times of crises such as food shortages or trauma as these are associated with increased morbidity and mortality.

Guidelines for the identification and management of malnutrition have been published by various international and non-governmental organizations. These include Medicines Sans Frontiers' [8], the World Health Organization [9, 10], and UNHCR/UNICEF/WFP/WHO [11]. In addition, food security, nutrition, and food aid are included in the minimum standards set by "The Sphere Project [12]" (Box 33.7).

**Box 33.7 The Sphere Project**

The Sphere Project (the name conveys the sense of universality of this initiative), launched in 1997 by the Red Cross and Red Crescent movement and several non-government organizations (NGOs), aims to improve the effectiveness and accountability of humanitarian assistance. Their Humanitarian Charter and Minimum Standards in Disaster Response set standards in several areas including provision of shelter, safe water and sanitation and food security (2004)

## 33.3.1 Food insecurity and malnutrition

Identification of food insecurity and malnutrition normally commences with a rapid assessment of the general situation. When people are not able to access adequate food to assuage hunger and to meet their physiological needs, they are termed as food insecure. Such food insecurity could be transit or chronic in nature. Transitory food insecurity results from temporary disruption of access to food due to disasters or any other compelling circumstances while chronic food insecurity results from unavailability of adequate food over a long period (Box 33.8).

**Box 33.8 Concepts of Food Security**

Chronic Food Insecurity is the result of a consistently inadequate diet due to problems of food availability, food access and/or food utilization. More than 200 million Indians are undernourished; and chronically food insecure.

**Transitory Food,** Insecurity in food among households who normally can meet their minimum dietary need but are not able to cope with natural disasters. About 35 million Indians are affected by recurrent disasters every year; they are victims of transitory food insecurity.

Interviews and focus group discussions are carried out with members of the general population, as well as community leaders to get information on food availability and access, food beliefs, estimated population size, possible increases in illness and death, and information about water, sanitation, and food crops. This information is most essential in planning an effective food support programme as the cause of poor access to food can be identified and addressed; and sustainable systems can be initiated that would streamline the access of the affected population to adequate food.

### *Measuring malnutrition*

*The most widely accepted practice is to assess malnutrition levels in children aged 6–59 months as a proxy for the population as a whole.* It is usually the young children between 6 and 59 months who are measured in nutrition surveys, because these young children are the first to show the signs of malnutrition in times of food shortages and they are the most severely affected. *In cases where the ages of children are not known or cannot be assessed easily, children measuring between the length/height of 65 cm and 110 cm are used to represent the children in the age-group of 6–59 months.* However, other groups may be affected to a greater extent or face greater nutritional risk. When this is the case, the situation of these groups should be assessed, although measurement can be problematic.

Malnutrition can be assessed by clinical signs and by anthropometry. Anthropometric measurements such as weight-for-height are used as an objective assessment of nutritional status, which quantifies the nutritional situation at one point of time and allows comparisons over time.

Information on child mortality and child morbidity assists in understanding the underlying causes of malnutrition and the relationship characterised between malnutrition and mortality to determine the focus on specific interventions. Child mortality rates are particularly important.

International guidelines stipulate that a representative sample should be used for surveys; adherence to national guidelines can promote coordination and comparability of reporting. Where representative data are available on trends in nutritional status, these are preferable to a single prevalence figure.

### *Weight-for-height in children*

The "weight for height" (WFH) index is most commonly used to detect acute malnutrition (wasting) in surveys. WFH in children is the best indicator to assess and monitor nutritional status of populations and is normally estimated by surveying children aged 6 to 59 months, using cluster sampling. It compares weight with the median weight of a sample of children of the same height.

The actual weight of a child is calculated as a percentage of the standard weight for a normal child of that height, or as a Z-score. Z-scores are the standards and a preferred mode of presenting anthropometric indicators in nutrition surveys (Table 33.1). Thus a Z score of < –3 and/or oedema indicates severe acute malnutrition [13]. Moderate acute malnutrition is indicated if the WFH is between 70% and 80% of the median, or between –3 and –2 Z scores. The term "global acute malnutrition" (GAM) refers to the total number of children with severe acute malnutrition plus those with moderate acute malnutrition, that is all those with WFH < 80% of median, or < –2 Z scores. In selective feeding programmes percentage of median can be presented in addition to Z-scores in survey reports if there is a specific need, e.g., if it is required as a programmatic tool in selective feeding programmes.

Until recently, United States National Centre for Health Statistics/ Centers for Disease Control (NCHS/CDC) and Prevention reference tables adopted by the World Health Organization [14] were in use, but now the recently launched WHO Child Growth Standards provide a new international standard [15].

When anthropometric measurements are used in conjunction with clinical observations, these together provide a very clear picture of malnutrition, including micronutrient malnutrition. WFH less than 70% of the median and/or oedema indicates severe acute malnutrition while pallor indicates anemia, and signs of night blindness or bitot's spot indicate vitamin A deficiency.

*Table 33.1* Classification of acute malnutrition in children [12]

| | Total malnutrition* | Moderate malnutrition | Severe malnutrition |
|---|---|---|---|
| Children 6.0-up to months | <–2 Z scores WFH** or 80% median and/or nutritional oedema | –3 to <–2 Z scores or 70%–80% median WFH | <–3 Z score WFH or < 70% median WFH and / or nutritional oedema |

* This is also called global acute malnutrition.
** Weight for height.

WHO has set emergency thresholds, above which nutritional intervention is indicated for the population. *A critical situation is reached when over 15% of the children surveyed have global acute malnutrition.*

There are no agreed anthropometric cut-offs for acute malnutrition in infants below six months, apart from the presence of nutritional oedema. The NCHS/CDC growth references are of limited use since they are drawn from a population of babies fed artificially, whereas breastfed babies grow at a different rate. This means that malnutrition will tend to be overestimated in this age group (WHO). It is therefore important to assess infant feeding practices, particularly access to breast milk, and any medical conditions in order to determine whether malnutrition in this age group may be a problem.

Delayed growth in height for age, i.e. "stunting", can be found in situations of chronic malnutrition. In this case, weight for age (WFA) may be a preferred indicator as this indicator captures recent undernutrition, which often results in disasters when there is poor access to adequate food due to the disruption in normal food supply chain.

### *Body mass index*

Body mass index (BMI) is measured as weight in kg/height in $m^2$ and is used for assessing the nutritional status of adults by assessing the degree of thinness. A ratio of ≥16–18 indicates moderate malnutrition and <16 severe malnutrition (Table 33.2).

### *Mid-upper arm circumference*

Where large numbers of children have to be screened, mid-upper arm circumference (MUAC) can be used to identify wasting. MUAC is a simple and practical tool which can be used by minimally trained workers for detecting the severely malnourished in the community and for achieving high programme coverage. MUAC measurements <115 mm in children of <5 years are indicative of severe acute malnutrition and are of value in predicting mortality. MUAC has also been used to identify malnourished adolescents, and adults including pregnant women, in need of admission to feeding programmes. A MUAC of <20.7 cm indicates severe risk [12].

Nutritional survey reports should always describe the probable causes of malnutrition. Explanation on probable causes of malnutrition helps to effectively address the root-cause and provide some tangible solutions to reduce the magnitude of malnutrition.

*Also, nutritional oedema should be reported separately.* Presence of nutritional oedema is an indicator of protein deficiency and thus needs special attention and care. Also, while assessing the nutritional status using weight for age, children having nutritional oedema are excluded as the presence of oedema may show higher weight of the child due to the fluid accumulation and retention, thus interfering with correct assessment of malnutrition.

Trends in mortality are important in the interpretation of nutrition data. Crude mortality rate (CMR) is the number of deaths in the population, for example per 1,000 per month, or per 10,000 per day. A doubling of CMR above the baseline indicates a public health emergency [12].

*Table 33.2* Summary of key malnutrition indicators [10]

| Malnutrition | Children <5 years old | | | Adults |
|---|---|---|---|---|
| | WFH (W/H)%of median NCHS/WHO reference values | WFH (W/H) in Z scores or SD's of the median NCHS/WHO reference values | MUAC | BMI |
| Moderate | 70–79% | –3 to 2 Z scores | 115 mm to <125 mm | 16 to <17 |
| Severe | — | < 3 Z scores or oedema | <115 mm | Less than 16 |

On-going nutrition surveillance should be a standard practice in every country so that a deteriorating situation can be identified early. This requires developing the expertise of fieldworkers to carry out data collection, and strengthening the ability of the programme managers to seek access to logistical, statistical, and nutritional expertise to analyse and interpret finding.

## 33.4 Nutritional interventions

In any emergency or disaster, the first and foremost need is assuaging (assessing) hunger. Providing food and other nutritional interventions to the disaster affected persons is one of the most important activities of the collective response of the humanitarian aid agencies.

For planning nutrition intervention, it is important to undertake the initial assessment and analysis of the emergency situation and focus on people's own food and income sources, and assess the quantity and type of food assistance required to maintain adequate nutritional status for the general population, as well as of the vulnerable groups (Box 33.9). Moreover, it is important to understand the underlying causes of malnutrition and analyse information provided through the anthropometric surveys. Information on the causes of malnutrition can be gathered from primary or secondary sources, including existing health and nutrition profiles, research reports, early warning information, health centre records, food security reports and community welfare groups, and can comprise both quantitative and qualitative information. An early assessment of nutritional status of the disaster-affected population helps to plan emergency response, the components of rations and the requirement for any additional selective feeding programme.

Decision-making should rely on an understanding of all the possible underlying causes of malnutrition as well as results from anthropometric surveys. In an acute crisis, however, decisions to implement general food distribution need not await the results of anthropometric surveys, as these can take up to three weeks. It should, however, be possible to use anthropometric survey findings to inform decisions on responses aimed at correcting malnutrition.

**Box 33.9 Essentials of planning**

It is important to consider factors, such as cultural acceptability of the food ration and the choice of suitable foods. Providing a diverse diet, with culturally appropriate foods that are rich in micronutrients, is a major food aid challenge. The participation of disaster-affected people in decision-making, programme design and implementation, helps to ensure that programmes are equitable and effective. Special effort should be made to ensure the participation of women and a balanced male and female representation within the assistance programme. Participation in the food aid / support programme may also serve to reinforce people's sense of dignity and worth in times of crisis. It generates a sense of community ownership, which can help ensure the safety and security of those who are receiving assistance, as well as those who are responsible for its implementation.

The standard for food aid requirements is based on WHO's planning estimate for a typical population.

Nutritional interventions, primarily consisting of feeding, fall into two main categories:

(i) General feeding programmes and
(ii) Selective feeding programmes

The objectives of the feeding programme should be realistic and should be achieved within a period determined in advance.

Figure 33.1, based on the Nutrition Guidelines; MSF, 1995 [8] helps to understand the seriousness of the situation and decide on the type of nutrition programme that should be started. Supplementary feeding programmes provide nutritious food in addition to the general ration. They aim to rehabilitate malnourished persons or to prevent a deterioration of nutritional status of those most at-risk by meeting their additional needs, focusing particularly on young children, pregnant women and nursing mothers.

*General feeding programs*

These are designed to meet the needs of the overall population, and should adhere to the minimum standards set by The Sphere Project (2004). In situations where *the ration provided by the aid agency is the sole food source,* ration size is planned in such a way that it meets an average daily energy requirement of 2100 kcal per person (adult). This ration size is designed to address hunger and prevent further deterioration of the nutritional status. Calorie requirements of ration per person are increased in conditions where malnutrition is present, heavy physical work is being carried out, or population is living at low atmospheric temperatures.

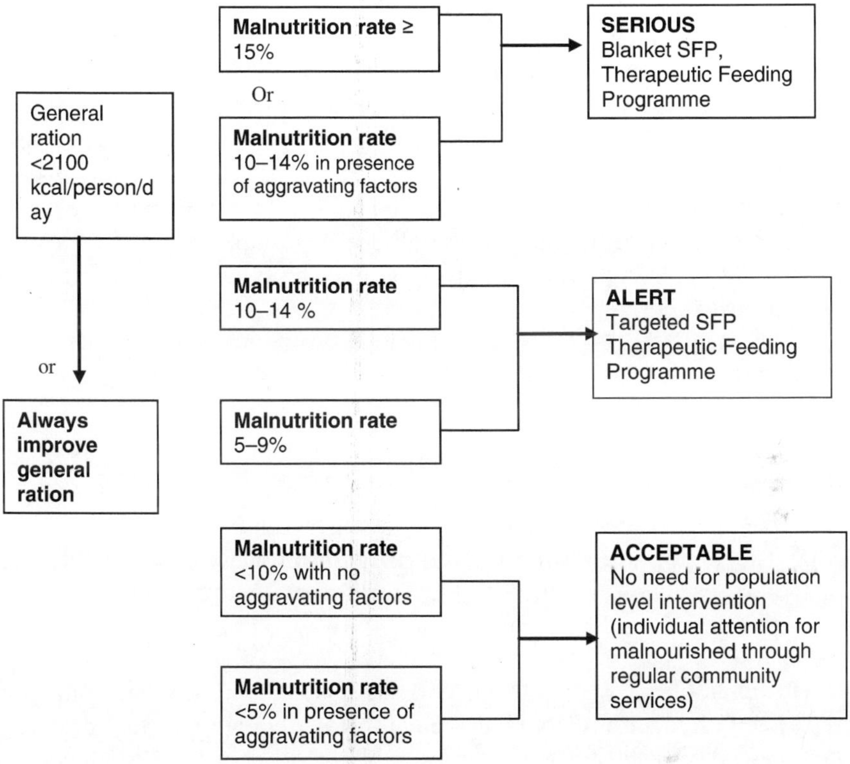


*33.1* Nutrition interventions and selective feeding programs.

The initial planning estimates of WHO for nutritional requirements for the general feeding programme and supplementary feeding programme are based on the following:

These feeding programmes are designed as a "safety net" to prevent further deterioration of nutritional status and reduce mortality.

*While for supplementary feeding programme, the nutritional requirement and the ration size would depend upon the nutrition gap between what is required vis-à-vis what the people are getting; for general feeding programme, the nutritional requirements of the daily ration include the following:*

- 2,100 kcal per person per day. (This is the basis used for population, irrespective of age group – Table 33.3.)
- 10–12% of total energy is provided by protein.
- 17% of total energy is provided from fat.

- Adequate micronutrient intake through fresh or fortified foods (refer Table 33.4).

In general rations, supplies are provided preferably as dry food rations, the basic commodities being cereals, pulses, and vegetable oil, to be prepared at home. As a short-term measure, rations may be provided as cooked meals.

In most emergency situations like the earthquakes, floods etc., the people get displaced and/or their house are damaged or destroyed. In the first few days following such disasters, on-spot cooking of food is nearly impossible, hence rations may be provided as cooked meals. As a short-term measure, the most appropriate foods are the 'High-energy biscuits' or similar 'Ready-to-eat' (RTE) foods, as these can be mobilized quickly and are logistically easy to distribute.

Reported difficulties with emergency food aid fall roughly into the following three categories:

1. The quantity of rations provided;
2. The quality of rations, particularly their micronutrient content and the appropriateness of foods in the ration; and
3. The coordination of food aid programming with the health and personal care components required for protecting the nutrition of people affected by emergencies.

However, biscuits and RTE need to be replaced by foods that would not only pacify hunger but would also be nutritionally appropriate. These can be replaced by a steady supply of a complete basket of food commodities in quantities sufficient to meet requirements. Thus, the dry food rations would include basic commodities such as cereals, pulses, and vegetable oil, which can be prepared at home. But, the unprocessed grains, though easy to procure, are not the ideal food choice in emergency situations because they need milling and cannot be consumed otherwise. Hence, foods like wheat flour/corn flour or the wheat–soya / corn–soya blends should be considered as an important part of the food basket as these can be cooked with minimal fuel and fuss.

Another advantage of these floors/blends is the ease with which these can be fortified with micronutrients, which are critical for meeting the micronutrient needs of the population groups. When foodstuffs like fruits and vegetables that provide naturally occurring essential vitamins and minerals to population groups are not available, the use of food fortified with micronutrients; following the principles outlined in Codex Alimentarius, should be the most appropriate alternative. At a minimum, the micronutrient fortification for all the processed grains can be undertaken with elemental iron and B vitamins, plus vitamin A.

Factors, such as cultural acceptability of the food ration and the choice of suitable foods, must be considered. There are many challenges in ensuring fair distribution of food aid. Food aid targeting should help identify the most vulnerable areas and households. This requires the use of various indicators, such as health status and food security, in addition to nutritional status.

In brief, commodity selection should consider the following:

- Local availability and market impact.
- Local acceptability and preparation.
- Fitness and nutritional composition.
- Fuel requirements for cooking.

*Selective feeding programmes (SFP)*

These aim to ensure that individuals in specific vulnerable groups receive adequate nourishment. Typically, such groups would include malnourished infants and young children and/or pregnant or nursing mothers. In SFP, the food rations either provide one or two food commodities to complement existing foods available and accessible to the affected population (for example, pulses and oil might be provided to complement locally accessible cereals), or provide specific foods as a supplement to the general ration, in order to cover the needs of particular groups. In SFP, the selection of food items to be included in the food basket is based on people's food and income sources and the availability and access to food.

Estimates of people's food and income sources include consideration of:

- Market and income opportunities.
- Foraging and wild food potential.
- Agricultural seasons and access to productive assets
- Sources of income and coping strategies

There are two types of selective feeding programmes:

- Supplementary feeding programmes (SFP) and
- Therapeutic feeding programmes (TFP).

The *Supplementary feeding programmes* aim to provide extra food *to the groups at risk in addition to the general ration.* The ration provided could be as a dry, take-home ration or a wet, on-the-spot feeding. These are of two types: *Blanket SFP* and *Targeted SFP*.

The blanket SFP provides a food and/or micronutrient(s) supplement to all members of a certain vulnerable group, regardless of their individual nutritional status in order to prevent a further deterioration in the nutritional status of those groups most at risk (usually children <5 years of age, pregnant women and nursing mothers).

The targeted SFP aims to rehabilitate those who are moderately malnourished. These could be infants, children, adults or older people and/or individuals selected on medical or social grounds, e.g. pregnant and nursing mothers and the sick. This is the most common type of SFP. As far as infants are concerned, breastfeeding, if possible, should always be encouraged. For older children and adults, in addition to the general food ration, the SFP should supply an extra 1000–1200 kcal/person/day (dry rations), or 500–700 kcal/person/day (cooked meal), as the need may be.

*Therapeutic feeding programmes (TFP)* generally target the severely malnourished, particularly infants and young children who are severely malnourished and critically ill with high rates of mortality. The TFP can either be implemented in special feeding centres or in a hospital or clinic or at the community level. TFP involves intensive medical and nutritional treatment. The management of severe malnutrition in children can take place through facility-based management and community-based therapeutic care.

*Facility-based management* refers to treatment in a hospital or a centre that provides skilled medical and nursing care where the affected infants and young children are treated under medical supervision. The priority in the first 1–2 days in such cases includes treating dehydration, infections, hypoglycaemia, fluid and electrolyte imbalance, and hypothermia. If the infant is being breastfed, this is encouraged to be continued. Once the child's appetite has returned (usually after 2–7 days), several weeks of rehabilitation follow and micronutrient supplements especially vitamin A (dosage specific for the age) is given. The children are then discharged to the care of their own families with weekly monitoring at the feeding centre [10].

*Community-based therapeutic care (CTC)* refers to diagnosing the condition, instituting treatment and monitoring the condition of child at home with some external input, such as the presence of a health worker/ trained community-based programme worker. Community-based therapeutic care includes treatment of severely malnourished child with vitamin/mineral supplements and/or Ready-to-Use Therapeutic Foods (RUTF). RUTFs are available as energy-dense pastes or biscuits, which are resistant to bacterial growth, unlike milk-based liquid products and are useful for treating severe malnutrition in children who have limited access to local family diets for nutritional rehabilitation. When RUTF is given to children with severe malnutrition, 150–220 kcal/kg/day should

**Box 33.10 Facility-based management**

Severely malnourished children in institutional setting are given F-75, a "starter formula", which is administered frequently - every 2-3 hours and in small amounts. Naso-gastric tube feeding may be required in this stage. Additionally, micronutrient supplements are given. Usually, the child's appetite returns to normal after 2-7 days. F-75 is gradually replaced with another formula F-100 or the "catch-up" formula. Both F-75 and F-100 are therapeutic milk products designed to treat severe malnutrition. F-75 contains 75 kcal of energy and 0.9 g protein per 100 ml, and F-100 contains 100 kcal of energy and 2.9 g proteins per 100 ml. Both are very high in energy, fat, and protein, and provide a large amount of nutrients. These are now used by all major humanitarian aid organizations to treat acute malnutrition. Ingredients include concentrated milk powder, food oil, and dextrin vitamin complexes. The formulas may be prepared by mixing with the local water supply. Sometimes 'Plump nut/peanut butter' is substituted for F-100. F-75 may be constituted using a cereal base in place of milk. However, it is important that child feeding should be accompanied with other components of child care such as social contact, simulation, play etc. Rehabilitation at institutional level should be followed by family level care and weekly monitoring at the institutional level.

be provided. This energy-dense fortified therapeutic food may be given in two-three doses depending upon the age, and severity of malnutrition. In case of moderate to severely malnourished children, anorexia may be a problem and hence the portion size of food has to be small.

**Box 33.11 Read-to-Use Therapeutic Foods (RUTF)**

RUTF have a similar nutrient composition to F100, which is the therapeutic diet used in hospital settings. But unlike F100, RUTF are not water-based, meaning that bacteria cannot grow in them. Therefore these foods can be used safely at home without refrigeration and even in areas where hygiene conditions are not optimal.

When there are no medical complications, a malnourished child with appetite, if aged six months or more, can be given a standard dose of RUTF adjusted to their weight. Guided by appetite, children may consume the food at home, with minimal supervision, directly from a container, at any time of the day or night. Because RUTF do not contain water, children should also be offered safe drinking water to drink at will.

The technology to produce RUTF is simple and can be transferred to any country with minimal industrial infrastructure. RUTF cost about US$3 per kilogram when locally produced. A child being treated for severe acute malnutrition will need 10–15 kg of RUTF, given over a period of six to eight weeks.

### *Ready-to-use therapeutic foods*

Ready-to-use therapeutic foods (RUTF) are high energy, fortified, ready-to-eat foods suitable for the treatment of children with severe acute malnutrition. These foods should be soft or crushable and should be easy for young children to eat without any preparation. At least half of the proteins contained in the foods should come from milk products. RUTF contains iron and F-100 does not contain this micronutrient.

*Nutritional composition of RUTF* [9, 16]

| | | |
|---|---|---|
| Moisture content | – | 2.5% maximum |
| Energy | – | 520–550 Kcal/100 g |
| Proteins | – | 10–12% total energy |
| Lipids | – | 45–60% total energy |
| Sodium | – | 290 mg/100 g maximum |
| Potassium | – | 1,110–1,400 mg/100 g |
| Calcium | – | 300–600 mg/100 g |
| Phosphorus (excluding phytate) | – | 300–600 mg/100 g |
| Magnesium | – | 80–140 mg/100 g |
| Iron | – | 10–14 mg/100 g |
| Zinc | – | 11–14 mg/100 g |
| Copper | – | 1.4–1.8 mg/100 g |
| Selenium | – | 20–40 µg |
| Iodine | – | 70–140 µg/100 g |
| Vitamin A | – | 0.8–1.1 mg/100 g |
| Vitamin D | – | 15–20 µg/100 g |
| Vitamin E | – | 20 mg/100 g minimum |
| Vitamin K | – | 15–30 µg/100 g |
| Vitamin $B_1$ | – | 0.5 mg/100 g minimum |
| Vitamin $B_2$ | – | 1.6 mg/100 g minimum |
| Vitamin C | – | 50 mg/100 g minimum |
| Vitamin $B_6$ | – | 0.6 mg/100 g minimum |
| Vitamin $B_{12}$ | – | 1.6 µg/100 g minimum |
| Folic acid | – | 200 µg/100 g minimum |
| Niacin | – | 5 mg/100 g minimum |
| Pantothenic acid | – | 3 mg/100 g minimum |
| Biotin | – | 60 µg/100 g minimum |
| n-6 fatty acids | – | 3%–10% of total energy |
| n-3 fatty acids | – | 0.3%–2.5% of total energy |

Children below 6 months should neither receive RUTF nor solid family foods. These very young infants need milk-based diets and their mothers to re-establish breastfeeding. These new methods of therapeutic feeding make it easier to care for moderately severely malnourished children at home, *who have no medical complications, are alert and have reasonable circumstances at home for rehabilitation. Children, who develop medical complications, become anorexic and develop pedal oedema, should be referred to an inpatient facility based management where trained staff can provide all the required medical and nutritional care.*

When families have access to nutrient-dense foods, severe malnutrition without medical complications can be managed in the community without RUTF, by means of carefully designed diets using low-cost family foods that are preferably prepared using fortified flour blends of cereals and lentils, and enriched with oil/butter/ghee. In addition, these children should be provided, appropriate mineral and vitamins as supplements.

## 33.5 Nutritional requirements

### 33.5.1 Energy requirements

The need for food assistance in the disasters / emergency situations has been discussed in details in the preceding sections. Table 33.3 presents the energy requirements for the different sections of population and has been adapted from "The Management of Nutrition in Major Emergencies, WHO, 2000" and these recommendations form the basis for deciding the food commodities to be given and the ration size.

*Table 33.3* Energy requirements for emergency-affected populations, developing country profile (demography and anthropometry) in kilocalories per day [10]

| Age/sex group (years) | Male[(a)] | | Female[(a)] | | Male and female[(a)] | |
|---|---|---|---|---|---|---|
| | % of total population per caput | Energy requirement | % of total population | Energy requirement per caput | % of total population | Energy requirement per caput |
| 0 | 1.31 | 850 | 1.27 | 780 | 2.59 | 820 |
| 1[(b)] | 1.26 | 1250 | 1.20 | 1190 | 2.46 | 1220 |
| 2[(b)] | 1.25 | 1430 | 1.20 | 1330 | 2.45 | 1380 |
| 3[(b)] | 1.25 | 1560 | 1.19 | 1440 | 2.44 | 1500 |
| 4[(b)] | 1.24 | 1690 | 1.18 | 1540 | 2.43 | 1620 |
| 0–4 | 6.32 | 1320 | 6.05 | 1250 | 12.37 | 1290 |
| 5–9 | 6.00 | 1980 | 5.69 | 1730 | 11.69 | 1860 |
| 10–14 | 5.39 | 2370 | 5.13 | 2040 | 10.53 | 2210 |
| 15–19 | 4.89 | 2700 | 4.64 | 2120 | 9.54 | 2420 |
| 20–59[(c)] | 24.80 | 2460 | 23.82 | 1990 | 48.63 | 2230 |
| +60[(c)] | 3.42 | 2010 | 3.82 | 1780) | 7.24 | 1890 |
| Pregnant | | | 2.4 | 285 (extra | 2.4 | 285 (extra) |
| Lactating | | | 2.6 | 500 (extra) | 2.6 | 500 (extra) |
| Whole population | 50.84 | 2250 | 49.16 | 2010 | 2080 | |

(a) adult weight: males: 60kg, female: 52 kg.

(b) population estimates for years 1, 2, 3 and 4 were not available from the United Nations so estimates were made by the interpolation of UN data for 0–5 years.

(c) Figures in the Table are for the energy requirements of light activity levels (1.55 × BMR for males and 1.56 × BMR for females).

For moderate and heavy activity levels, the energy requirements would need a revision and should be calculated as:

*Table 33.4* Vitamin and mineral requirements – safe levels of intake (summary)[a] [10]

| Age/sex group (years) | Vitamin A (μg retinol equivalent RE[b]) | Vitamin D (μg calciferol) | Thiamine (mg)[c] | Riboflavin (mg)[c] | Niacin equivalents (mg)[c] | Folic acid (μg) | Vitamin $B_{12}$ (μg) | VitaminC (mg) | Iron (mg)[d] Low (5–9%) | Iodine (μg) |
|---|---|---|---|---|---|---|---|---|---|---|
| 0 | 350 | 10.0 | 0.3 | 0.5 | 4.2 | 24 | 0.1 | 20 | 13 | 50–90[d] |
| 1 | 400 | 10.0 | 0.5 | 0.8 | 6.4 | 50 | 0.45 | 20 | 8 | 90 |
| 2 | 400 | 10.0 | 0.55 | 0.9 | 7.5 | 50 | 0.53 | 20 | 8 | 90 |
| 3 | 400 | 10.0 | 0.60 | 1.0 | 8.2 | 50 | 0.61 | 20 | 9 | 90 |
| 4 | 400 | 10.0 | 0.65 | 1.1 | 8.9 | 50 | 0.69 | 20 | 9 | 90 |
| 0–4 | 390 | 10.0 | 0.5 | 0.8 | 7.1 | 45 | 0.50 | 20 | 9 | 90 |
| 5–9 | 400 | 2.5 | 0.75 | 1.2 | 10.3 | 80 | 0.82 | 20 | 16 | 110 |
| 10–14 M | 550 | 2.5 | 0.95 | 1.6 | 13.1 | 150 | 1.0 | 25 | 24 | 140 |
| 10–14 F | 550 | 2.5 | 0.8 | 1.35 | 11.3 | 130 | 1.0 | 25 | 27 | 140 |
| 10–14 M/F | 550 | 2.5 | 0.9 | 1.5 | 12.2 | 140 | 1.0 | 25 | 26 | 140 |
| 15–19 M | 600 | 2.5 | 1.1 | 1.8 | 15.3 | 200 | 1.0 | 30 | 15 | 150 |
| 15–19 F | 500 | 2.5 | 0.9 | 1.4 | 11.9 | 170 | 1.0 | 30 | 32 | 150 |
| 15–19 MF | 550 | 2.5 | 1.0 | 1.6 | 13.6 | 185 | 1.0 | 30 | 24 | 150 |
| 20–59 M | 600 | 2.5 | 1.0 | 1.7 | 14.5 | 200 | 1.0 | 30 | 15 | 150 |
| 20–59 F | 500 | 2.5 | 0.8 | 1.4 | 11.5 | 170 | 1.0 | 30 | 32 | 150 |
| 20–59 M/F | 570 | 2.5 | 0.9 | 1.55 | 12.9 | 185 | 1.0 | 30 | 23 | 150 |
| Pregnant | +100 | +7.5 | +0.1 | +0.1 | +1.1 | +250 | +0.4 | +20 | 120 | +50 |
| Lactating | +350 | +7.5 | +0.2 | +0.3 | +2.7 | +100 | +0.3 | +20 | 17 | +50 |
| 60+ M | 600 | 3.2 | 0.9 | 1.4 | 11.9 | 200 | 1.0 | 30 | 15 | 150 |
| 60+ F | 500 | 3.2 | 0.75 | 1.2 | 10.3 | 170 | 1.0 | 30 | 15 | 150 |
| 60+ M/F | 540 | 3.2 | 0.8 | 1.3 | 10.9 | 185 | 1.0 | 30 | 15 | 150 |
| Whole population | 500 | 3.2–3.8[d] | 0.9 | 1.4 | 12.0 | 160 | 0.9 | 28 | 22 | 150 |

(a) Vitamin A requirements may be met by absorption of vitamin A itself (retinol) or provitamin A carotenoids, which have varying equivalence in terms of vitamin A activity. The requirement is expressed in terms of the retinol equivalent (RE) which is defined by the following relationships: 1ug retinol = 1.0mg RE; 1mg beta-carotene = 0.167 g RE; 1ug other provitamin A carotenoids = 0.084 mg RE.

(b) B-vitamin requirements are proportional to energy intake and are calculated: Thiamine: 0.4 mg per 1000 kilocalories ingested; Riboflavin: 0.6 mg per 1000 kilocalories ingested; Niacin equivalents: 6.6 mg per 1000 kilocalories.

(c) Iron requirements are based on the premise that in the developing countries, bioavailability of iron from the dietary sources is only 5–9%.

(d) The higher figure is used for developing countries because of the larger proportion of children under 5 years whose requirement is greater.

Moderate activity levels for males: 1.78 × BMR and for females 1.64 × BMR;

Heavy activity levels for males: 2.10 × BMR and for females; 1.82 × BMR.

## 33.5.2 Micronutrient requirements

Since the emergency programmes aim to cover the complete nutritional requirements of the target population, food fortification should be given active consideration. Food rations must be designed to meet these needs and to prevent micronutrient deficiency diseases. Table 33.4 gives the requirements of various micronutrients for different population groups. Levels of fortification, however, should be evaluated and adjusted according to bioavailability of the nutrient(s) in the diets of target populations.

Most countries in need of food aid do not have the capability to implement adequate food control procedures locally. Thus based on a realistic estimate of food intake, adequate levels of micronutrients at the point of consumption should be ensured, either through fortification or through supplementation. All required nutritional information must be provided through appropriate labeling. Also, it is important to monitor the levels of micronutrient, bioavailability, stability and shelf-life of fortified food used.

However, foods fortified with micronutrients may not meet fully the needs of certain nutritionally vulnerable subgroups such as pregnant and lactating women, or young children. For this reason UNICEF and the WHO have developed the daily multiple micronutrient formula shown in Table 33.5 to meet the daily recommended nutrient intake (RNI) of these vulnerable groups during emergencies [17, 18, 19].

*Table 33.5* The composition of multiple micronutrient supplements for pregnant women, lactating women, and children from 6 to 59 months of age [18–22]

| Micronutrients | Pregnant women | Children (6–59 months) |
|---|---|---|
| Vitamin A (μg) | 800.0 | 400.0 |
| Vitamin D (μg) | 5.0 | 5.0 |
| Vitamin E (mg) | 15.0 | 5.0 |
| Vitamin C (mg) | 55.0 | 30.0 |
| Thiamine (vitamin $B_1$) (mg) | 1.4 | 0.5 |
| Riboflavin (vitamin $B_2$) (mg) | 1.4 | 0.5 |
| Niacin (vitamin $B_3$) (mg) | 18.0 | 6.0 |
| Vitamin $B_6$ (mg) | 1.9 | 0.5 |
| Vitamin $B_{12}$ (μg) | 2.6 | 0.9 |
| Folic acid (μg) | 600.0 | 150.0 |
| Iron (mg) | 27.0 | 10.0 |
| Zinc (mg) | 10.0 | 4.1 |
| Copper (mg) | 1.15 | 0.56 |
| Selenium (μg) | 30.0 | 17.0 |
| Iodine (μg) | 250.0 | 90.0 |

Based on the detailed requirement for energy and micronutrients stated in Tables 33.3 and 33.5, the following figures for macro and micronutrients can be used for planning purposes in the initial stage of a disaster [10].

*Table 33.6* Recommended nutritional composition of a general food ration for the disaster affected population [10]

| S. No. | Nutrient | Mean population requirement |
|---|---|---|
| 1. | Energy | 2100 kcal |
| 2. | Protein | 10–12% of total energy (52–63 g) but <15% |
| 3. | Fat | 17% of total energy (40g) |
| 4. | Vitamin A | 1660 IU (or 0.5 mg retinol equivalent) |
| 5. | $B_1$ | 0.9 mg (or 0.4 mg per 1000 kcal) |
| 6. | $B_2$ | 1.4 mg (or 0.6 mg per 1000 kcal) |
| 7. | Folic acid | 160 mcg |
| 8. | $B_3$ | 12.0 mg (or 6.6 mg per 1000 kcal) |
| 9. | $B_{12}$ | 0.9 mcg |
| 10. | Vitamin C | 28.0 mg |
| 11. | Vitamin D | 3.2–3.8 mcg calciferol |
| 12. | Iron | 22 mg (low-bioavailability, i.e. 5–9%) |
| 13. | Iodine | 150 mcg |
| 14. | Magnesium* | 201 mg |
| 15. | Zinc* | 12.3 mg |
| 16. | Selenium* | 27.6 mcg |
| 17. | Vitamin E* | 8.0 mg alpha – TE |
| 18. | Vitamin K* | 48.2 mcg |
| 19. | Biotine* | 25.3 mcg |
| 20. | Pantothenic acid* | 4.6 mcg |

* provisional requirements

It may however be noted that the above mentioned requirements of various nutrients are based on a reference population as given in the following table:

*Table 33.7* Reference population [12]

| S. No. | Group | % of population |
|---|---|---|
| 1. | 0–4 years | 12 |
| 2. | 5–9 years | 12 |
| 3. | 10–14 years | 11 |
| 4. | 15–19 years | 10 |
| 5. | 20–59 years | 49 |
| 6. | 60+ years | 7 |
| 7. | Pregnant | 2.5 |
| 8. | Breastfeeding | 2.5 |
| 9. | Male/Female | 51/49 |

As the demographic structure of different populations varies, this will affect the nutritional requirements of the population concerned. For example, if 26% of the affected population is aged under five, and the population consists of 50% males and 50% females, the energy requirement is reduced to 1,940 kcal.

Energy and protein requirements should be adjusted for the following factors [12]:

1. The demographic structure of the population, in particular the percentage of those under five years of age and the percentage of females (this may change in populations affected by HIV/AIDS);
2. Mean adult weights and actual, usual or desirable body weights – Requirements will increase if the mean body weight for adult males exceeds 60kg and the mean body weight for adult females exceeds 52 kg;
3. Activity levels to maintain productive life – Requirements will increase if activity levels exceed light (i.e. 1.55 × Basal Metabolic Rate for men and 1.56 × Basal Metabolic Rate for women);
4. Average ambient temperature and shelter and clothing capacities. Requirements will increase if the mean ambient temperature is less than 20°C;
5. The nutritional and health status of the population – Requirements will increase if the population is malnourished and has extra requirements for catch-up growth. HIV/AIDS prevalence may affect average population requirements.

Whether general rations should be adjusted to meet these needs will depend on current international recommendations.

*If it is not possible to incorporate this kind of information into the initial assessment, the figures in the table above may be used as a minimum in the first instance.*

## 33.6 Addressing food security

Normal food production and consumption must resume as early as possible and effort should be made that nutrition intervention with community becoming dependent on outside help indefinitely, is discontinued as much as possible. Addressing food security is therefore crucial. Food security depends principally on three variables: availability of food, access to food and a nutritious diet, and proper use of food to ensure maximum nutrition and hygiene.

The humanitarian aid agencies along with NGOs, work towards food security through the capacity building initiatives, which provide cash for work or cash as well as food for work. These projects enable communities to build up their assets by working on specific projects. Projects involving cash or food in exchange for work help the communities, not only financially and nutritionally, but also increase their self-reliance. These projects can lead to infrastructure improvements, such as the rebuilding of roads and bridges, improvements in irrigation and drainage, tree planting, and building health posts and schools. Disadvantages may include a possible negative impact on the health of children whose mothers are enrolled in food for work schemes.

While these may increase the level of preparedness of the community for future food shortages, they need to be appropriate for the local agricultural environment and culture. Box 33.12 presents details of food security measures taken in Gujarat.

### Box 33.12 Addressing food security: WFP experience in Gujarat

The District of Kachchh, in the western most part of the State of Gujarat, suffered a continuing drought for the last two years. On the 26 January 2001, a severe earthquake hit the district causing widespread devastation. These factors caused a high degree of food insecurity in the district.

Immediately after the earthquake, International Federation of Red Cross and Red Crescent Societies, the World Food Programme, Save the Children and Oxfam conducted a survey to determine the prevalence of acute malnutrition in the District of Kachchh. Its focus was to use the anthropometric measurements of weight and height as the prime determinants of the level of acute malnutrition in the district and to establish baseline nutritional data, which could be used to determine the impact of the earthquake and to target and plan assistance. This survey collected quantitative information on the prevalence of diarrhea and respiratory infections, breastfeeding and the effect of the earthquake on food intake; to support the anthropometric data, through a questionnaire.

The survey targeted children aged between 6 and 59 months as a proxy for the rest of the population. Anthropometric measurements were taken from a total of 798 children randomly sampled throughout the District of Kachchh. A caretaker of each child was also interviewed to obtain basic information on the prevalence of diarrhea and respiratory infections, food intake since the earthquake, level of breastfeeding and registration at Anganwadi Centres (child development centre at village level).

The nutritional index of weight for height, the statistical description of Z-scores and international reference values (NCHS) were used to interpret the anthropometric data collected by this survey. Based on the survey report, food assistance in the form of India-mix (fortified blended food containing wheat, full-fat soya, sugar and 11 critical micronutrients) was provided to all the ICDS beneficiaries through the Anganwadi workers. ICDS system was useful in identifying and establishing contact with the beneficiaries. After over 8 months of intervention, a repeat survey was undertaken to see if there was any impact of the food-assistance. The results were very encouraging as it helped to not only stall deterioration of nutritional status but in fact helped to improve when compared to the baseline indicators as assessed immediately after the earthquake.

The post-phase survey, following 8 months of intervention, presented the following status:

*Overall malnutrition (weight for age) among children 6–59 months decreased by 9.9%*

- percent reduction higher in girls (14.1%) compared to boys (6.3%) in both age groups
- percent reduction higher in older children (36–59 months).

*Moderate malnutrition*

- Percent reduction in moderate malnutrition was 11.3% in the total sample
- reduction higher amongst younger children 6–35 months
- reduction was higher in girls than in boys in both age groups

*Rural-urban differences in malnutrition*

- overall malnutrition was higher in rural areas compared to urban areas (baseline versus post-phase survey)
- reversal of trends observed in the rural and urban areas in the post-phase.

An improvement over baseline seen in the rural areas was attributed to the concerted efforts in rural areas.

## 33.7 Types of disasters and disaster management in India

*(a) India: a country prone to natural calamities*

The Asia-Pacific region experiences nearly 60 per cent of the world's natural disasters. India, on account of its geographical position, climate and geological setting, is the worst-affected theatre of disaster in the South Asian region. India is adversely affected by drought and floods, earthquakes and cyclones year after year.

*(b) The cost and consequences of disasters*

The cost of natural disasters in India, in terms of human life, loss of property and assets and loss of shelter and livelihoods, is immense. Between 1980 and 1999 the total number of people killed in disasters was 110,131. Between 1988 and 1997, disasters affected 24.79 million every year in India. In 1998, 9,846 people died and 34.11 million people were affected by disasters. Between 1985 and 1995, disasters caused an annual economic loss of around US$ 1,883.93 million.

The economic loss from January 2001 earthquake alone was huge, the official estimate putting the number of human lives lost at 30,000 and the economic loss at US$ 10 billion [23]. According to estimates of the industry and business bodies, Confederation of Indian Industries (CII) and Federation of Indian Chambers of Commerce and Industry (FICCI), the damage to buildings and construction and related cost was Rs 120,000 to 150,000 million. The loss of infrastructure amounted to Rs 30,000 million. The damage to big factories was valued at Rs 15,000 million [24].

*(c) Disaster management in India*

Approach to disaster management in India has been primarily reactive and relief centric. Now, there is a paradigm shift to move from providing assistance to adopting a holistic and integrated approach with emphasis on prevention, mitigation and preparedness. These efforts are aimed to conserve developmental gains and also minimize losses to lives, livelihood and property.

In India the focus of 'Disaster Management' is shifting and the present approach comprises: prevention, mitigation and preparedness in pre-disaster phase, and response, rehabilitation and reconstruction in post-disaster phase.

The National Disaster Management Authority (NDMA), headed by the Prime Minister of India, is the apex body for disaster management in India. The setting up of the NDMA and the creation of an enabling environment for institutional mechanisms at the State and District levels is mandated by the Disaster Management Act, 2005. NDMA as the apex body is mandated to lay down the policies, plans and guidelines for Disaster Management to ensure timely and effective response to disasters.

Thus, various ministries at the central government level have been specifically identified and entrusted with the task of managing different types of disasters.

The responsibility to cope with natural disasters is essentially that of the State Government. The role of the Central Government is supportive in terms of supplementation of physical and financial resources.

The Chief Secretary of the State heads a state level committee which is in overall charge of the relief operations in the State and the Relief Commissioners who are in charge of the relief and rehabilitation measures in the wake of natural disasters in their States, function under the overall direction and control of the state level committee. In many states, Secretary, Department of Revenue, is also in-charge of relief. State Governments usually have relief manuals and the districts have their contingency plan that is updated from time to time.

The Government of India is a member of various international organisations in the field of disaster response and relief. While, as a policy, no requests for assistance or appeals are made to the international community in the event of a disaster, assistance offered suo moto is accepted. Linkages exist with the following UN organisations:

(a) UN Office for Coordination of Humanitarian Affairs (UN OCHA), which is responsible by UN General Assembly mandate for all international disaster response.
(b) United Nations Development Programme (UNDP), responsible for mitigation and prevention aspects of disaster management.
(c) UN Disaster Assessment and Coordination (UNDAC) System.

In most disaster and complex emergency situations that require international humanitarian assistance, the UN Resident Coordinator represents the Office for the Co-ordination of Humanitarian Affairs (OCHA), and its primary function is to facilitate and ensure the quick, effective, and well-coordinated provision of humanitarian assistance to those seriously affected by the complex emergency in question. This assistance includes: assessing and addressing humanitarian needs, humanitarian advocacy, and information dissemination. It also aims at strengthening national and regional disaster response capacity in disaster prone countries. Government of India however, as a policy does not take food aid for managing the disasters as it considers itself capable of mobilizing resources and providing the necessary food aid to the populations affected by any disaster.

*Way forward*

Nutritional status of individuals determines the ability to cope with the effect of natural disasters. Women and children are more prone to nutritional deficiencies because of their unique nutritional needs. Women are especially vulnerable when they are pregnant or breastfeeding, and some cultures, have household food hierarchies. This physical and biological difference heightens their vulnerability and their initial response to natural hazards [25]. Social norms and given roles (related to the expected behaviour of women) compounded by inequitable distribution of aid and resources caused by social hierarchies, leads to higher morbidity and mortality amongst women and children during disasters.

Hence for effective and preventive management of disasters, it is important for aid-agencies to be sensitive and focus on timely and adequate food aid for these vulnerable groups.

However, though women are disproportionately impacted by disasters and swift environmental changes, they also have contributed to curbing the impacts of disasters [26]. Women's knowledge and responsibilities related to natural resource management have proven to be critical to community survival and hence efforts must be made towards actively building the capacity of women and adolescent girls in planning for preparedness for disaster management. They would be the right resources to identify those in need of food aid within their communities and become powerful allies to reduce the impact of disasters on health, nutrition and survival of the communities.

## References

1. World Health Organization (2002). *Disasters and emergencies. Definitions Training Package*. WHO/EHA PanAfrican Emergency Training Centre, Addis Ababa. Retrieved August 10, 2006, from www.who.int/disasters/repo/7656.pdf

2. United Nations International Strategy for Disaster Reduction (UN/ISDR) (2004). Terminology: Basic terms of disaster risk reduction. Retrieved June 4, 2006, from www.unisdr.org/eng/library/lib-terminology-eng-p.htm
3. NOJI E (1997). Public Health Consequences of Disasters, New York, Oxford University Press.
4. Disaster Management in India – A Status Report, Ministry of Home Affairs, National Disaster Management Division, August 2004 p. 3.
5. JOSE RODRIGUEZ LL, VOS F, BELOW R, SAPIR DG (2009). Annual Disaster Statistical Review: Numbers and Trends 2008, Centre for Research on the Epidemiology of Disasters (CRED), Brussels.
6. *Natural Hazards Observer* **21**(5) May, 1997.
7. Displacement, loss of buying power and erosion of coping and caring capacities, limit people's access to health services and often contribute to an overall increase in morbidity and mortality.
8. MÉDICINS SANS FRONTIÈRES (1995). *MSF Nutrition Guidelines.*
9. World Health Organization (1999). Management of severe malnutrition: A manual for physicians and other senior health workers.
10. World Health Organization (2000). *The management of nutrition in major emergencies.* Geneva: WHO.
11. UNHCR/UNICEF/WFP/WHO (2003). Food and nutrition needs in emergencies.
12. The Sphere Project. (2004). Humanitarian charter and minimum standards in disaster response.
13. YOUNG H, BORREL A, HOLLAND D, and SALAMA P (2004). Public nutrition in complex emergencies. *Lancet*, **365**, pp. 1899–1909.
14. World Health Organization (1987). Global nutritional status, anthropometric indicators. Geneva, Switzerland: WHO Nutrition Unit, Division of Family Health.
15. World Health Organization (2006). *The WHO Child Growth Standards.*
16. http://www.who.int/child-adolescent-health/New_Publications/NUTRITION/CBSM/ tbp_4.pdf
17. UNICEF/UNU/WHO (1999). Composition of a multi-Micronutrient supplement to be used in pilot programmes among pregnant women in developing countries. Report of a Workshop. New York, UNICEF.
18. FAO/WHO (2005). Vitamin and mineral requirements in human nutrition, 2nd ed. Geneva, World Health Organization.
19. Institute of Medicine (2001). Food and Nutrition Board Dietary reference intakes. Application in dietary assessment. A report of the Subcommittee on Interpretation and uses of dietary reference intakes and the Standing Committee on the Scientific Evaluation of Dietary Reference Intakes. National Academic Press, Washington D.C.
20. www.searo.who.int/... Nutrition_for_Health_and_Development_WHO_UNICEF_statement_emergency.pdf
21. FAO/IAEA/WHO (1996). Trace elements in human nutrition and health. WHO. Geneva.
22. WHO. Prevention and control of iodine deficiency in pregnant and lactating women, and in children less than two years old. Report of a consultation. Geneva.
23. GUPTA HK, RAO PN, RASTOGI BK and SARKAR D (2001). *Science*, **291**, pp. 2101–2102.

24. Disasters: Background & Perspective by Vinod C Menon and Shirish Kavad – published in www.infochangeindia.org/200310045981/Disasters/Backgrounder/Disasters-Background-Perspective.
25. CANNON T (2002). Gender and climate hazards in Bangladesh. *Gender and Development*, **10**(2), pp. 45–50.
26. AGUILAR L (2004). Climate change and disaster mitigation: Gender makes the difference: IUCN. Switzerland.

# 34

# Nutrition for the aged

*Kumud Khanna* and *Seema Puri*

**Kumud Khanna** is the Director of Institute of Home Economics and the Head of Department of Home Science, University of Delhi. Dr. Khanna is PhD in Community Nutrition from Harvard University, Washington, USA. She has over thirty five years of teaching and research experience. Her research interests include geriatric nutrition, clinical nutrition and public health nutrition.

**Seema Puri** is an Associate Professor at Institute of Home Economics, Delhi University. She is PhD in Nutrition from Delhi University and has undergone specialized training in Social Gerontology. She has over twenty five years of teaching and research experience. Her research interests include geriatric nutrition, bone health, nutrition and HIV/AIDS.

## 34.1 Introduction

Population ageing is having profound effects on society. It is the most significant result of the process known as demographic transition. Reduction in fertility results in a decline in the proportion of young in the population. Reduction in mortality means a longer life span for individuals. Population ageing involves a shift from high mortality / high fertility to low mortality / low fertility and consequently an increased number of old people in the population. India is undergoing such a demographic transition. Its influence is being felt at every level, from family life and living arrangements, employment, the provision of health services and pension systems, to the state of economy. Ageing will need to occupy the increasing attention of policymakers in the twenty first century.

## 34.2 Definition of old age

It is difficult to precisely define ageing. Ageing is an inevitable, irreversible and progressive phenomenon and is the last phase of human life cycle. Ageing has also been defined as a progressive loss of adaptability with the passage of time so that the individual is less able to react adaptively to challenges from the external or internal environment. Bagchi [1] has stated that ageing implies predictable, progressive, universal deterioration in various physiological systems - mental and physical, behavioural and biomedical. At the same time, ageing can also involve psychological growth in capacities for creativity, prudence, wisdom and experience.

The age at which one's productive contribution declines and one tends to be economically dependent can probably be treated as the onset of the aged state of life. It is usually regarded as synonymous with pensionable age or age at retirement. In India, retirement from active life is equated with old age. In modern India, retirement age is fixed at 60 years in most Government jobs. In academic research too, retirement age is often taken as an index of aged status. For all practical purposes people above 60 years are considered to be "senior citizens". A three-fold classification given by William and Anderson [2] is generally used to distinguish the older adult population:

(a) 'Young-Old' is the age group between 60 and 74 years, living in relatively healthy and vigorous state and are retired but remain productive to the extent that they can support themselves without being too heavy a burden on their families and the State.
(b) 'Old-Old' comprises the aged between 75 and 84 years, in which they remain active, but the majority needs a range of supportive health and social services.
(c) 'Oldest-Old' are 85 years or older, generally dependent on the family and need a comprehensive programme of supportive health and social services.

## 34.3 Greying of nations

The demographic transition, commonly known as greying of nations reveals that the number of elderly is on the rise, which has intensified the concern for this vulnerable section of the population. Changes at both the lower and upper ends of the population distribution will give rise to an explosive growth of the elderly (persons aged 65 and above) and especially the oldest old (persons aged 80 and above) population. Figure 34.1 presents the population pyramid which indicates a significant projected increase in population in over 60 years age – infact almost double of the 1995 figures.

United Nations Demographic Estimations has forecast that the number of people of 60 years and above worldwide is likely to go up from 427 million in 1985 to 1,171 million in 2025, an increase of over 174 per cent [3]. These percentages are and shall remain higher in the coming decades in the more developed regions of the world than in the less developed regions. However, unlike developed regions where decline in fertility began in the last century, the less developed regions have just started fertility decline and therefore currently account for most of the increase in the world's elderly population. In every region, however, the population over 75 years will increase at an even faster rate and those over 80 years will increase fastest of all. In most regions, the proportion in the oldest group will be more than double.

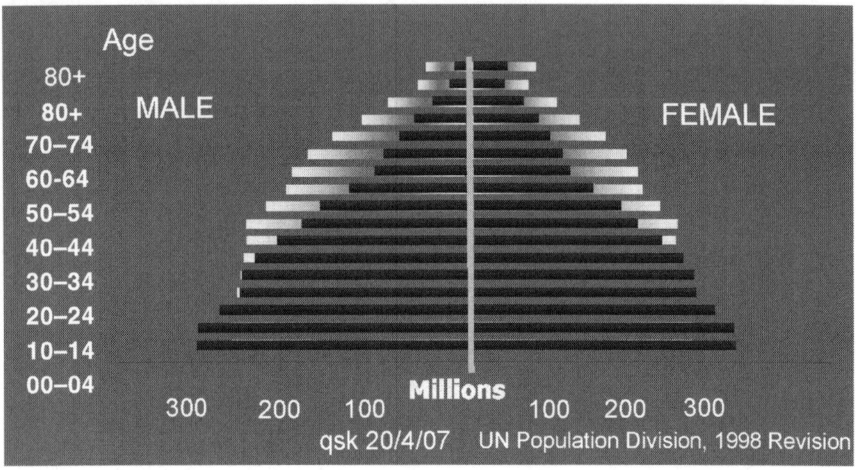


*34.1* The world population is ageing. Population pyramid in 1995 and 2025.

## 34.4 Characteristic trends of ageing in India

India already ranks second population-wise, in the world, and has the largest proportion of the world's elderly population in absolute numbers. The Census of India, conducted every 10 years, has been the major (rather only) source of information on the age structure of the population. The last census report revealed the ageing population to be 76 million in 2001.

The United Nations defines a country as 'ageing' where the proportion of people over 60 years reaches 7 per cent. With 7.5 per cent of the total population being over 60 years old India has progressed from being a mature society (elderly population between 4 to 7%) to becoming an ageing society (ageing population more than 7%).

*Fast growth rate* – The number of persons aged 60 years and above in India has increased at a faster rate as compared to the growth rate of the population of all ages (total population) both in rural and urban areas. It has increased from 12 million in 1901 to 19.6 million in 1951 to 76 million in 2001, constituting 7.5 percent of the total population [4]. Further, the total number of elderly persons is projected to be around 300 million by

2051, comprising 17.3 percent of the population (Table 34.1).

*Table 34.1* Size of ageing population in India (Census, 2001) [4]

| | *Size* | *%* |
|---|---|---|
| 1961 | 25 | 5.6 |
| 1971 | 33 | 5.9 |
| 1981 | 43 | 6.5 |
| 1991 | 57 | 6.8 |
| 2001 | 76 | 7.5 |

This demographic shift in the ageing population amounts to a revolution in both demographic and cultural terms and have been brought about partly by socio-economic factors like better nutrition and living conditions and partly by improvement in health care.

*Life expectancy* – As a result of improved health care facilities and standard of living, life expectancy of Indians is going up. The average Indian, who lived for 32 years in 1947, today has longevity of 62 years which may further go up to 75 years by the year 2015. At 60 years, males can expect to live up to 76 years while females have 18 years more after 60 years [5].

*Age structure of the population* – The number of elderly persons declines with increase in the age. According to Census data (2001), about 7.5 percent of the elderly population belongs to the age group 60+ and about 2.9 percent of them were in the 70+ age group. Less than 1 percent of the elderly persons were 80 years and above. In comparison, the respective figures for 1961 stood at 5.6 percent for 60+, 2.0 percent for 70+ and 0.5 percent for 80+ age groups (Table 34.2) [4]. Thus, the young old have been increasing at a much faster pace than the old-old in India, whereas globally maximum growth is recorded in the latter and not in the former category of elderly.

*Table 34.2* Age structure of ageing population – millions (%). [5]

| *Age Structure* | *1961* | *2001* |
|---|---|---|
| 60+ | 24.7 (5.6) | 76.6 (7.5) |
| 70+ | 8.6 (2.0) | 29.3 (2.9) |
| 80+ | 2.4 (0.5) | 8.0 (0.8) |
| 90+ | 0.5 (0.1) | 1.2 (0.2) |
| 100+ | 0.09 (0.02) | 0.2 (0.02) |

In India, in the next several years, the old-old will represent a notable segment exerting their own influence on morbidity, disability and mortality in the aged. The population of old-old will produce great stresses on the basic communities, especially within families. Among the likely consequences of an increase in the old-old category, two should be mentioned. First, the probable increase in the number of frail or dependent persons due to increased frequency of handicaps and disabilities in later life and second, the increased difficulties to be overcome by families who are eager to play their traditional caring role.

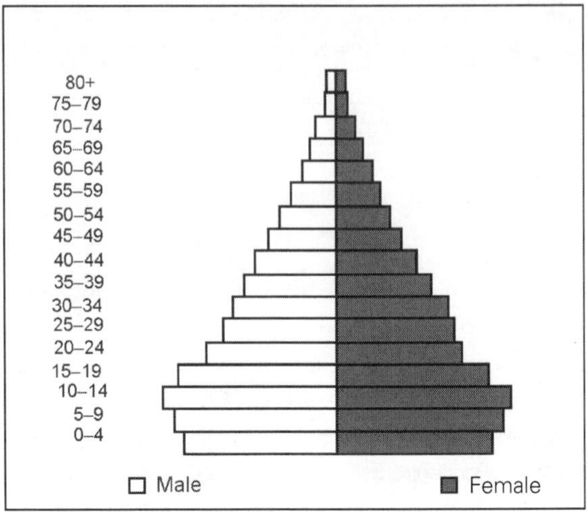


*34.2* Age Pyramid for India, 2001.

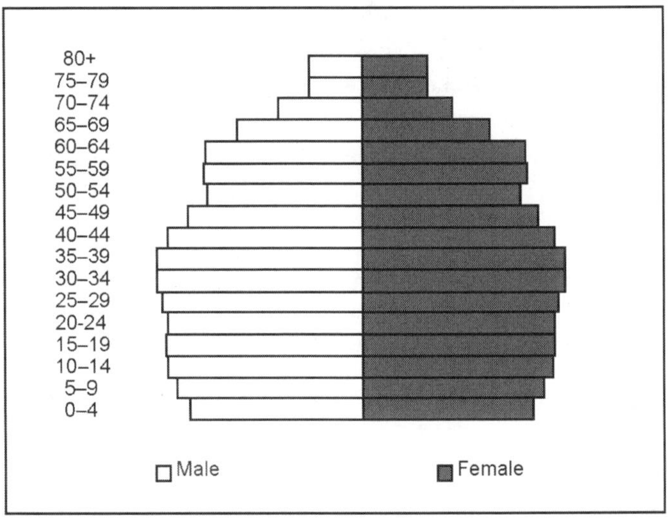


*34.3* Age Pyramid for India, 2051.

*Feminization of old age* – Another feature of the demographic transition with serious, long-term implications is the increasing number of elderly females. Women make up the majority of the older population in virtually all countries. The "feminization" of old age is already advanced in the developed world and is growing even faster in the developing countries.

India is one of the few countries in the world where men outnumber women at all ages till about 70 years. Only in the very old age group, 80 and over, are there more women in the population than men. This phenomenon among the older people is of importance as female life expectancy is higher than that of males. It also gives an indication of

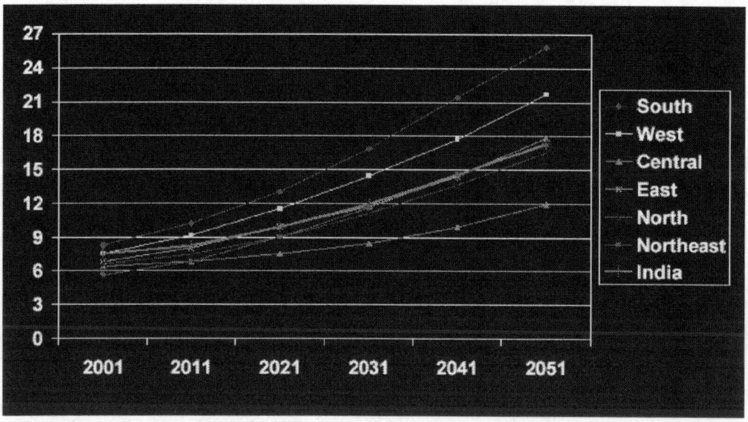


*34.4* Regional difference in the proportion of elderly (60+), 2001–2051 (Census 2001) [5].

widowhood or widowerhood. More than 54 percent of Indian women over 60 years of age live without a spouse as compared to 15.5 percent of older men [5].

As women have a longer life expectancy than that of men and in most cases, their husbands are several years older, a large proportion experience a prolonged period of widowhood, social isolation and declining health coupled with financial difficulties and dependence on others, i.e. family members, community, charitable and philanthropic organizations.

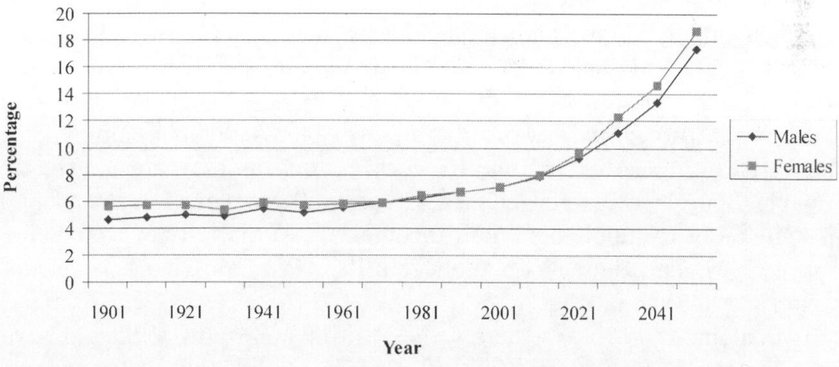


*34.5* Percentage of elderly 60 and above by sex, 1901–2051.

*Socio-economic transition in India* – Along with the changes in the demographic profile, the country is also undergoing a changing social, cultural and economic milieu. Urbanization, accompanied with a breakdown of joint family system, increased migration from rural to urban areas to abroad, and loss of traditional values have left the elderly alone and lonely, often economically helpless. Increasing economic burden on the young family is resulting in greater desolation for the elderly. More and more young women are joining jobs, leaving the elderly to fend for themselves. Job competition poses further demands on the young couple, leaving still less time for social interactions with the elderly.

*Family structure* – Industrialization and urbanization have brought great changes to family structure in this century. The extended family that existed in feudal society has changed to the nuclear family. This has affected the position of the elderly in the family as well as the family's capacity to take care of the aged.

The traditional Indian family structure used to provide the required environment for comfortable living of the elderly. The extended family usually consisted of two generations living together wherein the elderly used to have a different status in the household. In recent years, there has been a significant shift from the patriarchal family towards a nuclear family. Again, with rapid urbanization and industrialization and increasing frequency of full time and part time paid work by both spouses, traditional family support systems for the elderly are also considerably strained. Various survey findings in this direction conclude on the deteriorating status of the elderly in the transient Indian family structure [6]. They observed that change in living arrangements, family structure and mode of sudden retirement adversely affects the old, and further, that the old people are in increasing proportions losing the status and security which they enjoyed in the traditional Indian family structure.

*Economic situation* – Inadequate financial resources have been reported to be a major problem facing the elderly. Financial problems are more common among widows and among elderly in nuclear families. They also indicated economic insecurity to be having some bearing with the social strata of class and caste. In India, older people have to depend mostly on their own earnings/savings or on their own family. People employed in the agriculture sector continue to work as long as they are physically capable. In urban areas, retired men, i.e. after 60 years of age, may take up part time jobs to supplement their income. A vast majority of women are housewives, and depend on their families. Women's work is hardly quantified and monetized.

In contemporary Indian society, the position and status of the old have been undermined by several factors such as:

(a) Decline in the institution of the joint family;
(b) Changing values as reflected in growing individualism arising from urbanisation, westernisation and according high priority to the needs of the immediately family;

(c) Fewer children due to acceptance of small family norms by the middle and upper classes;
(d) Participation of women in employment in cities, leaving the old unattended during the day;
(e) Migration of younger members for alternative sources of livelihood;
(f) Acute paucity of accommodation in urban areas, exorbitant rents and high cost of living which act as a strong disincentive to bring old parents to live with the children;
(g) Complexities of modern life and fast pace of social change;
(h) Economic dependency status of old people in the absence of old age social security benefits [7].

## 34.5 Physiological ageing

Ageing is a normal biological process. The human growth period terminates at around 30 years of age, when senescence begins. Senescence is the organic process of growing older and displaying the effects of increased age. Advancing age is accompanied by progressive physiological changes in functions of most organs; the rate of change varies among individuals and among organ systems. As people age, there also tends to be a concomitant increase in the presence and number of chronic conditions such as hypertension, cardiovascular disease, osteoporosis, diabetes and dementia among others. These further compromise the quality of life in old age.

Ageing is associated with a decline in many body functions, an accompanying change in structure, loss of lean mass and a relative increase in fat mass over time. While earlier these changes were considered to be intrinsically due to ageing, research over the past several decades has increasingly ascribed them to age-related disuse, inactivity and degenerative diseases.

*Changes in body composition* – Some of the most dramatic changes seen with age are in body composition. Lean body mass declines over the adult age span and the decline accelerates beyond 80 years. Sarcopenia, a deficiency of flesh or muscle, strongly influences muscle strength, gait and balance, contributing to the increased risk of falls and frailty in older persons. Sarcopenia develops even in healthy, successfully ageing adults and does not depend on the onset of disease. Its multifactorial etiology includes biological changes of ageing, disuse atrophy secondary to declining physical activities and in some cases, protein or energy undernutrition or catabolic disease processes such as congestive heart failure, rheumatoid arthritis, hyperthyroidism, Parkinson disease, and chronic infection.

Fat mass increases twofold between 20 and 60 years of age, followed by progressive decline. High fat mass is a risk factor for many diseases affecting older persons, including coronary heart disease, high blood pressure, diabetes, gallstones, osteoarthritis, and cancers of the breast and prostate. Increased obesity, especially distributed in the abdominal area, is associated with insulin resistance, which in turn causes diabetes and may also play a role in hypertension and hyperlipidaemia.

A positive energy balance, i.e. energy intakes exceeding energy expenditure, can explain the increase in body fat mass through middle age. Conversely, negative energy balance is the primary cause of loss of body fat in old age. Since protein balance is closely linked to energy balance, this negative energy balance may also be the cause of loss of body protein in old age even when a protein-adequate diet is consumed.

Consequent to these changes in body composition, alterations in body weight are also observed. Body weight increases during adult life until 50–59 years, after which it is seen to decline, particularly in the next two decades. Further, a reduction in lean body mass and decline in body weight leads to a decrease in basal metabolic rate, as age increases. Coupled with a decrease in physical activity, it leads to a reduction in energy requirements and consequently in the quantum of the food to be eaten.

*Changes in bone health* – Ageing is typically associated with a loss of bone and total body calcium. Women at all ages have lower total bone mass or total body calcium than men. Over a lifetime, women lose about 40 percent of their skeletal calcium, approximately one half in the first five years after menopause and the remainder at a slower rate thereafter. The implications of poor bone health in older persons are related to an increased fracture risk and the effect on their functional ability and quality of life. In most cases hip fractures result from an injurious fall in persons with osteopenia. Prevention of hip fracture thus requires attention to both fall-related risk factors and bone density. Nutritional factors associated with traumatic hip fractures include protein-calorie malnutrition, alcohol abuse, osteomalaecia, low BMI, low muscle mass and strength, low levels of body fat, and low amounts of soft-tissue padding over the greater trochanteric region [8].

*Immune function* – Considerable evidence indicates that ageing is associated with altered regulation of the immune system which contributes to the increased incidence of infectious, inflammatory and neoplastic diseases observed in older persons and to their prolonged post-illness recovery periods. The illness patterns in the elderly reflect both a deterioration of immune function and increased incidence of upper respiratory infections, tuberculosis and cancer. Several investigators have suggested that the nutritional status of older persons may be less than optimal, thereby contributing to immunological changes. Many macro- and micronutrients such as protein, zinc and vitamins E, C, and $B_6$, have been shown to play a regulatory role in immune system maintenance.

*Neurological and cognitive function* – On an average the brain loses 5–10 percent of its weight between the ages of 20 and 90, besides undergoing other changes like decrease in surface area and increase in number of plaques and neurofibrillary tangles. Neurological functions most commonly affected are cognition, gait, coordination, sensations and daily living tasks. Mental impairment and dementia a result of chronic degenerative brain disease, have a particularly severe impact on autonomy and independence.

Depression, not an inevitable consequence of ageing, is fairly common in older adults. It may be associated with failing health, loss of independence, social isolation, financial concerns, grief over death of near and dear ones etc. Depression can affect appetite, dietary intake, digestion, weight status, fatigue and the overall sense of well being.

It is generally accepted that dementing illnesses and depression have a strong genetic background. Nevertheless, nutrients can have either a disease-accelerating or protective effect. Also, nutrition can have an impact on brain function by impairing energy supply; affecting neurotransmitter synthesis and intermediary metabolism; enhancing, or protecting from oxidative stress; and influencing cytokines. Mental symptoms such as cognitive impairment, emotional irritability or other neurological signs are well known in case of vitamin deficiencies.

*Sensory losses* – Sensory losses affect people to varying degrees and at different ages. Age related alterations to the sense of taste, smell and touch can lead to poor appetite, inappropriate food choices and lower nutrient intakes. While decreased sensitivity to taste (dysgeusia) and smell (hyposmia) are commonly attributable to old age, other causes include medications, diabetes, liver and kidney disease, hypertension, dementias or zinc or niacin deficiency. Approximately 25 percent of adults over 65 years of age have a reduced ability to detect one or more of the four basic tastes (sweet, sour, salty and bitter) due to a reduction in the number and function of the taste buds in the tongue. Sensitivity to bitter and sour taste lasts longer than to sweet or salty taste. Furthermore, the olfactory bulbs in the brain begin to shrivel which reduces the ability to smell. This further makes food taste even blander.

### 34.5.1 Hearing loss and vision loss is also seen in old people to varying degrees.

*Oral health* – Diet and nutrition can be compromised by poor oral health. Loss of teeth, dry mouth (xerostomia), faulty dentures or even no dentures significantly alters the type of food eaten. The diet may be soft and mashy and raw vegetable and fruits, hard to chew foods are avoided. Consequently, a deficiency of vitamins and minerals as well as fibre may arise.

*Gastrointestinal tract changes* – After the age of 50, there is a reduction in salivary secretion and a reduction in ptyalin content. Hence the digestion of complex carbohydrates is affected. Dysphagia or difficulty in swallowing may also increase the risk of aspiration pneumonia. Gastric pepsin secretion as well as acid secretion decreases, gastric volume is reduced. Delayed emptying of the stomach is seen in elderly. Intestinal motility is reduced due to atrophy of gastrointestinal tract musculature. Such changes in the alimentary tract lead to altered food intake and avoidance of many foods. Constipation and flatulence are common complaints among the elderly.

## 34.6 Pathological ageing

Coupled with the age related physiological decline is the imposition of chronic degenerative diseases in old age e.g. hypertension, cardiovascular disorders, diabetes and cancers. In fact, multiple morbidities are very commonly found in this age. Furthermore, "clustering" of these diseases towards the terminal part of life is a common phenomenon.

*Coronary heart disease and stroke* – Coronary heart disease and stroke have become the major causes of death and disability among both ageing women and men. CVD age related changes are highly variable and impacted by environmental influences such as smoking, exercise and diet. Proper food intake, particularly reduced intake of total and saturated fat and increased intake of plant food, is a cornerstone in preventing and managing coronary risk factors protecting against arterial damage.

*Cancer* – The five most deadly cancers worldwide are also the most common in terms of their incidence. Together they account for about 50 percent of all cancer cases and deaths.

Among men, the leading eight killer sites are lung, stomach, liver, colon-rectum, oesophagus, mouth/pharynx, prostate and lymph nodes. In women, the leading killer sites are breast, stomach, colon-rectum, cervix, lung, ovary, oesophagus and liver. Analysis of the risk factors involved in the development of major cancers shows that a few factors dominate-tobacco, diet, alcohol, infections and hormones; fortunately, all lend themselves to preventive action [8].

*Osteoporosis and bone fractures* – Osteoporosis and associated bone fractures are one of the major causes of disability and death that result in enormous medical expense the world over. The number of osteoporotic fractures increases exponentially with age. In India, unlike the senile osteoporotic fractures of the West, the high fluoride, low calcium dietaries and post-menopausal loss of bone density may be contributing factors for developing osteoporosis [9].

Women are more prone because their bone loss accelerates after menopause. While estrogen deficiency is the primary cause, especially in elderly women, factors such as diet, physical activity and smoking are closely associated with osteoporosis. Lifestyle modifications, particularly increased calcium intake and physical activity, could over time have an important preventive impact on fracture rates.

In order to live longer and healthier lives, it would therefore not only be necessary to delay the process of physiological ageing but also to prevent/delay the imposition of pathological ageing (in the form of chronic degenerative diseases) on an individual, while maintaining a good quality of life. While lower morbidity would reduce mortality, compression of morbidity into a lesser time frame would ensure a life with minimum disability and frailty, a life of dignity and independence.

## 34.7 Nutrition and ageing

Nutrition fits into the two ageing domains of gerontology and geriatrics. *Gerontology*, the study of normal ageing, derives from science, psychology and sociology. *Gerontologic nutrition* focuses on health promotion, risk reduction and disease prevention in older persons. Geriatrics is the study of chronic diseases frequently associated with ageing, including their diagnosis and treatment. Medical nutrition therapy for older adults is often called *geriatric nutrition.*

In ageing, nutrition may play multiple roles. Firstly, as a primary prevention, role of nutrition should be emphasized in health promotion and disease prevention. It is a good strategy to combine healthy eating with physical activity. As secondary prevention, nutrition involves risk reduction and slowing the progression of chronic nutrition related diseases like hypertension, cardiovascular disorders, diabetes, osteoporosis and cancer to maintain functionality and quality of life. Tertiary prevention includes medical nutrition therapy of various diseases, often in a hospital setting.

Nutrition is coming to the fore as a major modifiable determinant of chronic disease and age-related decline. Scientific evidence increasingly supports the view that alterations in the diet have strong effects, both positive and negative, on health throughout life. Most importantly, dietary adjustments may not only influence present health but may determine whether or not an individual will develop diseases like cancer, cardiovascular disease and diabetes much later in life. Researchers have evaluated the influence of various diet patterns on ageing changes and length of life in both experimental animals and human epidemiological studies. Several concepts have emerged from these studies.

*Energy* – Studies on experimental animals have established that calorie restriction is an important measure for prolonging life span. Animals fed diets restricted in kilocalories yet adequate in protein, vitamins and minerals beginning at weaning and continuing through adulthood live 40 percent longer than those given unlimited access to food. Chronic diseases such as heart and kidney disease also appear at a later age in energy restricted animals. However, such studies have not been replicated in human subjects.

Basal metabolic rates decrease linearly with age due to the changes in body composition. Energy requirements generally decrease with age because of changes in body composition, decrease in basal metabolic rate (BMR) and a reduction in physical activity. Energy needs decrease approximately 3 percent per decade. WHO (2002) has recommended that since low levels of physical activity and unchanged levels of energy absorption typically accompany older age, lower energy intakes are required to prevent obesity. The energy requirements of old age appear to be 1.4 to 1.8 multiples of the BMR to maintain body weight at different levels of physical activity [8]. Levels of physical activity that result in energy requirements in the higher end of the range are desirable for reducing morbidity and mortality. Translated into quantitative estimates, an intake less than 1500 kcals daily may result in micronutrient deficiencies and also give rise to health problems in the elderly.

**Box 34.1 Recommended daily nutrient intakes (WHO, 2002) [8]**

Energy – 1.4–1.8 multiples of BMR to maintain body weight at different levels of physical activity.

Protein – 0.9–1.1 g/kg

Fat – 30 en% in sedentary older persons and 35 en% for active older persons. Saturated fats should not exceed 8 en%.

Riboflavin – 1.3 mg for men and for 1.1 mg for women.

Folate – 400 µg

Vitamin $B_{12}$ – 2.5 µg

Vitamin C – 60–100 mg

Vitamin A – 600–700 µg retinol equivalents

Vitamin D – 10–15 µg

Vitamin E – 100–400 IU

Vitamin K – 60–90 µg

Calcium – 800–1200 mg (in the presence of adequate vitamin D nutrition)

Iron – 10 mg assuming there are no excessive iron losses

Selenium – 50–70 µg

Zinc – High Zn availability (50+%) men 4.2 mg; women 3.0 mg

Moderate Zn availability (30%) men 7.0 mg; women 4.9 mg

Low Zn availability (15%) men 14.0 mg; women 9.8 mg

In India, ICMR (1990) have also given lower energy requirements for elderly as compared to young adults, based on their age and activity levels [10]. Requirements of other nutrients have not been specifically outlined for older persons even in the Proposed Recommendations (2008-09) [11].

*Proteins* – As people age and experience a loss of skeletal tissue mass, stores of protein in skeletal muscle may be inadequate to meet the body's needs, making dietary protein intake more important. Decreased food intake and sedentary lifestyle along with reduced energy expenditure become critical risk factors for malnutrition especially for insufficient intake of protein and micronutrients. WHO (2002) has therefore suggested that protein intakes of 0.9–1.1 g/kg body weight per day may be considered beneficial for healthy older persons. Lower intakes would, however, result in depletion of muscle mass and sarcopenia and excess amounts could unnecessarily stress the kidneys [8].

*Carbohydrates* – An abundant intake of carbohydrates is needed to protect protein from being used as a source of energy. Current dietary guidelines [12] recommend that approximately 45–65 percent of total daily calories should come from carbohydrates. Emphasis should be placed on increasing the intake of complex carbohydrate sources such as legumes, whole grains, vegetables and fruits to provide fibre, phytochemicals and essential minerals and vitamins. Since constipation is a serious concern for many older adults, increasing dietary fibre intakes is essential.

*Lipids* – In relation to this aspect, one can relate a high fat intake, particularly saturated fat and cholesterol to increased morbidity and mortality risk. Besides obesity, a high fat consumption has been linked to CHD, stroke, certain cancers and even Alzheimer's disease. Hence reduction in fat and energy intake from a younger age will contribute immensely to healthy ageing.

Current dietary recommendations propose 25–35 percent energy to come from fats with most from polyunsaturated and monounsaturated sources and intakes of cholesterol should be less than 300 mg/day [8, 12]. To meet the total fat recommendation of 20 to 35 percent of calories, most dietary fats should come from sources of polyunsaturated and monounsaturated fatty acids. The consumption of saturated fats should be minimized and not exceed 8 percent of total energy. Sources of omega-6 polyunsaturated fatty acids are liquid vegetable oils, including soybean oil, corn oil, and safflower oil. Plant sources of omega-3 polyunsaturated fatty acids (linolenic acid) include soybean oil, canola oil, walnuts, and flaxseed. Eicosapentaenoic acid (EPA) and docosahexaenoic acid (DHA) are omega-3 fatty acids that are contained in fish and shellfish. An optimal ratio of n-6 to n-3 fatty acids in the diet is believed to be ≈4:1. Plant sources that are rich in monounsaturated fatty acids include vegetable oils (e.g., canola, olive, high oleic safflower, and sunflower oils) that are liquid at room temperature and nuts.

A relatively new concern with respect to monounsaturated fatty acid consumption involves the concentration of trans-fatty acids in the diet. Elaidic acid (trans 18:1n-9) is the principal trans fatty acid in the diet.

Trans-fatty acids are formed during the hydrogenation process, a process that converts vegetable oils to a semisolid state. Major sources of trans-fatty acids in the diet are baked products, processed foods, and margarines rich in hydrogenated fat or oil. There is evidence that increased trans-fatty acid consumption, in contrast with consumption of saturated fat, increases plasma concentrations of lipoprotein (a), an independent risk factor for CHD. They also have a deleterious effect on the plasma lipoprotein profile, elevating LDL-cholesterol and reducing HDL-cholesterol concentrations.

*Minerals* – Whereas overt mineral deficiencies are less common in healthy adults, sub-clinical nutrient deficiencies can develop. Poor mineral status in older persons may be attributed to inadequate intake, physiological changes that may affect the need of such nutrients and medications.

Ageing is typically associated with a loss of bone and total body calcium more so in women. It has been suggested that in the presence of adequate vitamin D nutrition, calcium intakes in the range of 800–1200 mg/day will result in both a beneficial effect on bone mineral density of the femur, neck and lumbar spine and a reduction in fracture rates. Potential benefits of high calcium intakes and various other health-related measures, e.g. reduced blood pressure and decreased risk of a colon cancer, may also be important, although data are insufficient to know for certain [8]. Iron requirements in women decrease after menopause, while those of men remain similar. Iron deficiency anaemia in old age is most likely to be related to blood loss from disease and medications or decreased absorption caused by medications or hypochlorhydria rather than inadequate intakes.

Zinc status is especially important for older persons, who need to maintain their full immunocompetence. Intakes of zinc in older adults decrease in relation to decrease in energy intake and maybe much below the required levels. Zinc deficiency is associated with impaired immune function, anorexia, loss of sense of taste, delayed wound healing and pressure ulcers has given the recommended intakes for dietary zinc for people over 65 years of age as 4.2 mg/day for men and 3.0 mg/day for women (high Zn availability (> 50%); 7.0 mg/day for men and 4.9 mg/day for women (moderate Zn availability – 30%); 14.0 mg/day for men and 9.8 mg/day for women (low Zn availability – 15%)[8].

Sodium intakes are often associated with hypertension. Therefore it is prudent to limit dietary sodium to approximately 2–4 g/day.

*Vitamins* – Several vitamins have been ascribed with significant anti ageing contributions. Antioxidant vitamins like vitamin E, C and carotenoids are known to display disease prevention properties for a number of diseases ranging from cardiovascular disease and cancer to cataracts and macular degeneration. B group vitamins play an important role in maintaining cognitive ability and neuromuscular integrity as age advances.

It is thought that requirements of vitamin A are high in old age due to the possible role of provitamin carotenoids in disease prevention, e.g. cancer, cardiovascular disease. However, concern has also been expressed about a low margin of safety for preformed dietary vitamin A in older persons. Based on these considerations, it appears that 600–700 µg RE/day represents an adequate intake for older men and women.

Inadequate vitamin D intake can also lead to bone loss and increased risk of osteoporosis. There are many reasons for vitamin D malnutrition in older persons including low exposure to sunlight, poor skin response to sunlight, and decreased absorption or decreased hydroxylation of vitamin D. Studies have shown that 1.2 g of elemental calcium and 20 µg of vitamin D/day significantly reduced the risk of hip fractures in older women [13]. According to US dietary recommendations, it appears that older persons need 10–15 µg vitamin D per day to ensure optimal bone health [14].

Vitamin E is of interest as a protective antioxidant and membrane stabilizer. In addition, vitamin E intakes have been associated with a protective effect against cataract and cancer, Alzheimer's disease and cardiovascular disorders. However, further research is needed to determine the adequacy of current vitamin E recommendations for older persons. Most of the interest in vitamin E requirements has centred on the possible beneficial effects of pharmacological doses (60–400 IU/day) of the vitamin, which could not be achieved through an otherwise healthy diet.

High vitamin C blood levels and/or intakes have been associated with a lower prevalence of senile cataract, higher high-density lipoprotein cholesterol concentrations and lower incidences of coronary artery disease [15]. However, it appears that older persons do not have different vitamin C requirements to younger people and that an intake level of 60–100 mg/day is adequate [8].

Recently, a new marker of folate status-homocysteine levels-has come into widespread use. There is great interest in the role of homocysteine as an atherogenic agent and the possibility that tissue folate deficiency could play an indirect role in atheromatous disease. Data from the Framingham Heart Study among older people demonstrated that serum homocysteine levels are correlated with dietary folate levels, and that serum homocysteine levels are high at dietary folate intakes of <400 µg/day [16]. Large-scale intervention studies will be needed to show that administration of folate at this level or above will in fact diminish the risk of vascular disease.

*Antioxidant nutrients* – The role of antioxidant nutrients in preventing free radical damage has been well documented. Although a wide variety of antioxidants in foods contribute to disease prevention, the bulk of research has focussed on antioxidant nutrients like vitamin E, vitamin C, carotenoids and selenium. Green leafy vegetables and fruits are rich in these nutrients and hence most nutritionists emphasize a liberal intake of these foods in old age.

Besides its anti–ageing properties, vitamin E is known to afford protection against cancer ischemia, cataract, arthritis and certain neurological disorders. The protective effects of vitamin C extend to cancer, coronary artery disease, arthritis and ageing. Carotenoids, including B carotene, and selenium are associated with reduced risk of certain cancers. However, the general consensus is that liberal servings of fruits and vegetables are more beneficial than antioxidant pills or medication [17, 18].

*Phytochemicals* – In addition to the recognized essential nutrients, there are many other food components-collectively known as phytochemicals-about which little is known but whose biological effects can lower the risk of major health problems such as cancer and heart disease. Their effects may be hormonal, anti-inflammatory, anti-microbial, anti-oxidant, anti-mutagenic or anti-angiogenic (Table 34.4). Phytochemicals, mostly phenolic acids and flavonoids, are found in garlic, onion, ginger, oats, soyabean, tea, certain herbs and spice and red wine. The presence of these anti-oxidants in such foods may be the reason for the anti ageing properties associated with them.

**Box 34.2 Phytochemicals in foods**

- *Carotenoids* in orange/green vegetables, red wine: antimutagen antioxidant, anti-carcinogen, immuno-enhancing.
- *Flavonoids* in green/yellow vegetables, soy: antioxidant, anticarcinogen, estrogen, immuno-modulating.
- *Polyphenolics* in berries, oregano: antioxidant, antibacterial.
- *Catechins* in green tea: antimutagen, anticarcinogen.
- *Isothiocyanates and indoles* in cruciferous vegetables: antimutagen.
- *Allyl sulphides* in garlic, onions: cholesterol lowering, anticarcinogen, antibacterial.
- *Curcumin* in turmeric: anti-inflammatory.
- *Non-digestible carbohydrates* in vegetables and fruits: cholesterol lowering, stimulates growth of microbial flora

*Water* – Maintenance of fluid balance is essential for normal physiologic functions at all ages. Dehydration in older adults can be caused by impaired sense of thirst, decreased fluid intake, decreased kidney function or increased losses due to increased urine output from medicines like diuretics. It often goes undetected but can present itself as falls, confusion, and decline in consciousness, weakness, fatigue etc.

It is important to obtain essential nutrients through a food-based approach and not be dependent on vitamin and mineral supplements. The traditional nutrient based approach is limited in that it does not take into account the environmental, socioeconomic and lifestyle context of eating, nor does it adequately address the chemical complexity of foods and the interactions and synergies, whether between different foods or individual food components. On the other hand, the food-based approach extends beyond nutrients and food groups; they include the way foods are produced (agriculture), prepared (cuisine), processed and developed (industry). They are therefore culture sensitive.

## 34.8 Dietary guidelines for older persons

In view of the increasing older population worldwide, many agencies including the WHO [8] and US Departments of Agriculture and Health and Human Services [12] have outlined dietary guidelines for older persons. WHO (2002) has emphasized the inclusion of healthy traditional vegetable and legume-based dishes where meat and nuts may be used only as condiments. The use of herbs and spices is encouraged but the consumption of traditional dishes/foods that are heavily preserved/ pickled in salt is to be limited. The guidelines recommend a prudent selection of nutrient-dense foods such as fish, lean meat, liver, eggs, soy products (e.g. tofu and tempeh) and low-fat dairy products, yeast-based products, fruits and vegetables, herbs and spices, whole grain cereals, nuts and seeds. Moreover, nuts, seeds, beans, olives and fatty fish would also cater to the fat intake. Where refined fats are necessary for cooking, selection from a variety of liquid oils including those high in n-3 and n-6 fats (canola, soyabean and olive oil) is desirable. There is also a strong focus on increasing variety in foods to be eaten as well as preserving healthy traditional food related practices. As the dependence on easily available ready to eat foods in increasing, the rapidly growing processed food industry and fast food chains should make concerted efforts to shift from the ready availability of high fat convenience foods to meals which are low in animal fat and high in nutrients and phytochemicals. Box 34.3 presents WHO (2002) food-based dietary guidelines for older persons.

The key recommendations for Older Adults as part of the Dietary Guidelines for Americans (2005) include consumption of vitamin $B_{12}$ and vitamin D through fortified foods or supplements. Consumption of sodium should be restricted to 1500 mg, while potassium intakes should be minimum 4700 mg/day [12].

Besides regular physical activity, recommendations also caution against starting a weight loss programme without medical consultation. It also warns against eating or drinking raw or unpasteurised milk, egg or meats.

**Box 34.3 Food-based dietary guidelines for older persons (WHO, 2002) [8]**

- Emphasize healthy traditional vegetable- and legume-based dishes with meat and nuts to be used as condiments.
- Limit consumption of traditional dishes/foods that are heavily preserved/pickled in salt and encourage the use of herbs and spices.
- Introduce healthy traditional foods or dishes from other cuisines (e.g. tofu in Europe and the tomato in Asia) to increase the variety of foods consumed.
- Select nutrient-dense foods such as fish, lean meat, liver, eggs, soy products (e.g. tofu) and low-fat dairy products, yeast-based products (e.g. spreads), fruits and vegetables, herbs and spices, whole-grain cereals, nuts and seeds.
- Consume fat from whole foods such as nuts, seeds, beans, olives and fatty fish. Where refined fats are necessary for cooking, select from a variety of liquid oils, including those high in n-3 and n-6 fats. Avoid fatty spreads.
- Enjoy food and eating in the company of others. Avoid the regular use of celebratory foods (e.g. ice cream, cakes and pastries, mithai and confectioneries)
- Encourage the processed food industry and fast-food chains to produce ready-made meals that are low in animal fats and high in nutrients and phytochemicals.
- Eat several (5-6) small non-fatty meals. This pattern appears to be associated with greater food variety and lower body fat and blood glucose and lipid levels, especially if larger meals are eaten early in the day.
- Transfer as much as possible of one's food culture, health knowledge and related skills to one's children, grandchildren and the wider community.
- Be physically active on a regular basis and include exercises that strengthen muscles and improve balance.
- Avoid dehydration by regularly consuming, especially in warm climates, fluids and foods with high water content.

## 34.9 Ageing in the development agenda

Till a decade ago, ageing did not figure as a priority in the development agenda. With the increasing numbers of older persons, planners and policy makers have woken up to the fact that suitable initiatives need to be undertaken to deal with this group. A time line of these key events is outlined below (Box 34.4).

The Vienna International Plan of Action on Ageing, adopted by nearly 125 countries of the world at the First World Assembly on Ageing held in Vienna in 1982 was the first formal commitment towards concern for the elderly. This plan identified particular areas of concern for ageing persons and provided a starting point for approaching the subject in a systematic manner by recognizing the multiple dimensions of ageing. The primary aim of this plan was to strengthen the capacities of countries to deal effectively with the ageing of their populations and with the special concerns and needs of their elderly. It also aimed to promote an appropriate international response to the issues of ageing through action for the establishment of the new economic order and increased international technical cooperation, particularly among the developing countries themselves [19].

**Box 34.4 Key events, 1982–2002**

1982 First World Assembly on Ageing, Vienna - International Plan of Action on Ageing
1991 United Nations Principles for Older Persons
1993 World Conference on Human Rights, Vienna Assembly
1994 United Nations International Conference on Population And Development, Cairo
1995 United Nations Social Development Conference, Copenhagen
1997 Fourth International Conference on Health Promotion, Delhi
1999 United Nations International Year of the Older Persons
1999 Macao Plan of Action on Ageing for Asia and the Pacific
1999 National Policy of Older Persons, Govt. of India
1999 National Council for Older Persons, India
2000 Year of the Older Persons, India
2002 Valencia Forum - Research Agenda on Ageing for the 21st Century
2002 Second World Assembly on Ageing, Madrid - Madrid International Plan of Action on Ageing, 2002
2002 Asia Pacific Seminar on Regional Follow-up to the Second World Assembly on Ageing, Shanghai - Regional Implementation Strategy for the Madrid International Plan of Action on Ageing, 2002
2007 The Maintenance and Welfare of Parents and Senior Citizens Act, Govt. of India

The UN International Year of the Older Persons in 1999 ensured that continuing attention was focussed on the elderly. The Macao Declaration and Plan of Action on Ageing for Asia and the Pacific endorsed by Governments in the region, in 1999, addressed seven areas of concern relating to ageing and older persons - a significant one being health and nutrition. The Research Agenda on Ageing for the 21st Century, a joint project of the United Nations Office on Ageing and the International Association of Gerontology, was submitted to the Second World Assembly on Ageing through the Valencia Forum in April 2002. It identified major priorities and critical arenas for research exploration. Salient among the priorities was research on healthy ageing and quality of life issues.

Focus on older persons continued even at the Second World Assembly on Ageing held in Madrid in April 2002. A life course approach to deal with ageing issues was recommended. The Shanghai Regional Implementation Strategy for the Madrid International Plan of Action on Ageing and the Macao Plan of Action on Ageing for Asia and the Pacific [20] also reiterated the need to ensure quality of life at all ages for a healthy old age by promoting a life course perspective on health and ageing, through such measures as promoting good nutrition, healthy lifestyle and avoidance of risk factors.

*National Policy for Older Persons* – In India, the concern for senior citizens has gained momentum only recently. The year 2000 was declared as the Year of the Older Persons in India, soon after the UN International Year of Older Persons in 1999. After several years of deliberation, the

Ministry of Social Justice and Empowerment released A National Policy for Older Persons in the year 1999. The policy provides a broad framework for inter sectoral collaboration and cooperation both within the government as well as between governmental and non-governmental agencies. The policy has identified a number of areas of intervention: financial security, health care and nutrition, shelter, education, welfare, protection of life and property etc. for the wellbeing of older persons in the country. Amongst others, the policy also recognizes the role of the NGO sector in providing user friendly affordable services to complement the endeavors of the State. The policy also emphasizes the importance of family in providing vital non-formal social security for older persons. To facilitate implementation of this policy, the participation of Panchayati Raj institutions, State Governments and different Departments of the Government is envisaged with the coordinating responsibility resting with the Ministry of Social Justice and Empowerment, Government of India [21].

*National Council for Older Persons (NCOP)* has been constituted by the Ministry of Social Justice and Empowerment in May 1999 to operationalise the National Policy on Older Persons. The objectives of the NCOP are as follows:

- Advice the government on policies and programmes for older persons.
- Provide feedback to the government on the implementation of the National Policy as well as on specific programme initiatives for older persons.
- Advocate the best interests of older persons.
- Provide a nodal point at the national level for redressing the grievances of older persons at an individual level.
- Provide a lobby for concessions, rebates and discounts for older persons both with the Government and private sector.
- Represent the collective opinion of older persons to the Government.
- Suggest steps to make old age productive and interesting.
- Suggest measures to enhance the quality of inter-generational relationships.
- Undertake any other work or activity in the best interest of older persons.

*The Maintenance and Welfare of Parents and Senior Citizens Act* was passed by the Parliament in 2007. The bill has a clause for punishment to those who abandon their parents or relatives whose property they have inherited or would get as their legal heirs. The bill provides for setting up of a tribunal in each district for helping the old in distress. It also has a provision for establishment of old age homes which should be the last resort for the poor and the childless [22].

## 34.10 Initiatives in old age care

Other initiatives taken by the nodal Ministry, the Ministry of Social Justice and Empowerment, Government of India, include getting the instructions issued from the Ministry of Health to all State Governments to ensure separate queues for older persons at all stages, getting the instructions issued from the Hon'ble Chief Justice of High Courts and Lower Courts for expeditious disposal of cases involving older persons and setting up of a telephone help line with the help of an NGO, Agewell Foundation, in Delhi.

Certain ongoing schemes of the Ministry were revised during 1998–99 to facilitate implementation of the National Policy. The one-time construction grant for old age homes/multiservice centres for older persons under the Scheme of Assistance to Panchayati Raj Institutions/Voluntary Organizations/Self-help Groups has been enhanced from Rs 5 lakhs to Rs 30 lakhs for eligible organizations. An Integrated Programme for Older Persons has been formulated by revising the earlier scheme of assistance to voluntary organizations for programmes relating to the welfare of the aged. The strategy involved in this scheme includes awareness creation and sensitization of children and youth towards older persons, reinforcing the Indian family tradition of providing special care and attention to the elderly, organizing the older persons into coherent self help groups and making productive use of older persons. Under this scheme, financial assistance upto 90% of the project cost is provided to the NGO for establishing and maintaining old age homes, day care centres, mobile medicare units and for providing non institutional services to older people [22].

## 34.11 Initiatives by the voluntary sector

HelpAge India is the biggest NGO working for the benefit of older persons. Some of their initiatives include formulating a plan of action for implementation of the policy. Key features of the plan included pension for all poor aged especially widows, microcredit schemes to reach all villages, financial security for daily wage earners, healthcare at doorstep of all elderly, promotion of healthy ageing, home care services for all aged persons, incentives to elderly to pursue education, media to play a more positive and expanded role.

Several Governmental and non-governmental agencies have established day care centres and old age homes, some free of charge and some on a pay and stay basis. More than half of the 1000 old age homes nationwide and over 125 day care centres have been supported by HelpAge India. The Mobile Medicare Unit Programme is directly implemented by HelpAge India to provide basic essential at the doorsteps of needy and underprivileged elderly.

## Way forward

With a growing number of individuals surviving to enjoy their "renaissance years", there has been considerable interest in ensuring a good quality of life in healthy old age. In our efforts to provide a better quality of life to the elderly it is imperative to strengthen their economic security. Provision of old age pension or other social security benefits may be a step in this direction. To promote the concept of productive ageing, policies and programmes should be planned to utilize the expertise and skills of the elderly and maximise their contribution to the family and community at large.

Special efforts need to be directed towards provision of health and nutrition support for the elderly. Assistance to elderly persons living alone or disabled with regard to food, medical aid, banking, paying bills etc. should be considered. Facilities like home catering services, meals on wheels etc. may be encouraged for elderly unable to prepare meals for themselves. Access to medical care for the elderly should be ensured. Setting up of geriatric units/special clinics/mobile medical units/health camps in the area should be given priority. Dieticians and doctors who are sensitized about the special needs of the elderly would prove more effective in elderly care.

An integrated approach may be adopted by opening day-care centres for the elderly. Such centres could be located in each colony and provide facilities of recreation (TV, newspapers, magazines), religious activities (satsangs, discourses, group tours), basic medical care and referral as well as health and nutrition counselling services to the elderly women. Income generating activities, training programs, awareness creation campaigns etc. could also be initiated at these centres.

## References


1. BAGCHI K (2001). *Biological Changes in Ageing.* New Delhi: Public Lecture.
2. WILLIAMS SR and ANDERSON SL (1993). *Nutritional Assessment and Therapy in Patient Care* 7th ed. St Louis: Mosby, p. 457.
3. VIJAYAKUMAR S. (1999). Population ageing in India. *Research and Development Journal*, **5**(2), p. 3.
4. Registrar General of India (2001). Census of India. Ministry of Home Affairs, Government of India. www.censusindia.net/results/resultsmain.html. Accessed 12 May 2008.
5. IRUDAYARAJAN S (2006). Personal Communication.
6. IRUDUYARAJAN S, MISHRA US, SARMA PS (1999). India's elderly burden or challenge. New Delhi: Sage Publications India, **19**, p. 211.
7. BOSE AB (1994). Policies and programmes for the ageing in India. In: Department for Economic and Social Information and Policy Analysis. The Ageing of Asian Populations. New York: United Nations.

8. WORLD HEALTH ORGANISATION (2002). Keep fit for life. Meeting the nutritional needs of older persons. Geneva: WHO and Tufts University.
9. PURI S (2001). Nutritional concerns of older persons. In: Chaudhary A, ed. Active Ageing in the New Millenium. New Delhi: Anugraha India, p. 110.
10. Indian Council of Medical Research (ICMR) (1990). Nutrient requirements and recommended dietary allowances for Indians. A report of the expert group of the ICMR. Hyderabad: NIN.
11. NARASINGHA RAO BS and SIVAKUMAR B (2009). Nutrient Requirements and Recommended Dietary Allowances. In: Textbook of Human Nutrition 3rd edition, Bamji M, Krishnaswamy K, Brahmam GNV (eds.), Oxford and IBH Publishing Co.
12. U.S. Department of Health and Human Services and U.S. Department of Agriculture (2005). Dietary Guidelines for Americans, www.healthierus.gov/dietaryguidelines Accessed 15 December 2009.
13. DAWSON-HUGHES B et al (1991). Effect of vitamin D supplementation on wintertime overall bone loss in healthy postmenopausal women. *Annals of Internal Medicine*, **115**, pp. 505–512.
14. Institute of Medicine (1997). Dietary Reference Intakes for Calcium, Phosphorus, Magnesium, Vitamin D, and Fluoride. pp. 250–287.
15. FREI B (1991). Ascorbic acid protects lipids in human plasma and low-density lipoprotein against oxidative damage. *American Journal of Clinical Nutrition,* **54**, pp. S1113–S1118.
16. SELHUB J et al. (1993). Vitamin status and intake as primary determinants of homocysteinemia in an elderly population. *Journal of the American Medical Association*, **270**, pp. 2693–2698.
17. PURI S (1999). Dietary Antioxidants and Ageing – A Review. In: Diet and Ageing – Exploring Some Facets. Bagchi K, Puri S, (eds.). New Delhi: Society for Gerontological Research and HelpAge India, p. 95.
18. BAGCHI K and PURI S (1998). Free radicals and antioxidants in health and disease. *East Med J WHO*, **4**(2), p. 253.
19. WORLD HEALTH ORGANISATION (1998). Women, Ageing and Health – Achieving health across the life span. Geneva: WHO.
20. UNESCAP. Shanghai Regional Implementation Strategy for the Madrid International Plan of Action on Ageing and the Macao Plan of Action on Ageing for Asia and the Pacific http://www.unescap.org/esid/psis/ageing/strategy/toc.asp Accessed 15 December 2009.
21. Ministry of Social Justice and Empowerment (1999). Govt of India. National Policy for Older Persons.
22. Helpage India (2008). Senior Citizens Guide.

# 35

# Nutrition related non-communicable chronic disorders

*Kamala Krishnaswamy* and *Avula Laxmaiah*

**Kamala Krishnaswamy,** MD, is the former Director of the National Institute of Nutrition, India and former President of the Nutrition Society of India. Dr. Krishnaswamy is currently on governing and advisory boards of several institutes and chairperson of project advisory committees. She has carried out a number of research studies in the fields of diet-cancer interactions, nutrient-drug interactions, environmental toxicology, non-communicable chronic diseases and vitamin B complex deficiencies.

**Avula Laxmaiah** MBBS, MPH, is Deputy Director (Scientist 'E') at the National Institute of Nutrition, India. Dr. Laxmaiah is an epidemiologist and is involved in national nutrition monitoring through the National Nutrition Monitoring Bureau (NNMB).

## 35.1 Introduction

The current concerns in nutrition include not only undernutrition and its consequences but also many chronic diet related problems. Such disorders may have their origins in fetal (prenatal) and child malnutrition as well as intake of energy dense foods and physical inactivity in later life. The diet related chronic disorders are of global concern and contributing to rising health care costs [1]. In India, underweight and stunting due to number of macro and micronutrient deficiencies are common among children, adolescents and pregnant women [2]. These disorders have a cascading effect on diet related non-communicable diseases. In most nutrition circles, therefore, the need for a common agenda is often reiterated particularly in terms of lifestyle changes and physical activities to prevent disorders at both ends of the spectrum. Of this, diet, physical inactivity, personal risk behaviours are of prime importance [3]. The rising epidemic of obesity and insulin resistance, particularly in developing countries is the forerunner of almost all chronic non-communicable diseases and calls for an integrated package of interventions [4]. The metabolic programming of undernutrition in utero directly influences the development of diseases such as diabetes, coronary artery disease, hypertension, stroke and cancer [5]. Intrauterine undernutrition permanently alters structure, physiology, metabolism and function leading to enhanced risk of chronic non-communicable diseases in later life. The ageing phenomena as well as ailments such as arthritis, gallstones and cataract are also related to obesity and dietary intake of nutrients and phytonutrients. In fact, the origins of most of these disorders may be related to our genes as they are programmed to palaeolithic/hunger-gather society diets and activity patterns. The current diets and activities are not matched to our genes.

## 35.2 Prevalence of non-communicable diseases at global and national level

Non-communicable diseases (NCD) are not infectious or contagious. NCD may result mainly from lifestyle factors including risk behaviours of individuals and genetics. The important diseases are obesity, diabetes, hypertension, coronary artery diseases, chronic obstructive pulmonary diseases (COPD), mental problems, cancer etc. As per the World Health Organization (WHO) estimates, non-communicable diseases account for nearly 59% of the 57 million persons, who died in 2002 [6]. In the same year, deaths due to non-communicable diseases also outstripped deaths due to both communicable diseases and injuries, and were the leading cause of chronic illnesses world wide, accounting for nearly 47% of the 1.49 billion years of healthy life years 'lost' due to illness, as measured in disability adjusted life years (DALY) and to 46% global burden of disease.

It is further said that the burden of NCDs is expected to increase to 57% by 2020, of which 50% will be due to cardiovascular problems and 79% of all deaths worldwide will be attributable to chronic diseases in developing countries. In India, chronic diseases contribute to 53% of deaths and 44% of DALYs [7] (Table 35.1). It is evident that NCDs, particularly cardiovascular diseases, diabetes and hypertension are increasing through out the country particularly in urban India.

## 35.3 Cardiovascular diseases

Compared to all other ethnic groups, South Asians have an excess risk of coronary artery disease. The burden of cardiovascular diseases is 3–4% in rural and 8–10% in urban India. The prevalence of stroke in India is considered to be 203 per 100000 populations above the age of 20 years [7]. In 2001, heart disease and stroke were the leading cause of death in both high and low middle-income countries, accounting for 19% and 21%

*Table 35.1* Deaths and DALYs (Estimated) by cause in India [7]

| Cause | Deaths | DALYs |
|---|---|---|
| Cardiovascular diseases | 29 | 11 |
| Cancer | 7 | 4 |
| Chronic respiratory diseases | 7 | 3 |
| Diabetes | 2 | 1 |
| Other chronic diseases | 8 | 25 |
| Communicable diseases pre-natal and maternal conditions and nutritional deficiencies | 36 | 42 |
| Injuries | 11 | 14 |

respectively and cardiovascular diseases are the major contributors to mortality and morbidity in the South Asia region [8]. WHO estimates the cause specific mortality rate due to cardiovascular diseases will be the highest by 2020 in India. About 2.6 million Indians are predicted to die due to coronary heart diseases, which constitute 54.1% of all cardiovascular deaths. Nearly half of these deaths are likely to occur in young and middle aged individuals (30–39 years) [9]. The Global Burden of Disease (GBD) study has revealed that about 52% of the cardiovascular deaths occur below the age of 70 years in India as compared to 23% in developed countries [10].

### 35.3.1 Hypertension

A meta-analysis of data available shows a prevalence rate of 16.5% in urban and 15.7% in rural India [11]. Indian Council Medical Research study (1994) [12] reported that the prevalence of hypertension among men and women in urban areas of New Delhi was 25% and 29%, while it was only 13% and 10% among men and women respectively in rural areas. It ranges between 20% and 40% in urban and 12–17% in rural India [13]. The prevalence of hypertension worldwide was 972 millions in 2000 and will be 1.56 billion in 2025, with equal numbers in men and women [14]. According to National Nutrition Monitoring Bureau (NNMB) surveys carried out in 9 States during 2005–06 in India [15], the prevalence of hypertension (≥140 mm of Hg systolic blood pressure (SBP) and/or ≥90 mm of diastolic blood pressure (DBP)) was 25% and 24% among rural men and women, respectively. However, it was highest in the State of Kerala (men: 50.9%; women: 46.8%) Orissa (men: 40.9%; women: 42.4%), Maharashtra (men: 31.4%; women: 13.7%) and lowest in Gujarat (men: 14.2%; women: 10.4%) and Tamil Nadu (men: 17.8%; women: 46.8%).

### 35.3.2 Obesity and overweight

Recent estimates suggest that there are one billion overweight/obese people in the world. The problem is of a serious nature even among children and adolescents. The rates are far higher in middle and low-income countries. In South Asia, one-third of the urban adult population is classified as overweight and obese and is also increasing among South Asian children. The prevalence of overweight and obesity as per the National Nutrition Monitoring Bureau has doubled among men from 2.3% to 4.1% and women from 3.4% to 6% [16] over a period of two decades in rural areas (1975–79 to 1996–97). The prevalence of overweight/obesity among adolescents in urban areas ranged from 6% to 25% in various urban cities of India [17].

The Sentinel Surveillance system for cardiovascular diseases in Industrial populations in North Indian cities like Delhi, Lucknow, Ludhiana, the prevalence of overweight and obesity was 41%, 37% and 15% respectively [18], while in central Indian cities, it was 20% and 36% in Nagpur and Pune, respectively. In South Indian cities such as Bangalore, Trivandrum and Coimbatore, it was 48%, 38% and 27%, respectively.

Serial epidemiological surveys in Rajasthan have shown the prevalence as 60% during 1994 [7], 63% during 2001, and 79% during 2003 using the criteria (waist–hip ratio (WHR): Men >0.9, females: >0.8). Several studies also revealed that Indians in general, have higher body fat percent even at lower body mass index (≤25) [19, 20].

### 35.3.3 Diabetes

The prevalence of diabetes has risen more rapidly in South Asia than in any other region of the world. By the year 2030, India will have the highest number of persons with diabetes (79.4 millions) [21]. All community-based studies have documented rising prevalence of diabetes in all parts of India. Both diabetes and impaired glucose tolerance (IGT) increases with age. The sentinel surveillance project [18] documented 10% overall prevalence of diabetes from 10 regions of the country among 20–69 years. The Indian Council of Medical Research documented 58.3 million cases in 1998 and by 2004 it could have accounted for 1.15 million years lost due to disease and 2.26 million DALYs [11]. The prevalence of metabolic syndrome as reported by various workers varies from 10 to 40%, which is strongly associated with diabetes. Diabetes, if it is untreated or not well-controlled results in CVD, hypertension, kidney damage, eye disorders, gangrene, peripheral neuropathy and vascular disorders.

### 35.3.4 Cancer

The patterns of cancer vary greatly across the globe. In 2002, there were about 11 million cases worldwide of which 7 million died and it is estimated that this number will escalate to more than 16 million, with 10 million deaths by the year 2020 [22]. Almost 70% of these may be in developing countries with 5% of global resources. The overall incidence of cancer though low, is higher in urban India as compared to rural India. The calculated figures from ICMR (2001) registries show that in urban males the incidence rate is 113 per 100,000 and in urban females 123 per 100,000 while, in rural areas it is 46 and 58 per 100,000 in males and females, respectively [23]. The major cancers are tobacco related (lung, oral cavity, larynx, pharynx and oesophagus) in men while oral, oesophagus, lung (related to tobacco), breast and cervix in women. The prevalence of oral cancers are the highest and in recent times colon and prostate cancers are also increasing. The breast cancers in women are higher in urban India, while cervical cancers predominate in rural India.

## 35.4 Nutrition transition and NCDs

Several developing countries have conflicting goals of preventing undernutrition, obesity and diet related disorders [3]. Due to diverse public health control measures adopted, high rates of fertility, mortality and famines leading to undernutrition in vulnerable segments are now being replaced by low fertility, reduced mortality and increased life span [24] (Figure 35.1).

The demographic transition is resulting an increase in young adults as well as a substantial increase in the proportion of elderly population. However, the quality of life has not improved in all segments. The demographic changes accompanied by urbanisation, economic growth, technological innovations, mechanisation coupled with reduced physical activity and higher leisure time of sedentary nature have compounded the scenario. Migration from rural and tribal to urban agglomeration exposes people to adverse nutritional environment, inactivity and stresses, which are responsible for epidemiological and nutritional transition [25, 26].

## 35.5 Macronutrients

Dietary changes create an altered energy balance. The starchy foods of low calorie value with high fibre and micronutrient poor diets are being replaced with calorie dense, fatty, salty and low fibre and micronutrient/ phytonutrients poor diets with more animal foods, which are loaded with saturated fats. The children in urban areas are becoming obese due to both lack of physical activity as well as easy availability and access of *junk* food, which consists high energy, fat, sugar and salt and carbonated beverages, which promote fat deposition.The dangerous triad of stunting

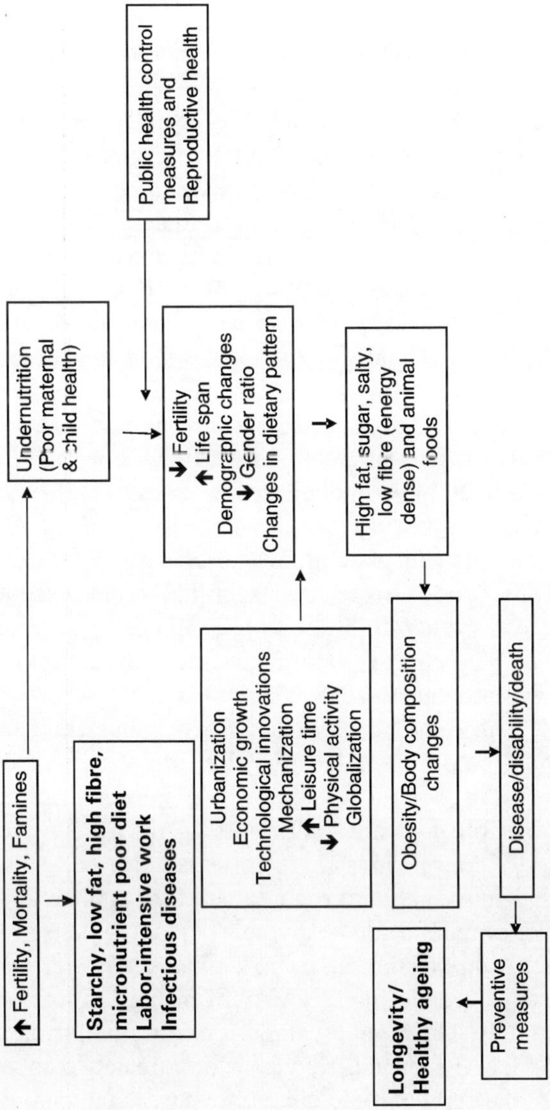


*35.1* Nutrition transition and NCDs.

due to malnutrition in early ages, availability of energy dense foods at a later date and sedentary habits escalate the problems of obesity and changes in body composition with specific reference to fat deposition promoting insulin resistance and diet related non-communicable diseases. Trace elements such as Mg and Ca were significantly lower for Asian Indian vegetarians than for the white Caucasians vegetarians [27]. Nearly 95% of ethnic South Asians in the UK, whose random blood glucose level indicated high risk of diabetes had vitamin D deficiency. However, the clear cut implications of micronutrient deficiencies on the metabolic syndrome and cardiovascular diseases are not clear, especially for South Asians and further studies may be required with sufficient duration.

The latent predisposition to chronic disorders appears to be related to our ancestral diet of Palaeolithic or Hunter-gatherer society [28]. The principal defect appears to be related to a quick insulin response based on the low glycemic index for the current foods. This response earlier conferred survival benefits in "Fasting and Famine" situations of our ancestors and favoured lipogenesis and glucose conversion to storage lipids. The gatherer foods are more bulky while the hunted foods are high in animal protein (lean mass). The foods were rich in complex carbohydrates, mono and polyunsaturated fatty acids (MUFA and PUFA), micro and phytonutrients, fibre and low in cholesterol, saturated fats and sodium. The quality of fat was apparently better with a lower omega 6/ omega 3 ratio than the current fats which are more saturated and relatively higher in omega 6 fats. The foods were also minimally processed. Potassium in the diets was invariably high due to plant foods of diverse nature. The high protein (19–35% energy) would have reduced the lipids. The carbohydrate content was around 22–40%, which are much lower than current intakes of 60–70%. Further, their physical activity was much higher. Thus our genes are sculpted or programmed to Palaeolithic diets. The modern diets are more refined and are high in glycemic index (insulinogenic), are low in fibre and micronutrients as they are more refined. The diets are energy dense foods (high in sugar, fat) and salt. Such diets coupled with sedentary habits promote insulin resistance and adiposity. Further the intake of animal foods apparently is more dense in saturated fats and cholesterol due to the nature of animal feeds and are diametrically opposite to our ancestral dietary pattern of high intake of lean protein from forest animals. The rapid escalations of obesity in tribes indicate acculturation to modern diets and life styles which are detrimental to human health and result in several chronic diseases. Nutritional studies in hunter-gatherers indicate that they would have had better folic acid and vitamin $B_{12}$ status. Vascular problems such as coronary artery disease, stroke and peripheral vascular disease can be mitigated by folate and Vitamin $B_{12}$ found in plant foods such as vegetables, fruits and beans and milk respectively. The wild plants grown in natural soils rich in micronutrients is a nature's gift for mankind to provide the necessary vitamins and minerals as against the current practices of intensive agriculture, usage of artificial fertilisers and pesticides. Industrial effluents further complicate the problems (Table 35.2).

*Table 35.2*

| Hunter-Gatherer diets | | Current diets | | |
|---|---|---|---|---|
| Bulky | | Palatable | | |
| Low energy density | | Energy dense | | |
| Slowly digested | | Rapidly digested | | |
| Protein | ↑ | Protein | | ↓ |
| Fat | ↓ | Fat | ↑ | |
| Unsaturated fats | ↑ | Saturated fats | ↑ | |
| Complex carbohydrates-fibre | ↑ | Refined foods | ↓ | |
| | | Fibre | | |
| Vitamins / minerals | ↑ | vitamins/minerals | | |
| Glycemic index | ↓ | Glycemic index | ↑ | |
| Na/K ratio | ↓ | Na/K Ratio | ↑ | |
| Calcium | ↑ | Calcium | | ↓ |

## 35.6 Risk factors for diet related NCDs

Diet and lifestyles (modifiable factors) are important determinants of NCD. While age, sex and genetic factors cannot be altered (non modifiable factors), it is possible to change the risk profile by altering the diet and physical activities. Equal priority should be given to the control of nutritional deficiency diseases as well as NCDs. The risk factors for chronic disorders (Box 35.1) are high blood pressure, high concentrations of blood cholesterol and triglycerides, overweight and obesity, physical inactivity and tobacco use. These lead to metabolic abnormalities of insulin resistance and inflammatory state, which are further perpetuated by high intake of energy dense foods and high salt intake. Poor nutrition during pregnancy, infancy and early childhood further deteriorate the situation. High plasma concentrations of the amino acid homocysteine have been associated with atherothrombotic disease. High homocysteine concentrations are thought to impair endothelial function, increase oxidative stress, impair methylation reactions, and alter protein structure. Although some studies have shown improvement of vascular surrogate end points, homocysteine-lowering treatment has not yet been associated with a significant reduction of cardiovascular events. Studies that have examined the relationship between plasma homocysteine and arterial stiffness parameters have shown heterogenous results. There were ethnic differences for plasma folate and

**Box 35.1 NCDs – important risk factors**

- High blood pressure
- High blood concentrations of lipids – ↑cholesterol / Triglycerides (TG) / ↓High Density Lipoprotein (HDL)
- Overweight / obesity – Truncal / central distribution
- Inadequate intake – low micro & phyto nutrients, fibre present in fruit and vegetables
- High intakes of energy dense foods – fat / sugar
- High intake of salt
- Reduced physical activity – home, school, work, transport, recreation
- Excess use of tobacco & alcohol
- Poor maternal / fetal / early infant / child nutrition (altered structure / physiology / metabolism)
- Glucose intolerance (Insulin resistance)

vitamin $B_{12}$ (in particular lower levels in Indians); there was no evidence that homocysteine plays a role in different ethnic groups differently for ischemic heart disease (CHD) in Singapore and in particular to the Indians [29].

## 35.7 Overweight and obesity and dietary factors

The rising trend in obesity and overweight is part of the global epidemiological transition and is a public health threat and a serious burden on the public health expenditure. Though short-term measures are available for treatment, none of them are sustainable and it is essential to prevent the disorder. Obesity is simply defined as a condition of abnormal or excess fat or adipose mass, which impairs health and productivity. World over data clearly indicates that body mass index and abdominal obesity is increasing in epidemic proportions, which are important risk factors for type 2 diabetes, the metabolic syndrome and cardiovascular disease (CAD) [30–31]. WHO's expert consultation has also agreed that Asian Indians have higher health risks even at lower BMI, and consists more body fat and health risks, than the European populations. The obesity epidemic appears to be more in developing countries and especially in poor socioeconomic groups. The levels of BMI are the indicators for risk of morbidity, mortality and suggest priorities for interventions. The abdominal fat is a greater risk for development of metabolic syndrome.

Overweight and obesity are independent risk factors for insulin resistance, type 2 diabetes, cardio-vascular diseases and some cancers of gastrointestinal tract, breast and ovary, arthritis, gall stones as well as psychosocial consequences (Table 35.3). Morbidity due to obesity is universal with several systems being affected. Thus obesity demands the attention of all health care workers and there is a drain on health care costs. It needs preventive care as the consequences are cost prohibitive.

*Table 35.3* Health consequences of overweight and obesity

| Cardiovascular problems | Cancers |
|---|---|
| Ischemic heart disease (CHD)<br>Stroke<br>Hypertension<br>Cardiomyopathy<br>Deep vein thrombosis | Breast (post menopausal)<br>Endometrial<br>Ovary<br>Colon<br>Oesophagus, Stomach<br>Kidney |
| **Endocrine** | **Metabolic disorders** |
| Type 2 diabetes(NIDDM)<br>Infertility<br>Polycystic ovarian syndrome<br>Reproductive hormone disturbances | Dyslipidaemia<br>Insulin resistance<br>Metabolic syndrome<br>Inflammation<br>Hyperuricaemia<br>Gout |
| Pulmonary<br>Sleep Apnoea<br>Breathlessness<br>Asthma<br>Pulmonary embolus | Gastrointestinal<br>Gastro-oesophageal reflux<br>Gall stones<br>Non alcoholic fatty liver |
| **Others** | |
| Osteoarthritis<br>Low back pain | Increased anaesthetic risk<br>Fetal defects |

Though there are certain endocrine and metabolic disorders, which result in obesity, the major aetiological factor appears to be a positive energy balance. Energy dense foods or excess energy intake per se with very little physical activity and energy expenditure results in increased body weight and body composition changes with accumulation of fat in abdominal region and truncal areas. In recent times, the food intake appears to be more or less stable while the physical activity levels are reducing at all levels from childhood to adults. Energy cannot be created or destroyed, but can be converted to different forms. A small increase in food intake over a period of time results in gain in weight. There is convincing evidence that sedentary living coupled with energy dense foods, sugary drinks and fast foods promote obesity in all sections of populations. With added disadvantage of being under nourished at an earlier age the problems multiply. Sedentary behaviours, such as television viewing and working on computers or leisure time activity, which do not involve any physical activity, contribute to positive energy balance. Apart from CVDs and diabetes the serious consequences of obesity are certain types of cancers (Table 35.3). The origins of obesity can be traced back to fetal undernutrition, which programs the individual to higher risks of obesity in a later life. There is enough evidence now to suggest that exclusive breastfeeding and longer duration of breastfeeding prevent obesity and related disorders later [22]. Human milk is a natural source of all nutrients. The bioactive constituents of human milk (leptin) could modulate energy metabolism.

## 35.8 Blood lipids (Dyslipedaemia)

Cardiovascular diseases are caused by narrowing of blood vessels due to atherosclerotic fatty deposits and plaque formation associated with inflammatory deposits. Immune cells and their inflammatory activity and smooth muscle cell proliferation of arterial walls following endothelial damage resulting in platelet adhesions and reactivity and monocyte/macrophage infiltration are the major events in the process of atherosclerosis. The oxidised lipids formed in the lesion perpetuate the process. Micro thrombi and plaque instability lead to obstruction, haemorrhage and rupture.

Epidemiological, clinical, metabolic and experimental studies consistently indicate that high intake of saturated fats, trans in hydrogenated fats and dietary cholesterol enhance blood cholesterol, triglycerides including low and very low density lipoproteins and insulin resistance which in turn damage the endothelium leading to arterial lesions and higher blood pressure. Various investigations have shown that the intake of saturated fatty acids (SFA) is a significant independent predictor of fasting and post-prandial insulin concentrations [32]. The protection provided by HDL cholesterol is also an important factor and has emerged as a predictor. Refined carbohydrates increase triglycerides and decrease HDL. Among fatty acids, the saturated fats are harmful, while mono and polyunsaturated are protective [33]. The long chain omega 3 fats as in fish (EPA & DHA) have several beneficial effects (decrease lipids, blood pressure, inflammation and stabilizes plaque) [34]. Evidence from experimental studies has also indicated the benefit of long chain n-3 PUFA (fish oil) over n-6 PUFA (safflower-seed oil) in preventing insulin resistance, but convincing evidence from human studies is lacking. Supplementation with long chain n-3 PUFA appears to improve insulin sensitivity in subjects with impaired glucose tolerance [35]. It has been shown that an imbalance in dietary n-6 and n-3 PUFA may be important for the development of insulin resistance and dyslipidaemia in South Asians [36]. In vegetarian Asian Indians, a higher intake of n-3 PUFA could be obtained by the addition of several low cost vegetarian dietary items containing n-3 PUFA (GLV, *rajmah, bajra*, black gram). The bioactive components in fruits and vegetables lower atherosclerotic process to reduce cardiovascular accidents and also have some anti-tumour activities to prevent some of the tumours [37].

## 35.9 Metabolic syndrome

The metabolic syndrome is a group of conditions that put one at risk of developing heart disease and diabetes mellitus (Box 35.2). Metabolic syndrome is widely prevalent in Asia and India (30%) in particular and is associated with a higher risk of CVD and diabetes [38]. Insulin resistance is central to the syndrome and it may also be associated with fetal and childhood malnutrition and subsequent changes in growth pattern and fat accumulation which begins as early as two years or even at birth [39]. Genetic factors may also operate at different levels. High waist/hip ratio (WHR), elevated triglycerides, reduced HDL, high blood pressure and elevated fasting glucose levels are typical of this syndrome (Table 35.4). Dietary aberrations and poor physical activity are the determinants of the syndrome.

**Box 35.2 Criteria for clinical diagnosis of metabolic* syndrome**

1. Abdominal obesity (Excessive fat tissue in and around the abdomen)
2. Atherogenic dyslipidemia (high triglycerides, low HDL cholesterol and high LDL cholesterol)
3. Elevated blood pressure
4. Insulin resistance and glucose intolerance (the body can't properly use insulin or blood sugar)

** Presence of any 3 factors considered diagnostic for metabolic syndrome*

*Glucose intolerance (Insulin resistance)*

Glucose Intolerance (Insulin resistance) occurs when the body's ability to process glucose becomes impaired. The rise in the blood glucose levels in the fed state (after meal) stimulates the pancreas to produce more insulin that is necessary in the metabolism process to assimilate and store the available glucose. Impaired glucose tolerance occurs when the pancreas either does not release enough insulin or the cells become resistant to the insulin. Insulin resistance (or impaired glucose tolerance) is classified as a fasting glucose level of 110 mg/dl to <126 mg/dl.

## 35.10 Hypertension

High blood pressure is a risk factor for CVDs and strokes. Several studies have related high sodium intake and blood pressure (BP). In tribals who do not take salt, even age associated increase in blood pressure is not observed. In many populations sodium excretion in urine and blood pressure are related [45]. Increased potassium intake in the diet lowers the blood pressure levels. Vegetables and fruits supply adequate amounts

*Table 35.4* Cut-off levels for risk factors of non-communicable diseases

| Indicators | Level (mg/dL) | Interpretation | References |
|---|---|---|---|
| Total cholesterol (mg/dl) | <200 | Desirable/Normal | 40 |
| | 200–239 | Borderline high | |
| | >240 | High | |
| Low density lipoprotein (LDL) (mg/dl) | <100 | Optimal LDL cholesterol | |
| | 100–129 | Near optimal LDL level | |
| | 130–159 | Borderline high LDL level | |
| | 160–189 | High LDL level | |
| | >190 | Very high LDL level | |
| HDL cholesterol (mg/dl) | <40 | Low | |
| | 40–60 | Normal | |
| | >60 | High | |
| Serum triglycerides (mg/dl) | <150 | Normal | |
| | 150–199 | Borderline | |
| | 200–499 | High | |
| Waist circumference for Asians Indian (cms) | ≥ 90 cm | Men | 41 |
| | ≥80 cm | Women | |
| Body mass index (BMI) = [Weight (kg)/Height (m)$^2$] | <16.0 | III degree CED | 42 |
| | 16.0–17.0 | II degree CED | |
| | 17.0–18.5 | I degree CED | |
| | 18.5–20.0 | Low Normal | |
| | 20.0–25.0 | Normal | |
| | 25.0–30.0 | Over weight | |
| | ≥30 | Obesity | |
| Body mass index (BMI) = [Weight (kg)/Height (m)$^2$] | <18.5 | Underweight | 43 |
| | 18.5–<23.0 | Normal | |
| | ≥23.0–<27.5 | Increased risk | |
| | ≥27.5 | High risk | |
| Diabetes mellitus | <110 mg/dl | Normal | 44 |
| | ≥ 110 to <126 | Impaired glucose tolerance | |
| | ≥126 | Diabetes Mellitus | |

of potassium and can counteract the effects of sodium, if consumed in smaller amounts. A balanced diet also provides calcium and magnesium, which lowers blood pressure. From a health point of view vegetables and fruits with dairy products minus the fats would provide the much needed minerals. The dietary approaches to stop hypertension (DASH) [46] diet of reduced salt, weight reduction diets high in fruits and vegetables, low in dairy fat, high in whole grains, poultry, fish, nuts and low in fats, sugar and sugary beverages are comparable with antihypertensive drug effects. Urbanisation is one of the important factors for nutrition transition and emergence of obesity, the metabolic syndrome and cardiovascular diseases. Urbanisation is variable within the developing regions; almost three fourths of the population in Latin America and Caribbean, and 38% in Africa and Asia [47]. The rural to urban migration in many of the developing countries exposes migrants to urbanized diets and life styles. Studies done in Brazil and India have shown that many of these migrants living in urban slums have become obese and are affected by non-communicable diseases [48].

## 35.11 Fetal and childhood malnutrition

According to Barker's hypothesis [5], intra uterine growth retardation (IUGR), premature delivery and subsequent rapid postnatal catch up growth is associated with higher risk of coronary heart disease, stroke, diabetes and hypertension. A thrifty phenotype hypothesis that emphasises fetal undernutrition leading to altered metabolic programming is perhaps a better explanation in resource poor developing countries because abundant food supply later in life leads to maladaptive increase in weight and increases the risk of non-communicable diseases [49]. Several studies have shown that Asian Indian babies born small and with low birth weight had higher systolic blood pressure and adiposity at 8 years of age [50].

**Box 35.3 David Barker's hypothesis**

Professor David Barker and his colleagues working in Southampton have shown that fetal nourishment before birth and nutrition in infancy determine the patterns of fetal and infant growth, programme the development of risk factors such as raised blood pressure, fibrinogen concentration, and factor VIII concentration and glucose intolerance and hence are key determinants of coronary heart disease.

Even cancer mortality due to breast, uterus, and colon is higher in stunted children with accelerated growth [51]. Underweight and stunting can lead to tracking of risk factors for NCDs which are associated with an increased risk of chronic heart disease, stroke, diabetes etc. There are evidences to show that the risk of adult obesity increases if the individual suffered from undernutrition during the childhood [52]. In many countries, the urban poor and illiterates have high prevalence rates of overweight [53]. Unhealthy dietary practices worsen the situation. The factors that influence the incidence of non-communicable diseases are presented in Table 35.5.

## 35.12 Vegetables and fruits in the diet

Urged by scientific evidence, dietary guidelines of all countries strongly recommend that vegetables and fruits be consumed daily in sufficient

*Table 35.5* Risk for non-communicable diseases

| Diseases | Increased risk | Decreased risk |
|---|---|---|
| Obesity | • Energy dense foods<br>• Sugar sweetened soft drinks<br>• Physical inactivity<br>• Adverse socio-economic conditions<br>• Heavy marketing strategies | • High intake of fibre<br>• Fruits and vegetables<br>• Physical activity<br>• Exclusive breast feeding |
| Cardiovascular diseases | • Abdominal obesity and obesity<br>• Saturated and trans fatty acids/ Dietary cholesterol/ Myristic acid<br>• High sodium<br>• Unfiltered boiled coffee<br>• High alcohol | • Linoleic and alpha linoleic fatty acids / fish (EPA-DHA), Oleic acid<br>• Plant sterols, nuts,<br>• Dietary fibre<br>• Whole grains cereals<br>• Potassium<br>• Fruits and vegetables<br>• Low intake of alcohol<br>• Physical activity |
| Cancer | • Obesity/Overweight<br>• Salt preserved food (fish)<br>• Preserved red meat<br>• Very hot drinks<br>• High intake of alcohol<br>• Aflatoxins<br>• Tobacco consumption | • Vegetables and fruits<br>• Physical activity |
| Type 2 Diabetes | • Overweight/Obesity/ abdominal obesity<br>• IUGR<br>• Maternal diabetes<br>• Physical inactivity | • Dietary fibre<br>• Vegetables and fruits<br>• Physical activity |

quantities to provide micronutrients and phytonutrients that are thought to promote human health and combat both micronutrient deficiencies as well as pathogenesis of several chronic disorders (Box 35.4). Fruits, vegetables, grains, legumes, nuts, and tea are rich sources of phytonutrients. Vegetables and fruits are widely recognised as miracle foods for promotion of health and prevention of chronic diseases due to their bioactive constituents by varied mechanisms. The Joint FAO/WHO Expert Consultation (2004) on Diet, Nutrition and the Prevention of Chronic Diseases recommends the intake of a minimum of 400 grams of fruit and vegetables per day, excluding starchy tubers such as potatoes, for the prevention of chronic diseases including heart disease, cancer, type 2 diabetes and obesity. World Health Report 2002 indicates that 2.7 million lives could potentially be saved each year if fruit and vegetable consumption could be sufficiently increased.

Vegetables and fruits are low in calories, bulky with fibre, with a high satiety factor and therefore are of great value to reduce calorie intake and prevent obesity, a forerunner of all diet related chronic disorders. Some of these reduce lipids and glucose absorption due to their fibre content. The active constituents influence the aetiopathogenis of cardiovascular diseases, cancer, cataract, osteoporosis, diabetes, chronic obstructive pulmonary diseases, arthritis and diverticulosis. Non-starchy vegetables, complex carbohydrates probably decrease mouth, pharynx, larynx, oesophagus and stomach cancers [54]. Allium vegetables with organosulfur compounds modulate the activity of several metabolizing enzymes that activate or detoxify (glutathione S-transferases) carcinogens and inhibit the formation of DNA in several target tissues.

Red meat contains high saturated fat and collagen, which leads to collagen sensitization and consequent production of anti-collagen antibodies in susceptible individuals leading to inflammatory arthritis. Alcohol consumption causes cancers of the oral cavity, pharynx, oesophagus and liver, and a small increase in the risk for breast cancer. Chinese style salted fish, salt preserved foods and high salt increases the risk for nasopharyngeal cancer and stomach cancer [54]. In the developing world, tobacco consumption is rising by 3.4% per year. Major health effects of smoking, the most common use of tobacco, include an increased risk in hypertension, lung cancer and cardiovascular diseases [55].

**Box 35.4 Commonly available phytonutrients**

- Flavonoids (Polyphenols)
- Carotenoids
- Isoflavones (Phytoestrogens)
- Lignans (Phytoestrogens)
- Inositol Phosphates (Phytates)
- Isothiocyanates, Indoles and Saponins
- Phenols, Cyclic Compounds and Sulfides

## 35.13 Prevention and control of NCDs

The epidemiological transition in India from infections to chronic, non-communicable diseases has created different challenges for our public health system. It is therefore essential to encourage health-promoting behaviours, which include healthy diets and physical activity as well as avoidance of tobacco and stress management to impact NCDs. A population-based strategy of healthy diets across the life span has to be adopted in primordial and primary prevention for those at risk. Complementary to this, measures have to be taken to detect chronic conditions through early screening and initiate optimal treatment of the disease (secondary and tertiary prevention). These diseases are lifestyle related, have a long latent period and need specialized infrastructure and human resource for treatment.

### 35.13.1 Policies

Developing countries like India are facing a double burden of diseases, namely chronic energy/protein deficiency and obesity, leading to several non-communicable diseases. Therefore, a comprehensive policy addressing all risk factors including fetal/child malnutrition is crucial. A multi-sectoral, multi-pronged and multidisciplinary approach with a strong public/private partnership will provide an enabling environment and reduce the risks by improving morbidity, mortality, and impact healthcare costs. A life course approach is needed for successful primordial and primary prevention. There should be concordant policies on health, food, agriculture, nutrition, education, industry and commerce, urban rural development, social welfare and information technology.

The food label is one of the most important and direct means of communication of product information between buyers and sellers. It is the primary means by which consumers differentiate between individual foods and branded to make informed purchasing choices. In the Indian context, where overweight, obesity and the resultant non-communicable diseases are assuming epidemic proportions, consumption of unhealthy foods can be discouraged to a large extent by effective food labelling practices, which give ample scope for the consumers to make informed choices.

The government needs to work along with private sector and civic societies to make available, affordable and accessible healthy choices and options for physical activity. A good leadership and functional alliances will provide an enabling environment to upgrade education, knowledge and skills among all sectors (Figure 35.2). The community should be empowered to actively participate. A public health cadre with carrier opportunities and restructuring of health care system for effective functioning are required.

The Government of India and many other countries have already launched several National programmes to prevent and control non-communicable diseases. In India the important programmes are; the National Cancer Control Programme (1984), National Program for the Prevention and Control of Diabetes (1987), National Program for the Prevention and Control of Cardiovascular Diseases, and Stroke (2006).

### 35.13.2 Strategies

*Diet*

Strategies to promote health mostly focus on production, preservation,

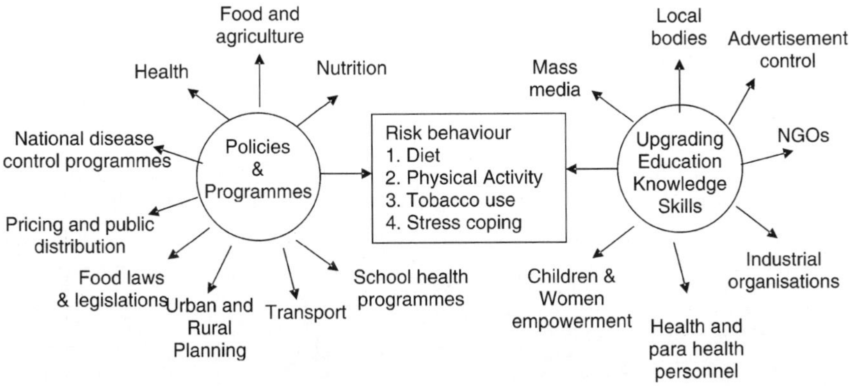


*35.2* Public health interventions.

processing, value addition and making available, accessible and affordable healthy choices. Therefore, focus should be on the availability of the healthy foods with mandatory labelling patterns on every food product released to the market for sale.

It is evident that integrated approaches to both undernutrition and over-nutrition can reduce the burden of non-communicable diseases to a greater extent. Integrated multi-sectoral, multifaceted and multidisciplinary approaches have to be evolved to prevent and control the already escalating obesity and related morbidities. Active measures to promote physical activity both at individual, community and at group level (schools, industries and offices) must be encouraged. Recreational activities, which promote physical activities, must receive more attention. More walking and cycling paths to promote safe activities are required. The strategy is to promote physical activity at workplaces and schools where people spend a lot of their time daily. The school children act as change agents. Trim and Fit programmes for students have to be initiated to reduce obesity and improve physical fitness. Greater involvement of parents in this programme is needed, as the home environment contributes largely to the moulding of habits of the children. Comprehensive workplace health promotion programmes are effective in improving the health status and productivity of employees. Therefore, 'National Workplace Health Promotion Programme' has to be initiated to encourage organizations to conduct and sustain workplace health promotion programmes that will achieve desired health outcomes. Training courses and education initiatives have to be carried out to equip management with the knowledge and skills to conduct and promote a healthy lifestyle at their workplaces. Tobacco in all its forms must be censured and tobacco farms should be diversified to other commercial crops as one of the important control strategies.

*Maternal and fetal nutrition*

Maternal nutrition is an important determinant of birth weight. In India almost one in three babies are of low birth weight and therefore it is essential to build the nutrition of adolescent and pregnant mothers with healthy diets consisting of macro and micronutrients particularly of iron, folate, iodine, vitamin A, zinc, calcium, magnesium and vitamin $B_{12}$. During pregnancy, attention is required to fulfil calorie, protein and micronutrient requirements to promote 10–12 kg body weight gain and lactation to support the growth of the foetus and infant. The type of fatty acid (oleic acid/ DHA being beneficial) in the diet during pregnancy and lactation are known to influence the plasma cholesterol and cognition in infancy and childhood. Exclusive breast-feeding and prolonged breast-feeding can reduce the risk of obesity and related disorders later. Energy dense and micronutrient rich complementary foods to promote growth and development must be ensured to prevent dual burden of diseases and to avoid irreversible changes in brain growth, prevent stunting and obesity in adult life.

## 35.14 Actions

Greater political commitment and strong leadership in the public health sector is required to ensure the prevention and control of non-communicable diseases. Advocacy can be broadened to raise awareness and encourage the policy and institutional changes necessary for creation and strengthening of existing health infrastructure for tackling of non-communicable diseases.

The health care providers need to lobby and accord high priority to the following:

All the interventions must be culture and region specific and utilize local resources

1. Define national goals and objectives and target populations for advocacy to control non-communicable diseases, including health as well as non-health sectors.
2. Establish and strengthen existing policies for the prevention and control of non-communicable diseases
3. Ensure reduction of risk factors as an integral part of National health development plans, paying special attention to the needy population.
4. Establish national multisectoral body or mechanism for planning, guiding, monitoring activities for prevention and control of non-communicable diseases.

**Box 35.3 Healthy practices**

- Achieve energy balance and appropriate weight for height.
- Achieve good nutrition during pregnancy and lactation.
- Exclusive breastfeeding for 6 months and introduction of complementary foods at 6 months.
- Prevent stunting and promote growth in children and adolescents (linear growth and muscle mass) by ensuring consumption of adequate good quality proteins and micronutrients.
- Increase consumption of fruits and vegetables, legumes, whole grains and nuts.
- Limit energy intake from total fat, shift fat consumption from saturated to unsaturated
- Consume unsaturated fats with appropriate fatty acids.
- Eliminate trans fatty acids (bakery products and sweets).
- Limit intake of free sugars and salt.
- Restrict alcohol and avoid tobacco.
- Encourage physical activity.
- Be aware of fattening trajectory (adiposity rebound in malnourished children)
- Promote complex carbohydrates and fibre rich diets.

5. Build capacity for intersectoral collaboration involving all government sectors and other stakeholders, such as professional association, community representatives, and non-governmental organisations.
6. Establish separate units for tackling of non-communicable diseases in the Ministry of Health and Family Welfare and different levels of health systems.
7. Develop and implement an evidence based plan for health promotion and prevention of non-communicable diseases.
8. Establish mechanisms for early detection and screening for common non-communicable diseases such as hypertension, diabetes, and certain cancers.
9. Develop training programmes to strengthen capacity for building health systems

State governments, regional and local institutes have the responsibility and specific role to convert the above mentioned strategies into action. Persons at several levels need to be empowered with knowledge and skills. Village Panchayats, NGOs, self-help groups, women working groups, labour unions, teachers and health and para-health professionals must be involved for proper implementation of appropriate actions.

Canteens, restaurants, and other public catering establishments must be encouraged to serve healthy foods. The healthier choice symbol on packed food should be encouraged for easy consumer recognition. Restaurants, food courts, and fast food centres have to be encouraged to offer more vegetables and fruits and less salt, sugar and fats to their customers.

## 35.15 Childhood and adolescent nutrition

Nutritious diet is essential to achieve full genetic potentials of growth and development during these periods. Adolescents need appropriate health education and supplementary nutrition for micronutrient deficiencies and healthy pregnancy outcomes to prevent intrauterine growth retardation and low birth babies. In order to avoid adiposity, linear growth, muscle and bone mass have to be built up during childhood and adolescence. Tracking of risk behaviours and unhealthy dietary practices in time and providing appropriate education to them may be useful for prevention of NCDs. Faulty dietary habits have to specially receive due attention. Thus, a life cycle approach prevents an obesogenic environment including regulation of inactive TV viewing, long hours of computer work and sedentary leisure time activities to prevent clustering of risk factors of metabolic syndrome.

*Adulthood*

Diet, physical activity, avoidance of tobacco and alcohol are major issues for prevention and control of NCDs. It is important to practice relaxation technique (yoga etc) to avoid stress. It is evident that the way we are born and grow and the food we eat, the drinks we take, the way we play, move around, the work we do and the stress of life, all have an important role to play in the initiation, promotion and progression of NCDs.

*Education*

Public awareness programmes must target all age groups and simple messages on diet and physical activity and harmful effects of tobacco must receive great attention. Both dietary and physical activity guidelines should be widely published through mass media approach and information technology (web-based guidelines). Media has a strong impact especially on children and adolescents, and hence unhealthy foods should not be advertised. Education can play a critical role in awareness building and policy implementation. A wide reach and an active partnership of media can go a long way in promoting health and wellbeing of the individuals.

## 35.16 Community-based programmes for primary prevention

A National Healthy Lifestyle Campaign programme should be under taken to educate the people on the importance of healthy lifestyles to provide a supportive environment for healthier eating. Health education and promotion will provide information to the public on the benefits of a healthier lifestyle. Measures have to be taken to provide an environment conducive for the adoption of healthy habits. As the population becomes more educated, they are more aware and better informed on health choices resulting in higher interest in adoption of correct preventive practices.

## 35.17 Health education and role of mass media

It is necessary to provide skills and environmental cues for the public to effect the appropriate behaviour changes by establishing health promotion cells. Social marketing strategies have a strong place in information, education and communication. The primary tool for control of non-communicable diseases is comprehensive and active awareness of the population about the risk factors and practicing the preventive measures. Research studies evaluating the effectiveness of health education in India and elsewhere have shown successful results among the youth and adults [56, 57].

## 35.18 Secondary and tertiary prevention

Diabetes and hypertension are major risk factors for cardiovascular diseases. To improve early detection of the chronic conditions of diabetes, hypertension and hypercholesterolemia, a 'community health screening' programme targeted at >35 years population needs to be developed. The population based strategy aims at relatively modest reductions in the risk for each individual, but the cumulative benefits to the community are large since there are many more persons in the mild or moderate risk category factor than in the higher risk category. The two strategies are not mutually exclusive but should be synergistically complementary to each other. Low-cost case-management strategies are also required for persons who manifest disease. Such technologies are already available but await widespread dissemination and application.

## 35.19 Conclusions

The global epidemic of NCDs due to faulty lifestyles is a serious matter of concern and warrants immediate attention of all concerned. The rapidly increasing incidence of these diseases is affecting the poor and disadvantaged populations disproportionately, contributing to widening health gaps between and within countries. Developmental, demographic, economic, health and nutritional transitions result in altered dietary habits and sedentary life styles. The risk factors require to be addressed in totality by comprehensive policies and well-structured programs involving multiple sectors through multifaceted strategies. The plans should focus on overall mapping of the epidemics of non-communicable diseases and analysing their technical, social, economic, and behavioural determinants as basis for providing guidance on policy, programme, legislative and financial allocation that are needed to support the prevention and control of communicable diseases. Exposure of individuals and populations to the common risk behaviours for non-communicable diseases, such as tobacco consumption, unhealthy diet, physical inactivity, and alcohol should be reduced. Health care for non-communicable diseases should be strengthened by developing appropriate guidelines and healthy diets on cost effective basis [58]. It is also essential to prioritise research issues for prevention and control of non-communicable chronic diseases.

## References

1. The World Health Report (2002). Reducing risks, promoting healthy life. Geneva, World Health Organization.
2. National Family Health survey (NFHS 3) 2005–06. International Institute of Population Sciences, Bombay.
3. World Health Assembly 57.17 (2004). Global strategy on diet and physical activity. Geneva: World Health Organization.
4. Nutrition in Developmental Transition (2006). Proceedings of Symposium organized by NFI-WHO (SEARO).
5. BARKER DJ (2007). The origins of the developmental origins theory. *J Intern Med.*, **261**(5), pp. 412–417.
6. WORLD HEALTH ORGANIZATION (WHO). Health situation in the South East Asia 1998-2000. New Delhi, WHO regional office.
7. REDDY KS, SHAH B, VARGHESE C, RAMADOSS A (2005). Responding to the threat of chronic diseases in India. *Lancet*, **366**(9498), pp. 1744–9.
8. GHAFFAR A, REDDY KS, SINGHI M (2004). Burden of non-communicable diseases in South Asia, *BMJ*, **32**(8), pp. 807–810.
9. EZZATI M and LOPEZ A (2003). Estimates of global mortality attributable to smoking in 2000. *Lancet.* **36**(2), pp. 847–852.
10. LOPEZ A, MATHERS C, EZZATI M, JAMISON D, MURRAY C (2006). *Global Burden of Disease and Risk Factors.* Oxford University Press, New York, and Washington DC, World Bank.
11. INDIAN COUNCIL OF MEDICAL RESEARCH (2006). Assessment of Burden of Non-Communicable Diseases..
12. ICMR (1994). Task force project on Collaboration study of coronary heart study.
13. GUPTA R (2004). Trends in hypertension epidemiology in India. *J Hum Hypertens.*, **18**(2), pp. 73–8.
14. KEARNEY PM, WHELTON M, REYNOLDS K, MUNTNER P, WHELTON PK, HE J (2005). Global burden of hypertension: analysis of worldwide data. *Lancet*, **365**(9455), pp. 217–23.
15. NATIONAL NUTRITION MONITORING BUREAU (NNMB 2005–06). Diet and Nutritional status of population and prevalence of hypertension among adults in rural areas, NNMB Technical No. 24, National Institute of Nutrition, *ICMR*, Hyderabad.

16. NATIONAL NUTRITION MONITORING BUREAU (NNMB 2001). Second Repeat survey. Diet and Nutritional status of population. NNMB Technical No. 18, National Institute of Nutrition, *ICMR*, Hyderabad.
17. LAXMAIAH A, BALAKRISHNA N, VIJAYARAGHAVAN K, NAIR VM (2007). Factors effecting overweight among urban Adolescents in Hyderabad, Andhra Pradesh. *Obesity* **15**, pp. 1384–1390.
18. WHO Project on Sentinel Surveillance of Indian industrial population, 2001–03.
19. DEURENBURG YM, SCHMIDT G, VAN STAVEREN WA, HAURVAST JG, DEURENBURG P (2000). The paradox of low body mass index and high body fat percentage among Chinese, Malahys, and Indian in Singapore. *Int. J Obes Metab Disord*, **24**, pp. 1011–1017.
20. MISRA A (2003). Body composition and the metabolic syndrome in Asian Indians; a saga of multiple adversities, *Natl Med J India*, **16**, pp. 3–7.
21. WILD S, ROGLIC G, GREEN A, SICREE R, KING H (2004). Global prevalence of diabetes. Estimates for the year 2000 and projections for 2030. *Diabetes Care*, **27**, pp. 1047–1053.
22. WORLD CANCER RESEARCH FUND/AMERICAN INSTITUTE FOR CANCER RESEARCH (2007). Food, Nutrition, Physical Activity, and the Prevention of Cancer: A Global Perspective. Washington, DC: AICR.
23. INDIA COUNCIL OF MEDICAL RESEARCH (2001). National cancer registry programme, New Delhi.
24. MISRA A and KHURANA L (2008). Obesity and metabolic syndrome in developing countries, *J clinical Endocrinol Metab*, **93**(11), pp. S11–S30.
25. WORLD HEALTH ORGANISATION (1998). The World Health Report: Life in the 21st Century: a vision for all. Geneva: *World Health Organisation.*
26. HOFFMAN DJ (2001). Obesity in developing countries: causes and implications. Food, Nutrition and Agriculture. A Publication of the FAO food and nutrition division. Available at http://ftp.fao.org/docrep/fao/003/yo600m/y0600m04.pdf.last accessed in November 2008.
27. KELSAY JL, FRAZIER CW, PRATHER ES, CANARY JJ, CLARK WM, POWELL AS (1998). Impact of variation in carbohydrate intake on mineral utilization by vegetarians, *Am J Clin Nutr.*, **48**, pp. 875–879.
28. Evolutionary Aspects of Nutrition and Health: Diet, Exercise, Genetics and Chronic Disease (World Review of Nutrition and Dietetics) AP. *Simopoulos.*
29. HUGHES K and ONG C (2000). Homocysteine, folate, vitamin $B_{12}$, and cardiovascular risk in Indians, Malays, and Chinese in Singapore, *J Epidemiol Community Health*. **54**(1), pp. 31–34.
30. MISRA A and VIKRAM NK (2003). Clinical and pathological consequences of abdominal obesity and abdominal adipose tissue depots, *Nutrition* **19**, pp. 457–466.
31. YUSUF S, HAWKEN S, OUNPUU S, DANS T, AVEZUM A, LANAS F, MC QUEEN M, BUDAJ A, PAIS P, VARIGOS J, LISHENG L (2004). Effect of potentially modifiable risk factors associated with myocardial infarction in 52 countries (the INTER HEART study): case control study, *Lancet*, **36**(4), pp. 937–952.
32. MARON DJ, FAIR JM, HASKELL WL (1991). Saturated fat intake and insulin resistance in men with coronary artery disease, *Circulation*, **84**, pp. 2020–2027.
33. GHAFOORUNISS A and KRISHNASWAMY K (1998). Diet and Heart Disease, National Institute of Nutrition.
34. ZHANG J, SASAKI S, AMANO K, KESTELOOT H (1999). Fish consumption and mortality from all causes, ischemic heart disease and stroke: an epidemiological study. *Preventive medicine* **28**, pp. 522–29.

35. GIACCO R, CUOMO V, VESSBY B, UUSITUPA M, HERMANSEN K, MEYER BJ, RICCARDI G, RIVELLESE AA (2007). Fish oil, insulin sensitivity, insulin secretion and glucose tolerance in healthy people: is there any effect of fish oil supplementation in relation to the type of background diet and habitual dietary intake of n-6 and n-3 fatty acids? *Nutr Metab Cardiovasc Dis*, **17**, pp. 572–580.
36. GHAFOORUNSS A (1998). Requirements of dietary fats to meet nutritional needs and prevent the risk of atherosclerosis – an Indian perspective, *Ind J Med Res*, **10**(8), pp. 191–102.
37. KRISHNASWAMY K (2004). Newer roles of vegetables in the prevention and control of problem of over nutrition and chronic degenerative diseases. In: *Nutrition and Vegetables*. Nath P, Gaddagimath PB and Dutta OP (eds). Dr. Prem Nath Agricultural Science Foundation, Bangalore, pp. 162–180.
38. MISRA A, MISRA R, WIJESURIYA M, BANERJEE D (2007). The metabolic syndrome in South Asians: Continuing escalation & possible solutions, *Indian J Med Res* **12**(5), pp. 345–354.
39. YAJNIK CS (2002). The life cycle effects of nutrition and body size on adult adiposity, diabetes and cardiovascular disease. *Obes Rev.*, **3**, pp. 217–224.
40. FEEMAN et al (2001). Guidelines for diagnosis and treatment of high cholesterol, *JAMA* **28**(6), pp. 2400–2402.
41. MISRA A, VIKRAM NK, GUPTA R, PANDEY RM, WASIR JS, GUPTA VP (2006). Waist circumference cutoff points and action levels for Asian Indians for identification of abdominal obesity, *International Journal of Obesity*, pp. 106–111.
42. JAMES WP, FERRO-LUZZI A, WATERLOW JC (1988). Definition of chronic energy. *Eur. J. Clin. Nutr.*, **42**, pp. 969–981.
43. WHO Expert Consultation (2004). Appropriate body mass index for Asian populations and its implications for policy and intervention strategies *The Lancet*, 36(3), pp. 157–163.
44. The Expert Committee on the diagnosis and classification of diabetes mellitus. Report of the Expert Committee on the diagnosis and classification of diabetes mellitus. *Diabetes Care Suppl*, **25**(1), pp. 5–20.
45. REDDY KS and KATAN MB (2004).Diet, nutrition and prevention of hypertension and cardiovascular disease. *Pub Health Nut*, **7**(1), pp. 167–186.
46. SACKS FM et al (2001). Effects on blood pressure of reduced dietary sodium and the dietary approaches to stop hypertension (DASH) diet. *New Engl J Med.* **34**(4), pp. 3–10.
47. FOOD AND AGRICULTURAL ORGANISATION (2004). Globalisation of food systems in developing countries impact on food security and nutrition. Food and nutrition paper. United Nations; FAO.
48. SAWAYA AL, DALLAL G, SOLYMOS G, DE SOUSA MH, VENTURA ML, ROBERTS SB, SIGULEM DM (1995). Obesity and malnutrition in a shantytown population in the city of Sao Paulo, Brazil. *Obes Res*, **3**(2), pp. S107–S115.
49. PRENTICE AM (2003). Intrauterine factors, adiposity, and hyperinsulinemia, *BMJ*, **32**(7), pp. 880–881.
50. BAVDEKAR A, YAJNIK CS, FALL CH, BAPAT S, PANDIT AN, DESPANDE V, BHAVE S, KELLINGRAY SD, JOGLEKAR C (1999). Insulin resistance Syndrome in 8 year old Indian Children: small at birth, big at 8 years, or both? *Diabetes*, **48**, pp. 2422–2429.
51. WHO/FAO (2002). Diet, nutrition and the prevention of chronic diseases. Report of a joint WHO/FAO Export consultation. WHO Technical Report series 916, WHO/FAO, United Nations.

52. DELISLE H (2005). Early nutritional influences on obesity, diabetes and cardiovascular disease risk. International Workshop, 6–9 June 2004, Montreal University, Quebec, Canada. *Maternal and Child Nutrition*, **1**(3), pp. 128–129.
53. MENDEZ M and POPKIN B (2004). Globalization, urbanization and nutritional change in the developing world. In FAO. Globalization of food systems in developing countries: impact on food security and nutrition, pp. 55–80.
54. KEY TJ, SCHATZKIN A, WILLETT WC, ALLEN NE, SPENCER EA, TRAVIS RC (2004). Diet, nutrition and the prevention of cancer, *Public Health Nutr.* **7**(1), pp. 187–200.
55. WHO Report on the Global Tobacco Epidemic, 2008.
56. POEHLMAN ET and HORTON ES (1989). The impact of food intake and exercise on energy expenditure. *Nutr Rev.* **47**(5), pp. 129–37.
57. DOWSE GK, GAREEBOO H, ALBERTI KG (1995). Changes in population cholesterol concentrations and other cardiovascular risk factor levels after five years of the non-communicable disease intervention programme in Mauritius. *Br Med J*, **311**, pp. 1255–1259.
58. WORLD HEALTH ORGANISATION (2008). Prevention and control of communicable diseases: implementation of the global strategy. *Executive Board Provisional Agenda,* Document No A53/14, WHO 16 January 2008.

# 36

# Planning result-oriented public health nutrition programs: theory and practice

*Ashi K. Kathuria*

**Ashi Kohli Kathuria**, MSc (Food and Nutrition), is the senior nutrition specialist at the World Bank, New Delhi. She has extensively provided strategic and technical leadership to large public health and nutrition programmes in India. Her areas of interest include programme development, monitoring and evaluation, policy and advocacy work, and sector assessment and analyses. Prior to her position at the World Bank, Ms. Kathuria was deputy director at USAID, New Delhi, office of social development, and among other guided USAID (India) work in the maternal and child health and nutrition, education, women's empowerment, workforce development, and disaster preparedness and response.

## 36.1 Introduction

Public health program planning in its early days related largely to the planning of public health infrastructure and systems. It was undertaken almost exclusively by public health professionals. Today, it has evolved into a notably specialized and comprehensive field that integrates cutting edge public health science, social science theories, principles of management, and social dynamics and interactions. It engages a range of stakeholders in the process, including the program participants[1] and incorporates their perspectives during each stage of program planning.

Two major advances in international development over the past decade have had significant directional implications for public health program planning and management. One is the focus on development results and their effective measurement; the other is the emphasis on collaboration within the development community for policy coherence, technical cooperation and aid harmonization. Several international initiatives have

1. The term program participant refers to the people who benefit from the services and is distinct from program person. It is synonymous with the often used term, 'beneficiaries', but is the preferred term used throughout this chapter. This is in recognition of, and to highlight, the fact that no program would be possible without the participation of the people who are expected to benefit from the program.

led to these directions. The Millennium Declaration marked the beginning of an unprecedented era of collaboration for development; and the Millennium Development Goals (MDGs) are probably the best known and most ambitious global commitments to results-based development. The agreed MDGs, targets, and indicators provide the basis for measuring progress and the effectiveness of aid. The Monterrey Consensus (2002), the Rome Declaration (2003), the Paris Declaration (2005) and the Managing for Development Results global initiative further underscored the shared responsibility of all stakeholders in achieving development results[1].

To improve the effectiveness of international aid and to better demonstrate development results, many international agencies, donors and countries adopted practices referred to as Managing for Development Results (MfDR) or Results Based Management (RBM). MfDR or RBM makes results central to all phases of the development process. It aligns program development, implementation, monitoring and evaluation with results, and uses results as the basis of learning and decision-making [2, 3]. All public health nutrition program planning efforts must be responsive to this context. They should ensure a strong result focus during all stages of planning and seek to build partnerships and foster collaboration.

In the specific context of public health nutrition, several events have underscored the need to invest in, and to accelerate action, to improve nutrition. Starting with the MDGs, the critical role of nutrition in human development has been highlighted. Improving nutrition will contribute to the achievement of six MDGs – directly to MDG 1, 4 and 5 and indirectly to MDG 2, 3, 6 (see Box 36.1 for the contribution of nutrition to each of these MDGs). The 2008 *Lancet* special series "Maternal and Child Undernutrition" highlighted the significant contribution of undernutrition to mortality and disease. It demonstrated that interventions to address maternal and child undernutrition and save millions of lives are available. The Lancet also pointed out the low priority accorded to nutrition by donors and developing countries [4]. The "Copenhagen Consensus 2008"[2] ranked five nutrition interventions amongst the top ten most cost-effective development interventions [5]. This is far higher than interventions in any other sector, and demonstrates the highly cost-effective nature of nutrition interventions. Following these events, higher commitment to improve nutrition is emerging from the international agencies, bilateral agencies, private foundations, civil society and the private sector. Consensus is also emerging on a global "Framework of Action" to scale-up action to address malnutrition. This framework outlines key considerations, principles, and priorities for action to address malnutrition [6].

2. The Copenhagen consensus summarizes the views of a panel of leading economists, including five Nobel Laureates, on the top ten development investments.

**Box 36.1 Nutrition's contributions to the attainment of MDGs [19]**

**Goal 1 – Eradicate extreme poverty and hunger**

- Malnutrition erodes human capital, reduces resilience to shocks and reduces productivity (impaired physical and mental capacity).

**Goal 2 – Achieve universal primary education**

- *Malnutrition reduces mental capacity.*
- Malnourished children are less likely to enroll in school or more likely to drop out.
- Current hunger and malnutrition reduces school performance.

**Goal 3 – Promote gender equality and empower women**

- *Better-nourished girls are more likely to stay in school and to have more control over* future choices.

**Goal 4 – Reduce child mortality**

- *Malnutrition is directly or indirectly associated with more than 35% of all child* mortality.
- *Malnutrition is the main contributor to the burden of disease in the developing world.*

**Goal 5 – Improve maternal health**

- Maternal health is compromised by an anti-female bias in allocation of food, health and care.
- Malnutrition is associated with most major risk factors for maternal mortality.

**Goal 6 – Combat HIV/AIDS, malaria, and other diseases**

- Malnutrition weakens resistance to infections.
- Undernutrition reduces malaria and diarrhoea survival rates.

The aforementioned developments have important implications for public health nutrition program planning. One, program planning for public health nutrition programs must focus on the most cost-effective, proven interventions; they must include robust monitoring and evaluation systems to measure and document results. Two, it must build in mechanisms to test effectiveness of the delivery approaches. This will contribute to a better understanding of the 'how' of the delivery of nutrition interventions, an area less understood than the 'what' of nutrition interventions. Finally, it must incorporate strategies to advocate for and build commitment for nutrition, within the organization as well as amongst a range of external audience, including leaders and opinion makers, policy makers, and programmers.

This chapter attempts to bring to the reader a comprehensive discussion of the key elements of program planning, some prominent theories and conceptual frameworks used in planning public health programs, and guide them through the various steps in a program planning cycle. It does not offer a blue-print or prescription for program planning, since program planning can happen in many different ways and there is no 'one best way" to plan public health nutrition programs. Instead, by bringing together the academic and the practitioner perspectives on program planning, the chapter hopes to help the reader understand and apply the theories, concepts and tools of program planning to develop nutrition programs that have a higher potential for achieving their intended results.

The chapter is organized into five sections. The first section provides the background; the second provides an overview of program planning and its nature; the third discusses some of the widely used frameworks, concepts, theories and tools for program planning including two frameworks specifically applicable to nutrition program planning. The fourth section takes the reader through the steps involved in program planning. Illustrations and practical examples from nutrition programs are used across all sections to make the connections between theory and practice. The last section concludes with a few points for further reading, thought and discussion.

## 36.2 Program planning – an overview

### 36.2.1 Definitions

Planning has been defined in several ways. It refers to the management function that involves envisioning the change desired to improve a situation or to resolve a problem, setting goals and objectives, and after examining several options in a rational manner, making choices about the best route for achieving the intended change, laying out the course of action, planning to proceed with these in a logical, preset manner and establish a means to measure the attainment of those desired improvements [7].

The term 'program' refers to an organized and structured set of strategies and actions to deliver some prioritized services or interventions to address a problem, improve a specified situation, bring about the intended change, or achieve the desired result. Program planning serves as a bridge between and among theories, measurement sciences, substantive content and actual practice of public health [8]. It often involves working backwards through the entire chain starting with the intended result that the plan is to achieve. After having identified the result, planners identify the actions and processes required to be undertaken to produce that result, and thereafter the inputs or resources needed to carry out those actions.

Although some texts draw distinctions between a program and a project (generally programs being more complex and large with respect to geographical coverage and reach, duration, planned results and resource levels, as compared to projects), throughout this chapter (unless specified otherwise) the term 'program planning' encompasses project planning, as the principles, concepts and steps discussed are applicable to both.

Of the many approaches to planning, the one that is almost universally applied to the planning of public health programs is 'rational planning'. Rational planning is based on a cause and effect relationship and involves an analysis of the problem to be addressed (including the full set of conditions and associated factors that cause, enhance or limit it); the use of scientific knowledge and theories to find the most effective intervention or mix of interventions to address the problem; and the application of systematic, logical sequence of thoughts and actions to improve the problem of concern. Planners set goals, consider alternatives, implement programs, monitor results and evaluate the program [9].

## 36.2.2 The nature of planning

Program planning involves many steps but it is not a linear process and the steps may not be sequenced. It is an iterative process involving to and fro between various steps. These steps are sequenced in the diagrammatic representation in Fig. 36.1 for ease of exposition, but it is important to remember that these steps may not be linear.

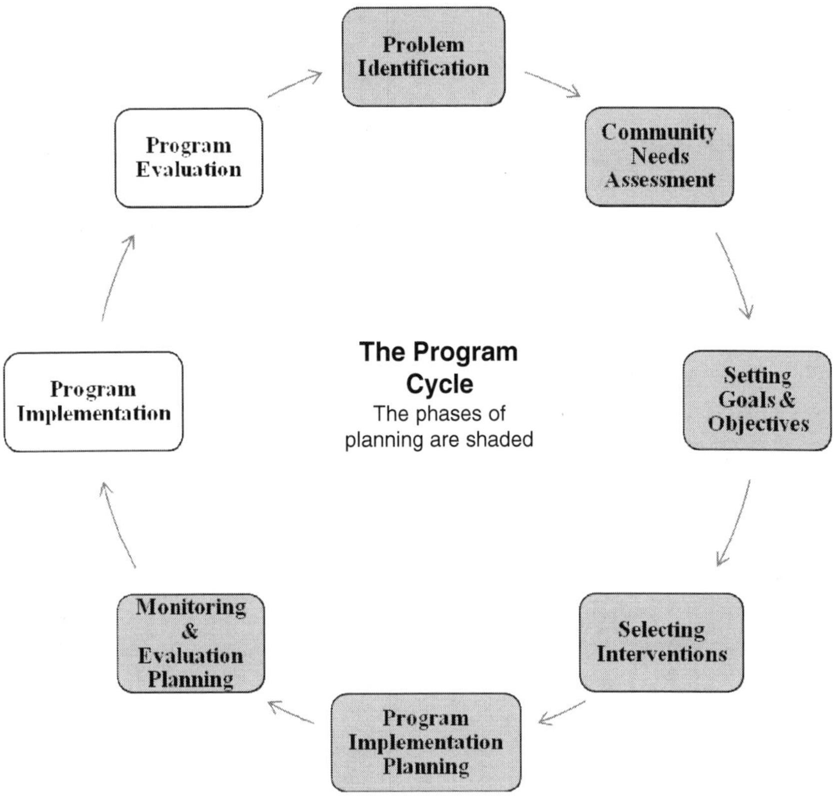


*36.1* Steps in program planning

The starting point for the program planning process may differ depending on the need and context of the planning effort, particularly the circumstances that triggered the planning. For example, if program planning is initiated in response to a community needs assessment during which health problems to be addressed have been prioritized, then a number of steps related to the problem identification that would otherwise be necessary, would not need to be undertaken. Similarly, if planning for a new national nutrition program is initiated in response to a national strategic priority or a policy to address a nutrition problem highlighted by a large survey, then again problem identification has already taken place. If planning is related to an ongoing program, the first step would then be to review the learnings from the earlier implementation experience and the findings of any evaluation that might have been conducted.

Program planning is also a continuous process and does not necessarily end when a program gets into the implementation phase. Good planning is, in fact, cognizant of, and responsive to, events, situations, and new learnings that occur during the life of a program that might trigger a reconsideration of options. A change in policy, an increase or decrease in the resources available to the program, a change in its context, implementation experience, availability of new knowledge and so on are examples of situation that may require a change of course, or a revision of targets or the intervention mix or the manner of service delivery. Good planning also factors in the information flowing back to the program through various feedback loops such as program monitoring data or through feedback received from the program personnel and participants, or findings and recommendations of the evaluation.

Planning, program implementation and evaluation have a cyclical relationship [9]. Good program planning not only draws up the program implementation plans but also builds in plans and resources for evaluation, and is informed by evaluation findings. Similarly, evaluation should focus on how to improve the effectiveness of programs and should, during the evaluation process, consider the program planners' perspectives. The program cycle (Figure 36.1) shows the cyclical nature of planning and evaluation.

### 36.2.3 Factors that prompt nutrition program planning

The need for program planning may be prompted by several factors that result in highlighting a nutrition problem of concern, an opportunity to address a known nutrition problem, a policy or governmental mandate, or a combination of all of these. A nutrition problem could be highlighted through the findings of nutrition and health surveys, such as the national Demographic Health Surveys (DHS) conducted periodically in several countries, the District Level Household Surveys (DLHS) in India, or other sub-national or even local surveys. Routinely collected hospital/other health system statistics may also be indicative of a nutritional problem, e.g., number of cases of diabetes, night blindness during pregnancy, low birth weight and underweight children. It is also possible that an existing and known nutrition problem might find a strong champion to take up the cause and become the advocate for developing a program to address the issue [9]. Governmental priorities and mandates, policy recommendations and budgetary allocations are important triggers for program planning [9]. Further, international commitments – for example the adoption of the MDGs, donor priorities, the announcements of grants and requests for proposals, civil society interest and so on – could provide the impetus for program planning.

Public health nutritionists must be alert to situations that may offer the opportunity to address a nutritional problem, and take leadership in actively pursuing options and resources for programs to improve nutrition, build champions to advocate for evidence-based policies and programs.

Against this backdrop, the next section discusses the basic concepts underlying rational planning and introduces some planning tools and frameworks used in the planning of public health programs.

## 36.3 Theory, concepts, frameworks

The purpose of this section is to provide the reader an understanding of the theory and concepts fundamental to developing results-oriented programs and familiarize them with some program planning tools that help the planner to keep the focus on results during the planning process. The section includes a description of the 'program theory'; two generic program planning frameworks widely used in public health program planning, the 'logical framework' and the 'results framework'; and two nutrition-specific conceptual frameworks – 'the nutrition cause and intervention framework'; and 'the life cycle framework'. While the theoretical concepts are covered in this section, the development of the program theory through an example is discussed in Section 36.4, entitled 'Steps in Program Planning'.

### 36.3.1 Program theory

The program theory is the conceptual framework that shows how a program intends to address the problem and bring about the desired change [10]. It hypothesizes the relationship between the nutrition problem (in the instance of a nutrition program) and the proposed set of actions to address it, identifies the various causal factors, and describes how the program actions interact with the causal variables to produce the desired change. Thus, it forms the backbone of 'theory-driven' program planning and program evaluation efforts.

However, program development is often undertaken on the basis of broad cause-effect relationships, and does not make explicit the detailed program theory. There are compelling reasons to develop and articulate the program theory during the development phase of the program. During the planning stage, it provides a rigorous conceptual framework to assess logic and plausibility of the full chain of events that begins with the problem and its causes, the assumptions and the feasibility of the interventions and program action and ends with the intended change that the program expects to achieve. A well-articulated program theory serves as a simple, yet comprehensive tool, for communicating the program's logic, intentions and desired results with different stakeholders [9], seeking their inputs for verifying the planners' understanding of the problem, assessing the feasibility of interventions, and finally in strengthening their belief in the program. It puts the program plan on a firmer footing, thereby strengthening the support base for the program [9] which is necessary for program implementation and resource mobilization. During implementation, it is a good communication tool to develop a shared understanding of the program logic amongst the program staff, contributing to better implementation [9]. During evaluation, the articulated program theory presents to the evaluators an accurate view of the program from the planners' perspectives.

The program theory has been described in several ways, e.g., the 'logic model', 'program model', 'outcome line', 'theory of change' and 'action theory' [11]. The common feature underlying all of these descriptions is that they map and describe the model of how a program is supposed to work and the process through which program components are presumed to produce the desired effect [10]. Two models of the program theory are described here: (a) the Rossi, Lipsey and Freeman program theory; and (b) the Logical Model.

### *The Rossi, Lipsey and Freeman program theory*

The Rossi, Lipsey and Freeman model of program theory has three inter-related components – the impact theory, the program's organizational plan, and the service utilization plan [11]. The organizational plan and the service utilization plan are together referred to as the process theory (Figure 36.2).

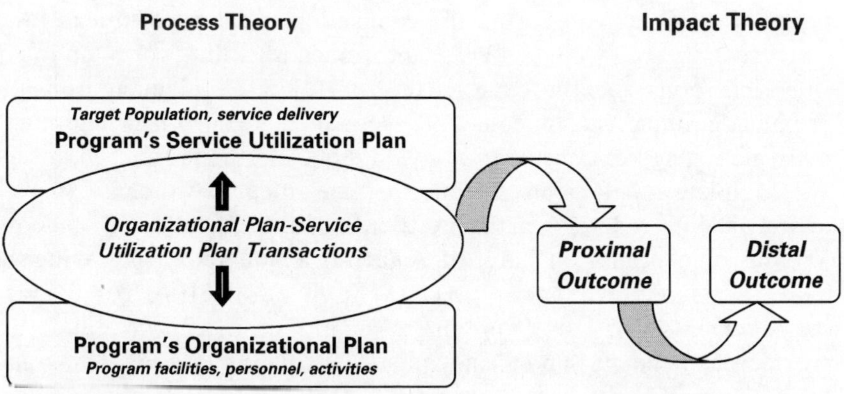


*36.2* Overview of program (*Source*: Adapted from P.H. Rossi et al [11]).

The *impact theory* explains the causal and effect relationship between the program's activities and its intended results. It describes the assumptions around this cause–effect relationship and how the program activities will result in improved conditions to address the problem. The cause–effect relationship could be direct, e.g. when a certain program activity can affect some intermediate condition and lead to the improved outcome [11]. It could also involve a sequence of outcomes leading to the intended change. In this chain of events, direct outcomes are referred to as proximal or immediate outcomes and the outcomes that follow later are the intermediate outcomes and the distal outcomes. The achievement of distal outcomes is dependent on the successful attainment of the proximal outcomes [11].

The cause–effect relationship, in its simplest form has a single pathway. However, in practice, often this relationship is complex and there are multiple pathways leading to the intended change [10]. The cause–effect relationship is often influenced by certain factors, referred to as moderating factors or moderators – influencing either the program-proximal outcome relationship, or the proximal-distal outcome relationship, or both – which could either enhance or constrain the causal linkage [10]. Moderators could be qualitative variables, such as gender, motivation, socio-economic status, or quantitative variables, such as program coverage, the number of contacts [10]. Given the significant influence that moderators could exert on the achievement of a program's intended outcomes, during program development it is crucial to identify the various moderators and the possible influence of these on outcomes, so that these could be addressed to the extent possible.

To illustrate the impact theory, let us assume that a program for pregnant women intends to reduce the prevalence of anemia during pregnancy. It delivers three interventions: (1) dietary counseling; (2) counseling regarding the benefits of iron–folate supplements during pregnancy; (3) distribution of the prescribed number of iron–folate tablets, including treatment dose for anemic women. Assuming that the program is implemented well, the counseling is expected to lead to an increase in the knowledge of pregnant women regarding consumption of iron rich foods and the benefits of iron-folate supplementation, the proximal or immediate outcomes. These immediate outcomes in turn will motivate women to consume improved diets and the prescribed dosage of iron–folate supplements, the intermediate outcome, which is expected to bring about a reduction in the prevalence of anemia, the distal outcome. The pre-conception iron status of women is a moderator. Improving the iron status of adolescent girls through counseling for dietary improvements and iron supplements could significantly reduce the prevalence of anemia in pregnancy (distal outcome). Figure 36.3 diagrams the path to outcomes in this example.

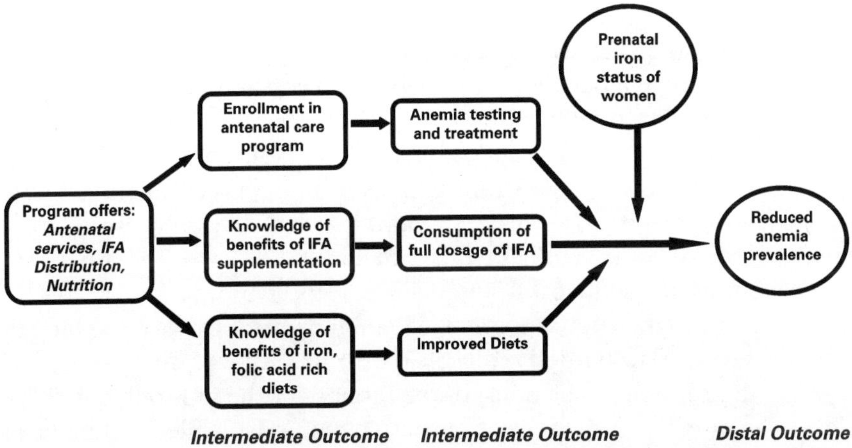


*36.3* Impact theory of the "prevention of anemia in pregnancy" example showing sequence of outcomes and moderator

The Rossi, Lipsey and Freeman theory has been further nuanced by Issel. Issel describes three sets of inter-related relationships – the causal theory (describing the causal linkages), the intervention theory (describing the intervention–causal linkages) and the effect theory (describing the linkages to outcomes) [9]. The effect theory is akin to the impact theory described above. This model is helpful in a step-by-step construction of the impact theory, and is used in Section 36.3 to take the reader through a systematic development of the program theory.

The *process theory* describes the transactions that take place between the program and the participants to actuate the cause–effect relationship – on the program side by the organizational plan and on the participants' side by the service utilization plan. The organizational plan describes the functions, activities, resources (human, financial, and physical) of the program and their organization to deliver the program services [11]. The service utilization plan focuses on the program's service delivery aspects that relate to the program participants – their perspectives, motivation, experiences, socio-cultural background, and so on [11]. The process theory is a good framework to guide the planning of program processes in a manner that integrates the perspectives of the program organization and that of the program beneficiaries or participants.

### *The logical model of program theory*

The 'logical model' or the 'logic model' is another popular tool used to represent the program theory or the logic on which the program produces its presumed effect. It links outcomes (both, short and long term) with program activities and the theoretical assumptions of the program. It is a systematic, visual depiction of the relationship among the resources to deliver the program, the planned activities and the changes or results that are expected to be achieved [12].

The basic logic model consists of five elements – inputs or resources, activities, outputs, outcomes, and impact. Resources include the human, financial, organizational and community resources available to a program to dedicate to performing the activities that will help achieve the intended results. The program activities are the processes, tools, events, technology and actions needed to deliver the program interventions to achieve the intended results. Outputs are the direct products of program activities and may include, for example, the targets for the services to be delivered by the program (e.g., the number of counseling sessions to be held) or the targets for the program coverage (e.g., the number or percent of participants to be enrolled). Outcomes are the specific changes in program participants' behavior, knowledge, skills, status and level of functioning [12] (e.g., increase in numbers or percent of mothers exclusively breast feeding their babies for six months]. These five elements are linked through a chain of reasoning or 'if–then' statements or assumptions (Figure 36.4).

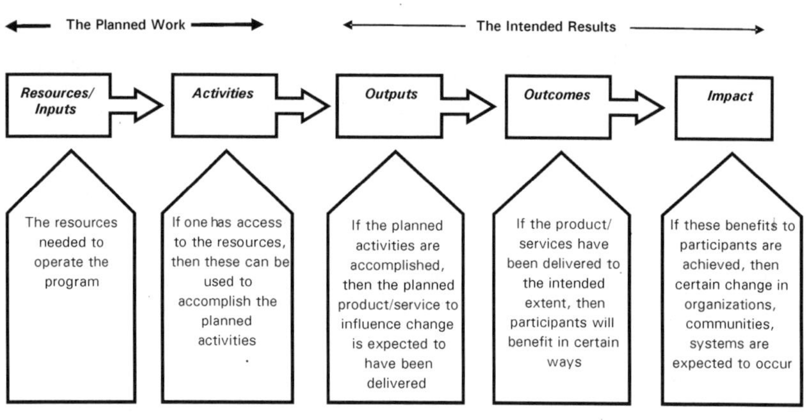


*36.4* The logical model

Outcomes could be short-term, generally those that can be attained within a 1–3 year timeframe, and long-term, those that are attainable in 4–6 years. Impact is the fundamental intended change that the program hopes to achieve as a result of the program activities, and is generally expected over a 7–10 year period [12].

Although there are differences in the logic model representation of the program framework and the program theory described earlier, there are overlaps and consistencies. The logical model's inputs and activities overlap with the process theory; and the outputs, outcomes and impact of the logic model overlap with the impact theory. The prominent difference is that in the logic model all program activities are drawn together without differentiating between the interventions and the activities that will lead to the outcome and other supportive activities, whereas this distinction is clearly made in the process theory [9]. Some believe that because the logic model lays a relatively higher emphasis on inputs and activities, the program rationale may not receive the due attention [9]. In the program theory, on the other hand because of the distinct process and impact theory, both aspects get strong emphasis. Program planners and evaluators must view the above approaches as tools that help to think through and develop plausible programs that have a strong scientific rationale, assess needs and gaps, and develop the entire program and select the one that best suits them.

*Program planning frameworks*

(a) Logical framework

The logical framework (also referred to as 'logframe') is one of the core techniques used widely during the entire project cycle from program planning, through implementation and monitoring to eventually, the evaluation. It is a "cause and effect" model of the program's interventions to bring about the intended results and draws together all key components of the planned project or program into a clear set of statements and communicates in a simple and concise manner, the essential elements of a complex program. At the same time it helps to organize thinking, relate activities and investments to expected results, set a framework for monitoring and evaluation, performance indicators, allocate responsibilities and communicate concisely and unambiguously with all key stakeholders as well as achieve stakeholder consensus [13].

A logframe is a 4 × 4 matrix with a hierarchy of objectives — the project structure, indicators of performance, means of verifying the indicator and important risks and assumptions along the horizontal axis and the goal, purpose, outputs and activities along the vertical' axis (Figure 36.5). The framework uses the if-then logic to work through the matrix and check the logic. Starting at the activities level, the if-then logic means that if we undertake the activities and the assumptions hold true, this will lead to the outputs. If the outputs are produced, and if the assumptions hold true, then the purpose will be achieved. If the purpose is achieved and the assumptions hold true, then the program will contribute to the goals [14].

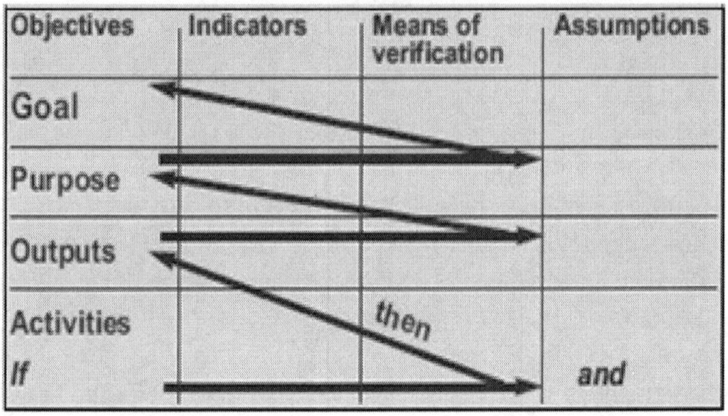


*36.5* The Logical Framework – The 'If'/ 'And'/ 'Then'/ Logic that underlies the logframe approach [14].

Developing the logframe is a collaborative process and a participatory 'team approach' involving program management, staff and all key and primary stakeholders is critical in the development of a good logframe. Stakeholder's commitment and ownership are as important as the technical design, quality and intended results. A logframe is a living document and can be modified during the program implementation as required following a team process [14].

(b) Results framework

The Results framework is a conceptual tool for planning and performance measurement that has been adopted by many development organizations in response to the focus on RBM and the heightened emphasis on development results [15]. The Results framework is a generic term to describe a strategic planning, management and results measurement tool [16]. It is based along the lines of the logical model and is used in many contexts – at the program level, organizational level, country level and the global level. It is used not only to define the results to be achieved but to also describe the context in which results are planned to be achieved, measured and monitored [17].

At a program or project level, the results framework displays the program logic that explains how the development objective is to be achieved, including causal relationships and assumptions underlying these [18]. It diagrams the logical cause-effect relationships between various activity outputs at the bottom, intermediate results or outcomes in the middle, and the strategic development objective at the top [3]. In a results framework, the logical sequence through which a development intervention transforms a set of inputs into specific outputs, outcomes and impacts is depicted through a 'results chain'. The results chain is a plausible causal relationship that described how certain inputs will likely lead to intended outcomes. They form the 'storyline' underlying the program and explains visually the problem(s) that the intervention is trying to address, the desired objective(s) to be achieved, the intermediate results that are critical for achieving the objective(s), and the required arrangements to measure progress towards these objectives. The results framework, thus, facilitates planning, execution, monitoring and evaluation of a development intervention [17].

The distinctive feature of the results framework is that it puts the higher order development objective and intermediate outcomes centre-stage, and is less concerned about defining and measuring the inputs, processes and outputs; whereas in the traditional project approach there is equal emphasis on monitoring all elements of the log-frame hierarchy. A potential danger with this approach is that by concentrating on the higher-order results, their linkages with project activities may become overly vague or disconnected and might compromise activity implementation monitoring. To mitigate this risk, it is suggested that programmer's devote time and attention to also align individual program activities into the overall results framework [3].

*Nutrition-specific planning frameworks*

Nutrition is a complex interplay of many factors, and the determinants of nutrition often lie across many sectors. Many of the nutrition problems seen in a particular target or age group might have their origin in another phase of life. Thus, any nutrition program planning efforts must take into account the various inter-related causes leading to the problem at hand and examine the problem from the perspective of its origin. This is essential to make rational decisions and to identify the most appropriate and effective interventions to address the problem. Two widely accepted frameworks that most public health nutritionists will be familiar with, are presented here as possible frameworks to guide the analysis of the key determinants of the problem and the influencing factors, select the critical intervention points and identify the most appropriate mix of interventions to address the problem.

(a) The nutrition conceptual framework

The conceptual framework presented in Fig. 36.6 (adapted from the UNICEF nutrition framework) is a good tool for the analysis of the causes of child undernutrition, and to select suitable interventions. The framework shows that the immediate causes of undernutrition are inadequate 'food and nutrient intake' and 'infections/disease'. These are influenced by three underlying causes – access to food, maternal and child care practices, and lack of sanitation, hygiene and health services. Income, poverty and its various contributors and the social, political and economic contexts are the major basic causes that contribute to malnutrition. The framework also lays out effective nutrition interventions at each of the levels. Direct nutrition interventions such as infant and young child feeding and caring practices, micronutrient interventions and household hygiene and sanitation address the immediate causes of malnutrition (these are also the short routes to improving nutrition). Agricultural interventions, poverty reduction, education , women's empowerment, health systems improvement are interventions to address the underlying causes (these are the longer routes to improve nutrition but are by no means less important).

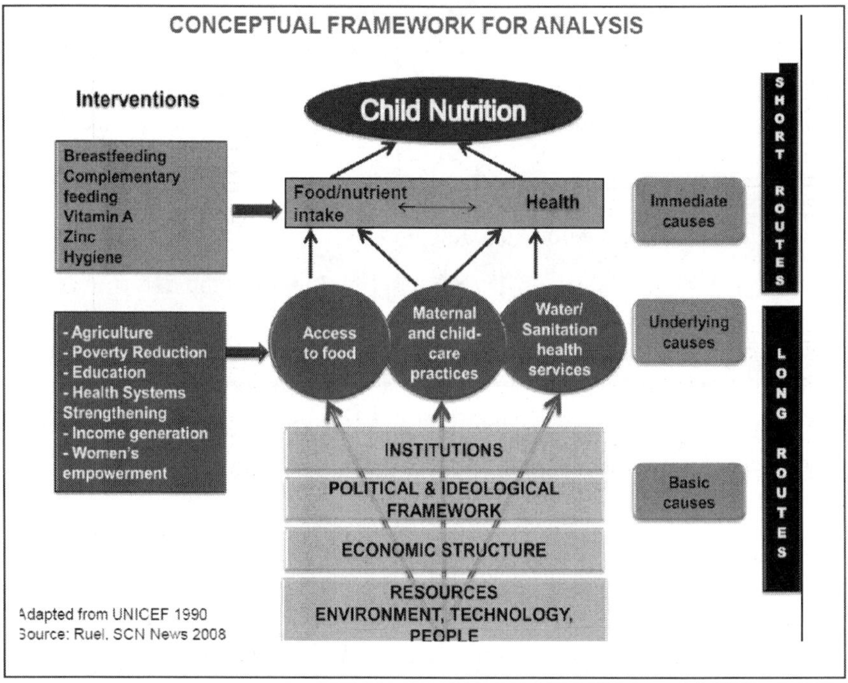


*36.6* Conceptual framework for analysis

While using the malnutrition causal framework, an analysis of the immediate causes (the direct determinants) and the factors at the underlying and basic levels, in the specific context of the particular community is important. There is increasing evidence of the strong association between the poor status of women and higher rates of child malnutrition; this is understood to be one of the key contributors to the high levels of malnutrition in South Asia [19]. Therefore, issues that relate to power equations, gender inequality, low female literacy, and social exclusion are important factors to consider, especially since they constrain the abilities of households, mothers and caregivers to access services and practice appropriate behaviors important to achieving optimum nutrition. It is likely that they strongly moderate the program-outcome pathway and must be fully explored during the community needs assessment.

(b) Nutrition life cycle framework

Examining the nutritional problems through the life cycle approach during planning of public health nutrition programs provides many benefits. First, it highlights the specific nutrition needs, problems and vulnerabilities unique to each of the life cycle stages, thus helping design suitable ways and means to promote good nutrition throughout the life course, taking into consideration the specific nutritional issues and vulnerabilities of that stage [20]. For example, for optimum nutrition during infancy, early and exclusive breast feeding, timely and appropriate complementary feeding, prevention and treatment of infections, continued breast feeding during illnesses, micronutrient supplementation, growth monitoring and promotion are essential for optimum nutrition. Second, health and nutritional problems that manifest during a particular life cycle stage may not wholly depend on the nutritional intakes and status during that particular phase, although nutrition during the specific period may also be compromised or may have also its own unique problems. Nutrition status during an earlier life stage may continue to interact with and affect the nutrition outcomes of the present life stage [20]. For example, better nutrition during pregnancy improves intra-uterine growth, improve birth outcomes, and results in better nutrition for the newborn. Similarly appropriate nutrition during the first two years of life improves physical growth and development, including cognition and brain functions and affects adult height and improved cognitive function. The life cycle approach helps one analyze and consider the relative benefits of intervening in a life stage earlier to the one which presents the nutritional problem, or in both, to achieve the maximum nutrition benefit. It thus helps weigh the criticality of extending the intervention to include another life cycle phase, and select appropriate intervention and approach mix against the consideration of benefits, costs, resource levels, the program time period and so on.

## 36.4 Steps in program planning

This section guides the reader through the preparation for planning, the phases of program planning and the key elements to be considered by the planning team in each phase. For this purpose, the planning process has been organized into six phases – problem identification, envisioning and defining results, selecting interventions, implementation planning, monitoring and evaluation planning and finally planning for program ending. While the phases are distinct, it does not mean that planning would move in a linear manner from one phase to the next. As highlighted earlier, planning is an iterative process that involves going back and forth between the various steps and phases. The development of the program theory is taken up through the example of a hypothetical public health nutrition program, a program to reduce the prevalence of anemia in pregnant women living in a remote tribal area.

## 36.4.1 Getting ready for program planning

Prior to initiating active program planning phases, some preparatory actions are required. These include, putting together a planning team, identifying stakeholders and partners, outlining the planning approach and process, establishing timeline and so on.

*The planning team*

Program planning is best done as a team effort. For nutrition program planning, a team of planners could include the public health nutritionist, health and social science professionals/experts, government representatives, civil society representatives, community members, communication experts, members of the business community, advocates for nutrition. While the decision on who to have on the planning team, how large a planning team to have, and what kind of structure to adopt for the team is very contextual, criteria such as the type of skill mix and expertise needed, engagement of other partners, agencies, and stakeholders – the scope and boundaries for their engagement, the mix of external and internal members on the planning team need to be very carefully considered. Many of these considerations will depend on the internal expertise, experience and capacity of the organization undertaking the planning, the budget allocated or that could potentially be mobilized for the planning effort. The choice of the team leader is another critical consideration. Because many critical technical decisions will need to be made during the planning process, ideally the team leader should bring strong technical skills and leadership qualities to steer the process [9].

*Partnerships*

The program planning phase is the most appropriate phase for forming partnerships, engaging stakeholders, and building ownership towards the program [14]. The exploration and mapping of who is doing what in terms of public health nutrition, or who is interested in doing something to improve the nutrition problem is important. Actively seeking partnerships or ways in which other existing or upcoming programs can complement the program being planned is crucial for coordinated efforts, synergy of purpose, harmonization of strategies and optimal utilization of resources. It is also worthwhile to identify and involve a champion or advocate who will lend weight to the planning team, influence decision makers within an organization or in the larger arena [9].

*Program planning plan and the guiding principles*

Before initiating the planning, the planning team should draw up the program planning plan. This includes, outlining the approach and the process to be followed, establishing timelines, assigning roles and responsibilities, and estimating and securing resources required for the planning effort. Making choices and decisions will be required throughout the planning process, including situations where consensus may not emerge and hard choices would need to be made. Therefore, it is a good practice for the planning team to agree on some key principles to guide decision making. Examples of possible guiding principles are, involving stakeholders in all stages of planning and decision making, the option that is of the maximum benefit to the participants will be preferred over other options all other things being equal, and so on. Such a decision making framework with pre-agreed criteria is a very helpful tool during the planning process.

With these basics in place, the planning team is ready to initiate the planning process outlined in Fig. 36.1 and discussed below.

## 36.4.2 The planning process

*Problem identification and statement*

An accurate understanding of the health problem to be addressed, its dimensions, the causal chain leading to the problem, including the contributing or protective factors, forms the basis for the need of the program, and the foundation upon which the program is built. The problem forms the basis for envisioning the intended change or result for determining the interventions and mechanisms for their delivery, and for measuring the change in the situation as a result of the program. Three key elements of the problem identification phase are information gathering and exploration, prioritization, and articulation of the problem.

*Information gathering and exploration*

One of the key elements of identifying the problem is to collect as much information as possible about the nutrition-related issues in the setting of the proposed program. This involves, first and foremost, searching for the existing data, both qualitative and quantitative from all possible sources, such as literature, survey reports, medical records, data from existing programs and projects – large and small, public and others (NGO, donor-supported, public–private partnership programs) [9] . Planners should carefully review the existing information to identify critical gaps in information that need to be filled through primary data collection and to inform the decision about the type and scope of the community health/ nutrition assessment – frequently referred to as community needs assessment – to be undertaken.

*Community Needs Assessment (CNA)*

The CNA could serve as the starting point for program planning. If the problem is already well understood, then it is a means to verify the problem and assess community needs. In the context of public health nutrition, CNA provides a realistic measure of the situation of nutrition in the particular community, the key problems and their causes, including the factors (moderators) that enhance or limit the problem [21]. For example, the community members' initial awareness about nutrition, what they think and feel about a particular situation, prevalent feeding and caring practices, infant feeding practices are important determinants or contributing factors to the situation of nutrition in the community. In addition, the CNA provides valuable insights in to the health and social aspects that could add to, or undermine the success of the program, e.g., factors like preventive health services, socio-economic conditions, gender and power relations, and motivation to participate.

Not only is the information from a CNA valuable, the process is itself of great value. It provides the opportunity for communities, or their representatives, to get engaged in identifying problems and needs, prioritizing the most important ones, setting goals and objectives and finding solutions to the problem [21]. It also provides the community groups or sponsor agencies the opportunity to assess current programs and policies, the resources available and to identify what may be further required of the programmer and the communities to change things. For the planning team, the CNA serves as an opportunity to identify the different stakeholders and understand their interests.

A CNA can be conducted in many different ways (Box 36.2 for some possible approaches to conducting a CNA). It is important to remember that the CNA may not be a one-time effort and it may be necessary to go back to the community to get stakeholder involvement, and to ensure that the program as being planning is indeed responsive to the problem and the community needs [9].

**Box 36.2 Possible approaches for conducting a Community Needs Assessment**

*A CNA may be conducted using different approaches and processes. For example, existing data can be used, surveys can be designed and conducted, key informants can be interviewed, community foray can be organized, and focus group discussions can be held. Observational data is a relatively inexpensive and unobtrusive manner of gathering information, especially to understand community characteristics, their organization, traditions, and so on. For example, walking through a village weekly market may provide a good sense of who does the food shopping and makes decision about what is to be bought – the men or the women? Do men and women interact freely with each other? This information, for instance, will inform decisions about the critical target audience for a nutrition education program and whether to conduct joint or separate sessions for men and women. Depending upon the time and resources available to the planning team, any of these approaches or a combination of sorts can be used. A series of 2-3 stakeholder workshops that bring together representatives from across the relevant community constituencies, e.g., men and women, community leaders, opinion makers are often used as an efficient way of determining community needs. No matter whichever approach is followed, it is important to have information on the magnitude of the problem, the causative factors specifically as they pertain to the problem in that context, population characteristics, attitudes and behaviors.*

*Problem analysis and prioritization*

The process of prioritization and decision making to select the problem(s) to be addressed can be both overwhelming and challenging - overwhelming, because it requires organizing, analyzing large amounts of information collected from multiple sources, which may not always be consistent with each other; challenging, because of the potential for lack of consensus arising from the varied interests of the different stakeholders and possible biases of particular team members, especially towards their area of expertise. It is usually helpful to first, involve as many stakeholders as possible and involve communities in the prioritization of the problem, and second, to adopt a framework of rational criteria for decision making. Some criteria, such as the magnitude of the problem, its severity, the availability of effective interventions and so on, are useful to consider during prioritization (Box 36.3 for a description of some of the criteria to consider during prioritization).

**Box 36.3 Possible criteria for prioritization of public health nutrition problems**

**Magnitude of the problem**

From the public health nutritionist's view, the magnitude or the size of the problem is its relative deviation from a normally acceptable level or norm (the normative need), reflected through measures such as mortality rates, prevalence rates, relative risks, or through quality measures such as QALYs and DALYs. From the community's perspective, the expressed need coming out of the CNA reflects the magnitude in terms of the relative demand for or utilization of services. It is possible that the normative need and the expressed need are not consistent and it may be challenging to give full consideration to both during prioritization.

Severity or the importance of the problem: This should be carefully considered, since at times the most severe problem may affect only a small proportion of the population. It is possible, as is generally the case with nutritional problems that the problem is silent until the damage is done. For instance, underweight and stunting in children might not be noticed unless very severe but results in permanent damage to physical and mental growth; micronutrient deficiencies such as anemia, iodine deficiency disorders are not visible until very late.

**Potential effectiveness of the interventions**

Problems with causes that have a higher potential to being modified through an intervention might receive a relatively higher priority over others on this criteria. Technically effective nutrition interventions for most of the public health nutrition problems, especially undernutrition are known. The Lancet series on Maternal and Child Undernutrition (2008) has laid out a comprehensive set of efficacious solutions that have been shown to work under all contexts.

**Potential availability of resources**

The approximate estimated costs of addressing the different problems and how these match with the available or potentially available resources is another consideration. This criterion could determine the number of problems that would be feasible for the program to address. Yet other criteria related to costs of the program and the program's potential to address the problem are cost-effectiveness, cost- benefit ratios and costs per program participant.

**Organizational priorities and comparative advantages**

The prioritized problems and actions to address them must be aligned to the strategic priorities of the organization undertaking the planning and should preferably be able to capitalize on its comparative advantages.

It is helpful to develop a prioritization matrix with the prioritizing criteria against the X-axis and the problem against the Y-axis. Scoring each of the identified problems against the criteria in the matrix (which can be assigned weights according to their relative importance in the given context), or simply assigning a high/low value and then prioritizing on the basis of the scores is one rational way to prioritize problems [8]. It is important to remember that such a matrix serves only as a framework for decision-making and is not a mathematical calculation tool. Planning teams can design their own prioritization tools or mechanism to suit their needs.

Problem analysis and prioritization is not a linear process, and the need to re-prioritize may emerge as analysis progresses. It is possible that a problem initially thought to be of high priority might either not be amenable to change, or might not be within the program's scope, or that it is not politically or culturally feasible, or that verification with stakeholders or through the CNA indicates differently [9].

### *Developing the causal theory*

The first step in developing the causal theory is to get an accurate understanding of the health problem, its dimensions, the causal chain leading to the problem, including the main causative factors and influencing factors contributing to or limiting the problem. This is essential to clarify the causal links and determine vital pathways that can be modified with known interventions. One helpful way is to diagram the problem and the full causal chain, including the influencing factors. The chain diagram provides the framework to link the causative factors to the program's interventions. It is in fact, a good idea to diagram several of the top ranked problems [9]. Doing so will expose the problems for which one or more causal factors that may exist are not within the scope or manageable interest of the program, thus helping further prioritization.

While developing the causal chain it is important to draw upon the scientific evidence base, at the same time draw upon the CNA and the specific context and environment of the problem. In the instance of public health nutrition, while there is a good evidence base for a large number of the problems, it is imperative to verify the operating causative factors in the context in which the problem is situated, and identify the socio-cultural and other factors that either contribute to the known causes or offer a protective effect.

It is also important to examine the causes of the nutrition problem, particularly in the instance of maternal and child undernutrition, from the malnutrition causal framework and the life-cycle framework described earlier in Section 36.2. The former will help explore which particular aspect(s) of the immediate causes of nutrition – food insecurity, lack of appropriate care, lack of health services, are the most pervasive, which ones might be affecting specific socio-economic groups and so on. The life-cycle framework will help understand the origin of the problem and examine the relative effectiveness and benefits of the intervention points.

Once the casual diagram is completed, it must be shared with different stakeholders and the program population for a reality check. This is a crucial step. If the diagnosis of the problem and its causal chain is not accurate, no matter how good the interventions and their implementation, the program will not produce the intended effect [9].

The development of the causal chain for problem in our example of the high prevalence of anemia is illustrated in Fig. 36.7. The causal chain shows the causes for the high prevalence of anemia, the influencing factors and moderators.

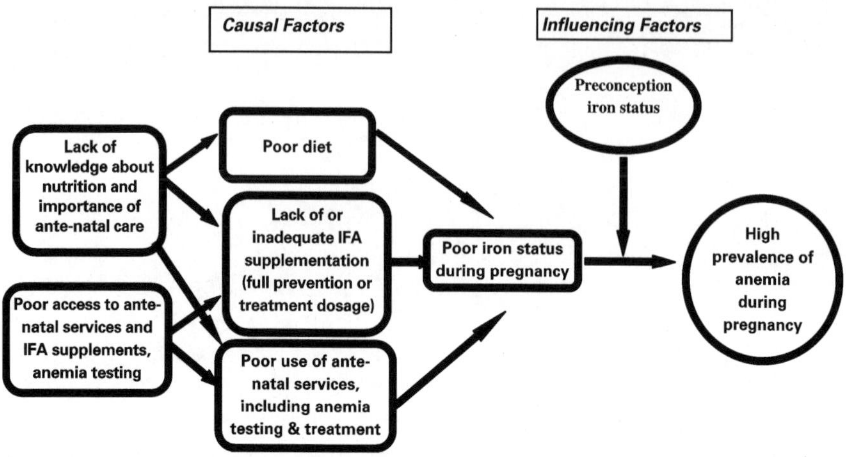


*36.7* Causal chain of the anemia in pregnancy example

### *Formulating the problem statement*

There is no one prescribed way to state the problem. This can be done in innumerable ways, as long as it explains the causes of the problem with all the linkage such that it facilitates choosing the appropriate intervention and intervention point. Issel provides a very comprehensive template for the problem statement that facilitates directly linking causal statement to the different elements of program design and evaluation [9]. Using a slightly modified version[3] of this template, the problem statement for the high prevalence rates of anemia in pregnancy example could be articulated as follows:

The high prevalence of (anemia) among (pregnant women in tribal villages of India), indicated by (the low hemoglobin concentrations of < 12 g), is caused by (low intake of dietary iron, lack of access to ante-natal services and to iron-folate supplements), and is influenced by (poor pre-pregnancy iron status, lack of knowledge about benefits of iron-folate supplementation).

Issel's template helps to provide the framework that link each aspect of the problem statement to the program development and to the program evaluation. For example,in the above problem statement, the high prevalence of (*Health problem*) part of the problem statement directly relates to the *goal* for the program to be kept in mind during program development and to the outcome evaluation; the among *(population/community*) part defines the 'targeted participants' for program development purposes and the 'intervention group' during evaluation; the indicated in (health outcome indicators) part of the statement are the 'outcome indicator/s' selected during program development and their achievement is assessed during evaluation;

[3] This modified template uses the term 'influencing factors' to collectively reflect the terms 'mediating factors' and 'antecedents' used by Issel in the context of the causal theory, since this text uses the terms 'moderating' and 'mediating' factors as described in the Rossi, Lipsey, Freeman model as factors operating between the proximal and distal outcomes.

the is caused by (causative factors) and is influenced by (influencing factors) part of the statement helps determine the interventions during program development and represent the outcomes during evaluation.

Once the problem statement is defined, the next step is to envision the change in respect of the problem that the program intends to bring about, and set concrete goals and objectives for the program.

### 36.4.3 Envisioning and defining results

*Setting goals and objectives*

This step of program planning focuses on envisioning and defining the results that the program intends to achieve, setting goals and objectives, selecting indicators, and setting targets. In many texts, setting goals and objectives is suggested as a step that follows selection of interventions and the development of the logical model or the program impact theory. However, given the centrality of results to program planning, beginning with the desired vision of change and articulation of the goals and objectives is useful. This approach aids in the selection of interventions and the further development of the program with an eye on the planned results. However, just as in other aspects of planning, setting goals and objectives is a non-linear and iterative process. Goals and objectives flow from the health problem, and are linked to the interventions and program activities. Therefore, on one hand while objectives and targets may drive the choice of interventions, on the other they may need to be adjusted or revised based on the interventions, e.g. their feasibility, dosage, intensity, and such other factors.

Goals are broad statements of the desired status of nutrition or health to which the program results contribute. In terms of the results framework and the results chain order, goals correspond to the highest order of results at the top of the chain and are expected to be achieved over a long term horizon. Objectives correspond to the outcomes; and several objectives may contribute to the achievement of a goal [17]. For example, improved maternal nutrition (objective) and child nutrition (another objective) and several others such as those related to prevention and timely treatment of infections, improving sanitation and hygiene contribute to reducing child mortality (goal). Goal statements are not necessarily made in measurable terms.

Objectives are specific measurable statements of desired change, generally in an outcome such as the knowledge, behavior, biochemical parameter or another intermediate outcome such as policy, but could at times be related to process changes that the program intends to bring about. Well-defined objectives clearly state what will change, by how much or to what extent, and by when [9]. They guide the further development of the program, serve as the programmer's framework for decision making and resource allocation, and provide a structure for program evaluation [22].

Program objectives are derived from the analysis of the problem and can be stated in many different ways. It could be stated in terms of increasing or decreasing, improving or reducing a certain outcome, or it could be stated in terms of maintaining current levels, if a deteriorating trend calls for maintaining current levels, or in terms of a level of achievement (e.g. reducing by 10 percent). No matter how the objective is stated, it must address the what, by when, and by how much of the intended change in relation to the problem [9].

### *Selecting indicators*

Indicators are measurable parameters that directly or indirectly measure program outcomes, outputs and processes. They are used to track program performance and determine the success or failure of a program. Given their importance in measuring and judging program performance, indicators must be selected with great care. An indicator must be relevant and meaningful, i.e., it must be closely related to the effect or to the key process that it measures and must also be meaningful to program personnel; it must be sensitive to showing change within the timeframe of the objective or outcome, else it could dilute or not capture the intended change; it should be feasible to collect data on the indicator at a reasonable cost; standardized tools must either exist (or be developed and standardized) for data collection; and finally certain indicators might be mandated by some donors/funding agencies [9, 14].

Objectively Verifiable Indicators (OVIs) are standards against which change can be measured. They set targets in terms of Quantity, Quality and Time (QQT). Indicators should be specific, usable, measurable, sensitive, cost-effective, and available. Two acronyms are widely used to characterize good indicators – SMARTER which refers to **S**pecific **M**easurable **A**chievable **R**ealistic **T**ime-Bound + **E**njoyable **R**ewarding, and SPICED which refers to **S**ubjective, **P**articipatory, **I**ndirect, **C**ross-Checked, **E**mpowering, **D**iverse [14].

### Box 36.4 Types of indicators [14]

**Direct and proxy indicators**

Direct indicators are those that relate to directly observable change. These are simply a more precise, comprehensive and operational restatement of the respective objective. Indirect or proxy indicators are used when the expected changes are not directly observable like the quality of life, organizational development; or if the costs of measuring direct indicators is not justified; or if they are measurable beyond the life span of the activity. Proxy indicators may be used instead of, or in addition to direct indicators.

**Cross-Sector indicators**

Sector-based or technical indicators must be balanced by the inclusion of other more cross-sector indicators; for example relating to social issues, gender, the environment, and capacity building.

**Formative and summative indicators**

Formative indicators are set with a time-frame to be measured during part of, or across the whole of, an activity; hence, they are really synonymous with milestones. Summative indicators are used to measure performance at the end.

**Qualitative and quantitative indicators**

Quantitative indicators measure magnitude of change in quantitative terms. These are not able to capture change that is difficult to quantify. Qualitative indicators capture qualitative data and may not be straightforward. Process indicators are usually qualitative and assess the how of activities or processes. For example, how technologies were developed and adopted, how income was generated, and who was involved. These may at times be subjective and can be verified with end-users and participants, but may still be less than fully objective. It is best to have a mix of quantitative and qualitative indicators.

*Setting targets*

Targets are numerical values that depict the level of desirable change in an objective or an indicator as a result of the program. A target normally has two parts. One part states the magnitude of change and the other states the date or time period by which the change will be achieved [9]. Estimating and assigning numerical values to the magnitude of expected change is a complex task and informed judgments are required to set realistic and achievable targets. Estimations should be based on a rational basis, such as, trend analysis that can be undertaken through literature review, drawing upon experience from similar programs, examining the magnitude of the effect of the intervention from efficacy or effectiveness trials, using objectives set by a state or national plan or a combination of some of these bases. Some possible ways to make rational decisions pertaining to target setting are briefly discussed below.

When the current state of health or nutrition is to be maintained, then it is best to use the current baseline as the target. Another method is to use prescribed norms or targets, e.g., those prescribed by national goals or planning documents. Depending upon where the existing parameter value of the target population lies in relation to the national value, this method can also be nuanced to better suit the program. For example, if the target population lies far below the national target, then a reasonable percentage of the national target (chosen against considerations of intervention intensity, its efficacy and the other parameters discussed earlier) could be used. If disaggregated data for the national value is available, then many other options could be used, such as 50 percent of the best or the target of the middle ranking, and so on depending on where the target population lies in relation to the national or sub-national values. For setting multi-year program targets, the cumulative value of estimated annual change (based on some of the above parameters) may be used to determine the program targets. Another option is to calculate the target that would be required to demonstrate a statistically significant magnitude of change, although this method could lead to selecting highly ambitious targets [23, 9]. A set of options for setting targets for objectives suggested by the Public Health Foundation, USA in Box 36.5 can be helpful in selecting an appropriate method for setting targets.

**Box 36.5 Possible methods to use in setting targets for objectives**

- Use an absolute percentage to indicate a "reasonable" change over the period. For example, an absolute decline of 1% of the current level adds to 10% over the decade. Be careful to calculate the % for the numbers from the beginning of the decade or it will be a compounded percentage achieved (as below).
- Use a compounded percentage to both indicate a "reasonable" change over the period but one which becomes less than the absolute. For instance, a decline of 1% each year from the previous year over the period of a decade is actually 9.6% $(1-(.99)^{9})$ and not 10% as above. Reverse this calculation to obtain the annual percentage change if you have a total that you'd like to achieve by the end of the decade.
- Use the current U.S. rate as the challenge point. This works when the state or community rate is worse than the U.S. rate and within a distance achievable. This works when the jurisdiction is deemed "like the U.S." or average in some way.
- Use the median values of one's peers. The Community Health Status Indicators (CHSI) Project has generated 88 peer groupings of counties that share similar characteristics. These characteristics include factors that are thought to influence community-level health. This target works when the U.S. rate is too high or too low for the type of jurisdiction. For instance, southern states tend to have more poverty and so to compare health outcomes to the U.S. rate is too much of a challenge.
- Adopt the Healthy People 2010 targets for the indicators. When the jurisdiction cannot decide and when its current levels are similar to the U.S., the actual Healthy People targets may be very appropriate as well as ready and easy to use.
- Calculate the "better than the best" (used in Healthy People 2010) - setting a target better than the current status of the best population group in the state.
- Calculate the "best of the best" (Allison 1999) - benchmarking against the top 10% in any area of the U.S.
- Calculate what's achievable based on clinical or community trials. For instance, breast and colon cancer deaths can be reduced by 30-40% of the peak in breast cancer in the mid 1980's and by the same amount in colon cancer today. Consideration needs to be made in how quickly intervention (in this case, screening) will affect the death rate and how effectively the intervention will be launched in the community.

*Source*: Public Health Foundation (11/00), Setting Target Levels for Objectives.

It is important to involve the stakeholder in setting objectives and targets. This builds ownership, creates a better understanding of the program, and gets their commitment. If it is not possible to develop these with the stakeholders, a final reality check with them is essential.

### 36.4.4 Selecting interventions

*The intervention package*

Interventions are the actions that are undertaken to alter the causal pathway to effect the desired change. These may exert their effect by either directly acting on the cause, by altering the influencing or moderating factors. The causal statement provides the starting point for selection of interventions. For each problem with all its causes, influencing factors and moderating factors, there will be several interventions to choose from [9]. Therefore, selecting the most feasible, and the most cost-effective intervention or set of interventions, usually referred to as intervention package, is required. Several criteria useful in making the right choice of interventions include: the efficacy of the intervention which indicates the strength of the cause–effect relationship; the feasibility of the intervention and its delivery (technical, administrative, social, geographical and political); its adaptability, e.g., to be tailored to the specific target age groups, cultural and linguistic settings; the cost as assessed by cost–benefit ratios, cost-effectiveness, or costs and benefits [9, 24].

The efficacy and effectiveness of several nutrition interventions is known. A list of effective nutrition interventions to address the major public health nutrition problems for which a strong evidence base exists have been presented in the 2008 Lancet Series on Maternal and Child Nutrition [4]. Box 36.6 presents a list of these interventions. Another set of prioritized interventions, the short routes and the long routes to improving nutrition from "Repositioning Nutrition: a Call for Reform and Action" is presented in Box 36.7 [25]. Nutrition program planners can select the most appropriate interventions package in the specific context of their program and the problem.

*The intervention dosage*

The term intervention dosage refers to the amount, strength and duration of the intervention [9]. As related to nutrition interventions, dosage could be measured in terms of milligrams or micrograms of a specific nutrient or micronutrient administered over a specified number of days, or it could be specified in terms of the number of days, or hours of nutrition education, or weeks of counseling and so on. The dose-response can influence outcome, therefore the dosage of the intervention exposure needs to be carefully considered. For some interventions, such as vitamin A or iron supplementation, well established protocols specify the intervention dosage. However, for interventions such as nutrition education or counseling, a critical component of most nutrition program intervention packages, the knowledge base on dose-response is not yet conclusive and requires more research [26]. Given this situation selecting the dosage may be a difficult task. Nevertheless, decisions will need to be made regarding

**Box 36.6 Interventions that effect maternal and child undernutrition. [4]**

| Sufficient evidence for implementation in all 36 countries | Evidence for implementation in specific, situational contexts |
|---|---|
| **Maternal and birth outcomes** | |
| Iron folate supplementation | Maternal supplements of balanced energy and protein |
| Maternal supplements of multiple micronutrients | Maternal iodine supplements |
| Maternal iodine through Iodisation of salt | Maternal deworming in pregnancy |
| Maternal calcium supplementation | Intermittent preventive treatment for malaria |
| Interventions to reduce tobacco consumption or indoor air pollution | Insecticide-treated bednets |
| **Newborn babies** | |
| Promotion of breastfeeding (individual and group counselling) | Neonatal vitamin A supplementation |
| | Delayed cord clamping |
| **Infants and children** | |
| Promotion of breastfeeding (individual and group counselling) | Conditional cash transfer programmes (with nutritional education) |
| Behaviour change communication for improved complementary feeding* | |
| Zinc supplementation | Deworming |
| Zinc in management of diarrhea | Iron fortification and supplementation programmes |
| Vitamin A fortification or supplementation | Insecticide-treated bednets |
| Universal salt iodisation | |
| Handwashing or hygiene interventions | |
| Treatment of severe acute malnutri-tion | |

* Additional food supplements in food-insecure populations.

the number of educational contacts, activities, length of contact, duration of the intervention, type of communication channels to be used and so on. Review of prior nutrition education program experience, advice from social science, especially behavior change experts, identifying a suitable theory are some of the ways that can inform the decision making regarding intervention dosage.

*Further developing the program impact theory/effect theory*

This section builds upon the causal theory developed in the previous section to further develop the intervention and the impact theory.

The intervention theory explains how the interventions affect the causal

**Box 36.7 Routes to better nutrition [25]**

| *Demand-side behavior change* | *Supply-side incentives* | *Demand-side incentives* |
|---|---|---|
| | *Long routes* | |
| • Primary health services (such as family planning) and infectious disease control<br>• Safe water and sanitation<br>• Policies on marketing breast milk substitutes<br>• Food and agricultural policies to increase supply of safe and healthy food, or of healthier foods<br>• Food industry development and market incentives (disincentives) for developing healthy (unhealthy) food<br>• Fruit and vegetable production<br>• Parks, bike paths, recreation centers | • Economic development (incomes of the poor)<br>• Participatory programs and policy development<br>• Employment creation<br>• Fiscal and food price policies to increase poor peoples' purchasing power for the right kind of foods<br>• Marketing regulation of unhealthy foods | • Improving women's status<br>• Reducing women's workload, especially in pregnancy<br>• Increasing women's education |
| | *Short routes* | |
| • Community-based nutrition and health services (community growth promotion programs, community Integrated Management of Childhood Illnesses [C-IMCI])<br>• Facility-based nutrition and health services (health and nutrition services, and antenatal care)<br>• Micronutrient supplements<br>• Micronutrient fortification<br>• Targeted food aid<br>• Biofortification | • Conditional cash transfers<br>• Microcredit cum nutrition education<br>• Food supplementation<br>• Micronutrient supplements<br>• Food stamps<br>• Targeted food aid | • Maternal nutrition, knowledge, and care-seeking during pregnancy and lactation<br>• Infant and young child feeding<br>• Weight control education<br>• Hygiene education<br>• Promoting healthy life styles (increase physical activity; consume more fruits and vegetables and less salt, sugar, and fat, and so on) |

*Source:* Repositioning Nutrition as Central to Development: A strategy for Large Scale Action, World Bank, 2006

factors, including the influencing factors and how they interact with them, and includes a description of the relationship between the intervention and the outcome [9]. The articulation of the intervention theory enables planners to fully understand the relative ability of interventions to significantly alter the key causal factors in the specific context of the program situation, identify any factors that may be outside the manageable interest or the purview of the program and prioritize, and refine the intervention or the intervention package. It helps program staff to understand the rationale for the intervention; and during evaluation it presents to the evaluators the planners' view of the cause–effect framework [9].

Given the multiple cause–effect linkages and cross-cutting relationships that exist in real-life situations, developing the cause–effect theory can be a complex task [11]. It requires drawing on the literature and existing knowledge, using intuition, creativity with logical thinking and reasoning to contextualize the established causal relationships to the program situation, and realistically assess the risks and assumptions [11, 9]. Stakeholder engagement is particularly valuable – it brings to the table new ideas, exposes perspectives and experiences that might otherwise be missed, and provides the necessary logic and reality check. It could be helpful to get some expertise and experience in developing program theory, e.g. a researcher or evaluator to help develop a valid, plausible and well-articulated program theory.

In order to develop the intervention theory, planners need to identify and transpose next to the causes and/or influencing factors, one or more interventions (selected on the basis discussed earlier) that will interact with and alter that specific causal pathway. This exposes the points of interventions, their relative effects, and the points at which weak or no causal linkages exist and forms the basis of selecting the most appropriate and effective interventions that the program will undertake.

Taking the earlier example of reducing anemia prevalence in pregnant women, the intervention theory transposed against the causal theory developed earlier is diagrammed in Fig. 36.8.

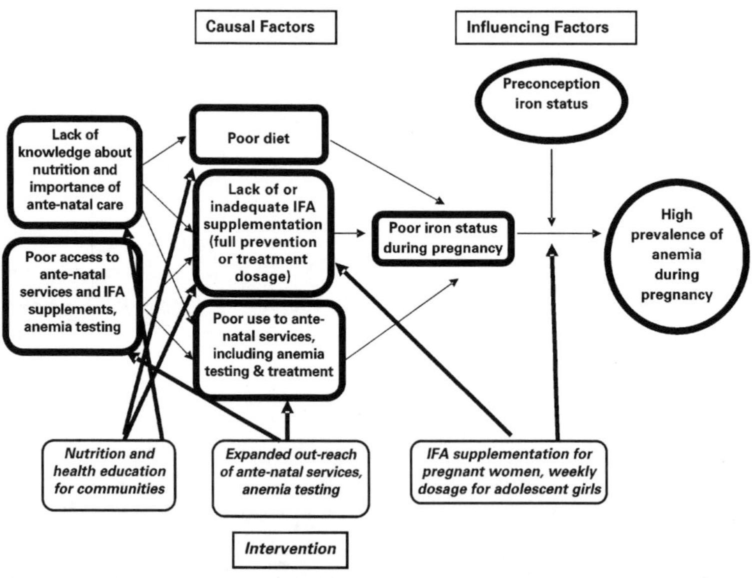


*36.8* Intervention theory showing points of altering of causal chain and influencing factors

The next step is to articulate the impact theory. The impact theory specifies the relationship between proximal, intermediate and distal outcomes or the expected impact. This requires identifying the operating moderating factors that influence the relationship between the proximal and distal outcomes, and the actions that the program will take directly, or leverage from existing program to positively impact the relationship. The impact theory for the prevention of anemia in pregnancy example is diagrammed in Fig. 36.3.

As developing the three sets of relationships is an iterative process, the articulation of the impact theory may require going back to the causal theory or even to the CNA to theorize which of the interventions will be effective in the specific context of the particular community or program. Once the program theory is articulated, it must be reviewed and validated with stakeholders. At this point goals, objectives and targets must be reviewed to better judge if these are attainable or to consider any revisions that might seem necessary [11].

The strength and the validity of the program intervention can be only as strong and valid as the impact theory. If the cause and effect relationship is not valid or very weak, no matter how well and careful planned and implemented, the program will not lead to the anticipated result [10]. A valid impact theory must be supported by evidence that the cause and effect relationship assumed actually exists. This evidence can come from research, prior program experiences, efficacy or effectiveness trials. If none of these is available, then a smaller operations research could be considered prior to developing a large-scale program.

### *Planning for program implementation*

The best and most effective interventions, if not delivered as conceived, in the planned dosage, in the right manner, at the right time, in the right sequence, at the right place will not lead to the desired results. The strongest of the cause–effect relationship might theoretically exist, yet if that interaction is constrained in the actual transaction that will put the theory into practice, expected results will not be achieved. Thus robust plans for program implementation are crucial to develop and test prior to the full-scale implementation of the program. Planning for program implementation essentially means detailing the 'process theory' of the program. The section below describes key aspects of developing the service utilization and the organisation plan – the two key elements of the 'process theory'.

#### (i) Developing process theory

A useful starting point is to use the program process theory framework to define the various aspects of the service utilization plan and the organizational plan [9]. Implementation planning includes planning for implementation structures, arrangements, resources – human, physical, financial, the logistics, and so on (components of the organizational plan) that will deliver the planned interventions in the planned dosage and manner to the program participants in a way that recognizes and responds to their needs, motivates them to participate in the program and utilize the services for the duration required for the effect to be produced (components of the service utilization plan).

(a) Service utilization plan – Developing elements of the service utilization plan to feed into the development of the organizational plan is a logical good practice, although much back-and-forth between the two is to be expected. For example, human resources – a key element of the organizational plan – can only be appropriately assessed once the program's participants or target clients, place of delivery, ways of reaching out to them and the activities have been finalized, which are all elements of the service utilization plan. Taking the example of reduction of the prevalence of anemia in pregnant women, the service utilization plan will delve into questions such as: What will motivate pregnant women in the particular community setting that the program is expected to target to enroll in and attend ante-natal clinics? What are the barriers and constraints to their participation or in taking iron–folate tablets? It will outline appropriate measures that respond to these issues and factor these into program development. For example, the constraints identified are distance to clinics and resistance by family elders and men. The responses could be either provision of services nearer home or provision of transport/transport costs to address the distance issue, and counseling of family elders and men about the importance of antenatal care for the health and well being of the mother and the baby. One of the first and foremost aspects of the service utilization plan is defining the target population, setting eligibility criteria for participation (if it is not targeted to the entire population), determine ways to maximize the inclusion of those who are eligible for services (e.g., through outreach communication, enrollment drives and so on), and minimize the inclusion of those who do not need the services (e.g., through screening methods) [9]. Both, inclusion into the program of those who do not need the program services and will not benefit from them, and under-inclusion of those who need the program services and would benefit from them, amount to sub-optimal provision services to the target group and could undermine the effect of the program. There are also implications for resource use and any further economic analysis undertaken during evaluation or otherwise [9].

The social marketing theory and its 'four Ps' – product, place, price and promotion, is one useful way to apply to developing aspects of the program participant perspectives of their interaction with the program

[9]. As applicable to nutrition programs, the 'product' is the service to be delivered, the 'place' is the most appropriate place for service delivery from the participants' viewpoint, the 'price' relates to the constraints and barriers of the participants in accessing the program services (just as the price of a product would take into account the purchasing power constraints of the buyer), the 'promotion' is about creating awareness of the services, and motivation and incentives to utilize the services until the duration of the program [9].

Analysis of social dynamics and cultural aspects such as power equations, women's status, literacy levels, gender, linguistic preferences, and environmental issues need to be considered during the development of the service utilization plan. It is possible that while developing the service utilization plan, one might need to revisit the CNA findings or consult program participants or community representatives.

(b) Organizational plan – Having determined these aspects, an organizational plan that is responsive to the service utilization plan can be developed. Again taking the example of the reducing the prevalence of a*nemia in pregnant women program*, the organizational plan will delve into questions such as the kind of personnel, their organization, skills and capacities required to perform the program functions and deliver services, e.g., enrolling pregnant women into the program, counseling them, questions about when, where, which screening tests and by whom will be undertaken to screen anemic women. What will be the protocols for iron-folate distribution? What are the follow-up mechanisms needed? Will the program be delivered at clinics or at outreach centers? Some of the key components of the organizational plan that are important to consider during planning include the organization and delivery of the program interventions and activities, the organization and management of program resources – human, physical, financial and time, policies and systems including management, administrative, financial, logistics systems, monitoring and information systems. While estimating the financial resource requirement and planning for monitoring and management information systems is discussed in subsequent sections, the salient points pertaining to the other aspects are discussed here.

(i) *Activity implementation plan* – Planning for the delivery of program interventions and carrying out the program activities in an organized timely manner should take into account the information obtained from the service utilization plan. The terms intervention and activities are sometimes used interchangeably, but here they are used as distinct from each other. For example, nutrition education is the selected intervention in a certain program However, in order to conduct nutrition education successfully, several activities will need to be performed –

activities not only to deliver the education session but activities that will motivate the participants to come for the sessions. Listing the key activities that need to be performed, their sequencing and frequency, the responsible person, the timing and the timeline for their being undertaken and completed are critical aspects of planning related to activities. A detailed implementation plan that shows the activities, when these will be initiated and concluded, who will be responsible for the activity is a good planning tool. A separate timeline or a PERT chart could also be useful tools to plan, manage and monitor activities as well as timelines.

(ii) *Physical and material resources* – These include the physical infrastructure or the facilities to house the program offices, the office furniture, equipment, supplies, including computer software, required to run the program offices. On the program delivery side, it includes facilities such as the centers from which services are to be delivered, their location, furniture and equipment including equipment associated with service delivery or screening (e.g., for nutrition programs these may include weighing scales, height boards, mid-upper arm circumference tapes), the supplies, including registers and records and the supplies to be delivered to the participant (e.g., micronutrient supplements, supplemental food), communication material (e.g., videos, print material, flip charts), and the logistics and supply chain to ensure an uninterrupted supply. Planning for physical resource planning, especially the aspects that relate to the program's interface with the participants, should take account of the information from the service utilization plan.

(iii) *Human resources* – Human resources are the most critical of all program resources and usually forms the largest proportion of the program cost. Planning for human resources includes anticipating and planning for need for the number and type of personnel, types of expertise, skills, experience and capacities required, organization and location of personnel, associated teams and/or hierarchies, their recruitment and retention, training, performance, accountability, motivation, incentives and rewards. If the program has a role for volunteers, the specific roles for them, their recruitment and training, incentives, their motivations should be planned for separately as these are likely to be different from the regular program staff. Similarly, if the program plans to associate personnel from an existing program, its rationale and feasibility should be carefully assessed, in terms of how much can be realistically expected from them, their skill sets, and whether it potentially creates competing priorities. Personnel needs should also be thought of in terms of the program leadership and management functions, as well as the support functions for the program – technical support, and administrative support including financial and procurement. An organizational chart is a good tool to depict how personnel are organized into work groups or teams, the relationship of these work groups, the chains of authority and responsibilities, the reporting relationships, and so on. It also shows how the program is located within the organization as the cross support from other programs and the like can be depicted in the organization chart.

(iv) *Policies, protocols and systems* – Integral to good implementation is the development and adoption of sound policies, systems, operations manuals that will guide program personnel and operations. Some of the key policies and systems pertain to human resources – their recruitment, remuneration and benefits, performance, training, incentives; administration, finance management and procurement; communication and information systems. It is very likely that the organization doing the planning or to implement the program already has the necessary policies and systems in place and new ones do not need to be developed for the program. However, these should be reviewed in term of the program's need. For example, the organization's policy might be to have all staff located at determined centralized levels. The service utilization plan demands that service providers deliver services at the community level, thereby making it impossible for some service providers to be located at centralized locations. Under circumstances such as the one arising in this example, existing policies might need to be modified or special exceptions will be required. The need to develop specific protocols and operations manuals for the program must be examined in earnest. These are necessary to ensure that the program maintains fidelity to its design and is delivered in a standardized manner as conceptualized.

Assessing and testing the organizational and service utilization plan is important. Are these appropriate to not only operationalize the impact theory but relate appropriately to the actual situation and circumstances of the program and the participants it serves? Are the procedures and functions well defined and adequate for the purpose, viewed both from the perspectives of the program managers as well as the program participants? Such questions are helpful to assess the implementation plan. If the program being planned is large and complex and, especially if it is trying new approaches for implementation, it is wise to run a pilot-test for implementation at a small scale before implementing the program at full scale. The learning from the piloting should be used to revise or modify the implementation plan. Similarly any new material resources, protocols or operational guidelines must be pre-tested. Pre-testing can be done in several ways – having focus group reviews, testing in the community where the program will operate, seeking expert opinion and comments.

Figure 36.9 shows a graphic display of the program theory – the impact and the process theory, including elements of the organizational plan and the service utilization plan, for the prevention of anemia in pregnancy example.

## 36.5 Estimating and securing financial resources

### 36.5.1 Developing budgets

After having determined all the requirements of a program, the cost of each of the items has to be estimated. A budget is the tool to estimate the financial requirements of the program by translating all of the program's activities and plans into monetary terms. Thus, a budget is like the program plan expressed in terms of money [27]. Budget formats or templates may vary by the type of budget, or the requirement of the program sponsors/ funding agencies. Budgets may be called for by line-items and cost categories, by program components or objectives, year-wise or for multiple years [27]. Regardless of the format required, in terms of developing budgets, it is useful for the planner to develop annual line item budgets for each program component. These can then be computed, transcribed and presented into the required format. A component wise budget offers the advantage of planning different scenarios and based on component priorities to trim or expand the budget as necessary. Similarly, annual budgets allow for tracking expenditures against the year's budget.

In terms of cost categories, there are at least two major categories – personnel and non-personnel. Personnel costs include salary, benefits and allowances of the staff, and consultant costs. Non-personnel costs generally include travel, equipment, supplies, rent, communication, transportation and other categories that may be specific to the program activities. A third category – indirect costs – is sometimes included by many funding agencies. Indirect costs cover a share of the cost of utilities, equipment, facilities that are shared across many programs. Different agencies have a different formula for calculating indirect costs, so this should be taken directly from the agency to be requested for funding [27].

To cost each item in the program, it is necessary to review each activity and the implementation plan against the timeline. This provides more realistic estimates since some costs are not required from the beginning of the program, and may be phased in later, or some activities may be planned only for certain duration of the program. Once all the items are outlined,

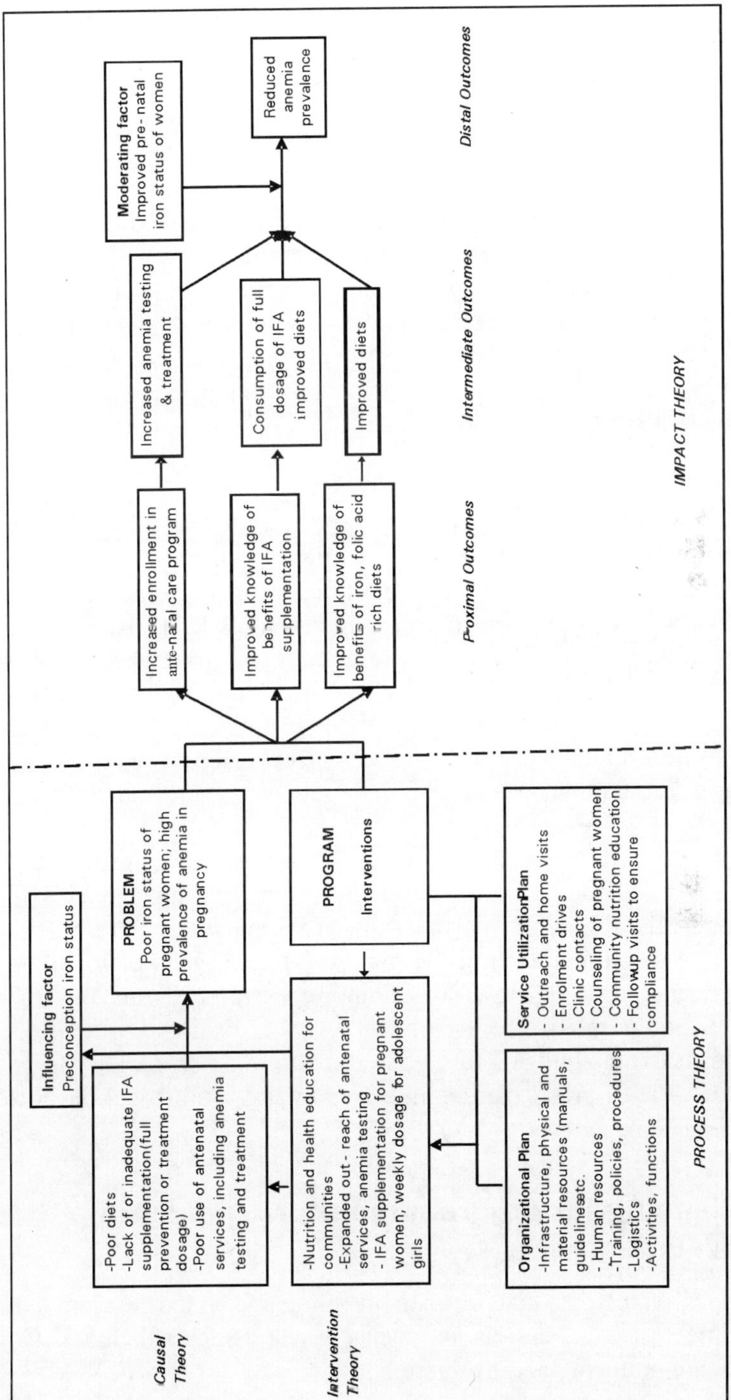


36.9 Program Theory (Anemia in pregnancy program example).

per unit costs should be estimated and multiplied by the number of units and number of months or years for recurring expenditures and once for one-time costs. When planning multi-year budgets, annual salary raises and cost escalation need to be factored in. The budget must also include the cost of evaluation and monitoring. Precision and specificity are important in budgeting. Thus, obtaining real estimates from the right source, e.g., from personnel department for personnel, distributors for equipment, supplies and so on contribute to developing more realistic budgets. Under-budgeting and over-budgeting should be avoided; the former may constrain program activities and the latter may lead to under-spending. It is also important that costs be reasonable – this is generally an important criterion during the review of budgets by the funding agency or program sponsor. Calculating and presenting per participant cost is generally a good strategy with some justification if these are high.

### 36.5.2 Budget justification

Budget justification or budget narrative is often required to be provided along with the budget. This explains the rationale for including the items and how they are necessary for the planned activities [27]. Because the budget is the financial summary of the program plan, it is important that there is consistency between objectives, activities, implementation plans and the budget. There should be no surprises in the budget, nor should any activities be left unbudgeted. Calculation errors can prove very costly; therefore it is prudent to have an appropriate review and clearance system in place.

A plan to raise the required resources that identifies options and strategies for mobilizing resources, such as the funding agencies to contact, fund-raising events, partnerships, seeking internal resources should also be developed during the planning phase. This plan should also identify budget scale-down or trimming options, if the required resources cannot be mobilized. One of the ways of dealing with budget uncertainties is to plan budgets for two or three funding scenarios – high, medium, low – with prioritized components being retained in the low funding scenario.

## 36.6 Planning for program monitoring and evaluation

Result-orientation requires that program planning include the development of appropriate systems to assess and measure results. This includes two key aspects – monitoring and evaluation.

### 36.6.1 Monitoring

Monitoring, or to be more accurate, process monitoring, is the on-going, almost real-time activity of collecting data about the implementation of the program, its analysis, and use at different levels of the program to assess implementation and take timely corrective action when necessary [9]. A robust monitoring system that generates reliable, timely data on the right indicators serves as a critical managerial or oversight tool to ensure that during implementation, the program is delivered within the parameters established during the planning [9]. Program monitoring relates to the assessment of the organizational plan and the service utilization plan (the process theory). It provides the necessary information to alert program personnel about aspects of the organization plan or the service utilization plan that are not working as expected, and make decisions to modify or revise those aspects to make the program more effective [9]. Thus, the monitoring system forms an ongoing loop to feed into the implementation planning or re-planning necessary to make changes that might be required to improve the processes, outcomes and results, in addition to serving as a management tool to address issues of accountability.

The monitoring process, ideally, is a two-way flow of information. This two-way flow requires that data collected at a particular level, in addition to being used at that level, flows upward (all of the data or at least some part of it), is collated and analyzed at designated levels to translate the data into meaningful information, and feedback on performance, specifically including aspects of follow-up or corrective actions to be undertaken flows back. In practice, many times the downward information flow, referred to as the feedback loop, is weak or at times non-existent. Often, in the absence of formalized systems for data analysis and use, data although collected and sent up is not adequately utilized. This is a huge lost opportunity to actually assess the program implementation, take corrective action to ensure that the program indeed functions to deliver the services as planned.

In planning for a monitoring system, one of the first questions to be addressed is what all should be monitored? While there is no prescribed set of activities that are a must to be monitored, a general rule of the thumb is to map out critical activities and processes that relate to the expected outputs or process objectives [28] are closely associated with intervention delivery in the manner and dosage planned, and track coverage of target participants. Once the critical set of activities have been selected, the planning team must identify the set of outputs, inputs and processes that are critical to track, and select appropriate indicators or specific measures relating to these. In other words, the team should complete the results framework by working further down the results chain from the objectives and outcomes that were outlined in the section "setting goals and objectives". Thereafter, one must consider how the data on these measures or indicators will be collected (e.g., the data source and quality, periodicity of its collection, the tools for data collection and recording) [14], how and where will the data flow, be processed and analyzed (e.g., when and where which set of data will be analyzed and processed to turn it into meaningful information), and finally how it will be used (e.g., data interpretation and corrective action). Developing these systems during planning will ensure that appropriate resources are allocated for monitoring and the system guides program managers and staff to effectively track implementation and take corrective action on a real-time basis to support the achievement of results. Program planners might want to consider incorporating other forms of monitoring such as participatory monitoring, community-based monitoring, social audits, community reviews. These offer great value in terms of stakeholder engagement, holding program providers accountable, self-correction, empowering communities, and building partnerships and capacity [14]. Depending on the decisions on the choice of the monitoring mechanisms selected, costs of monitoring must be budgeted for.

### 36.6.2 Evaluation

Program evaluation is the systematic process planned to measure the program's effect against its stated objectives; or to examine aspects of how the program was implemented in relation to what was planned; or both.

Program planning and evaluation are inter-related and cyclical [9]. Evaluation planning will determine the purpose, scope, design, type of the evaluation to be conducted, and the quantum of resources required (human and financial). Evaluation provides the loop to feed learnings and insights from the program into the next planning cycle [9]. While it makes intuitive sense to give due consideration to evaluation planning and budgeting adequately for evaluation, in reality this is often not the case. Some of the reason that evaluation planning is an afterthought include competing priorities for resources (resources allocated for evaluation could mean those many resources less for implementation), lack of expertise, apprehensions in the minds of programmers and other stakeholders of evaluations, since these are often seen as judging a program's performance, the rush to complete planning and begin implementation, and so on. With the focus on RBM and results management, several funding agencies and program sponsors now require evaluation plans as part of the proposals. It is suggested that the planning team build into the planning process time for and resources for key evaluation planning activities such developing the evaluation plan, the evaluation design, development of tools and their testing, and the conduct of the baseline (either prior to implementation or as soon as implementation begins).

Some key aspects that should be considered by the planning team while thinking of the program's evaluation plan include: the purpose of the evaluation (e.g., requirements of the program, needs of the different stakeholders), how the evaluation findings will be used (e.g., to improve the program, inform policy), what type of evaluation methods will be desirable (e.g., quantitative, qualitative, participatory or a mix), what kind of evaluation design to consider (e.g., pre-post, comparison against a counterfactual), the evaluation team (e.g., internal or external evaluators), the costs, and many others. It could be useful to involve a person with evaluation expertise on the team for a full consideration of these issues. Involving stakeholders in the consideration of, and decisions on these issues helps in making evaluation an integral part of planning, addressing to an extent apprehensions of 'being evaluated', feeding evaluation findings to be considered into future planning.

Evaluation of the process theory as well as the impact theory is desirable to fully assess if a program was successful in bringing about the desired change. Impact or outcome evaluation measures the program impact. It is also important to understand how these impacts were achieved (or not achieved). For instance, if the impact evaluation determines that the program did not have the intended impact, it would be crucial to understand if indeed the program was delivered in the planned manner, the interventions delivered in the planned dosage for the planned duration, the coverage achieved. These aspects, the subject of the process evaluation, will help determine whether the effect theory was incorrect, or if implementation failure led to or contributed to the programs' failure [9]. Program failure could have its roots either in the impact theory or in the process theory (see Fig. 36.10) [9]. Qualitative research will answer questions such as the quality of program transactions, capacity of program staff, and relevant social, institutional and governance issues. In order to enable evaluators to better understand issues, problems, what worked and so on from the perspectives of the different stakeholders qualitative methods complement quantitative evaluation techniques. A combination of quantitative and qualitative methods offers many advantages – it helps to explain, contradict or confirm findings from quantitative surveys, capture new unanticipated perspectives, enables data triangulation, and fully understand the range of factors (e.g., social, political, cultural institutional, governance) that help to explain the outcomes [29,30].

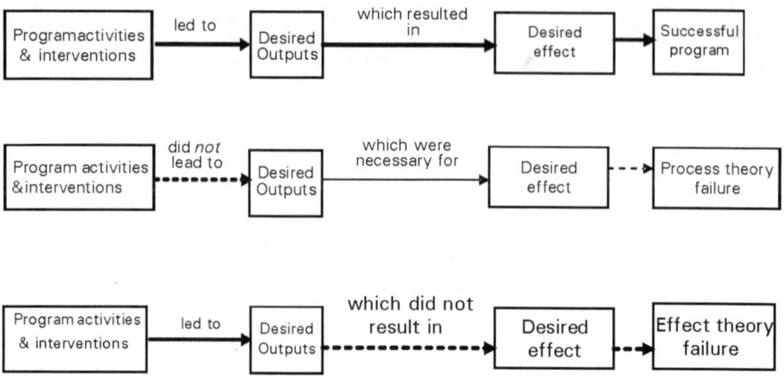


*36.10* Causes of program failure [9].

## 36.7 Planning for program ending or termination

All development programs have time limits dictated largely by the program funding cycle, and at the end of the cycle, the program must either end or, depending on funding availability, roll over to another funding cycle. Because program termination has consequences for the sustainability of the program impact, the program participants, it is imperative that program planners articulate an explicit strategy and plan for its withdrawal in an orderly and responsible manner. This is best done during the program design phase, or early in the life of a program, so that it allows time for proper preparation and deliberate actions over the life of the program to protect and sustain program gains and outcomes once it ends.

Two key terms 'Exit' and 'Graduation' are used in the program withdrawal or ending context. 'Exit' refers to the withdrawal of all externally provided program resources from an entire project or program area. 'Graduation' refers to the withdrawal of program resources from specific program sites or activities that according to certain pre-determined criteria or benchmarks [31]. The *exit strategy or graduation strategy*, describes how the program intends to withdraw its resources while assuring that the outcomes achieved do not erode and that further progress towards the program goals continues. Ideally, the exit strategy sets in place a system whereby the benefits expand beyond the original beneficiaries and their communities [31].

Developing an exit strategy requires the following: Identifying approaches to be used for different program components; selecting criteria for graduation (of communities) and exit (of the program from the region); setting benchmarks for assessing progress toward meeting the criteria; establishing a time line, recognizing flexibility may be required; identifying action steps, dedicating resources; developing mechanisms for periodic review of the progress of and learnings from strategy implementation and for possible modification of the exit plan [31].

Possible approaches for program exit include *phase down*, *phase over* and *phase out*. Phase down, the gradual reduction of program inputs, is the preliminary stage to both phase over and phase out. Phase over refers to the transfer of program responsibility to another entity that could either be an existing organization (community-based, civil society, NGO, governmental) or one especially formed by the program to take over its functions. This approach is appropriate when a core set of program activities will need to be continued beyond program exit. Phase out refers to the withdrawal of program inputs (service provision, other resources, technical assistance) without making explicit arrangements for the program's continuation. This approach is generally considered when the change produced is of a self-sustaining nature, and once achieved outside inputs can be discontinued, but the impact of the program continues, e.g., behavior changes related to health, nutrition and child caring practices can become permanent without requiring continued efforts or activities, provided communities see the benefit of adopting these [31]. The choice of the most appropriate exit approach for a program will depend on the type of program activities, the program environment, the time-frame for exit, and the available human, institutional, financial and physical resources.

It is important to identify the exit approach either during program planning or early in the life of the program for many reasons. If program responsibilities have to be phased over to community groups, community-based organizations, governmental or quasi-governmental bodies, either existing ones or to be created during the life of the program, their engagement with the program early on will be critical. A realistic assessment of their capacities and systematic building up of these will need to be undertaken during the life of the program. In some cases, legal empowerment of the organization created might be needed.

Another aspect to consider is the determination of the criteria to be used to trigger program exit. The criteria could be based on time limits (program exit to happen after a pre-determined time frame), achievement of program outcomes or impacts (as determined by achievement of pre-determined targets), and progress toward the identified graduation process (as determined by achievement of graduation related milestones). Many program situations call for using a combination of criteria from each of the three groups [31].

Another important aspect of the exit plan, especially when a phase-over approach is adopted is the generation of resources through alternative means, such as establishing the organization or service as a business, using a revolving credit or business model, seeking community contributions if economic situation of households permit, establishing user fees or charges for services, and seeking alternative institutional (external) support from government or private donors, fund-raising events and so on.

## 36.8 Conclusion

Several international initiatives over the past decade, the Millennium Declaration and the adoption of the MDGs, the Monterrey Consensus (2002), the Rome Declaration (2003), the Paris Declaration (2005) and the Managing for Development Results global initiative have underscored two points that are highly relevant for public health nutrition program planning. One is the imperative to demonstrate results, and the other is the focus on partnerships, collaboration, and harmonization of efforts to achieve development results. The discussion through the chapter situated program planning in this context and maintained a results-oriented approach with the engagement of stakeholders through its various sections. It also brought together the theory and practice of planning programs that focus on results – their measurement and achievement. The discussion of the theories, concepts, frameworks and tools for planning, built our understanding of the theoretical basis underlying results-oriented programs and their planning. The subsequent section that led us through the various steps of the planning process to develop a result-oriented program helped us meaningfully integrate results-orientation into the practice of public health nutrition program planning. The practical guidance in this section on setting objectives and targets, selecting interventions, planning for program implementation, measurement of results, the cyclical evaluation-planning linkage, and especially the use of a hypothetical nutrition program example, 'reducing the prevalence of anemia in pregnant women' to systematically articulate the program theory helped translate the theory of program planning into practice. Finally, planning for an exit strategy for the program during the planning or early in the life of a program, a crucial but often omitted step, highlighted that the program must deliver results within a defined time-frame and must use appropriate strategies to ensure that its impact is maintained and sustained.

### Points for further thought and discussion

The following points apply specifically in the context of planning of nutrition programs and relate largely to the 'how to' aspects of programming. The scope of the chapter did not permit a full discussion of these, but are critical for nutrition program planners to fully consider. Innovation and operational research related to these points within the program context is one specific aspect for consideration.

- The multi-sectoral nature of the causes of nutrition problems and the complexity of applying solutions that lie across many sectors, ministries or departments.
- Arising out of the above referred issue, and of great significance to

program planning, is the related question of convergence between the actions of programs that lie across various sectors in a manner that the problem of nutrition is addressed in a holistic manner.

- The role of social power equations, particularly gender and women's empowerment and comprehensively integrating these issues with technical solutions to address nutrition
- Strategies and approaches to effectively address the challenging task of behaviour change at scale. The intervention dosage for nutrition education or counseling - aspects such as length and duration of each session, the total number of sessions, especially from the perspective of retaining the interest and engagement of the participants.
- Conditional cash transfer programs to improve nutrition.

## References


1. SCHMITZ S. OECD, MFDR in the global context. In: Emerging Good Practice in MfDR, Source Book, 3rd Edition, 2008. Available at http://www.mfdr.org/Sourcebook/3rdEdition/SourceBook3FINAL.pdf Accessed December 19, 2009
2. OECD, The World Bank, Emerging Good Practice in Managing for Development Results, Source Book first issue, 2006. Available at http://www.mfdr.org/Sourcebook/1stEdition/MfDDRSourcebook-Feb 16 2006.pdf Accessed December 19, 2009.
3. DAC Working Party on Aid Evaluation, Results Based Management in the Development Co-operation Agencies: a review of experience, available at http://www.oecd.org/dataoecd/19/13/35350081.pdf Accessed December 19, 2009
4. The Lancet, "Maternal and Child Undernutrition," Special Series, January, 2008.
5. Copenhagen Consensus 2008, Results of the 2008 meeting. Available at http://www.copenhagenconsensus.com/Home.aspx Accessed December 23, 2009
6. BEZANSON K, ISENMAN P. Policy brief – Scaling Up Nutrition: A Framework of Action http://www.unscn.org/files/Annual_Sessions/2009_Brussels/Policy_brief_Final_Feb_14.pdf
7. MORESCHI JULIE M. Planning and Evaluating Nutrition Services for the Community. In Nutrition in Public Health: a handbook for developing programs and services, editor Edelstein S., 2nd ed. Sudbury, Massachusetts, USA: Jones and Bartlett Publishers, 2006
8. PEOPLES-SHEPS MARY D, FAREL A, ROGERS MARY M. Assessment of Health Status Problems, School of Public Health, University of North Carolina at Chapel Hill, revised 2001. Available at http://www.shepscenter.unc.edu/data/peoples/assessment.pdf (Accessed on December 12, 2009)
9. MICHELE IL. Health program planning and evaluation: a practical and systematic approach for community health, 2nd ed. Sudbury, Massachusetts, USA: Jones and Bartlett Publishers, 2009.
10. DONALDSON SE. Program theory-driven evaluation science: strategies and applications, New York, USA: Lawrence Erlbaum Associates, Taylor and Francis Group, 2007.
11. ROSSI PH, LIPSEY MW, FREEMAN HE. Evaluation: a systematic approach, 7th ed. Thousand Oaks, California, USA: Sage Publications Inc, 2004.

12. KELLOGG WK FOUNDATION. Logic model development guide, 2004. W. K. Kellogg Foundation website. Available at http://www.wkkf.org/
13. World Bank, The Logframe Handbook: A Logical Framework Approach to Project Cycle Management. Available at http://www.wds.worldbank.org/external/default/WDSContentServer/WDSP/IB/2005/06/07/000160016_20050607122225/Rendered/PDF/31240b0LFhandbook.pdf (Accessed on December 19, 2009).
14. Department for International Development UK, Tools for development: a handbook for those engaged in development, 2003. DFID website. Available at http://www.dfid.gov.uk/Documents/publications/toolsfordevelopment.pdf (Accessed on December 12, 2009).
15. Canadian International Development Agency, RBM Handbook on Developing Results chain. Available at http://www.acdi-cida.gc.ca/acdi-cida/ACDI-CIDA.nsf/eng/ANN-923135230-NYD. (Accessed on December 19, 2009).
16. USAID Center for Development Information and Evaluation, TIPS 2000, Number 13: Building a Results Framework. Available at http://pdf.usaid.gov/pdf_docs/PNACA947.pdf (Accessed on December 13, 2009).
17. World Bank, Resources for Staff – Results Framework. Available at the World Bank's intranet network. Accessed January 6, 2010.
18. Managing for Development Results, Emerging Good Practice in MfDR, Source Book, 3rd Edition, 2008. Available at http://www.mfdr.org/Sourcebook/3rdEdition/SourceBook3FINAL.pdf (Accessed on December 19, 2009).
19. Department for International Development UK, The neglected crisis of undernutrition: evidence for action, Available at http://www.dfid.gov.uk/Documents/publications/nutrition-evidence-paper.pdf. Accessed 28 December 2009
20. SHETTY P, (ed). Nutrition through the life cycle, Surrey, UK: Leatherhead Publishing and Cambridge, UK: Royal Society of Chemistry, 2002.
21. NNAKWE NR. Community nutrition: planning health promotion and disease prevention, Sudbury, Massachusetts, USA: Jones and Bartlett Publishers, 2009
22. PEOPLES-SHEPS MD, BYARS E, ROGERS MM, FINERTY EJ, FAREL A. Setting Objectives, School of Public Health, University of North Carolina at Chapel Hill, revised 2001.http://www.shepscenter.unc.edu/data/peoples/setting.pdf (Accessed on December 12, 2009).
23. Public Health Foundation. Setting Target Levels for Objectives. Available at http://www.phf.org/pmqi/HPtools/state/DE_setting_targets_for_objectives.pdf (Accessed on January 5, 2010).
24. PEOPLES-SHEPS M. Development and Selection of Interventions D. School of Public Health, University of North Carolina at Chapel Hill, revised 2001. Available at http://www.shepscenter.unc.edu/data/peoples/development.pdf. (Accessed on December 12, 2009).
25. World Bank, Repositioning Nutrition as Central to Development: A Strategy for Large Scale Action. Washington DC, USA, The World Bank, 2006.
26. OLANDER C. Nutrition education and the role of dosage, Food and nutrition service, USDA website. Available at http://www.fns.usda.gov/ORA/menu/Published/NutritionEducation/Files/LitReview_Dosage.pdf (Accessed on January 9, 2010).
27. PEOPLES-SHEPS M, FOSHEE V, BENDER D. Programming and Implementation, School of Public Health, University of North Carolina at Chapel Hill, revised 2001 http://www.shepscenter.unc.edu/data/peoples/programming.pdf (Accessed on December 12, 2009).
28. PEOPLES-SHEPS MD, ROGERS MM, FINERTY EJ. Evaluation: Monitoring Progress

Towards Achievement of Objectives, School of Public Health, University of North Carolina at Chapel Hill, revised 2001 http://www.shepscenter.unc.edu/data/peoples/evaluation.pdf (Accessed on December 12, 2009).

29. ROGERS BL, MACIAS K, JICK TD (1979). Mixing qualitative and quantitative methods: Triangulation in action. Administrative Science Quarterly 24 (4): 602–661.

30. GREENE JC, CARACELLI VJ, and GRAHAM WF (1989). Towards a conceptual framework for mixed-method evaluation design. Educational Evaluation and Policy Analysis 11 (3): 225–274.

31. ROGERS BL, MACIAS KE. Program graduation and strategies: a focus on Title II food aid development programs, Washington DC, USA, Food and Nutrition Technical Assistance project, Academy for Educational Development, 2004.

# 37

# Monitoring and evaluation of public health nutrition programmes

*Jerard M Selvam* and *Sheila C. Vir*

**Jerard M Selvam**, MD, is Professor and Head of the Department of Epidemiology at the Tamil Nadu Dr. MGR Medical University, Chennai. The author is postgraduate in Community Medicine from Madras Medical College in 1998. He has also completed a Fellowship programme on 'Public Health Field Leadership' offered by the Public Health Management Institute, Hyderabad in collaboration with CDC, USA. Selvam has served as Deputy Director in the World Bank supported Tamil Nadu Health Systems Project.

**Sheila C Vir,** MSc, PhD, is a senior nutrition consultant and Director of Public Health Nutrition and Development Centre, New Delhi. Following MSc (Food and Nutrition) from University of Delhi, Dr Vir was awarded PhD by the Queen's University of Belfast, United Kingdom. Dr. Vir, a past secretary of the Nutrition Society of India, is a recipient of the fellowship of the Department of Health and Social Services, UK, and Commonwealth Van den Bergh Nutrition Award. Dr Vir worked briefly with the Aga Khan Foundation (India) and later with UNICEF. As a Nutrition Programme Officer with UNICEF for twenty years, Dr. Vir provided strategic and technical leadership for policy formulation and implementation of nutrition programmes in India.

## 37.1 Introduction to Monitoring and Evaluation (M & E)

Monitoring and Evaluation (M&E) of development activities, such as public health nutrition, provides development managers, civil society and government officials with information for improving service delivery, learning from past experiences, formulating future strategy and plan as well as in providing information for allocating resources and in demonstrating result with reference to accountability to key stakeholders [1]. Monitoring and evaluation are two distinct sets of organizational activities, related but not identical [2]. M & E is an essential management tool to assist the project or the implementers of the programme to assess the progress that is being made against the defined objectives as well as to analyse the constraints and positive attributes for helping in making adjustments for ensuring efficient smooth progress and desirable impact. M & E therefore assist us to know when plans are working and when circumstances have changed. Plans are essential but they are not set in concrete or in a totally fixed mode. If they are not working, or if the circumstances change, then plans need to change too. It is aptly said that "*Getting something wrong is not a crime. Failing to learn from past mistakes because you are not monitoring and evaluating is ...*". Both monitoring and evaluation are geared towards learning from what one is doing and how one is doing it. Both focus on efficiency, effectiveness and impact (Box 37.1).

**Box 37.1**

*Efficiency*: assesses whether the input (in terms of money, time, staff, equipment etc) is appropriate in terms of the output. This is an important element of project prior to considering replicability and going to scale.
*Effectiveness* : measures the extent to which the development program or project achieves the set specific objectives.
*Impact* : assesses whether or not the project/program made a difference to the problem situation that was being addressed.

The cycle of monitoring and evaluation is presented in Figure 37.1. It is evident that monitoring and evaluation is best done when there has been proper planning against which to assess progress and achievements. Monitoring and Evaluation system (M & E) should be part of a planning process and an integral component in the implementation plan. Inclusion of monitoring and evaluation in the programme plan is often diluted at various levels due to reasons such as lack of appreciation of its significance, fear of being found at fault, lack of transparency and accountability by programme implementers, lack of knowledge and skills, resistance to change by entire programme team, fear of piracy by external evaluators etc [1]. It is therefore imperative that the stakeholders at different levels in the implementation of any public health or public health nutrition programme understand the significance and principles of M & E and ensure inclusion of M & E component in the stage of programme designing. This chapter focuses essentially on the significance, purpose, principles and design of M & E system for public health nutrition programs.

## 37.2 Monitoring

Monitoring is the process of continuous and periodic surveillance of the physical implementation of a programme. It pertains to a systematic collection and analysis of information as a project progresses and involves.

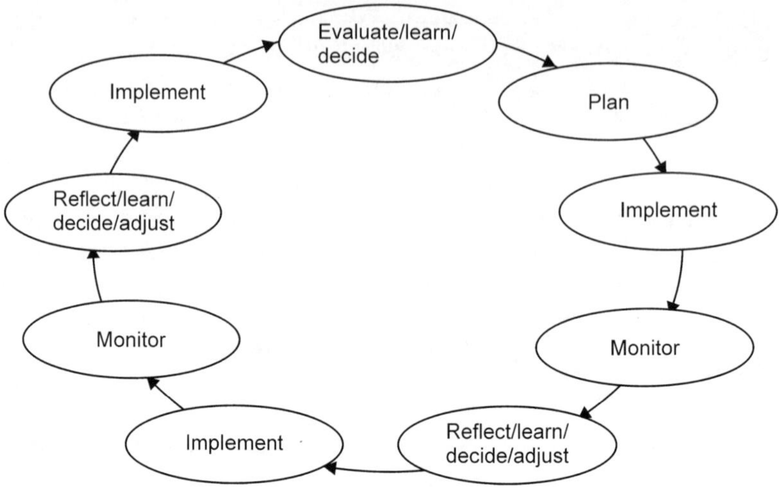


*37.1* Cycle of Monitoring and Evaluation [2].

It is essentially an organized and continuous process of following and keeping track of project/program to ensure that it is proceeding as per the plan and to modify it by making corrective actions when deviations occur. Monitoring is an internal function of any project or organization. Monitoring therefore envisages comparison of what is being achieved with what is intended to be achieved [3].

Monitoring is an invaluable tool for effective management and is closely related with programme implementation design (Figure 37.2). Monitoring involves establishing indicators of efficiency, effectiveness and impact, setting up systems to collect information relating to these indicators, collecting and recording the information including documentation of the project activities, analyzing the information and using the information to notify day-to-day management [2].

Monitoring is vital for the following reasons [2]:

- Ascertains that implementation is proceeding as planned;
- Facilitates one to reflect on where one is going and how one is moving towards the objectives/goals;
- Helps to identify problems and their causes;
- Suggests possible solutions to problems;
- Raises questions about assumptions and strategy;
- Provides with information and insight and encourages to act.

Monitoring is not an exclusive function of the programme implementers. Beneficiaries such as community plays a critical role in monitoring their own health services (Box 37.2).

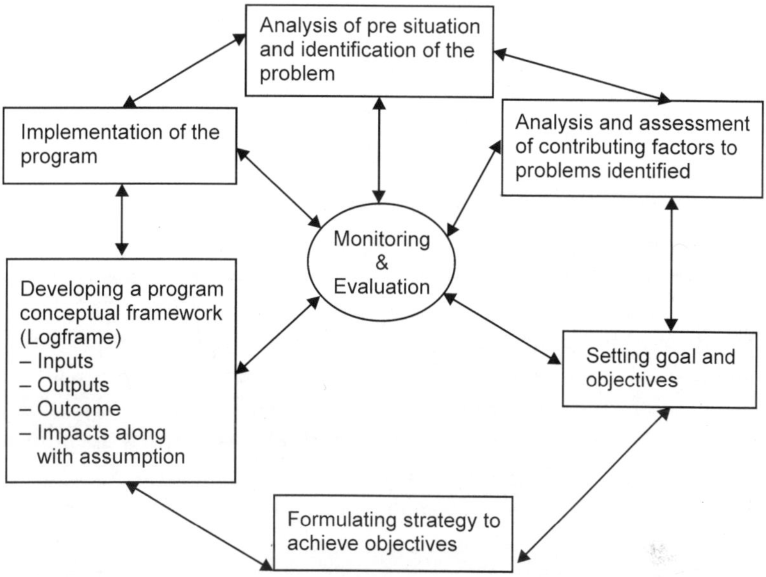


*37.2* Monitoring and Evaluation – integral component of a program.

**Box 37.2 Community-based monitoring**

A new approach introduced in recent years is 'community-based monitoring' of health services. This is one of the key strategies adopted by the National Rural Health Mission (NRHM) in India to ensure that the services reach those for whom they are meant, especially for those residing in rural areas, the poor, women and children. Community monitoring, an important aspect of promoting community led action in the field of health, is executed through the creation of 'Monitoring and Planning Committees' at Primary Health Centre (PHC), Block, District and State levels. The adoption of a comprehensive framework for community-based monitoring and planning at various levels places people at the centre of the process of regularly assessing whether the health needs and rights of the community are being fulfilled. Community monitoring reviews the progress to ensure that the work is moving towards the decided purpose, and the purpose has not shifted, nor has the work got derailed in any way. It helps to identify obstacles in the work so that appropriate timely changes can be made to cross the obstacles [5].

The ultimate purpose of monitoring is to see if the programme is heading in the right direction within the defined time frame and to assess the factors that are contributing to the progress or hindering implementation process as well as the expected outputs. Monitoring information is used primarily for management decisions. However, information needs to be verified first-hand by raising suitable questions such as the following:

- Whether the problem has been identified correctly and whether there has been a change in the problem?
- Are the interventions strategies appropriate for the defined target population and set objectives?

- Whether the indicators chosen are suitable?
- How efficiently the resources have been utilized?
- What are the strengths and weaknesses of the programmes?
- What updates need to be provided to the stakeholders?
- What can be further improved in the programme?

Monitoring therefore helps in identifying and documenting critical milestones, identifying new issues and/or unforeseen circumstances that may be obstacles and identifying necessary corrective measures such as strategy modifications and re-enforcement of positive aspects of the programme. The exercise entails identifying differences between knowledge and practice in order to take corrective actions. It is also equally important to verify whether resources are being used effectively (including cost effectiveness) to meet the set objectives [3]. Effective monitoring also contributes significantly in strengthening relationships amongst collaborators (donors, implementers and beneficiaries) and serves as a motivation to implementers and beneficiaries [1].

### 37.2.1 Designing monitoring system – logical framework approach

Monitoring system design should answer a range of questions such as are the program inputs and activities transferred into outputs that generate desired results. For designing a monitoring system for a public health program, it is important to take a formative viewpoint and establish a system that will provide useful information on an ongoing basis so as to improve what is being done and the process of how it is being done. The stakeholders involved in the process of programme designing therefore need to be guided to undertake the following tasks which are based on using the logical framework approach.

- Draw a logical framework (logframe) – Logframe helps to strengthen project design, implementation and evaluation.
- Generate a list of indicators for each of the following three aspects – efficiency, effectiveness and impact.
- Set up systems to collect information relating to these indicators and mode of collection of information.
- Examine information already collected/available to the project team or the organization.
- Decide on method of creating database computerized or manual.
- Storage & analysis of data and reporting (including format to be used).
- Timely feedback on information to facilitate day to day management.

Developing a logical framework is of paramount importance in conceptualizing a programme and facilitating in designing a comprehensive monitoring system. The 'Logical Framework' (logframe) is a tool to help in clarifying objectives of any project, program or policy as well as project activities, including implementation, monitoring and evaluation activities. Logical Framework Approach (LFA) helps to clearly state (a) what is being aimed to achieve and how it will be achieved; (b) how will you assess whether you are achieving the set objectives and the monitoring mechanism envisaged; (c) proactively analyse and present assumption and condition that are critical for success but are outside the direct control of the project/ program. Such an analysis includes assessment of risks for the project if the assumption fails or change. Logframe helps to identify most relevant indicators for measuring attainment of project outputs and objectives. Logframe is also an analytic tool that has the power to communicate a complex project clearly and understandably on a single sheet of paper. The logframe is entirely "objective-driven" since any action under a project should be aimed at achieving its objectives. It links project goals and objectives with project components and their respective inputs, processes, activities, outputs, outcomes and impact. The framework leads to identification of the performance indicators at each stage in this chain.

In addition, theory-based approach is also used which has similarities to logframe approach but allows a much more in-depth understanding of a programme or activity. This approach does not assume a simple linear cause and effect relationship [6]. The approach maps out determining or casual factors that are viewed as important for the success of the program/ project as well as how these factors interact. Using this approach, design of complex activities is mapped. This approach allows identification of critical success factors and assists in addressing unintended effects of the programme. Early feedback facilitates in prioritizing which issues to investigate in greater depth and what monitoring and evaluation techniques needs to be focused on. The disadvantage is that the approach can easily become rather complex if the scale of activities is large.

Logframe is developed by defining the goal and determining the purposes, outputs and the activities needed. It is a participatory planning tool whose effectiveness depends on how well it incorporates the full range of views of intended beneficiaries and others who have a stake in the project design [6]. The terms used in a logical framework are presented in Table 37.1.

*(a) The advantages and disadvantages of using logical framework are presented below [6]:*

*Advantages:*

- Helps to clarify objectives of any project, program, or policy and aids in the identifications of the expected causal links or the program logic in the programme chain viz. inputs, processes, outputs (including coverage or reach' across beneficiary groups), outcomes and impact.

- Summarizes design of complex activities.
- Leads to identification of performance indicators at each stage in this chain as well as risks which might impede the attainment of the stated objectives.
- Improves quality of project and program designs by clearly stating the objective as well as the performance indicators and assessing the possible risks.

*Table 37.1* Terms used in logical framework [7]

| | |
|---|---|
| Goal | Goal is the broader objectives or aims to which project will contribute. Objectives are statement of intentions. Objectives are derived from goals and should be SMART (Specific, Measurable, Attainable, Relevant, Time-bound) |
| Outcome | Describes the desired impact of the project changes in behaviour/ practices which is a result of programme activities. Right quality and quantity of outputs will result in producing desirable outcome. |
| Output | These are the project deliverables for meeting the purpose, i.e. all the goods and services delivered to the target population by the programme. The quantity and quality of output is important. Programme inputs have to be transformed into outputs. |
| Activities | For producing each output, a cluster of 5–10 activities may be required. The activities together form the set of actions planned for the project. Gantt chart is helpful tool for this. |
| Performance indicators | Describes how well the programme is achieving its objectives and it defines the quality standards of projects along with details. |
| Assumptions/risks | External conditions, situations, factors which play a role in influencing success of project/program. The achievement of aims depends on whether or not assumptions hold true and the risks do not materialize. The assumptions and risks are thus external conditions or the external logic that are outside the control of the programme. |

- Engages partners in clearly stating the objectives and designing activities.
- Serves as a useful tool to review the progress during implementation and take corrective action.
- Assists the preparation of detailed operational plans.
- Provides objective basis for activity review, monitoring and evaluation.
- Ensures that decision makers raise fundamental questions and proactively identify and analyse the assumptions and risks.
- Engages stakeholders in the planning and monitoring process.

It serves as an effective management tool, when used dynamically, to guide in the implementation, monitoring and evaluation tasks.

*Disadvantages of logical framework (logframe):*

- Restrains creativity and innovation, if rigidly managed.
- Risk of using the framework as a static tool that does not reflect changing conditions.

*(b) Development of Logframe Matrix*

*Logframe Matrix* is a participatory planning, monitoring and evaluation tool. The effectiveness and potential of the tool depends on the degree to which it incorporates the full range of views of intended beneficiaries and others who have a stake in the programme design [7, 8]. Developing a logframe aims at defining the means and ends as well as clearly stating the linkages between each level of aims. The better the means and end linkages between each level of aims, the better the programme design [8]. A logframe therefore presents purpose, activities and output of the project or the programme (Table 37.2). The following steps are involved in development of logframe.

- Identifying outputs and activities.
- Verifying the vertical logic.
- Identifying the risks and assumptions.
- Verifying the logic of the risks and assumptions.
- Determining the indicators of achievement and means of verification.

*Table 37.2* Logical Framework — a matrix of 4 columns and 16 boxes [7]

| Project summary (Objective hierarchy) | Performance indicators | Monitoring mechanism (Means of verification) | Assumptions/risks |
|---|---|---|---|
| **Goal** (Overall objectives, development objectives) | Indicators to goal achievement mechanism | Source of data for goal level performance | Risk regarding strategic impact |
| **Purpose** (project development objectives) | Impact indicators | Source of data for purpose level performance | Risk purpose to goal |
| **Outputs (results)** The products, services or results that must be delivered by the project for attaining objectives and purpose | Project output indicators | Source of data for output level performance | Risk output to purpose design effectiveness |
| **Activities** Actions taken by the project that are required for delivering of inputs | Input/resource budget by activities; monetary, physical, human resources for activities | Source of data for activity level performance indicators | Risk activities to output risk regarding implementation and effectiveness |

This matrix cross-references seven key areas of the project to ensure that the key questions are asked.

- Goal – what results are expected?

- Purpose – why is the programme being undertaken?
- Outputs – what are the deliverables?
- Activities – what will be done for delivering the outputs?
- Indicators of achievement – how will it be assessed whether the project has been successful?
- Means of verification – how will the reported results be checked?
- Risks and assumptions – what assumptions underlie the structure of the project and what is the risk that will prevail?

For example, a framework for monitoring a vitamin A fortification program and a framework for an adolescent anemia control program are presented in Tables 37.3 and 37.4. The logical framework tables cover activity in terms of provision of service, utilization, coverage and impact. It also raises the questions related to each activity, identifies the key indicators, outcomes to be measured and means of verification/data collection methods.

*Table 37.3* A framework for monitoring a vitamin A fortification program [9]

| Activity | Questions | Examples of key indicators | Data collection methods |
|---|---|---|---|
| Provision | Is the fortified food available in sufficient quantity?<br>Are the distribution/ sale outlets accessible to the population?<br>Is the quality of the food adequate? | Amount of fortified food produced (Crude and per Capita)<br>Number and location of sales / distribution outlets<br>Vitamin A content of fortified food | Food industry statistics<br>Production records and quality control reports<br>Commercial census<br>Government statistics<br>Food analysis using quantitative or qualitative assay methods |
| Utilisation | Is the fortified food being distributed? Purchased? | Sales and distribution of fortified food (crude and per capita) | Food industry statistics<br>Market survey |
| Coverage | What proportion of the target population is eating fortified foods? | Proportion of all children under 5 or post partum women regularly consuming sufficient amounts of fortified food | Household surveys |
| Impact | Did health and nutrition Improve? | Time trends in serum retinol levels Time trends In deaths and hospital admissions | Household surveys<br>Routine reporting data (if available) or special surveys |

The logical framework for Adolescent Anemia Control Programme presented below in two parts of Table 37.4. First section specifies goal, strategic results, including indicators and means of verification as well outcomes. In the second section of the table, for a selected outcome, details of outputs, inputs, indicators and means of verification are presented. (Table 37.4)

*Table 37.4a* Logical framework for Adolescent Anemia Control Programme in district A

| | | |
|---|---|---|
| Goal | The nutrition and health status of adolescent girls (10–19 years old) is improved through preventive and promotive interventions for the control of anemia in district A. | |
| Strategic results | The prevalence of anemia noted in 2010 is reduced by at least 30% in district A by 2012. Specifically:<br>• The *coverage* of the adolescent anemia control programme – comprising IFA supplementation (weekly), deworming (bi-annual), and IEC/BCC (through the project period) – is expanded to one million adolescent girls using school- and community-based interventions as delivery channels.<br>• The *prevalence* of anemia among school-going adolescent girls is reduced by at least 40% by 2012 through the delivery of IFA supplementation weekly through school system), deworming (bi-annual), and IEC/BCC (regular).<br>• The prevalence of anemia among out-of-school adolescent girls is reduced by at least 20% by 2012 through the delivery of IFA supplementation (weekly), deworming (bi-annual) and IEC/BCC (regular) using community-based interventions as the delivery channel. | |
| | **Indicators** | **Means of verification** |
| | • Percent adolescent girls covered by the school-based component of the adolescent anemia control program. | Middle and secondary school data |
| | • Percent adolescent girls covered by the community-based component of the adolescent anemia control program. | Secondary census data and survey report-the ongoing nutrition programme |
| | • Prevalence of anemia among adolescent girls benefiting from the school-based component of the adolescent anemia control programme | Baseline and final survey |
| | • Prevalence of anemia among adolescent girls benefiting from the community-based component of the adolescent anemia control program. | Baseline and final survey |

*Expected outcomes*

(i) Implementation of district-level advocacy, programme implementation, undertaken in school and community and knowledge management framework established.

(ii) The capacity of school-based programmes to provide services or the control of anemia among school-going adolescent girls is strengthened

(iii) The capacity of community-based programmes to provide services for the control of anemia among out-of-school adolescent girls is strengthened.

For each of these outcomes, following details need to be worked out – outputs, inputs, indicators and means of verification and important assumption and risks. The details of outcome (i) are presented below as an example (Table 37.4b).

Table 37.4b Outcome (i) – Implementation of district-level advocacy, programme implementation, and knowledge management frameworks

| Outputs under outcome (i) | Inputs/Activities | Indicators | Means of verification | Assumptions / Risks |
|---|---|---|---|---|
| *Output 1*<br>An advocacy strategy for the control of anemia in adolescent girls through school and community-based interventions. | Sensitizing key stakeholders' on importance of anemia control program using existing evidence.<br>Key stakeholders:<br>• Policy-decision makers, program planners, mangers of sectoral depts. (Education, /Social Welfare, Health/Rural Development (community-based organization), Tribal).<br>• Professional and academic bodies | • Number of key stakeholders sensitized on the importance of anemia control program using existing evidence.<br>• Issue of guidelines by the government authority for initiating/ accelerating implementation. | Minutes of meetings, reports / documents / guidelines | Election scheduled in three months time could result in education department and teachers being occupied with election duties |
| *Output 2*<br>A program strategy of the district authority for control of anemia in adolescent girls through school- and community-based interventions. | (i) Establishing a consultation process to facilitate development of a Plan of Action (POA). | • Number of blocks (smallest administrative units) with POA developed.<br>• Number of blocks which have launched the programme | District and block POA in place Field visit/joint reviews/minutes of meetings/ monthly monitoring reports. | |
| *Output 3*<br>A knowledge management framework of the state government to monitor and evaluate the implementation and effectiveness of the adolescent anemia control programme. | (ii) Designing of monitoring framework and undertake process /impact assessments. Timely dissemination of findings for timely action. | • Number of blocks which have completed assessments.<br>• Prevalence of Anemia (block-wise).<br>• % of girls who have consumed at least 40 tablets in a year (block-wise). | Reports (baseline/monitoring/impact assessments)<br>Field visits.<br><br>District level coordinating committee reviews | |

### *(c) Identification and selection of appropriate monitoring/evaluation indicators – using the logical framework tool*

In monitoring and evaluation, indicators are measurable or tangible signs to show what has been done or achieved. Indicators need to be appropriately selected in order to measure programme inputs, outcomes, process and impact. The logical framework tool helps to focus on appropriate indicators and through such selected indicators, the response to following questions can be obtained [2]:

- Who?
- How many?
- How often?
- How much?

Identification of appropriate indicators for monitoring is critical as it has the advantage of assisting in identifying, developing and taking timely corrections at the lowest to the highest level of implementation so that the goals of the intervention programmes are achieved. The critical indicators have to be examined at the peripheral level so that timely corrective decisions are taken and implemented without any delay or waiting for assessment by top level or external agencies. Monitoring indicators should therefore help in making quick decisions in a de-centralized manner at the lowest implementation level. Selection of indicators for evaluation follows the same principles. Identifying and selecting appropriate indicators for evaluation are expected to serve as "trigger points" for action as they will provide information that will be useful for mid-course corrections [1].

#### *(i) Characteristics of indicators*

Characteristics required of monitoring/evaluation indicators are presented in Table 37.5.

#### *(ii) Types of indicators*

Primarily there are two types of indicators: (a) Process, and (b) Impact indicators.

(a) Process indicators – these indicators monitor the implementation of actions and activities of the programme to see whether or not the intervention is functioning effectively. Examples for process indicators are presented below in Table 37.6.

(b) Impact indicators – these measure outcomes and impacts of a programme or a project. One of the major constraint often encountered is regarding lags between project implementation and impact or, in other words between the time of impact and the time it is feasible to collect data

*Table 37.5* Characteristics required of a Monitoring and Evaluation indicators [1]

| Required characteristic | Description |
|---|---|
| Simple | Selecting a simple indicator is not always an easy task. Each term of an indicator should be clearly and precisely defined. It may require finding a balance between the ideal (which may be complex and/or impossible to collect) and the practical |
| Measurable | Both quantitative and qualitative indicators should be measurable. Some indicators are directly measurable, e.g., height and weight, while other indicators need to be defined. |
| Valid | A valid indicator accurately reflects the situation it is intended to measure. A valid indicator in one area may be less so in another, therefore it may be inappropriate to transfer indicators from region to region or programme to programme. |
| Reliable | A reliable indicator will produce the same results every time it is measured, regardless of who collects the data. |
| Variable | Indicators to be useful, must show variation between subjects and over time. |
| Specific | Indicator should reflect changes for the specific situation concerned. |
| Feasible | Scope of obtaining the required data is feasible/practical. |
| Relevant | Indicator should contribute to the understanding of the phenomenon of interest. |
| Sensitive | Indicators must be sensitive to changes in the situation concerned over a period of time. |
| Acceptability | Indicator selected should have acceptability and it must be recognised that acceptability may vary among different populations. Some measures such as dietary intake are more widely accepted as compared to drawing venous blood. |
| Costs | Costs associate with the use of certain indicator. |

relating to impact. Examples of impact indicators recommended for Iodine Deficiency Disorders (IDD) control programme is presented in Table 37.7.

### *(iii) Clustering and selection of core indicators*

Clustering of indicators is essential to arrive at adequate and practical set of indicators by adhering to the following steps:

- Identify a limited number of indicators that adequately measure the outputs.
- Identify the data sources available and the type of data collection needed for each indicator.
- Construct a matrix listing the indicators, identifying their importance for programme monitoring and evaluation (high/low), the ease of obtaining data on the indicator (easy/feasible but requires effort/ difficult), and the cost of data collection.
- Prioritize indicators by importance, ease of obtaining data and cost.
- Based on the above, select a set of indicators.

*Table 37.6* Examples for process indicators in a vitamin A deficiency control programme [10]

*Supplement distribution programme*

- Percent coverage of at risk population by programme (e.g. capsules supplement) received and delivered per year per target population.
- Percent of the health centres/institutions etc. with sufficient supplement for coverage of the target population(s) for a 4–6 month distribution cycle.

*Fortification programme*

- Number of vitamin A fortified foods available in selected markets.
- Percentage of fortified foods available in market that meet specified levels of vitamin A.
- Percentage of households containing a specific vitamin A fortified food selected as suitable for consumption by target groups.
- Percentage of target group consuming a specific fortified food.

*Nutrition education/social marketing programs*

- Number of contacts for message delivery per week.
- Knowledge, attitude and practice (KAP) indicators of messages delivered and understood at the household level.
- Percentage awareness of consequences of vitamin A deficiency (VAD) and local vitamin A containing foods.
- Percentage of under 24-month-old infants consuming the recommended dietary intake (RDI) of vitamin A from foods or supplements.
- Feeding patterns for vitamin A rich foods, e.g., percentage of children under 3 years of age eating vitamin A rich foods 3 times a week.

*Horticulture programme*

- Percentage of homes in a district with a garden having pro-vitamin A containing foods.
- Percentage of schools in a district with gardens having pro-vitamin A containing foods.

*Table 37.7* Examples of impact indicators in an Iodine Deficiency Disorders (IDD) control programme [11]

- Median urinary iodine concentration (µg/l) among school-age children and pregnant women.
- Goitre rate assessed by palpation (%) among school-age children.
- Goitre rate assessed by ultrasound (%) among school-age children.
- TSH (mIU/l) levels among newborns
- Tg (µg/l) levels among school-age children.

- Group the selected indicators by source of data to determine the set of sources which can provide data on clusters of indicators.
- Make a final selection of a cluster of indicators and decide on a data collection plan in light of available logistical, human and financial resources and time.

A practical example is shown in Table 37.8. The core and optional indicators chosen by a working group on "Infant and Young Child Feeding" are presented in Table 37.8. The indicators that were finally agreed upon and selected were for only two critical age groups (infants, 6–23 months).

The selection of indicators was based on evidence of their positive association with child survival and/or nutrient intakes as well as feasibility of measurements. Details of these indicators are presented in Tables 37.9 and 37.10 [12].

*Table 37.8* Core and optional indicators for infant and young child feeding practices [12]

| Core indicator | Optional indicator |
|---|---|
| • Early initiation of breastfeeding<br>• Exclusive breastfeeding under 6 months<br>• Continued breastfeeding at one year<br>• Introduction of solid, semi-solid or soft foods<br>• Minimum dietary diversity<br>• Minimum meal frequency<br>• Minimum acceptable diet<br>• Consumption of iron-rich or iron-fortified foods | • Children ever breastfed<br>• Continued breastfeeding at 2 years<br>• Age-appropriate breastfeeding<br>• Predominant breastfeeding under 6 months<br>• Duration of breastfeeding<br>• Bottle feeding<br>• Milk feeding frequency for non-breastfed children |

*Table 37.9* Indicators to assess breastfeeding practices in infants [12]

| Core indicator selected | Measurement |
|---|---|
| • Exclusive breast feeding under 6 months | Infants 0–5 months of age who received only breast milk during the previous day |
| | **Total Infants 0–5 months age** |
| • Early initiation of breast feeding | Children born in the last 24 months who were put to the breast within one hour of birth |
| | **Total Children born in the last 24 months** |

## 37.3 Evaluation of programmes

Programme evaluation is a process of data collection designed to assess the effectiveness of the programme in attaining its originally stated objectives. Additionally evaluation also assesses and determines the extent to which the observed changes are due to the programme activities themselves and not from inputs and influences outside. Evaluation is the comparison of actual project impacts against the strategic plans that has been agreed to [2]. 'Evaluation is a systematic investigation of the worth or merit of an object' [13]. As per WHO, it measures the degree to which objectives and targets are fulfilled and the quality of the results obtained [13, 14]. Evaluation therefore looks at what one has set out to do, what has been accomplished and how it has been accomplished.

*Table 37.10* Indicators to assess feeding practices in children 6–23 months of age [13]

| Core indicator selected | Measurement |
|---|---|
| • Minimum acceptable diet | Breastfed children 6–23 months of age who had at least the minimum dietary diversity and the minimum meal frequency during the previous day<br>———————————<br>Total Breastfed children 6–23 months age<br>**and**<br>Non-breastfed children 6–23 months of age who received at least 2 milk feedings and had at least the minimum dietary diversity not including milk feeds and the minimum meal frequency during the previous day<br>———————————<br>Total Non-breastfed children 6–23 months of age |
| • Consumption of iron-rich or iron-fortified foods | Children 6–23 months of age who received an iron-rich food or a food that was specially designed for infants and young children and was fortified with iron, or a food that was fortified in the home with a product that included iron during the previous day<br>———————————<br>Children 6–23 months age |

Evaluation is a systematic process to assess *efficiency*, *effectiveness and impact* of the programme achievements based on the set objectives. There is clear distinction between effectiveness and efficiency of any intervention in public health programmes. Whilst *effectiveness* refers to the results obtained under real-world circumstances, *efficiency* refers to the results obtained relative to the resources expended [15]. In an overview of the effectiveness and efficiency of HIV prevention programs by D R Holtgrave *et al*, *'effectiveness'* was considered in terms of averting or reducing HIV-related risk behaviours or favourably modifying their determinants and *'efficiency'* of the intervention was viewed as implementing the intervention using a strategy at a minimal, cost-effective or cost-beneficial level of resource investment [16].

Evaluation should be developed during the design phase of the programme. The purpose of evaluation is to assess the achievement of the stated objectives of a programme, its adequacy, its efficiency and its acceptance by all parties involved [1]. The major purpose of an evaluation will depend on the type of approach and the typical focus questions arising out of it. This is highlighted in Table 37.11.

An evaluation helps to answer the following questions:

- Is the intervention correct or appropriate?
- Are additional interventions necessary to achieve the objectives?
- Is the intervention being implemented as planned?
- Is the strategy appropriate?
- Is the programme addressing the right problems?
- Are the outcomes and objectives being met?

*Table 37.11* Purpose and approaches to evaluation [17]

| Approach | Major purpose | Typical focus questions | Likely methodology |
|---|---|---|---|
| Goal-based | Assessing achievement of goals and objectives. | Were the goals achieved? Efficiently? Were they the right goals? | Comparing baseline and progress data; finding ways to measure indicators |
| Decision-making | Providing information | Is the project effective? Should it continue? | Assessing range of options related to the project context, inputs, process, and product. |
| | | How might it be modified? | Establishing some kind of decision-making consensus. |
| Goal-free | Assessing the full range of project effects, intended and unintended | What are all the outcomes? What value do they have? | Independent determination of needs and standards to judge project's worth. Qualitative and quantitative techniques to uncover any possible results. |
| Expert judgment | Use of expertise | How does an outside professional rate this project? | Critical review based on experience, informal surveying, and subjective insights. |

- Is the system in place?
- What are the lessons learned?

The evaluation process is important since it helps in assessing the work of the programme and also provides information that helps in redesigning the programme and increasing effectiveness of the programme management. Additionally, evaluation measures the productivity of available resources in achieving a set of clearly defined objectives and also the output or cost effectiveness. It checks whether the programme was implemented according to the detailed plan/design and verifies the problem thereby providing an opportunity for problem solving such as strategy modification. Evaluation is significant for other reasons such as maximizing the utilization of resources including re-allocation of priorities and resources on the basis of changing needs, identification of the strengths and weaknesses of the programme, providing information for planning and re-planning, providing learning opportunities and the right feedback to the various stakeholders. Thus it forms a basis for maintaining and/or improving the existing strategy and measures the effectiveness of the programme [1].

### 37.3.1 Phases of conducting evaluation

The following are the five phases of conducting evaluation [1]:

*(i) Planning the evaluation*

- Determine the purpose and type of the evaluation
- Review existing information in programme documents including monitoring information
- Describe the programme
- Develop/refine conceptual framework, assess strengths and limitations of the programme
- Put together an evaluation team including stakeholders

*(ii) Selecting appropriate evaluation methods*

- Identify evaluation goals and objectives
- Formulate evaluation questions and sub-questions
- Decide on the appropriate evaluation design
- Develop an evaluation schedule
- Develop a budget for the evaluation.

*(iii) Collecting and analyzing information*

- Develop data collection instruments.
- Pre-test data collection instruments.
- Undertake data collection activities.
- Analyze data.
- Interpret the data.

*(iv) Report findings*

- Write the evaluation report.
- Decide on the method of sharing the evaluation results.
- Decide on communication strategies in terms of the method to be adopted for presentation to different stakeholders involved in the programme.
- Share the draft report with stakeholders and revise as needed.
- Disseminate evaluation report.
- Meet with project stakeholders to discuss and follow-up on findings once the findings have been accepted

*(v) Implementing evaluation recommendations*

- Develop a new/revised implementation plan in partnership with stakeholders

- Monitor the implementation of evaluation recommendations and report regularly on the implementation progress
- Plan the next evaluation

## 37.3.2 Types of evaluation

Evaluation of programs is primarily of two types:

(i) formative evaluation; and (ii) impact or summative evaluation

### *(a) Formative evaluation*

Formative evaluation takes place during the life of a project or organization while summative evaluation is drawing lessons from a completed project or an organization that is no longer functioning. Evaluation theorist, Bob Stakes, has interestingly compared these two types of evaluation by the following description [13] – *"When the cook tastes the soup, that's formative; When the guests taste the soup, that's summative."*

The purpose of formative evaluation is to assess initial and ongoing project activities. It has two components namely

- *process or implementation evaluation*
- *progress evaluation*

Process evaluation begins during programme development and continuous throughout the life of the programme. Process evaluation addresses operational and implementation issues. It helps to assess whether the programme and its components are being conducted or implemented or operating as planned. It may occur once or several times during the life of the programme [13]. Process evaluations answer questions about how well a program is meeting administrative and procedural goals [18]. Results of process evaluation are presented in terms of output measures e.g. changes in users of services such as antenatal care, growth monitoring, and coverage of beneficiaries. Process evaluation provides information on inputs and how the inputs were transformed into outputs intended to contribute to the programme outcome.

The objective of progress evaluation is to assess progress in meeting the goals of the programme and the project. It involves collecting information to learn whether or not the benchmarks were met. The progress can be conveniently evaluated in the mid term when it is called mid-term evaluation. The mid-term evaluation, an assessment of the effectiveness and efficiency of a programme when it is half way through the planned period, gives an idea of whether the set objectives will be met within the project period [13].

*(b) Impact and summative evaluation*

The purpose of impact and summative evaluation is to assess a mature project's success or failure in reaching its stated goals. Impact evaluation gauges the extent to which the intervention has caused change in the desired direction at any given time. Impact evaluation is done at a set time, based on the requirements of programme or plan for review and re-plan. The evaluation reveals the outcomes, both positive and negative, resulting from the intervention and identifies intervention and external factors that are influencing the change. Summative evaluation is the final assessment done at the end of a project plan. Summative evaluation combines impact data with other relevant data to present a more complete scenario of operations and accomplishments of a programme. Summative evaluations focus on the goals of the program, both in terms of its impact on individuals and its impact on collaborating systems and the larger community [18]. Summative evaluation collects information about outcomes and related processes, strategies and activities that have led or not led to the defined goals. The results obtained help in identifying the extent of achievement of the programme lessons learned, positive and negative outcomes of the interventions, making decisions about continuation/termination of a programme and also to determine reformulation of strategy [13].

In addition, other evaluations methods used some times are spot checks and desk evaluation. '*Spot check evaluation*' is a brief ad hoc evaluation undertaken when there is an urgent need during programme implementation. It enables specific decisions to be made regarding the programme, provides a quick realistic picture of programme status as part of the accountability process and enables quick implementation of corrective measures. '*Desk evaluation*' which may be internal or external do not involve field visits but depend largely on secondary sources for information. Programme personnel or implementers using largely secondary sources of information do '*Self-evaluations*' or '*Internal evaluations*'. They are often subjective and mainly undertaken in small programmes [1].

## 37.4 Designing the evaluation

Designing the evaluation is the total process of stating the objectives, identifying questions, specifying a plan for collecting and analyzing data, reporting results, and getting the results used. It is to be noted that there is no perfect design. Each design has its own strengths and weaknesses. There are always trade-offs – time, costs, practicality; and it is important to acknowledge the trade-offs and potential weaknesses.

In general, the evaluation design consists of the following: evaluation questions and sub-questions, indicators and measures, data sources, defining sample size, data collection methods and instruments, methodology for data analysis and procedure for control of data quality.

Specification of the evaluation design requires a following thorough process since any design flow would limit the ability of evaluators to make solid conclusions about the intervention. Inappropriate design could render the entire evaluation exercise useless. Therefore, drawing a proper evaluation design matrix and paying attention to the specifics of questions, sub-questions, type of question, design, measures or indicators, criteria for normative questions is very crucial [19]. Table 37.12 presents an evaluation design matrix.

*Table 37.12* Evaluation Design Matrix [19]

| Questions | Sub-questions | Types of questions | Design | Measures of indicators | Criteria for normative questions |
|---|---|---|---|---|---|
| | | | | | |

| Data sources | Sample | Data collection instrument | Data analysis | Comments |
|---|---|---|---|---|
| | | | | |

As indicated in Table 37.13, common designs are based on the following three important types of questions:

(a) Descriptive
(b) Normative
(c) Cause–effect questions

*Table 37.13* Linkages between evaluation questions and design [19]

| Type of evaluation question | Evaluation design |
|---|---|
| Descriptive questions | Non-experimental;<br>quasi-experimental<br>or<br>qualitative approaches |
| Normative questions | Non-experimental; quasi-experimental,<br>or<br>qualitative approaches<br>Plus goals/standards/needs assessment |
| Cause–effect questions | Experimental, quasi-experimental, or<br>non-experimental with in-depth causal tracing |

### (a) Designs for descriptive questions

Descriptive questions generally use non-experimental designs. Non-experimental designs do not involve a comparison group that did not receive the intervention. They focus only on those who received the intervention. The common evaluation designs are as follows:

(i) *One shot* – A one-shot design is a look at the group receiving an intervention at one point in time following the treatment or intervention. This can be used to answer questions such as "How many women were treated?" or "How satisfied are the women with the services they received?"

(ii) *Cross-sectional* – Cross-sectional design shows a snapshot at one point in time but looks into sub-group responses. The sub-groups may be based on age, gender, income, education, ethnicity, or amount of intervention received. This design is often used with a survey method.

*(iii) Baseline and endline (Before-and-after)* – Before-and-after design looks at group characteristics before and after the intervention (also called the pre- and post-intervention characteristics). It is an assessment made at both baseline and_endline. There is no comparison group. For example, participants to a food-for-school program can be asked whether the program improved school attendance.

The design of this sort, however are subject to variety of biases or threats to validity. Before-and-after designs can be improved by gathering multiple data points before and after the program is introduced and by careful examination of other actors.

Baseline data is the information on which problem analysis is based. It is very difficult to measure the impact of the implementing programme if the baseline data on relevant indicators for measuring the impact is not available. The baseline data needs to focus on collecting general information about the situation. At times such data is available in official statistics. If the required information is not available from secondary sources then the information needs to be systematically obtained through a baseline survey keeping the focus on the relevant indicators for measuring impact.

It is very difficult to get baseline information after the work has begun and the situation has changed. There are ways of doing damage control; e.g. by gathering anecdotal information from those who were involved at the beginning or know what the situation was at the beginning of the project or through the records/written sources such as minutes, reports and so on.

(iv) *Time series* – Time series design looks for changes over time (either after or before and after the intervention) in order to discern trends. They can be simple time series designs or cross-sectional designs. For example, child mortality rates might be examined before and after an intervention, providing maternal nutrition supplements, to identify the trends in birth weights.

(v) *Longitudinal* – Longitudinal study is one in which repeated measures of the same variable are taken from the same people (or from a sample of groups in the same population). A panel design is a special type of longitudinal design in which a smaller group of people is tracked at multiple points in time and their experiences are recorded in considerable detail [19].

*(vii) Case studies* – The descriptive case study collects in-depth information over time to describe what implementation of the intervention looked like on the ground and why things happened the way they did. Rather than using large samples and following a rigid protocol to examine a limited number of variables, case study methods involve an in-depth, longitudinal examination of a single instance or event. It is a systematic way of looking at what is happening, collecting data, analyzing information, and reporting the results. It is a method of learning about a complex instance through extensive description and contextual analysis. The product is an articulation of why the instance occurred as it did, and what may be important to explore in similar situations. The product is a sharpened understanding of why the instance happened as it did, and what might be important to look at more extensively in future research. Thus, case studies are especially well suited toward generating, rather than testing, hypotheses. Case studies can generate a great deal of data that may not be easy to analyze [19, 20].

### *(b) Designs for normative questions*

The logic for normative questions is similar to descriptive questions, except that normative questions are always assessed against a criterion. The only difference between answering a normative and descriptive questions is that in normative questions goal, target or standard to be reached are specified and the actual findings are compared to that standard. Generally, the same designs work for normative questions as well as descriptive questions.

### *(c) Designs for cause–effect questions*

When answering cause–effect questions, evaluation design needs to address the question "What would the situation have been if the intervention had not taken place?" In order to evaluate impact, one or more types of the following designs may be considered (i) experimental design, (ii) quasi-experimental design, (iii) correlation design, (iv) case study design, and (v) non-experimental designs.

(i) *Experimental design* – The experimental design is the classic design or true experiment design. It is considered the strongest design for cause–effect questions. Experimental designs usually contain before-and-after measures for the comparison groups [19]. Random assignment is an essential component of experimental design. It is essential that comparison groups are comparable. One group is randomly assigned to receive the intervention and another randomly assigned group serves as the control group and does not receive the intervention. As long as there is equipoise regarding the benefits and harms of the intervention, potential for participants to benefit, and a means of informed consent, randomization is ethically acceptable. Experimental designs are the preferred method for outcome evaluations. The principal advantage is that a relatively high degree of confidence can be placed in findings of differences in outcomes between the two groups.

It is not always feasible, however, to use an experimental design. Firstly, experimental designs that minimize possible "contamination" of the experiment can be expensive. Secondly, the design may not be ethical or legal. For example, there can be an argument that it is unfair or a denial of equal protection of law to arbitrarily withhold beneficial program services from eligible participants who have a demonstrated need for treatment. One strategy that has been used to allay concerns related to defendants' need for, or rights to, treatment is to assign defendants to one of several different "categories" of treatment. For example, participants might be randomly assigned to a more intensive group (daily outpatient groups, assessment test and health education), or to a less intensive group (only assessment test and health education). This strategy ensures that all participants identified as needing treatment receive some services by falling into one of the groups. Experimental designs are generally more tenable only when participants provide a full and informed consent regarding their involvement in randomization procedures and other program evaluation activities. Evaluation procedures, including legal and ethical issues, should be carefully reviewed before an experimental evaluation design is implemented [20].

(ii) *Quasi-experimental design* – The quasi-experimental design is similar to true experiment except that the comparison groups have not been formed by random assignment. It is used to carry out evaluation when it is not possible to construct treatment and control groups using random assignments. Sometimes, a comparison group is created by matching key characteristics [19]. In public health, however, random assignment commonly either is not feasible or simply is not done. In such instances, Quasi-experimental-designs can be used for a scientifically rigorous examination of outcomes. Although these designs can improve inferential clarity, they cannot be relied on to yield unbiased estimates of the effects of interventions because the subjects are not assigned randomly.

One type of quasi-experimental evaluation is a pre-post design, in which outcomes obtained following discharge from an intervention programme are compared to those obtained prior to program participation. A drawback to pre-post designs is that they do not take into account other factors that influence the outcome measured.

Another type of quasi-experimental evaluation studies one or more comparison groups, rather than a randomly assigned control group. Using this design, results from the experimental and comparison groups are contrasted. Comparison groups consist of participants who do not participate in (or who do not complete) the intervention program. These groups are otherwise similar to program participants in key areas such as age, gender, ethnicity, employment, income, nutritional problem under study and other areas used as eligibility criteria in the program. It is often useful to "match" subjects in experimental and comparison groups to control for the problem of confounding variables introduced through non-random assignment. Using this approach, both groups' subjects are selected based on factors expected to affect outcomes [20].

(iii) *Correlation design* – Correlation design is often used when answering questions about relationships. Correlation designs can be used with data already available, or with new data. For example, to find out if having a higher education among women is related to lower maternal mortality, a correlation design could be used. However, correlation evidence alone cannot establish causality [19].

(iv) *Case study design* – A case study design is used when the intention is to gain an in-depth understanding of a process, event or situation. Case study method involves extensive description and contextual analysis to learn about a complex instance. It is especially useful when the intervention is relatively innovative or experimental or not well understood. The case study finding, present detail of why the instance occurred as it did as well as articulates what may be important to explore in similar situations. Evaluators considering the case study as a design for evaluation must first decide what type of evaluation question they have and then examine the ability of each type of case study to answer it. The crucial next step is in determining whether the methodological requirements of the chosen case study method can be met in the situation at hand. There are six types of case studies as detailed below.

*Illustrative case studies* are descriptive; they utilize one or two instances to show what a situation is like. The most serious limitation is with the selection of instances. The case(s) must adequately represent the situation or program. Where significant diversity exists, it may not be possible to select a typical site.

*Exploratory case studies* are condensed case studies, undertaken before implementing a large-scale investigation. Where considerable uncertainty exists about program operations, goals, and results, exploratory case studies serve to safeguard investment in larger studies. The greatest pitfall in the exploratory study is prematurity: the findings may seem convincing enough to be released inappropriately as conclusions. Other pitfalls include the tendency to extend the exploratory phase, and inadequate representation of diversity.

*Critical instance case studies* – This method is particularly suited for answering cause-and-effect questions about the instance of concern. The most serious pitfall in this application is inadequate specification of the evaluation question.

*Program implementation case studies* help discern whether implementation is in compliance with its intent. These case studies are also useful when concern exists about implementation problems. Extensive, longitudinal reports of what has happened over time can set a context for interpreting a finding of implementation variability. A requirement for good program implementation case studies is investment of sufficient time to obtain longitudinal data and breadth of information. Training and supervision is essential quality control for data collection and management.

*Program effects case studies* can determine the impact of programs and provide inference about reasons for success or failure

*Cumulative case studies* aggregate information from several sites collected at different times. The cumulative case study can be retrospective, collecting information across studies done in the past, or prospective, structuring a series of investigations for different times in the future. Retrospective cumulation allows generalization without cost and time of conducting numerous new case studies; prospective cumulation also allows generalization without unmanageably large numbers of cases in process at any one time. The techniques for ensuring sufficient comparability and quality and for aggregating the information are what constitute the "cumulative" part of the methodology. Opinions vary as to the credibility of cumulative case studies for answering program implementation and effects questions [20]. One authority notes that publication biases may favour programs that seem to work, which could lead to a misleading positive view [21]. Others are concerned about problems in verifying the quality of the original data and analysis [22].

(v) *Non-experimental design* – Non-experimental designs do not involve a comparison group that did not receive the intervention. The lowest level of evidence occurs with non experimental designs, which consist of case series and anecdotal reports. Although such studies can contain a wealth of useful information, they cannot support inference because they cannot control for factors such as maturation, self-selection, historical influences unrelated to the intervention, and changes in instrumentation [19].

Once the particular evaluation design based on the focus question is implemented, the next logical step is to undertake the programme efficiency analysis. The procedures employed in efficiency evaluation are often highly technical and the analysis is based on numerous assumptions [23, 24].

## 37.5 Programme efficiency analysis

For decision makers the reference programme is often the one that produces the most impact on the most targets for a given level of expenditure. This simple principle is the foundation for cost-benefit and cost-effectiveness analyses. These are tools for assessing whether or not costs of an activity can be justified by the outcomes and impacts [6]. The analysis estimates the efficiency of programme and projects. The economic assumptions are made explicit. It is useful for informing decisions about the most efficient allocation of resources. The information from such an analysis is useful for convincing policy makers and funders that the benefits justify the activity.

### 37.5.1 Cost-benefit analysis

Cost-benefit analysis measures both inputs and outputs in monetary terms [6]. The cost-benefit analysis is a management technique that has attracted the widest attention for application in the health field. The economic benefits of any programme are compared with the cost of that programme. The benefits are expressed in monetary terms to determine whether a given programme is economically sound, and to select the best out of several alternate programmes. The main draw back with this technique is that the benefits in the health field, as a result of a particular programme, cannot always be expressed in monetary terms. The benefits are generally expressed in terms of birth or deaths prevented or illness avoided or overcome [15]. Cost-benefit analysis is controversial because only a portion of programme inputs and outcomes may reasonably be assigned a monetary value. One must ultimately place a value on human life in order to fully monetize the programme benefits [23, 24]. As an example, the cost-benefit analyses of the outcomes of a nutrition education programmes would express in monetary terms as follows: i.e. focus on the difference between money expended on the nutrition education programme and the money savings from reduced expenditure for treating dietary-related diseases such as anemia, goitre, vitamin A related blindness, etc [25].

### 37.5.2 Cost-effective analysis

Cost effectiveness analysis estimates inputs in monetary terms and outcomes in non-monetary quantitative terms [6]. Cost-effectiveness analysis is seen as a more appropriate technique than cost-benefit analysis [23]. Cost-effectiveness analysis requires monetizing only the programme's cost, and the benefits are expressed in outcome units. For example, in a cost-effectiveness analyses of the outcome of a nutrition education programmes, the outcome would be expressed against the set goal in substantive terms [25]: 'A cost-effectiveness analysis of a nutrition education programme would focus on the estimation of money expended in relation to the improvement in the consumption of vitamin A rich foods by target groups'.

These analyses provide systematic approaches to resource allocation. From a conceptual point of view, perhaps the most significant value of efficiency analysis is that it forces evaluators and programme personnel to think in a disciplined fashion about both costs and benefits.

Three major types of efficiency analysis can be undertaken – ex-ante, ex-past or sensitivity. Efficiency analysis done either in the planning or design phases of a programme is called *ex-ante* analysis. Ex-ante analyses are not based on empirical information, and therefore run the risk of either under or over estimating the benefits of effectiveness. Most commonly, efficiency analyses of programmes take place after their completion, often as part of their impact evaluation. This is called *ex-post* analysis where the purpose is to assess whether the costs of the intervention can be justified by the magnitude of net outcomes. An important strategy in efficiency analysis is to undertake several different analyses of the same programme, varying the assumptions made which are open for review and checking. This is called *sensitivity analysis.*

Efficiency analysis may be impractical and unwise for several reasons [23]:

- The required technical procedures may be beyond the resources of the evaluation programme.
- Political or moral controversies may result from placing economic values on particular input and outcome measures. This may obscure the relevance and minimize the potential utility of an evaluation.
- Efficiency assessment may require taking different costs and outcomes into account, depending on the perspectives and values of sponsors, stakeholders, targets and evaluators themselves. This may be difficult for atleast some of the stakeholders to understand, and may obscure the relevance and utility of evaluations.
- It is a complex process to look at the stakeholders who are individuals or organizations directly or indirectly affected by the implementation and results of interventions programmes.
- In some cases, the data needed for undertaking cost-benefit calculations are not fully available. The analytic and conceptual models may be inadequate, and often untested underlying assumptions may lead to faulty, questionable and unreliable results.

## 37.6 Quantitative and qualitative techniques used in evaluation

Both quantitative and qualitative methodologies are used in evaluation depending on the type of evaluation. While impact or outcome evaluation is often quantitative, process monitoring and evaluation often use qualitative information. The relative advantages and disadvantages have been debated extensively in the evaluation literature. However qualitative procedures are difficult and expensive to use if the evaluation depends entirely on this alone. For example, it would be very difficult and expensive to build on qualitative observation in large-scale surveys [23]. The situations where quantitative and qualitative techniques could be used in evaluation are presented in Table 37.14.

*Table 37.14* Applications of quantitative and qualitative techniques [15]

| Quantitative techniques | Qualitative techniques |
|---|---|
| • Cost-benefit analysis | • Organization of the programme |
| • Cost-effective analysis | • Personnel management |
| • Input, process and output analysis | • Communication |
| • System analysis | • Management Information System (MIS) |
| • Network analysis | • Management by objectives |

The use of both qualitative and quantitative and multiple methods can strengthen the validity of findings if results produced by different methods are congruent and/or complement each other.

In summary, it is useful to remember the following points [25]:

- Both type of methodologies are important and have their own place.
- Qualitative methodologies are useful in monitoring and for undertaking process evaluation.
- Outcome/impact evaluation is often quantitative.
- Use of both type of methodologies strengthen validity of findings.

As stated above, the monitoring and evaluation process requires a combination of quantitative and qualitative information in order to be comprehensive. Some people find quantitative information comforting – it seems solid and reliable and "objective". They find qualitative information unconvincing and "subjective". It is a mistake to say, "Quantitative information speaks for itself". It requires just as much interpretation in order to make it meaningful as does qualitative information [2].

Quantitative measurements tell "how much or how many". This is the process of presenting and interpreting numerical data, which includes both descriptive statistics and inferential statistics. Quantitative measurement can be expressed in absolute numbers or as a percentage. It can also be expressed as a ratio [2].

Qualitative measurements tell how people feel about a situation or about how things are done or how people behave [2]. Qualitative research is an inquiry process of understanding a social or human problem based on distinct methodological traditions of inquiry. The researcher builds a complex, holistic picture, analyzes words, report detailed views of informants, and conducts the study in a natural setting. Qualitative data may be collected through open-ended questions in self-administered questionnaires, individual interviews, focus group discussions, or through observations during fieldwork [26].

### 37.6.1 Methods of data collection – quantitative and qualitative

There are various methods that could be followed for data collection when monitoring and evaluating public health nutrition programmes. These are primarily quantitative and qualitative methods. Quantitative methods include project records and reviews, population based surveys while qualitative methods include focus group discussions, observations, ethnographic surveys, social mapping, case studies etc. A few of the commonly used method such as records, surveys, observation, interviews and focus group discussions (FGDs) are presented below.

*(i) Records*

These are information routinely collected in nutrition projects, and the core of an ongoing monitoring system. It should be noted that information from records may be reviewed periodically. Another type of record is secondary data. For example, records from national or regional surveys regarding nutritional status, dietary intake, prevalence of micronutrient deficiencies, household income and expenditure can be obtained. Use of records can be a fast, inexpensive, and convenient way to obtain information. However, it requires a careful inspection of the original collection process, keeping in mind that the validity and reliability of the emerging findings will rest upon the quality of data collection skills [1].

*(ii) Surveys*

Surveys can cover an entire project population or a representative sample. They can include open or closed-ended questions. Open-ended questions allow respondents to answer in their own words while closed-ended questions require specific answers or selection from a set of possible answers. Survey data that is derived from open-ended questions, can give both quantitative and qualitative data. Surveys are a very popular method of collecting data and the reliability of such data depends on the sampling frame, quality of questions and care taken in administering the questionnaire. The surveys done at appropriate point of time in a project cycle can bring out useful data for inference and action. It can be done at baseline, midline and end line to keep a close track of the developments in the project [1, 27].

### *(iii) Observation*

Observations are one method used to assess time-use patterns and behaviours related to desired outcomes. Observation can also offer valuable insights into the social and physical context of the problem being addressed and the use of project inputs [1]. For example, in the field of nutrition, 24 hours feeding behaviour may be observed to learn valuable information. This can be done by one of the following methods:

- A single 24-hour recall
- Multiple 24-hour recalls or multiple diet records

*Single 24-hour recall* is the method of choice if the purpose of the study is simply to describe the average intake of a group. That is, it provides a mathematically accurate group mean. However, it does not provide a good estimate of an individual's usual intake for any individual member of the group.

In *multiple 24-hour recall* or multiple days of diet records method, a number of days of dietary intake are collected; the data begin to approximate an individual's usual intake. Thus, if enough days are collected on each individual, this could be an appropriate measure to use for research in which the individual's usual intake is the unit of interest. Generally, at least three days of diet data are required for the most stable nutrient, percent of calories from fat. Other macronutrients require more, and micronutrients such as vitamin C and vitamin A require many more days [28].

### *(iv) Key informant interviews*

A key informant interview involves a face-to-face meeting between a trained interviewer and a person who can provide an overview/big picture of knowledge, attitudes or practices of the group being monitored or evaluated. Key informants provide a broad view of the situation and this overview is critical in data collection. Similarly a focus group discussion involves group dynamics that allow participants to respond to one another's perceptions, generating new ideas and highlighting conflicting attitudes that might otherwise be inaccessible to an outsider [26, 29].

As mentioned above, an interview is a data collection method that involves oral questioning of respondents, either individually or as a group. It is suitable for use with illiterate people. It also permits clarification of questions through probing. Interviews are probably the most commonly used evaluation method. The tips to be an effective interviewer include [27, 28]:

- Be familiar with research material
- Be familiar with the interview guide
- Practice interviewing through role-playing exercises or pilot interviews
- Practice using the recoding equipment

The interviewer skills have an important influence on the comprehensiveness and complexity of the information that participants provide.

- The interviewer must be able to lend a sympathetic ear without taking on a counselling role; encourage participants to elaborate on their answers without expressing approval, disapproval, judgment or bias; keep track of the questions yet let the conversation develop naturally; and manage the interview while still respecting the principle of participant-as-expert.
- The core skills required establishing positive interviewer/ participant dynamics are rapport-building, emphasizing the participant's perspective and accommodating different personalities and emotional states.

*(v) Focus group discussions*

Focus group discussions (FGDs) are a qualitative method designed to use group dynamics and the flow of discussion to probe deeply into the images, beliefs, and concepts that people have about a particular subject. Ideally, people become involved in the discussion and react to one another's comments. It is not a group interview but a group discussion focused on a topic. These guided discussions are held with small groups of people who have similar characteristics. The discussions are led by a trained moderator who uses a question guide to introduce the topics of interest and probe for deeper discussion.

In the area of public health nutrition programmes, FGDs can be used for facilitating the following tasks [26–30]:

(a) Focus the evaluation and develop relevant evaluation questions by exploring in greater depth the problem to be investigated and its possible causes. It helps to focus on the topic of research and develop relevant research hypotheses by exploring in greater depth the problem to be investigated and its possible causes. For example, a district health officer had noticed that there were an unusually large number of cases of severe undernutrition in under-5-year children in a specific area in the district. The officer wanted to understand the reasons contributing to such situations. Three focus group discussions (one with leaders, one with mothers from the area and one with health staff from the area) were organised. The investigator hoped to identify potential causes of the problem through the FGDs and then develop a more intensive study, if necessary.

(b) Formulate appropriate questions for more structured larger-scale surveys. FGDs help in formulating appropriate questions. For example in planning a study of the incidence of childhood diarrhea and feeding practices, a focus group discussion showed that in the community under study, children below the age of 1 year were not perceived as having 'bouts of diarrhea' but merely 'having loose stools' that were associated with milestones such as sitting up, crawling, and teething. In the questionnaire that was developed after the FGD, the concept 'diarrhea' was therefore carefully described, using the community's notions and terms.

(c) Supplement information on community knowledge, beliefs, attitudes and behaviour already available but incomplete or unclear. FGDs help to understand and solve unexpected problems in interventions. In district X, a recent national (polio) immunization day (NID) showed widely different coverage for immunization per village (50–90%) and in a number of villages a marked decrease in the immunization coverage was observed compared to the previous year. Eight FGD were held with mothers, two in town, three in rural villages with decrease trend in NID coverage and three FGDs in villages with a high immunization coverage throughout. The FGD revealed that the overall concept of NID had raised confusion. Most people believed that the mass NID campaign strengthened the children's immunity against any (childhood) disease, including malaria and Respiratory Tract Infections. In the villages with a low NID coverage, there had been a high incidence of malaria in children immediately after the previous NID campaign and several children died. Mothers therefore, believed that the NID campaign was useless.

(d) Facilitate in developing appropriate messages such as for nutrition health education programmmes and also in exploring controversial topics and issues.

Qualitative data is in the form of description of events in words or transcripts of interview. In case of qualitative data, technique of handling of qualitative data emerging from focused group discussion is critical. For example to get the best results in case of focus groups discussions, one needs to ensure the following [30]:

- Ensure information provided adds meaning or value.
- Focus the analysis by concentrating on questions that meet the objectives of evaluation.

- Categorize information – identifying themes or patterns such as ideas, concepts, behaviour, interactions, incidents, terminology, phrases used. Organise information into coherent categories that summarizes and brings meaning to text.
- Identify patterns and connections within and between categories.
- Interpret the data – key points and important findings – attaching meaning and significance.

## 37.6.2 Process of data analysis

In the process of M & E, there is normally a large amount of information and data. Skills are required to effectively analyse the data. Figure 37.3 presents the process of data analysis which turns the detailed information into an understanding of patterns, trends, and interpretations leading to drawing and presenting conclusion. SWOT (Strengths, Weaknesses, Opportunities and Threats) analysis technique could be used for interpreting the data and drawing conclusions. Analysis is in fact the intuitive understanding of the key themes that come out of the information gathering process. Once the key themes are identified, it becomes possible to work through the information, structuring and organizing it. Then next step is to write up the analysis of the findings as a basis for reaching conclusions, and making recommendations.

The process involved in analysis is depicted in Fig. 37.3.

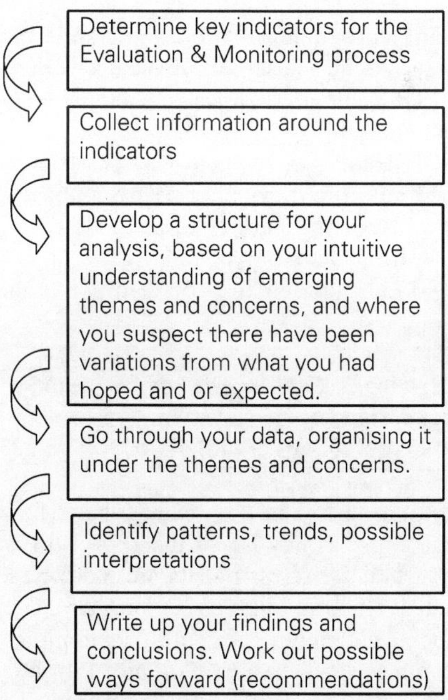


*37.3* Process of data analysis [2]

## 37.7 Monitoring and evaluation – decision making and moving forward

Monitoring and evaluation is of value when the implementers of a programme act on the information that emerges from the analysis of data collected. It is therefore critical to have a strategy and method for collecting, storing, reviewing, analyzing data as well as a timely information feedback system to facilitate management decision making. This cyclic tool is referred to management information system (MIS) and should be part of monitoring and evaluation. Once the findings, conclusions and recommendations from monitoring and evaluation process are in place, it is critical to follow the next set of steps for benefiting from the analytical findings [2].

- Share the findings with stakeholders.
- Review and reflect on the lessons learned. Draw out a list of options for actions.
- Identify programme elements that need to be addressed for improving efficiency, effectiveness and impact.
- Identify issues that are resistance for effective implementation and develop strategy to deal with resistance.
- Make effective decisions about how to move forward.

## References


1. The applied nutrition programme, "Monitoring and evaluation of nutrition and nutrition-related programmes – a training manual for programme managers and implementers". 1999. University of Nairobi and School of Nutrition Science & Policy, Tufts University.
2. SHAPIRO J (1996). Evaluation, Judgment Day or Management Tool? Olive.
3. BOSE AB (1986). Monitoring survival and Development of the young child.
4. Monitoring & evaluation – some tools, methods & approaches – The World Bank, 2004: www.nrhmcommunityaction.org.
5. Logical Framework Approach to project cycle management – LogFrame Handbook, 1997.
6. http://www.mindtools.com
7. PSI Logframe Handbook (2000). The logical framework approach to social marketing project design and management.
8. Monitoring vitamin A programs (1998). IDRC, Micronutrient Initiative, Ottawa, ON, CA.
9. Performance Monitoring Indicators – A handbook for task managers (1996). Published by Operations Policy Department, World Bank, Washington DC.
10. WHO (1996). Indicators for assessing vitamin A deficiency and their application in monitoring and evaluating intervention programmes. WHO / NUT/96.10.
11. Assessment of iodine deficiency disorders and monitoring their elimination – A Guide for Programme Managers (2007). Third Edition. WHO publication.
12. Indicators for assessing Infant and Young Child feeding practices (2008). WHO publication.

13. User-friendly Handbook for Project Evaluation (2002). (NSF 02-057).
14. LEVINSON JF, et al. (1999). Monitoring and Evaluation – A guidebook for Nutrition project Managers in developing countries. Published by Human Development Network, The World Bank.
15. PARK K (2007). Preventive and Social Medicine.
16. HOLTGRAVE DR, QUALLS NL, CURRAN JW, VALDISERRI RO, GUINAN ME, PARRA WC. (1995). An overview of the effectiveness and efficiency of HIV prevention programs. *Public Health Rep.* **110**, pp. 134–146.
17. http://www.civicus.org/new/media/Monitoring%20and%20Evaluation.pdf PACT's Evaluation Sourcebook, 1984.
18. www.ncbi.nlm.nih.gov/bookshelf/br.fcgi? book=hssamhsatip&part=A44942
19. International program for Development Evaluation Training – Building Skills to evaluate development Interventions (2007). Published by The World Bank Independent Evaluation Group & Carleton University.
20. LYNN D (1991). The application of case study evaluations. *Practical Assessment, Research & Evaluation*, **2**(9).
21. BERGER MA (1983). Studying Enrollment Decline (and Other Timely Issues) via the Case Survey. *Educational Evaluation and Policy Analysis*, **5**(3), pp. 307–317.
22. YIN RK (1989). *Case Study Research: Design and Methods.* Beverly Hills, CA: Sage.
23. ROSSI PH and FREEMAN HE (1993). *Evaluation: A Systematic Approach.* Sage Publications.
24. SØNBØ KI, EGGEN AE, THELLE DS (1991). Cost effectiveness of incremental programmes for lowering serum cholesterol concentration: is individual intervention worth while? *Br Med J.* **302**, pp. 1119–1122.
25. www.fao.org/docrep/w3733e/w3733e06.htm
26. www.idrc.ca
27. The teaching Module for Research Methodology and Bio-Statistics (2009). Department of Epidemiology, The Tamil Nadu Dr. M.G.R Medical University, Chennai, India.
28. http://www.nutritionquest.com/research/about_dietary_analysis.htm
29. http://www.bmj.com/cgi/content/full/320/7227/114
30. ELLEN TAYLOR-POWELL MARCUS RENNER (2003). *Analyzing qualitative Data.*

# District and village planning – a decentralised implementation approach in public health in India

*Shraddha Dwivedi, Madhulekha Bhattacharya* and *Ashish Mukherjee*

**Shraddha Dwivedi,** MD in Community Medicine, is Professor and Head of the Department of Preventive and Social Medicine at MLN Medical College, Allahabad.

**Madhulekha Bhattacharya,** MD in Community Medicine, is Dean of Studies and Professor & Head, Department of Community Health Administration at the National Institute of Health and Family Welfare.

**Ashish Mukherjee,** postgraduate in journalism and management, is currently Executive Director at the Centre for Development Finance (CDF) at the Institute of Financial Management and Research (IFMR), Chennai.

## 38.1 Introduction

Planning is an essential management function. It can be defined as a process of setting goals, developing strategies, and outlining tasks and schedules to accomplish the goals. The purpose of planning is to ensure efficient utilization of resources to achieve optimum outcomes. For promotion of effective and efficient delivery of health services to the community, public health planning is of utmost importance.

In India, soon after independence, a centralised approach to planning was adopted with a view to achieve rapid economic development. However, the centralised approach led to development of plans that had little relevance to local needs and did not promote community participation or generate a sense of ownership at the level of grass root implementation. Approaches to helping people have moved over the years from welfare based programmes to development based programmes. In the latter, the focus is on encouraging people to participate in activity and develop a sense of ownership at the level of grass root implementers with the failure of earlier vertical programmes and centralised approaches, decentralised and participative development of plans assumed importance. Numerous efforts have been made in recent times by the government to promote participative district planning approach. The 73rd and 74th Constitutional Amendment Acts, 1992 have accorded a constitutional status to the Panchayati Raj Institutions (PRIs) local bodies as the third-tier of government (Box 38.1).

The amendments have also devolved, both, administrative and financial powers to the local governance, i.e. Panchayati Raj Institutions or PRI. The District Planning Committees have the mandate to compile the action plans prepared by the panchayats and municipalities in the district and consolidate them into the Draft District Plan encompassing all sectors, such as, health, education, sanitation, roads, energy, housing, livelihoods, etc. The role of panchayats is central in the multi-sector development plan at the local level (Figure 38.1).

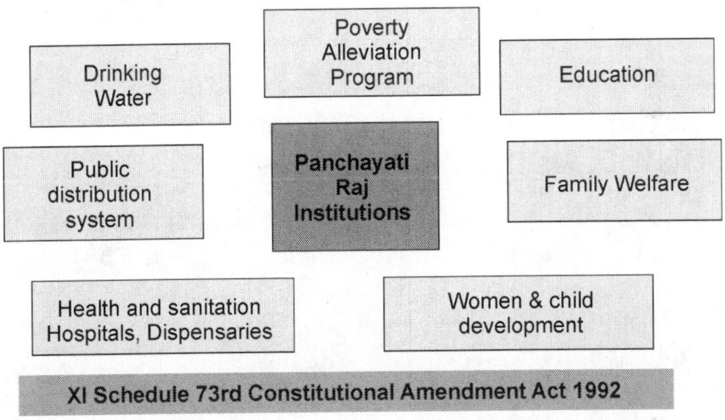


*38.1* Functions delegated to local body – Panchayati Raj Institutions (PRIs).

**Box 38.1 74th Constitutional Amendment Act and District Planning**

The 74th Constitutional Amendment Act mandated the establishment of the District Planning Committee (DPC) for consolidating plans. To facilitate the process the Ministry of Panchayati Raj addressed all the Secretaries of Panchayati Raj of the States on 30th May 2005 requesting them to constitute DPCs in their respective States if these had not been constituted. Their attention was also drawn to the meeting of the Committee of Chief Secretaries and Secretaries of Panchayati Raj Institutions (PRIs) in the states/union territories held on 11th April 2005 wherein the Ministry of Panchayati Raj had communicated that the States that had not constituted DPCs in accordance with Article 243ZD of the Constitution should do so before 31st October 2005 [2]. This led to almost universal constitution of the DPCs.

With reference to the District Health Care System, emerging key responsibilities of PRIs are as follows:

- Ensuring accountability, transparency, responsiveness, resource mobilisation, allocation
- Undertaking decentralised participatory planning
- Prioritizing of local needs
- Undertaking resource mapping
- Undertaking management, supervision, implementation, monitoring
- Involving community-opinion makers
- Conducting health education
- Providing and maintaining infrastructure and logistics
- Collecting and disseminating information-vital statistics
- Undertaking health communication, advocacy in locally relevant and acceptable dialect
- Ensuring inter-sectoral coordination-convergence of service delivery at village level
- Ensuring access to referral system and transport for reaching centres of referrals

## 38.2 National Rural Health Mission (NRHM) and District Health Action Plans

The National Rural Health Mission (NRHM) was launched throughout the country in April 2005, with a view to provide accessible, affordable and quality health care to the rural population. The Mission adopts a synergistic approach by relating health to determinants of good health, viz. segments of nutrition, sanitation, hygiene and safe drinking water. The key features in order to achieve the goals of the Mission include making the public health delivery system fully functional and accountable to the community, human resources management, community involvement, decentralization, rigorous monitoring & evaluation against defined standards, convergence of health and related programmes from village level upwards, innovations and flexible financing and also interventions for improving the health indicators.

Under the National Rural Health Mission (NRHM), a district has been recognized as the most important operational level for ensuring provision of primary health care. One of the key strategies of the NRHM policy is the preparation of need-based district health plans through intensive participation and consultation among the key stakeholders, which includes the PRI, civil society and the concerned government departments.

Each District Health Action Plan (DHAP) is expected to be tailored to the specific needs of each district. Health planning therefore aims at improving the health status of a given population while safeguarding equity and fairness of access, as well as, ensuring responsiveness of the health system to the perceived needs of a community. A district health action plan sets out the goals and strategies that would enable a district to best meet the health needs of its population and is expected to contain a situational analysis of the district, objectives and interventions, work plan, budgets and a monitoring and evaluation plan.

District health action plan integrates the various interrelated components of health to ensure quality of care and access to service with specific reference to various interrelated paradigm as mentioned below:

- *Resources* – health manpower, logistics and supplies, community resources and financial resources, voluntary sector health resources
- *Access to services* – public and private services as well as informal health care services; levels of integration of services within public health system
- *Utilization of services* – continuity of care, factors responsible for possible low utilization of public health system
- *Quality of care* – technical competence, interpersonal communication, and client satisfaction, client participation in management, accountability and redress mechanisms
- *Community* – needs, perceptions and economic capacities, PRI involvement in health, existing community organizations and nature of involvement in health
- *Socio-epidemiological situation* – local morbidity profile, major communicable diseases and transmission patterns, health needs of special social groups (e.g. tribals or *Adivasis*, migrants, very remote hamlets)

Many of the solutions for addressing problems at district level are likely to emerge from block level and village consultations. The district planning process therefore uses a bottom up approach. As the first level of integration, planning of health actions at village level is compiled in the block level action plans and these block level action plans are then consolidated into the district plan. Figure 38.2 presents an overview of the planning process. For this purpose, formation of planning teams and committees at various levels, that is, village, block and district levels have been envisaged.

Thus, the DHAP enables village, block, district and state level functionaries to identify the gaps and constraints to improve services with regard to access, demand and quality of health care. District health plan has been envisaged to be the principal instrument for planning, implementation and monitoring, through a participatory and bottom to up planning process. NRHM-DHAP is the cornerstone of all strategies and activities in the district.

District Missions and District Health Society have been set up in each district in all states for implementation of the programme, and District Missions have been entrusted with the task of development of the annual and prospective plans for the district.

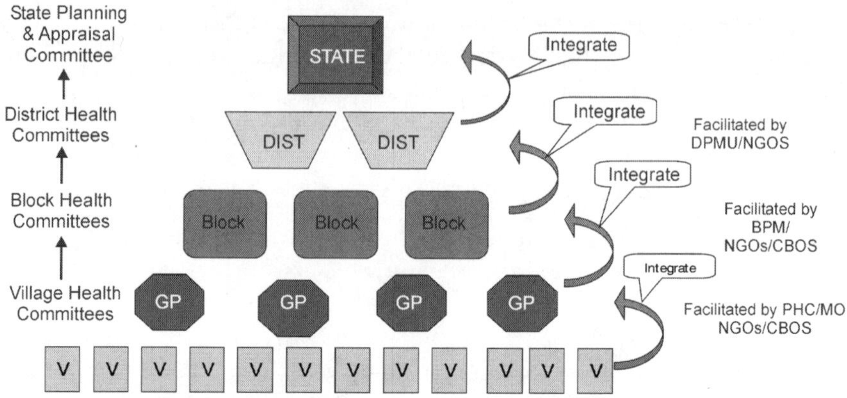


*38.2* Health and nutrition planning process – district health action plan (DHAP).

[V – Village, GP – Gram Panchayat, DPMU – District Programme Mangers of Health Unit, NGOs – Non-Government Organisations, BPM – Block Program Mangers of Health Unit, CBOs – Community-based Organisations, PHC – Primary Health Centre, MO – Medical Officer]

Some of the features of NRHM for increasing community ownership and accountability are as presented below –

## Village health planning

- Frontline community health worker known as ASHA (Accredited Social Health Activist) chosen through local consultative processes.
- ASHA accountable to Village Health Committee (VHC) or Village Health and Sanitation Committee (VHSC).
- VHSC to oversee implementation and monitoring of village health plan.
- Involvement of Block PRI in Block plan.
- Involvement of District PRI in District Health Mission and District Health planning process.
- Provision for Citizen's charter.
- Provision of Community Monitoring and Social Audit.
- Patient Welfare Committees (Rogi Kalyan Samitis) for community management of public hospitals.

Health sub-centres are expected to report on the performance to the lowest governance body of community (Panchayats), hospitals to the Patient Welfare society (*Rogi Kalyan Samitis)* and District Health Mission to the District Council (Zila Parishad).

For the preparation of a district plan, a planning workflow, as presented in Fig. 38.2, is advised to be followed. At the village level, the Village Health & Sanitation Committee (VHSC), a standing committee on health constituted in each village is responsible for the development of the village health plan. A VHSC ideally consists of about 6–8 members drawn from different strata, such as, the panchayat representative, ICDS worker (Anganwadi Worker), school teacher, respected elders of the village and the ASHA, a representative of non-government organisation (NGOs)/Community-based Organisation (CBOs)/Self-help groups (SHGs). The VHSC is entrusted with the task of collecting the basic village data in terms of population status, available resources from standpoint of health and information on burden of diseases, identification of foci of higher morbidities in the village and treatment seeking pattern of different segments of society. Rapid assessment and analysis of the situation is used as the basis for developing health interventions in meeting the health needs of the village population and reducing morbidities and mortalities, mostly owing to childhood diseases or maternal complications. The provision of safe drinking water, sanitation and nutrition of vulnerable groups, such as infants and children, adolescents, pregnant women and the aged, is also considered as an essential part of the plan.

These village plans are then collated at the *Gram Panchayat* level (a cluster of villages and hamlets under the local governance or panchayat. Depending on the size of the villages, one *gram (village) panchayat* (GP) may comprise a single village or a group of few villages). At this level, the GP chief (referred as *Gram Pradhan)* and selected members of the VHSC constitute the planning committee which is responsible for integrating the various village plans. The heath workers such as the ANM (auxillary nurse mid-wife) and MPW (male multi-purpose worker) are responsible for providing support to the village planning committee in conducting household survey and development of the village health plan.

The next level of consolidation is the cluster level or Primary Health Centre (PHC) level (one PHC normally covers a population of 30,000). The PHC level committee, comprising the PHC Medical Officer, representatives of the VHSCs and representatives of local civil society organizations, is responsible for over viewing the activities of the *gram panchayat* planning teams and consolidation of their plans to form the PHC plan. Ideally, at this stage the PHC medical officer is expected to identify resource requirements based on the assessment of the workload in the PHC area and include these in the PHC plan.

The PHC plans are consolidated into a Block Health Plan. Generally, there are about 2–4 PHC plans developed in a block. The Block level monitoring and planning committee comprising the *Block Pramukh* – (referred as *Adhyaksh* of the Block Panchayat Samiti), the Block Medical Officer, the Block Development Officer, NGO/CBO representatives, Block Program Managers of Health Unit (BPMU), wherever available, is responsible for finalizing the block health plans. As per the NRHM guidelines, additional human resources may also be contracted. In order to make the planning more intensive, organisation of public discussions and camps for interaction with key stakeholders are organised.

Finally, the block health plans are assimilated and consolidated to form the district health plan. A District Planning Team (DPT) is recommended to be constituted at the district level by the District Health Mission. DPT is responsible for monitoring the process of plan preparation at the various levels and formulation of the District Health Action Plan. The core members of the DPT team include the District Chief Medical Officer (CMO), Nodal Officers of the Health Department, District Programme Managers of NRHM (DPMU), and representatives of stakeholder departments, development partners and NGO/civil society organisations. The draft plan developed by the team is required to be presented before the District Health Society for approval and onward submission to the State National Rural Health Mission. For operationalising the concept of participative decentralised planning, strengthening of the district planning process assumes great significance. The advantages of district health action plans lie in the fact that:

- Planning is based on local evidence and needs
- Planners are in proximity and close contact of the target audience
- Area specific strategies are formulated to achieve health goals
- Higher interest and ownership of plans by health functionaries
- Mechanisms to partner with community suited to local social fabric is built in
- Cost-effective and practical solutions are expected
- There plans are outcome oriented and not budget-based plans

## 38.3 District Planning Development Cycle

The planning cycle is a sequence of steps which must be followed in deciding what is to be included in the plan [1]. Preparation of the plans at each level constitutes the stages of the planning cycle. The cycle seeks to answer the following questions:

*Where are we now?*

The first step in the planning process is to assess the current status of health and health-related needs and problems in the district. This requires carrying out a situational analysis with regard to health issues.

*Where do we want to go?*

Based on the situation analysis, the selection of priorities and identification of objectives and targets to be met in order to improve the health situation and/or service delivery in a district can be done. Objectives should be SMART (Specific, Measurable, Achievable, Realistic & Time bound).

*How will we get there?*

Details and organization of tasks or interventions to be carried out, by whom, during what period, at what costs and using what resources in order to achieve set objectives and targets.

*How will we know when we get there?*

As we progress with the project/program, we shall have to make an assessment whether we are moving in the right direction to achieve the desired objectives. This requires the development of Objectively Verifiable Indicators (OVIs) for monitoring progress and evaluating results. In heath programmes, indicators are generally depicted as rate, ratio or proportion.

The above questions form a planning cycle as represented in Figure 38.3.

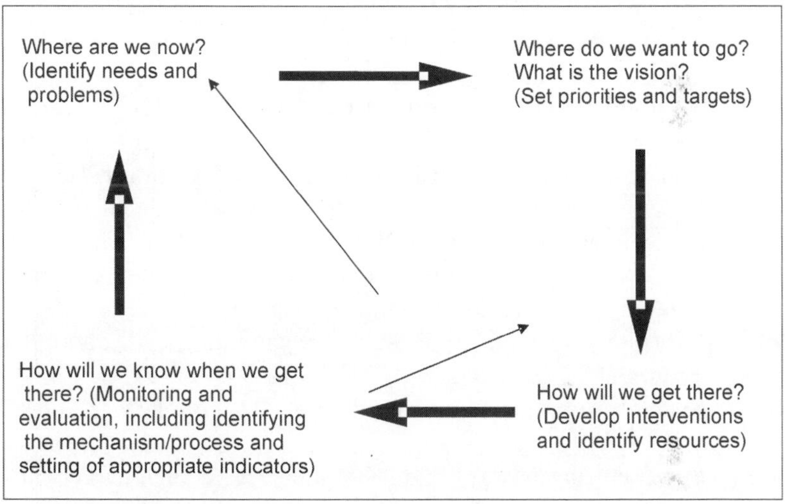


*38.3* The Planning Cycle [1].

As already described, a district plan includes situational analysis which identifies the existing health and health-related needs and problems, as well as an analysis of health service delivery problems. Recognising the fact that all issues cannot be addressed at one time, prioritization of identified problems is essential. This requires identification of objectives and targets to be met in order to improve the health situation and/or service delivery in a district. Accordingly, actions are prioritised and operation plans are prepared to address the identified issues which include assessment of resource requirements, planning implementation details and budget estimates. For effective implementation of the plan and for monitoring progress and outcome, monitoring and evaluation plans are developed in the beginning and included in the district plan.

Under the NRHM a district plan is encouraged to consider the following ten thematic areas so that important health related parameters are not over looked or missed out. These are expected to be incorporated in each of the plans starting from the village to the block level. Box 38.2 presents the format recommended to be used for the documentation of the NRHM district plans.

(i) Provision of quality service and achieving IPHS (Indian Public Health Standards) norms.
(ii) Support systems in terms of transport, human management, logistics, drug supplies, equipment gaps and infrastructure gaps.
(iii) Community participation initiatives like training and capacity building of front line workers.
(iv) Behaviour change communication and other community initiatives.
(v) Management, Administration and Governance like human resource availability, sector reforms etc.
(vi) Reproductive Child Health (RCH I now RCH II) program such as Maternal and Child Health and Mortality, other women issues and immunisation, also Pulse Polio Immunisation (PPI).
(vii) Disease control programs concerned with the local population as well as the National disease Control Programs like TB, Leprosy, Blindness, HIV and AIDS and other diseases in Integrated Disease Surveillance Program.
(viii) Nutrition and food supplies, water, sanitation and school health programs.
(ix) Special programs for urban areas, tribal populations and other vulnerable groups.
(x) Cross-cutting issues and a separate section such as gender and equity issues, private sector interventions which may need to be addressed with every issue in the above thematic areas.

**Box 38.2 The NRHM District Plan Presentation Framework**

- Profile of district
  - Brief history, geographical area, terrain, demographic data, types of habitations, social structure, etc.
  - Status of health indicators
  - Health infrastructure status
  - Human resource position
- Situational analysis
- Implementation/activity plan (should provide the need (justification) for the activity, operational modalities and expected output)
- Training needs/training plan
- Procurement plan
- Implementation arrangements
- Budget estimate

## 38.4 Development of a district plan – capacity building and situation analysis

Preparatory activities for the development of a district plan include constitution of district planning teams at various levels and orientation and capacity building of these teams. The team is responsible for disseminating government instructions pertaining to planning and work out a road map for action. The planning teams are therefore oriented on the objective of the exercise and the processes to be followed. Such orientations are undertaken by organising meetings at various levels – district, block and village levels. It may be noted that a key factor in the successful implementation of decentralised planning is capacity-building at the grassroots level. Therefore, in practical terms a substantial initial investment is required to train local people for conducting situational analysis at the lowest level of operation, i.e., village and based on these developing village plans. Some of the issues to be considered for successful village health planning are

- Community orientation to the role of VHCs and representation in it
- Village ownership of plan and participation in development
- Support to the village health plan by the civil society
- Monitoring of the plan by the VHSC
- Integration of the plan with the government system
- A gender sensitive leadership

Moreover, it is important that the following barriers to successful decentralised planning and implementation by the Village Heath and Sanitation Committee are recognised and taken into account right from the launch of the planning process:

- Lack of capacity to develop a need based heath and nutrition plan for the village.
- A long and formal process which needs simplification and hand holding of the VHSC members.
- Participation and ownership by villagers take time due to lack of understanding of the usefulness of the system.
- Lack of representation from all social classes especially marginalized/ vulnerable groups.
- Viewed as a government owned programme and hence lacking in credibility, resulting in lack of ownership.
- Lack of initiative of NGOs, and Self Help Groups to facilitate the planning process.

Besides capacity building, the planning teams are also required to be equipped with data and information for effective planning exercise. The NRHM guidelines in this respect provide a number of templates to facilitate in data collection. A number of sources of data are recommended to be – out of range from community and village level as well data sources from district level is also used to orient about indicators at the State and National level (Box 38.3). However, the Village Health & Sanitation Committee (VHSC) is the key unit which is responsible for the development of the village health plan and carries out household survey for collection of the basic village data. Discussions and application of Participatory Rural Appraisal (PRA) techniques, described below, is recommended for ascertaining the gaps in health service delivery and identification of village health needs. Box 38.3 shows the sources for gathering data and the planning process.

### Box 38.3 The data sources for decentralised planning

- Household surveys at village level.
- Facility surveys
- Eligible couple register village wise.
- Integrated Disease Surveillance Programme (IDSP)
- Routine reports from sub-centre to district level.
- District data available with the CMO and the District Magistrate.
- Reports under ICDS.
- State Annual Reports.

Data sources from district to orient about indicators at the state and national level

- National Family Health Surveys I, II, III.
- District Level Household Surveys I, II, III.
- Sample Registration System for vital statistics.
- Reports of National Sample Survey Organization (NSSO) on health.
- UNICEF/CARE/UNFPA/YBDO/World Bank/European commission/GTZ/NIPI/USAID etc. for health related studies done at local level.
- Special surveys by medical colleges/other organizations etc in the area on nutritional status, disease pattern and utilization of services.
- Multi-indicator coverage surveys.

**Desk review by the planning teams for**

(a) Assessment of functioning of the government system

- Compare district RCH/disease/utilization of services status with state average and NRHM objectives, at block level and village level data may be used for comparison.
- Map health care facilities/services available- staffing, infrastructure, proximity to habitation, population served etc.
- Map patient load and utilization rates of PHCs and CHCs.
- Review performance of National Programmes in the last year.
- Map the performance of the ANMs/MPWs
- Mapping of ASHA, TBA, AWW-ANM-LHV linkages – geographically sub-centre wise.
- Listing of NGOs – geographic outreach and focus of work.
- Community level groups existing in the district- block and activity wise.
- Last year's budget and expenditure analysis.

(b) Community assessment

- Resource mapping-service providers, communication facilities, drinking water sources, sanitation, nutritional status, levels of poverty.

- Understanding main health problems of women and children, providers used, perception of public health services and providers by focus group discussion.
- Main illnesses in the community, health care related expenditure, problems faced in referral and transport, perceptions about family planning and gender,
- Role of PRI in health related areas (water, sanitation).
- Understanding process of pregnancy, labour and post natal care, beliefs and practices –based on response to key informant interviews with elderly, TBAs.

(c) Understanding community participation and ownership

- Meeting with the village health and sanitation committee.
- Meeting at block level with PRI members to understand their perception of health
- Needs and role of PRI in addressing these needs.
- Meeting at district level with PRI members to understand their perception of health needs and role of PRI in addressing these needs.

(d) Additional information

- Have there been any special health related studies in the district by any other agency – government, international, NGO?

## 38.5 Village planning – understanding the community/ village situation – a shift from central to decentralised planning

This involves assessing the needs of the community from the following two perspectives:

1. Community's needs as perceived by members of community.
2. Community's needs as perceived by the service providers.

The only way to identify what the community feels its needs is to solicit their views and listen to them. One of the effective ways to ensure that the community accepts and acts on identified needs is by involving them in planning and decision making at all stages of service delivery. The community members should feel that the program is owned by them rather than the health worker or the government.

For effective assessment, it is essential to interact with a large number of people representing all socio economic groups in the village such that, in a short time, all the relevant information is collected. Thus, any method which encourages people's participation in expressing and analysing their views will be an effective method for assessing community's needs. This is known as Participatory Learning for Action (PLA). The PLA consists of a process of communication which enables active community participation in analysis of the situation and based on the analysis, plan, implement and monitor services relevant to their needs. The complete process involves.

1. Assessment of needs.
2. Analysis of problems.
3. Actions to be taken for correction.

It is referred to as the Triple A approach.

## Methods of PLA [5]

The following PLA methods are more commonly used and recommended:

1. The chapatti diagram
2. Village transect walk
3. Participatory mapping
4. The seasonality diagram
5. Relative ranking

(1) *The venn (chapatti) diagram.* These diagrams show relationships of various institutions, organizations, programs or individuals with each other and with the village as perceived by the villagers. The purpose of venn diagram is to examine the community's access to different services, that is to say how easily available are the services to them such as health centres, schools, balwadis, block development office, agriculture office, electricity office, irrigation etc. This exercise can be conducted by following steps:

- At the meeting place, a circle is drawn to represent the village.
- Participants cut papers in circles to represent services according to their availability in rendering the service e.g., a hospital may be represented by a large circle. They can arrange circles of different sizes as per their utility to them in descending order so that the sizes reveal their accessibility.
- The services close to the village are placed closer to the circle representing the village, and the services which are more difficult to reach in distance are placed farther away (Figure 38.4).
- Similar exercise, using the venn diagram is also undertaken for a specific service, e.g. care and services of pregnant women (Figure 38.5).

(2) *Village transect walk.* This is an observatory walk through the village living area, observing and making notes of the layout of the village, housing, drainage, backyards, infrastructure such as schools, shops, wells, health facility etc. This is a pre-requisite for mapping. This walk also helps to locate areas in the village which are in need of greater attention/ development. The village transect also gives a greater insight into the aspects of village life that are of a social nature such as caste, religion, customs, culture, health and interactions between various groups. Through

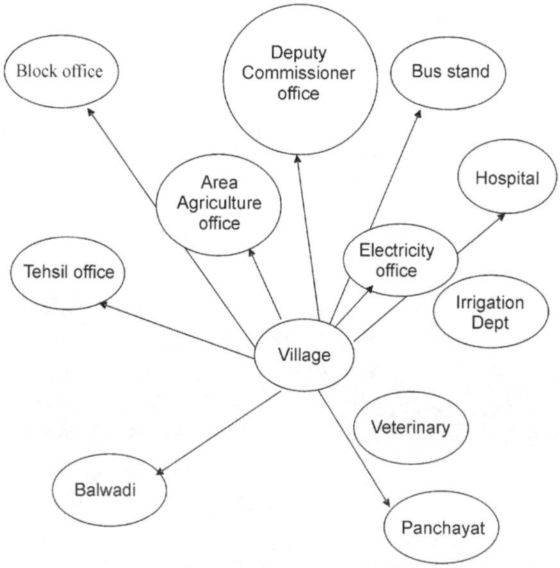


*38.4* Venn diagram – services available at a village level.

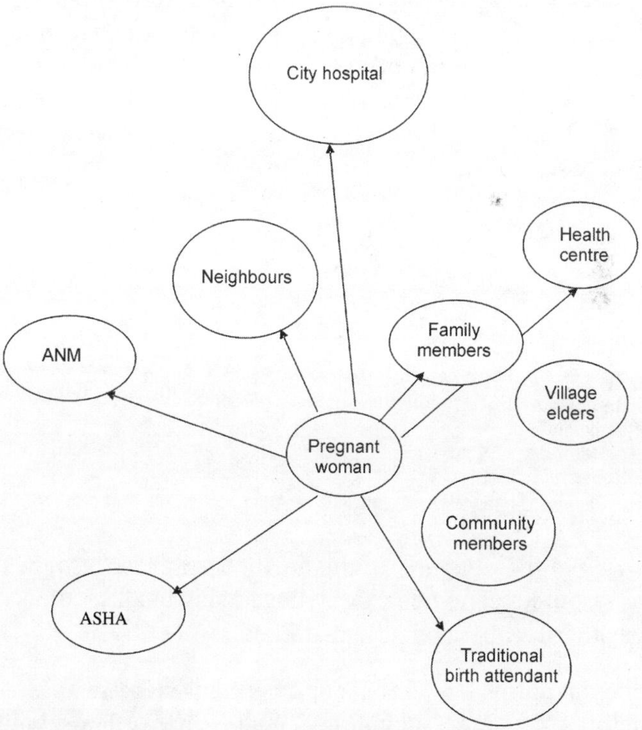


*38.5* Venn diagram – care and services to the pregnant women in a village.

this exercise, it is attempted to determine the ownership, type, productivity and present status of different resources from an area's geographical conditions by conducting the following activities.

- First, select persons from the community with good knowledge of the area's resources.
- Divide them into two groups, e.g. A and B. There should be a facilitator in each group who is responsible for conducting these exercises.
- In each group, start with a boundary of the area and set a distance e.g., 20 m, 30 m or 50 m (decided by the community). Collect information about all resources within that distance, including ownership, types, productivity, and uses. For example, Group A could begin on one side of the selected area and continue until they reach the other boundary, while group B could start at a different location as shown in the picture below. Usually, two groups take two opposite routes, one going vertically across the village and the other horizontally. Collect information about different resources on the basis of aforementioned parameters. For example, for water we would note canals, hand pumps, tube wells, public taps, ponds, irrigation tanks, etc. In this way, both groups will continue to gather information as they continue from one side of the area to the other.

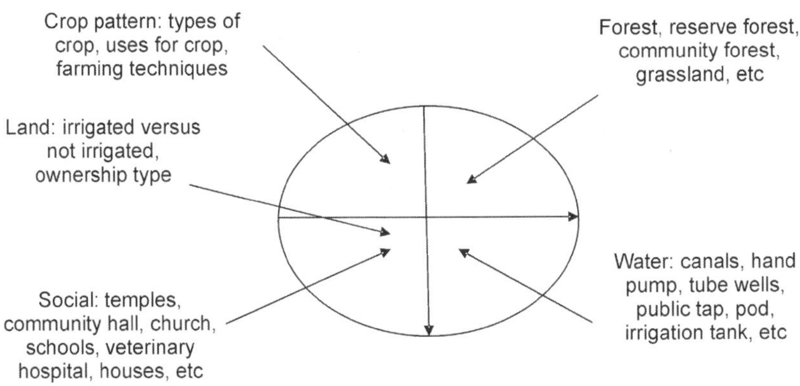


*38.6* Village transect walk.

(3) *Participatory mapping*. In this method villagers' groups undertake social and resource mapping of the village using chalks, coloured rangoli powder or other locally available materials.

(i) Social mapping – social mapping is an exercise to study social structures of an area, including elements such as households, castes, community centres (gathering places, temples, well, panchayat ghar, ration shop for PDS, veterinary centre, cooperative bank, health sub centre, shops, post office, bus stop etc), ratio of male / female and literacy status. The steps followed in social mapping are:

- This exercise is done in an open area.
- Facilitators must ensure participation by people from different castes and ages. Both men and women must participate.
- With the use of local materials such as coal, sandstone, and colored powder, participants are encouraged to map their local area.
- The map presents location of commonly used places, such as health centres, veterinary centres, ICDS Centres, schools, mahila mandal gathering places, panchayat etc.
- On the basis of participants' knowledge about the area, participants will create such a map.
- The facilitator must systematically collect and record information gained.
- It will aid in studying the socioeconomic status of the village. The habitation of different castes separately and together will emerge.

The exercise helps eventually in identifying names of the head of the family, the castes pattern and their habitations, number of men/women/ children and distribution of different age groups, their literacy status, main as well as other occupations, the livestock and grains and vegetables grown by the family in the land etc.

(ii) Resource mapping – resource mapping is a study and analysis of resources like water, forest, land etc. The existing situation is mapped and the resources available are analysed. Following method is followed for conducting resource mapping:

- In a community meeting, participants draw a map of their village using local materials.
- In this map, different resources are represented by using specific signs and materials.
- By using specific signs and materials, participants are encouraged to distinguish and classify specific types of resources. For example, different types of water resources include river, ponds, canals, tube wells, irrigation tanks, hand pumps, etc.
- By this method information on most aspects of rural life, resources within the community, location of various social and economic groups and houses of beneficiaries like pregnant mothers and children with diseases is put together in a visual map (Figure 38.7).

(4) *The Seasonality diagram.* This exercise helps to understand the seasonal problems related to disease prevalence, cropping pattern,

employment etc. Additional information on events such as needing a loan, grains for sustenance, festivals, sickness and weddings are collected. The activity is conducted as follows:

Represent each event with a different, locally available material, for example, a scarcity of food could be represented with a small quantity of such grains. Another example could be that during the rainy months of June and July, people have greater need for money due to lack of livelihood and may need loans. This could be represented by coins.

| | *Loan needed* | *Grains* | *Festival* | *Illness* | *Seasonal rainfall* | *Drought* | *Migration* | *Wedding* |
|---|---|---|---|---|---|---|---|---|
| January | | | * | ** | | | | |
| February | | | * | | | | | ** |
| March | | | * | | | | | *** |
| April | | | * | | | * | | |
| May | | | * | | | * | * | |
| June | *** | ** | * | * | ***** | | ** | |
| July | *** | ** | * | * | ***** | | ** | |
| August | | | * | | | | | |
| September | | | * | | | | | |
| October | | | * | | | | | |
| November | | | * | | | | | |
| December | | | * | ** | | | | |

Another seasonal exercise useful in health programmes is to analyse the months in which children suffer from diarrhoea or respiratory diseases. By this exercise, we can work with community to increase their understanding of courses and effort to be made to prevent and manage diarrhoea and acute respiratory infection.

(5) *Relative ranking.* This method indicates the priorities and the preferences of the people. It is a very useful method if the list of felt needs is long and prioritization as per their needs has to be done.

## 38.6 Village plan to district level plan

The understanding gained from this community needs assessment and the use of the triple A approach results in development of a plan for the village which can effectively use the resources of the community for the best result and ensure their participation to achieve the desired targets and goals related to health. Figure 38.8 shows the village level process and the collation of data up to the district level.

## 38.7 Conclusion

In conclusion it can be stated that the district health planning is now being followed under NRHM. All states use district planning as the base from which to formulate the Project Implementation Plan (PIP). Over the years,

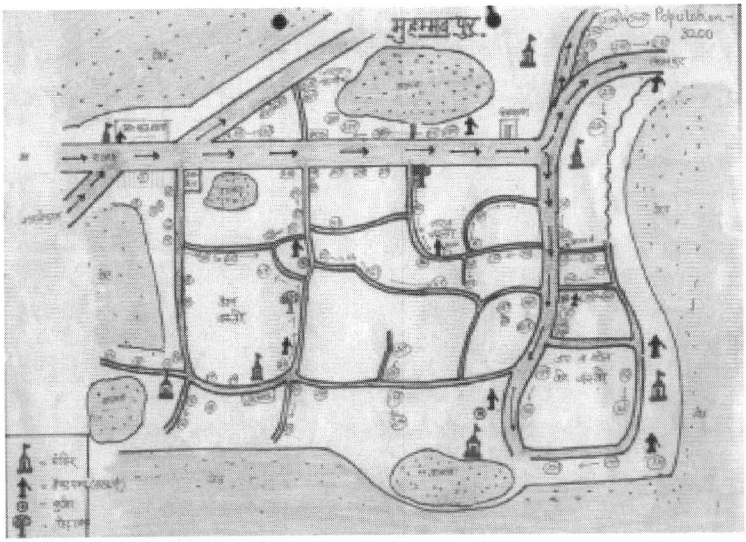

*38.7* Resource mapping at village level.

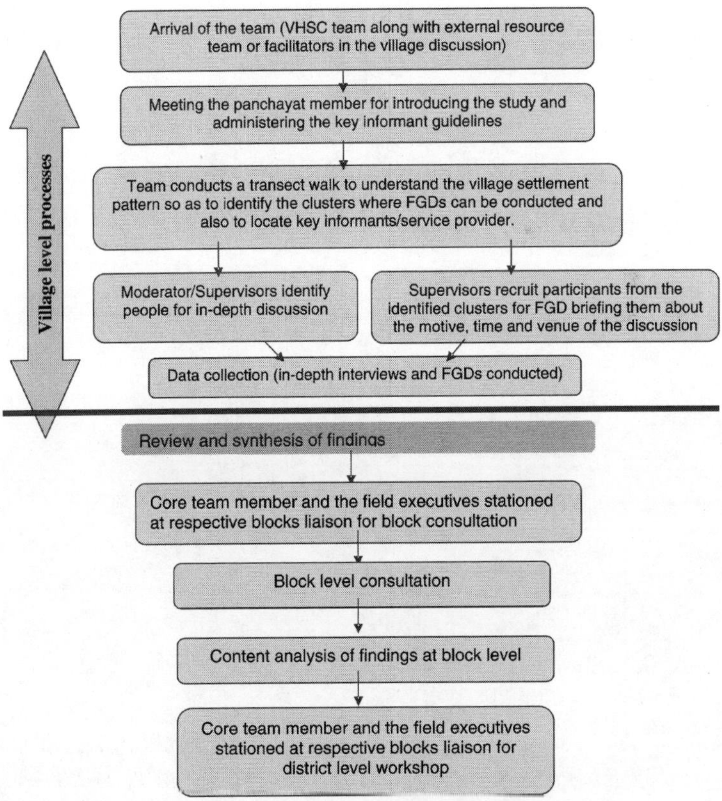


*38.8* Village level process and collation up to district level [3].

based on lessons learned, the district planning activity is continuously being refined and effort is being made to make the data base projections realistic. District plan of action also forms the basis for measuring achievements and for documenting the constraints faced in achieving the stated targets.

## References

1. District health management team training module: planning and implementation of health services, WHO Regional Office for Asia.
2. The State of Panchayats: 2007-08, An independent assessment. Volume I, Thematic report. Chapter 3a, pp. 117–134. Govt. of India, April 2008.
3. Broad Framework for Preparation of District Health Action Plans (2006). Ministry of Health & Family Welfare, Govt. of India.
4. Training of Auxiliary Nurse Midwives for "Building Effective Community Partnerships for implementing the Reproductive and Child Health programme" Facilitator's Guide. Ministry of Health & Family Welfare, Govt. of India.
5. CORD. CORD training manual, Book 1. CORD's Resource and Lead Centre, Sidhbari, Himachal Pradesh.

# 39

# Nutrition–Health education and communication for improving women and child nutrition

*Shubhada Kanani*

**Shubhada Kanani**, PhD, has been a faculty member in the Department of Food and Nutrition, the M.S. University of Baroda, Vadodara, India, for the last twenty two years. Her areas of expertise include nutrition anthropology, nutrition program management and evaluation, health systems research, gender sensitive nutrition research, and nutrition–health education communication. In particular, Dr. Kanani has been a trainer to build capacity in qualitative-participatory research, and behavior change communication interventions including methodologies such as Trials for Improved Practices (TIPS).

## 39.1 Introduction

One has heard these familiar lines: *Give a man a fish, and you feed him for a day; teach him how to fish, and you feed him for life.* This underscores the crucial importance of self-empowerment; and one of the most effective and long lasting empowering tools is knowledge. This chapter traces the beginnings of nutrition-health education, its critical importance in the prevailing nutrition scenario of the country and the emergence of the behavior change focus in program settings. This is followed by an overview of experiences and lessons learnt from major international and national projects. Key elements in the design of a successful behavior change intervention are described with the hope that readers can apply this knowledge in their own settings.

## 39.2 An operational definition of nutrition–health education

Although nutrition is a discipline distinct from health (including public health), in practice, nutrition services are most often linked to health services and commonly monitored in terms of both nutrition and health outcomes. Secondly, operationally speaking, education and communication programs for improving nutritional status are implemented under the umbrella of national health and development programs. Thirdly, nutritional improvements depend as much on addressing health disorders (for example, diarrhea) as they do on ameliorating nutrient deficiencies. Hence, integrating nutrition and health issues in education and communication efforts makes sense from both, the biological and programmatic perspectives. With this view, the term *Nutrition–Health Education (NHE)* refers to a systematic process, focusing on behavior change; that educates and facilitates people to understand the significance of optimal nutrition-health practices and to make the best use of available food–health and care resources with the ultimate goal of improving nutritional and health status.

This definition encompasses the importance of both knowledge and behavior change and keeps in focus the eventual goal, which is improving the state of nutrition and health. Thus, effective NHE is one that

- enhances knowledge regarding desirable nutrition-healthcare practices;
- positively influences attitudes and traditional beliefs;
- motivates vulnerable families to act on that knowledge for their own health and nutritional well being.

An important feature of good NHE is that it is culture and gender sensitive; for example, in a country like India, NHE should acknowledge girl child discrimination and women's constraints.

## 39.3 Why is nutrition–health education important?

Undernutrition, especially among women and young children from low socioeconomic strata has a multi-factorial etiology which includes the triad of food insecurity, infections coupled with poor access to health services and inadequate caregiving attention towards both, the woman and the child. NHE has the potential to address all these factors in an integrated manner. Secondly, NHE helps create demand for the available nutrition and healthcare services which often remain under-utilized simply because beneficiaries are not aware of them or their benefits. For example, educating women about the benefits of iron-folate tablets and how to manage side effects (if any) through effective NHE helps create a demand for these tablets and improves compliance. Thirdly, contrary to what is widely believed, NHE does show a positive and significant impact among vulnerable groups even in poverty situations – if designed, planned, implemented and evaluated properly by committed personnel.

How can NHE favorably influence nutrition–health-care practices in households [1]? Following are few examples with reference to nutrition:

- In poor communities, NHE can play an important role in educating families regarding best use of available resources.
- Even if calorie adequacy is ensured to some extent through increased income, effective NHE is often needed to bring about qualitative improvements in diets such as enhancing levels of several important micronutrients like vitamin A, iron and iodine.
- Due to strong traditional beliefs (rather than inadequacy of resources) foods are often withheld or given in inadequate amounts to infants or women. Feeding is discontinued during diarrhea. NHE has a strong potential to counter harmful beliefs and to change dietary practices.
- Urbanization, misinformation by health/medical practitioners and influence of mass media erode healthy traditional practices, like breastfeeding and encourage development of unhealthy lifestyles and food habits. NHE can help reverse such unfavorable trends and re-establish favorable practices.
- There is often an inability by parents or caregivers to *recognize* malnutrition (poor weight gain) in preschool children, especially 6–24 months of age. When moderately malnourished children (about 40% in India) escape notice, and are deprived of prompt attention in the early stages of growth faltering; many slip into severe malnutrition. NHE can help families and communities identify and recognize the 'invisible' problems of malnutrition so that timely remedial measures can be taken.
- NHE creates demands for services such as iron folic acid supplements, vitamin A supplements and other services.

Further, effective NHE which improves both awareness and practices can accelerate our progress towards achieving several of the Millennium Development Goals (MDGs) pertaining to not only child and maternal health but educational goals as well.

## 39.4 Shift in focus from nutrition education to behavior change communication

The beginning of modern nutrition education may be traced to the early attempts at prevention of protein energy malnutrition (PEM) in infants and children, primarily due to faulty complementary feeding. The need for nutrition education in developing countries gained international recognition in 1950 with the first report of the Joint Food and Agriculture Organization / World Health Organization (FAO/WHO Expert Committee on Nutrition, which emphasized the importance of nutrition education in the health sector. By 1958 the same committee reported, "Education in Nutrition is a necessary part of practical programs to improve human nutrition..." and recommended as channels for nutrition education, schools, maternal child health (MCH) and public health centers, community development and related programs as well as agricultural extension and home economics extension services. The 1960s saw an emphasis on audio-visual aids and the creation of programs such as the Applied Nutrition Programs (ANP), in which nutrition education was placed at a level of priority equal to that of other project activities, rather than being considered a casual adjunct to curative health [2].

### 39.4.1 From awareness to behavior change

Since the 1960s, and in particular, in the last twenty years, health programs, and along with them nutrition programs as well, evolved in many ways. One noteworthy change has been in the paradigm shift from viewing NHE activities as 'transfer of information to the intended beneficiary' to NHE which 'promotes and sustains behavior change based on the information imparted and knowledge given to the beneficiary'. For many years now, organizations have used the term "information, education and communication" (IEC) to refer to strategies to improve people's awareness and practices. However, in implementation of IEC activities, the attention has remained limited towards increasing awareness without enough focus on whether practices have indeed improved. Since the 1980s, as experience accumulated and better understanding of communication and behavior change theories developed, the term 'behavior change communication' (BCC) has been the preferred terminology instead of IEC. BCC builds on IEC, and emphasizes that communication should be strategic and guided by systematic processes and behavioral theories with the objective of influencing practice.

Strategic BCC programs use a systematic process to understand people's situations and influences on behavior. They develop messages that respond to people's concerns. They draw on behavioral theory, define clearly the specific objectives they want to achieve, integrate these objectives into their program plans, and use them as a basis for measuring success. Another important dimension of BCC programs is priority given to community involvement. Community participation can range from assisting with needs assessment, planning, implementing or evaluating activities to direct involvement in decisions about all aspects of program management, resource allocation, and assessing impact [3].

### 39.4.2 Social marketing – a major contributor to the behavior change focus

The term "social marketing" was first introduced in 1971 and described the use of marketing principles and techniques to advance a social cause, idea or behaviour [4]. With the emergence and application of the Social Marketing (SM) concept in the 80s and 90s, the significance and the means for behavior change promotion have been realized. SM is a systematic approach to solving problems, which is related to service utilization, product development and acceptance, and behavior adoption. Social marketing may involve both the selling of a commodity and the selling of an idea or practice; this also implies the promotion of a related attitude or belief which influences the nutrition or health practice.

Social marketing is distinguished by its emphasis on "non-tangible" products such as ideas, attitudes and lifestyle changes. The central tenet is that effective strategies are based on the needs and interests of the target consumer. Empirical consumer research is used to identify possible consumer segments, to understand their needs in the context of their lives, and for developing appropriate programs and communication strategies to meet their needs [5, 6].

Since the fundamentals of SM approach come from marketing principles, program management is often structured to reflect a marketing operation (e.g. health workers are trained to become better sales agents for the program, not just deliverers of services); and a result orientation of marketing implies that progress is measured in terms of outcomes, not mere coverage. Planners need to have a conceptual overview of how a social marketing intervention works (Table 39.1) [7].

*Table 39.1* Conceptual overview of a social marketing intervention [7]

| *Stage* | *Outcome* |
|---|---|
| (1) Planning research | Behaviour change objectives and other project goals defined |
| (2) Development of campaign strategy | Messages, materials designed, products and services established |
| (3) Prerequisite training and networking activities | Infrastructure prepared |
| (4) Project implementation activities | Social marketing campaign carried out |
| (5) Summative evaluation | Project outcomes assessed |

Four features of social marketing (SM) highlight the unique aspects of SM and distinguish it from other forms of NHE – two are related to objectives and two are related to techniques of SM [5].

Two major objectives of SM are aiming for change in behavior (not just imparting information) and creation of demand (concentrating on that half of the marketing equation that is often ignored – the people).

The behavior change emphasis encourages social marketers to beam their efforts on strategies that result in adoption of a desirable practice – whether it is at the household level (example, adding green leafy vegetables to complementary food of a toddler) or use of an available service (taking the regular supply of IFA from the health centre and consuming the tablets). Unless information is relevant to changing behavior, it usually does not find a place in SM approaches.

Behavioural change can be marketed to the individual directly (through direct action) or it can be facilitated by the provision of a new product or service (Table 39.2)

*Table 39.2* Marketing strategies for behaviour change objectives [7]

| *Health outcome* | *Marketing/promotion focus* | *Type of behaviour change objectives* |
|---|---|---|
| Family planning | Manufactured goods, e.g. condoms | Purchase and use |
| Personal hygiene reduces incidence of diarrheal diseases | Direct action | Skill and adherence |
| Immunisation to children | Service, e.g. administration of vaccine as per the schedule | Access and compliance |

In the case of family planning, the products to be marketed are the means, e.g. condoms or other contraceptives by which contraception behaviour can be altered. An ideal family planning social marketing campaign should have the dual task of promoting (through more effective distribution, pricing and promotional mechanisms) a family planning product as well as providing consumers with the knowledge and motivation to appropriately use contraceptives. Some behavioural change objectives do not require the marketing of a supportive good or service. For example, marketing personal hygiene is a question of individual knowledge, skills and motivations. In this case, the products to be marketed are knowledge and practices that will facilitate in taking direct actions to solve their problems [7].

Projects such as Brazilian breastfeeding campaign, contraceptive marketing efforts in Thailand and Bangladesh, social marketing of vitamin A rich foods in Thailand and social marketing of iron folic acid tablets to women in reproductive age group in Cambodia, Philippines are examples of well designed social marketing interventions [7–10]. Box 39.1 presents details of a social marketing intervention.

## Box 39.1 Social marketing – vitamin A rich foods [10]

The three year social marketing of vitamin A rich foods project was implemented in a district of north east Thailand between October 1988 and September 1991. The project used nutrition communication as its main approach for reaching 134 villages with a population of 122,000. The preliminary research (quantitative and qualitative) sought answers to four key questions:

- What is the vitamin A status and fat/oil consumption of people living in the target area?
- Who are the vulnerable groups for vitamin A deficiency?
- What potential strategies are available?
- Which strategies are feasible given existing cultural, economic and environmental conditions?

The findings revealed that dietary diversification, as a long term strategy, would need to focus on local production and consumption of vitamin A rich vegetables. With proper knowledge and motivation, community members, through social gardens could produce enough vegetables for the entire year which were drought resistant. The research also segmented the intended audience into primary, secondary and tertiary groups.

The social marketing strategy was used for a nutrition communication programme. The project design focused on gaining the support and confidence of national / local government administrators. New communication techniques were used to motivate the behaviour change process and there was influence from fields of marketing and advertising. It was recognised that while knowledge is important for change, there are a host of personal and environmental factors which play a role in the communication and behavior change process.

Formative research was used to design the communication programme (i.e., identify factors that could influence adoption of practices, define audience and their needs, selection of food items), select and pretest media, materials and channels as well as monitor educational program progress and evaluate the projects success. All factors contributing to behaviours – personal, community or environmental – were taken into consideration.

The campaign was implemented in three stages – first stage focused on creating and monitoring a nutrition information society. This was followed by ivy gourd as an image representing other vitamin A rich vegetables. The third stage entailed combining nutritional messages with concrete action programmes which was designed and carried out by community and local government collaborations. In the first stage, the focus was not only on 'why' a dietary or related practice needed changing, but on how this could be made feasible and acceptable. The second stage involved boosting the ivy gourd image. A social advertising approach was used. The communication strategy focused on fulfilling two specific behavioural objectives – raising community member's awareness about ivy gourd and getting them interested in it as a food item. In addition of mass media communication (radio, pamphlets/posters, newsletters, public address system, cassettes, direct manual, direct mail), community action programmes, school- and community-based activities were also organised.

Significant change in KAP (knowledge, attitude and practice) regarding consuming vitamin A rich foods was achieved. Ivy gourd was believed to be a food item of high nutritive value and was observed to be family and their children's favourite vegetable. Over 50% families actively grew ivy gourd. Results revealed that the project most successfully changed the usage of green leafy vegetables by lactating women, mothers of preschool children and school children. Positive impact was also observed among government officials and the community.

Demand creation is important because until we understand consumer needs; their view of 'good quality' in nutrition service or health care; and also cater to these needs, merely attending to the supply side will not help. When the importance of a service or a household practice is understood by the beneficiary and it is clearly perceived as meeting a felt need, then programs become more cost effective and behavior change is more rapid and visible.

Two techniques which are integral to SM include

- using a **feed forward approach** as popularized by Dick Manoff: an approach that minimizes "feed back shocks", that is, we first go to potential users of the messages or products being promoted to find out what they want, through formative research.
- focusing on **creativity** in message design and implementation strategy. Creativity is not just for message design where persuasive, captivating and memorable messages are the goal, but also developing program strategies through creative interpretation of research findings.

Box 39.2 presents four principles of SM in practice.

### Box 39.2 The marketing mix – the four P(s) of social marketing

SM conceives of the consumer as the centre of a process involving four variables: product, price, place, and promotion [5].

- A proposed **Product** (whether a commodity, idea, or health practices) is defined in terms of the users' beliefs, practices, and values. If the community perceives diarrhea in 1–2 year olds as a 'normal part of development' or looks for medicines to stop diarrhea rather than prevent dehydration, these concerns need to be addressed while encouraging the use of ORS packets when a child has diarrhea.

  A product can be positioned using several different strategies including pricing attributes (e.g., regular consumption of iron–folic acid tablets by mothers for health of foetus), benefits (e.g., contraceptives that prevent unwanted pregnancies), or attributes (e.g., low price). Positioning strategy also can be applied to health related behaviour change objectives and are best positioned in relation to target audience "resistance points". For example, for years breastfeeding was glamorized as the "ideal thing" to do whereas women viewed it as hard work. The successful media campaign in Brazil therefore positioned the media campaign with emphasis "breastfeeding is hardwork but is well worth that effort." An element of empathy was introduced in the message and was reinforced by health professionals and community-based mother support groups.
- **Price** can refer to a monetary expenditure, an opportunity cost, a status loss, or consumers' time. Even if a rural woman pays no money getting an ORS packet from the health centre, it does not mean that it costs her nothing. The day of travel to the centre to get her child examined by a doctor or nurse, the inconvenience to family, time taken to make the ORS at home, or the lack of conviction regarding usefulness of ORS may all seem too costly relative to perceived benefits. The price of a particular product is never fixed; it varies according to the target audience segment, and often according to the individual.

- The concept of **Place** refers to the channels through which products flow to users and the points at which they are offered. Product availability and distribution may involve not only retail and wholesale supply system, but also the efforts of health providers, volunteer workers, friends and neighbours. "Place" may be a store, a health centre, or even a person such as a traditional birth attendant who carries a supply of ORS.
- In any SM activity, **Promotion** requires more than simple advertising. It requires extensive consumer education to assure appropriate use of products. Motivational strategies are also essential in encouraging adoption of new ideas and social products. Correct ORS packet utilization or even educating households on how to make home-made ORS requires culturally sensitive and relevant promotional activities.

## 39.4.3 Focus on education for "optimal food intake" rather than "nutrient requirements"

Many countries have dietary guidelines expressed in scientific terms, with quantitative recommendations of nutrients and food components (Recommended Dietary Allowances – RDAs, Reference Nutrient Intakes – RNIs, or Recommended Dietary Intakes – RDI). However, such recommendations are commonly misunderstood and often applied inappropriately by both nutritionists and the public. Realizing the limitations of 'nutrient-based guidelines' for public education, the 'ICN Plan of Action', adopted in the 1992 International Conference on Nutrition (ICN) of FAO–WHO, included a significant section, 'Promoting appropriate diets and healthy lifestyles'. It stated, 'Governments are called upon ...to provide advice to the public by disseminating qualitative and/or quantitative dietary guidelines relevant for different age groups and lifestyles and appropriate for the country's population'. The ICN Plan of Action is notable for the absence of numerical targets for food and nutrient intakes. This indicates broader thinking among nutritionists, away from policies dictated by nutrient recommendations toward ones defined by prevailing public health issues and consumer needs. Subsequently to the ICN Plan of Action, Food-based Dietary Guidelines (FBDG) were developed by FAO–WHO after an international consultation in 1995 [11]. FBDGs are intended for use by the general public; and provide nutrition education and dietary guidance in terms that are understandable to most consumers. FBDGs are a practical way to assist people to reach appropriate nutritional goals, as they take into account customary dietary patterns and indicate modifications needed to address particular concerns; they are based on diets (foods) and not nutrients. These guidelines consider the total diet; they recognize the varied social, economic, agricultural and environmental conditions that affect eating patterns and acknowledge that various dietary patterns can be consistent with good health. They strive to ensure that they are easily understood by the people at various levels of literacy, refer to foods wherever possible, rather than nutrients and recommend use of educational approaches that avoid radical changes in current dietary practices, but rather build on existing practices.

According to FAO [12], the National Institute of Nutrition, India, initiated the process of developing FBDGs in 1997 and published and disseminated these guidelines in 1998. Some examples from these guidelines are as follows:

- Nutritionally adequate diet should be consumed through a variety of foods.
- Green leafy vegetables, other vegetables and fruits should be used in plenty.
- Cooking oils and animal foods should be used in moderation, and vanaspati/ghee/butter should be used only sparingly.
- Overeating should be avoided to prevent overweight and obesity.

### 39.4.4 NHE – holistic approach for addressing undernutrition

Over time, it was clearly evident by practitioners of NHE programs that NHE needs to be holistic; given the fact that malnutrition and disease have a multi-factorial etiology. The UNICEF conceptual model for childhood malnutrition (Figure 39.1) has accorded higher focus to NHE and has included all the three primary dimensions – food, health and care – for addressing undernutrition. This model set the stage for further development of NHE as an integrated intervention and not merely limited to influencing food or nutrient intake. As the UNICEF framework reveals, the immediate causes of malnutrition and death are inadequate dietary intake and/or disease which in turn are caused by conditions that affect (1) household food security; (2) health services and healthy environment; and (3) care for women and children, especially care of the girl child. The framework further reveals that the basic causes of undernutrition relate to poverty (poor availability of resources), social status (women's inferior status) and the government policies and priorities.

Thus, while NHE needs to have a clear focus on selected behaviors, it also needs to take into account the underlying and contextual factors influencing the behaviors and the problem being addressed.

## 39.5 Design and implementation of a nutrition health education program with a communications perspective

The acid test of successful NHE is that practices improve significantly in a majority of the vulnerable households in a sustained manner, and eventually become a 'norm' in the community. In the area of nutrition and

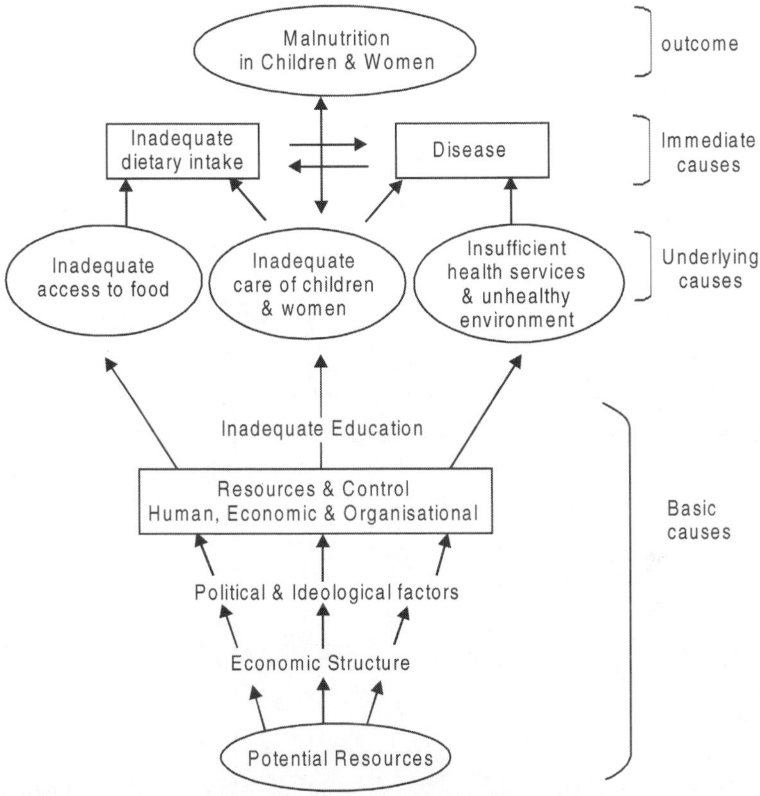


*39.1* The UNICEF conceptual model for childhood malnutrition [13].

health communication, many communication models and theories have been put forward. In this section is presented an adapted version of a simple and comprehensive model by Hubley (1993) [14] which gives four components of a communication process—these could be applied to any communication strategy. This framework has been found to be useful for imparting training on communication skills to grassroots functionaries and supervisors.

## 39.5.1 The receiver (audience)

It is absolutely critical to first become familiar with the belief systems, current practices, family and community environment of the intended audience. A method that will be effective with one audience may not succeed with another. Different individuals respond differently to the same message, one reason being differences in the characteristics of the receivers themselves. For example, a rural woman or adolescent will respond very

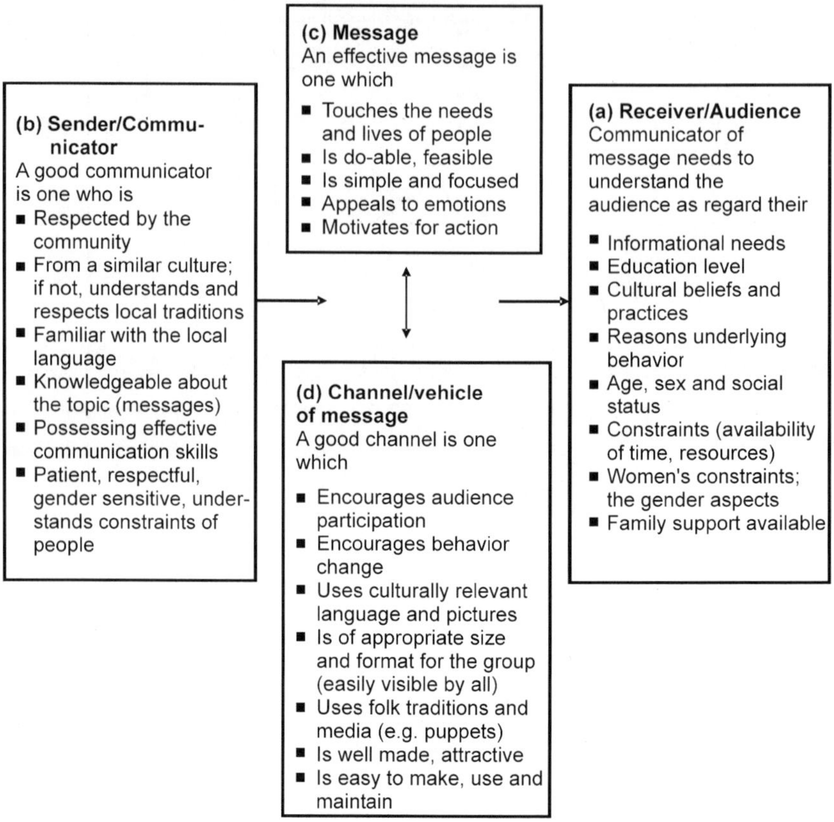


*39.2* Components of nutrition–health education communication [14].

differently to the same message compared to the urban counterpart. Similarly, less educated groups will receive a message differently compared to better educated groups. There are myriad differences among different ethnic groups from different regions; even in the same region or cultural group, among families at different socio-economic levels and so on.

Secondly, it needs to be realized that the recipients do not form a homogeneous group; and that audience segmentation is required.

Communications should be directed not only at the key beneficiary but also at the persons who influence the primary recipients of message in the family and community [14, 15]. Segmenting recipient groups or the target audience is important and it is critical to identify

- *The primary target audience*: those who will actually perform the new or modified nutrition–health practices.
- *The secondary audiences*: those who can be motivated to teach, support, and reinforce the practices and beliefs of the primary audience (e.g., health care providers, family and friends).

- *The tertiary audience*: decision-makers, financial supporters, and other influential people who can make the program a success.

Design a different communication strategy and different educational materials for each. Given limited time and resources, designate the audience segment most critical to program success. Using formative research, ensure that the following questions are answered:

- What are the behaviours of our audience groups and how can we describe them?
- What influences their behaviours? What are the underlying beliefs, gender issues?
- What is the role of culture, their family, and economic factors in determining behaviours?
- Which behaviour change messages will meet program needs as well as audience needs?

*Formative research* helps to understand the cultural, social, economic and political factors that influence beliefs and behaviors of the target groups. The results of formative research aid in establishing measurable objectives and realistic strategies for the communication program.

*Some commonly used methods for formative research include the following*

- *Focus group discussions (FGDs)* – They bring together eight to ten respondents typical of the intended target audience. A trained interviewer uses a prepared list of probing questions to collect information on vocabulary, attitudes and concepts related to the selected nutrition problem. Here the group atmosphere may stimulate more in-depth discussion than individual interviews do. Also insights into commonly held beliefs can be obtained relatively quickly.
- *Individual in-depth interviews* – They build on information gathered during other research efforts, to probe deeper into individual attitudes and concerns. They are useful when sensitive topics are addressed, when issues must be probed deeply, when individual rather than group responses are needed, or when it will prove difficult to gather respondents for a group meeting.
- *Participant observation* – The researcher participates in the daily life of the community he or she is studying- observing what is happening, listening to what people talk about, asking questions in various ways over a period of time.
- *Direct observation* – The researcher observes, but does not participate in an event. She usually has a checklist of behaviors to be observed and a recording format for the observations which may be unstructured or structured.

- *Informal conversations* – The researcher takes advantage of any opportunity to converse informally either individually or in small groups with the members of the community being studied.
- *Ethnographic studies* – They combine anthropological open-ended techniques to analyze how specific nutrition practices relate to the larger cultural context. An ethnographic study may employ several qualitative methods in a complementary manner to get a holistic picture of the nutritional problem.

*Analysis of formative research and setting objectives*

Analysis of the formative research results helps to identify the gap between the desired and the current behavior which is sought to be addressed through the NHE program. Define the expected behavior in as much detail as possible; specifying not only what the behavior should be but who is to carry it out and when. This in turn helps to set and refine the objectives. The objectives of NHE program could be related to improving understanding of a practice (cognitive) or improving the practice itself (behavioral). They must preferably be quantifiable and should cover the different dimensions of the communication effort such as exposure, knowledge, behaviour adoption and outcome. For example,

As compared to baseline, after 'y' months of implementation of NHE,

- X% more in the target audience will have heard a radio programme, or possess a growth chart, or have attended anganwadi sessions (**Exposure**).
- X% more in the target audience will state that children need to start on complementary foods at 6 months, or x% more will know where to obtain ORS packets (**Knowledge**).
- X% more of the target audience will report introducing their child to complementary foods at 6 months or will state treating child's episode of diarrhea with ORS (**Behavior Adoption**).
- Nutritional status due to the targeted nutritional problem will be reduced by X% in the target audience (**Outcome**).

## 39.5.2 The communicator (source)

A sender or communicator is the source of the message. S/he is the most important component of the communication program and may be the primary factor underlying the failure or success of the program. A poor message in the hands of a good communicator is better than an excellent message in the hands of a poor communicator.

The reason why the same individual responds differently to different communications is often because of the characteristics or attributes of the communicator. People are exposed to communications from many different sources and more likely to believe a communication from a source they trust, has high source- credibility. For example, a pregnant woman is more likely to believe and follow a village *dai's* (trained birth attendant) or Auxiliary Nurse Midwife (ANM) advice regarding her diet compared to a nutrition educator or health worker coming from another community or background.

If nutrition and health care program functionaries are not adequately equipped with the skills of how to communicate the messages, there is likely to be very limited impact on actual behavior change. In fact, managers, trainers, supervisors and functionaries need to reflect equally on their own behaviors and attitudes and change these first before reaching out to the community and make a difference. With training, practice and above all, an understanding and empathetic attitude, most of us can become reasonably successful communicators, provided the required effort is made.

### 39.5.3 The message

The message consists of what is actually communicated including the actual appeals, words, and pictures and sounds that the communicators use to get the ideas across. A message is a methodically designed communication for information and/or motivation. A nutrition communication message must be based on a thorough understanding of the behaviors underlying the nutritional or health problem. If the various audience groups are well understood; including the reasons underlying their behaviour, it is more likely that effective and focused messages, which are relevant to the audience, will be imparted.

Secondly, a well designed message addresses itself clearly to the problem to be dealt with. Messages should be *practice oriented* and *do-able*. More time, patience and perseverance will be required for changing the more complex behaviours (e.g. complementary feeding) than relatively simpler behaviours (e.g. initiating breastfeeding within an hour of birth).

Thirdly, a good message takes into account the resistance points to the desired action and has a motivational element. For example one reason why pregnant women may not increase their diet in pregnancy is because messages often do not take into account the resistance factors (why women believe it's harmful to increase food intake) or are unrealistic for the women to follow. Formative research as well as the process of pretesting of messages, including using a method called 'Trials for Improved Practices' or TIPS (see below) are useful to identify resistance points in the audience for each message as well as ways of overcoming them.

#### *Pretesting messages*

Pretesting is essential for ensuring that the content and the accompanying visuals are understood and culturally acceptable to the recipient groups.

Thus, once messages are drafted and a series of visuals are prepared, interviews are conducted with representatives of the intended audience in order to test the message and visuals. Pretesting helps project staff know whether the draft materials are understandable to the target audience. Through pretesting, it is possible to find out how well the message is communicated and the visual is understood by the recipient groups in terms of their understanding the symbols and pictures correctly; the content of the message and its relevance to their own lives and needs; whether there are unnecessary details.

Pretesting should be done before the materials are finalized so that they can be revised based on the audience's reactions and suggestions. Most materials must be pretested and revised several times. Each new or revised version is tested again until the material is well understood by, and acceptable to, the target audience. Pretest sites must be similar to those of intended audience for communication so that there are greater chances of the pretest predicting the responses of the audience.

Developing strategies to change behaviour require knowledge of not only how materials are acceptable to audiences (pretests) but also information about improved practices that are acceptable and feasible for families. All practices should be tested, ideally in people's homes, before they are recommended. This is done through Trials for Improved Practices (TIPS), which may be done simultaneously or before material pretest [16].

TIPS is a frequently used method for pretesting messages and recommended practices among mothers and caregivers; who are given a choice of recommendations for action, questioned about their reasons for that choice and then followed up (usually after 2–3 weeks) to see what actually happened after the trial period. In this way the proposed recommendations are tested in a real environment and information is gathered on their acceptability. This information helps program planners to set priorities among the many seemingly important nutrition practices and messages.

TIPS usually follows formative research in which the behaviors to be targeted for change have been decided; and counseling material has been prepared for each behaviour.

Table 39.3 below gives an example of a counseling guide that was prepared for TIPS prior to initiating an intervention to improve household dietary practices among pregnant and lactating women in Angarah block in Ranchi, Bihar [16]. The TIPS experience proved to be invaluable to design communication materials and strategies in this project.

*Table 39.3* A section of the counseling guide prepared to the TIPS process related to improving diets of pregnant women in Angarah, Ranchi

| *Behaviour change recommended* | *Benefits* | *Expected resistance* | *Response* |
|---|---|---|---|
| Improve quality of food eaten at home: | | | |
| (a) Eat at least one *katori* of *Saag* (50 g) four or more days of the week<br>(b) Eat an egg at least twice a week<br>(c) Eat ripe (not raw) pumpkin 2–3 times a week or<br>(d) Eat ripe papaya 1–2 times a week or more | • Woman's blood improves<br>• *Raataundhi* (Night blindness) can be prevented<br>• Woman gets strength, does not feel weak, tired, breathless<br>• Recovery from delivery is faster<br>• Lactate better<br>• Child's development–improves physical and mental | • *Saag* (green leafy vegetables –GLV) quantity not enough for family<br>• Eggs are expensive, not cooked frequently<br>• Ripe papaya, pumpkin are not available in market, are expensive | • *Saag (GLV)*, when plucked from vegetable gardens or the farms, should be plucked in more quantity to last for 2–3 days a week<br>• 1–2 *Kadchul* (tablespoon) should be left aside for the woman at mealtime<br>• Women should buy egg during the market visit and eat it there<br>• These foods not only benefit the woman but also the fetus; explain the benefits especially of *Saag*, ripe papaya, ripe pumpkin, egg |

## 39.5.4 The channel

This is also referred to as the communication method; the medium, the delivery system or a vehicle for communicating a message. There are basically three types of channels or vehicles to carry the messages [14]:

(a) Face-to-face ('interpersonal')
(b) Mass media
(c) Traditional/folk media

(a) *Face-to-face or interpersonal methods* include all those forms of communication involving direct interaction between the source and receiver: One-to-one counseling; small group counseling (less than 12 persons); intermediate group/lecture (between 12 and 30) and large group lecture/ public meeting (more than 30).

The advantage of face-to-face method is that it is possible to contact specific groups, make the advice relevant to their social needs, develop problem-solving skills and community participation. It creates opportunities for questions, discussion, participation and feedback. However, face-to-face methods are slower for spreading information in a population because of the need to mobilize field workers and travel to different communities to hold meetings. A communicator may be ineffective if s/he is "ill-informed, uses an unsuitable approach, or holds a status in the community felt to be inconsistent with his/her role". Further, as the size of the group increases, it is more difficult to have feedback and discussion. Many persons feel shy speaking out. Person-to-person education carried out by paid workers is often difficult to justify in terms of cost-effectiveness.

(b) *Mass media include broadcast media and print media* – It provides a rapid way to reach a very large (even non-literate) audience; makes good use of scarce manpower and can be inexpensive, at least in terms of cost per person reached. However, as mass media are broadcast to the whole population, it is not possible to make the message appropriate to the special situation of local communities, whose problems and needs may be different from the rest of the region. Mass communication cannot possibly have the required cultural, linguistic, and social sensitivity nor receive individual feedback that will help assure that messages are relevant, appropriate, and understood by the audience.

*(c) Traditional media* – This includes traditional forms of communication such as storytelling, drama, song, dance, proverb telling and puppetry. Community gatherings, religious meetings and ceremonies can also provide opportunities for NHE.

A well-planned NHE program will involve a carefully chosen mix of the following media.

Visual aids are a common tool used for communicating messages and the following are the key features of *a good visual aid.*

- Only one key action message is depicted on each visual; not more. Other related messages/explanatory notes may be behind the visual (e.g. back of a flash card) or in a separate guidebook.
- The visual has many pictures; is culturally appropriate and easily identifiable by the audience. If words and numerals be used, they are as few as possible and the size of the words is large enough for all in a group to be able to see clearly.
- Colours can be liberally used as they can increase the effectiveness of a picture and emphasize key points; provided they are appropriately used. However, if budgets are limited, even black and white or just two color visuals are effective if they are well made and used properly.
- More important than the visual itself is the proper use of the visual aid or other channels – for example, using it effectively to hold the group's interest, arouse curiosity; encourage questions and experience

sharing. The aid is held such that all can see it and adequate time is given to point out and explain the message given on the visual or multi-media/print channel.

## 39.6 Evaluation of NHE programs

Evaluation is defined as a systematic and scientific process determining the extent to which an action or set of actions were successful in the achievement of pre-determined objectives [14].

Evaluation involves assessing whether NHE resulted in making the difference that was planned and that the amount of effort required to produce the change was worthwhile.

Evaluation should be built into all phases of program planning, implementation, and management. Evaluation plans should be integrated into program planning phase for process evaluation and impact. Evaluation of NHE implies the objectives are defined precisely with details of specific outcomes expected under defined conditions.

Many evaluations show that program planners consistently underestimate time and effort needed to adopt a new practice. Thus, a well-planned NHE program may fail at the implementation level, hence continuous monitoring is essential. It is much better to change a program during implementation than await a retrospective analysis to find out where it went wrong and who was responsible for the failure – when it is too late.

NHE programs have a lot in common in the evaluation process of other nutrition–health programs. However, additionally, NHE process evaluation needs to consider whether in keeping with the behavioral objectives, the communicators (functionaries) are reaching the primary-secondary audience groups with communication strategies decided and at appropriate frequency; and the audience is attending the various program activities in sufficient numbers (coverage); understanding and implementing the messages in the desired manner.

Since an important function of process evaluation is to provide information about the match between program design and implementation as well as deficiencies needing attention, the results should be fed back to project managers and staff on a continual basis and prompt corrective action taken.

To conclude, both process and impact evaluation together provide a comprehensive picture of whether the NHE is being implemented in accordance with the objectives and whether impact is being achieved; what are the modifications required in the next phases to enable goals to be reached.

## 39.7 NHE in action – successful program experiences

When NHE programs are well designed, implemented with a strong BCC emphasis, they have shown results. An overview of some such programs is presented below.

### 39.7.1 The Nutrition Communication Project (NCP) of The Academy for Educational Development

An international project was implemented by USAID supported Academy for Educational Development (AED), with many international and country level partners including those in Government and NGOs [17]. Essential Principles for success in improving nutritional practices as analysed from the evaluation results of six country projects of NCP are as follows.

*Select specific action-based behaviors.* Experience shows that focusing on a limited set of very specific behaviors is key to improving nutrition. These behaviors must be practical for the target audience to implement – in terms of cost, time and compatibility with existing practices and beliefs.

*Give attention to coverage and maximize exposure.* Interpersonal, community and mass media channels must be maximally used to reach sufficient numbers of each different target audience to achieve impact. A combination of channels is usually most effective. Frequency of contact, and repetition of messages, is important.

*Create social support.* Nutritional habits are deeply imbedded in family tradition and local customs. Behavior change can be facilitated by identifying each of the groups of people that influence the target audience or can facilitate the behavior by contributing financial, emotional, or other essential support. Different messages and strategies are required for each.

*Aim for simplicity.* Most important is to begin getting the message out. Strategies should be simple to start with. New audiences and additional channels can be brought in gradually.

*Pursue a long-term effort.* Messages must be conveyed with enough saliency and for a long enough time that the practices being promoted become routine behavior, fully supported by social norms.

*Structuring interventions.* Nutrition social marketing offers a unique opportunity to integrate disparate health, population, and agriculture interventions.

*Capacity building.* Beginning with a short pilot phase (12 months or less) and limited goals can be a highly effective way to strengthen the capacity of implementing agencies and individuals and to build confidence.

*Monitoring.* Adequate monitoring (usually neglected) is an essential tool for understanding operational dynamics and for detecting what does and does not work in nutrition education interventions. Documentation of program inputs and implementation experience is essential to understanding program success and failures.

*Evaluation.* Projects do not always learn as much as they can about what works and what doesn't and under what circumstances. Systematic evaluation is critical to learn valuable lessons, to disseminate the success stories, to advocate for more resources and a higher priority to behaviour change interventions.

In addition, support and involvement of policy makers, government officials, program managers and other decision makers for strengthening nutrition communication programs by focusing on following actions is critical.

- Give nutrition communication higher priority and adequate resources, including staffing with well-trained program managers and health educators.
- Link nutrition interventions to other health and socio-economic development programs. Provide an adequate time frame and long-term commitment of personnel.
- Enlist help from universities and other groups with essential expertise that government and development organizations rarely keep in-house.
- Focus on the minimal per-recipient recurrent costs, rather than the cost-intensive start up, when making budget decisions.
- Remember that communication will be only part of the solution and that intersectoral collaboration and commitment of resources for development are also necessary.

### 39.7.2 NHE for behavior change based on the positive deviance concept

The term 'positive deviance' has been used to describe the performance (regarding health, growth and development) of certain children vis-à-vis the performance of other children in the community and families. It has been seen as a form of social, behavioral and physiological adaptability to nutritional status [18].

The application of the positive deviance concept implies that household level factors related to feeding, health and care-giving of children are identified in those families where children are growing well (at rates equal to or higher than the relevant growth standard for that region) – the positive deviants. This knowledge of determinants of positive growth in positive deviant children who live in the same impoverished environment as other malnourished children (for example, feeding and hygiene care practices) should be used to develop and implement education and communication strategies to rehabilitate other malnourished children.

Successful BCC interventions to improve child feeding practices and nutritional status based on the PD concept have been implemented in many countries, a few of which are illustrated here. One of the well known PD models is PD-Hearth model [19, 20]. In the intervened communities, small groups of mothers (4–5 or more) having malnourished children (below 2 or 3 years) met daily for 2–3 hours at the house of a volunteer mother (having a positive deviant or PD child) where they received nutrition-health messages and their child receives a well balanced meal. Nutrition Health messages and meal components were determined using information gathered from interviews with the mothers of PD children in the community who were well nourished despite their family's limited economic resources. These Hearth participants were then followed for a specified period (for example, six months) in their own home by the program village functionaries (known as "monitrices" in Haiti) who were women hired from each village and intensively trained to supervise the Hearth program. They also periodically weighed the children to evaluate their progress, and liaise between health centers/hospitals and the community.

The PD informed Hearth approach has been adopted to suit regional needs and conditions and also has been systematically monitored and evaluated; for example, in Haiti and Vietnam. In Haiti [18], where the program was known as Ti Foyer (Hearth) Community Based Nutrition Model, monitoring data indicated that a majority of children (above 50%) in intervened villages continued to gain weight as fast or faster than the international standard median, six months after participating in a Hearth program.

Similarly, technical deliberations held by CORE-PD-Hearth Expert group in 2002 [20], distilled the lessons learnt from several PD-Hearth interventions and the findings pointed out to the effectiveness of this model for improving child feeding – health care as well as growth velocity; though there were considerable variations between country experiences, as expected. The highlights from the "VISION Project" (Vietnam Study to Improve Outcomes In Nutrition), were presented; this was a partnership between Save the Children, Emory, AED, and the Research and Training Centre for Community Development in Hanoi, with support from USAID and the Linkages project. Research-based evidence pertaining to many of the important quality aspects of a successful PD/Hearth model in Vietnam revealed the following impact on children and women:

(i) Growth – Though overall, the intervention children did not show better growth than comparison children, children who were younger (less than 15 months old) and more malnourished (less than –2WAZ) at baseline had significantly better growth than similarly young, malnourished comparison children. Intervention children consumed more food and energy and had fewer respiratory illnesses than comparison children. More significant impact seen among younger children was believed to be due to 3 factors: high velocity of growth rate (weight gain/month) in infancy, high prevalence of growth faltering and hence greater impact, and the fact that it is easier to prevent growth faltering than reverse it.

(ii) Empowerment of women – Participant mothers reported increased knowledge and confidence in child feeding and care practices and increased sharing of advice with others (such as mothers-in-law, neighbours) as compared to comparison mothers.

The Vietnam project demonstrated that a message given through lecturing had no effect but a message based on dialogue and problem solving did produce a change. Peer reinforcement through dialogue was helpful. Many of the messages provided by trained health workers were not effective, since they wanted to "tell" what to do, rather than help people understand that the recipes and knowledge came from the community. Thus, it is important to involve the volunteer health workers in nutrition health education activities.

Some findings from the evaluations that negatively impacted on the program's success in Vietnam were long distance travel by care givers and children to the Hearth sessions (in some sites), workload of women restricting participation, less impact seen in scattered and dispersed communities as compared to more densely populated rural or urban areas, at times women not wanting to share their household food with others, meal prepared in the Hearth session replacing the home meal, the social stigma of being defined as a "negative" family. To take care of some of the limitations, several adaptations were made, with mixed success.

Overall, the PD-Hearth model has contributed to our understanding of what makes NHE and BCC work.

Another successful PD programme is reported from India – an initiative called *Kano Parbo Na*, meaning "Why can't we do it?" This programme was launched in West Bengal, India [21]. The project identified the feeding practices of mothers in the community with healthy children below 3 years of age (positive deviants) and transmitted messages related to these practices to other mothers through a community based approach using locally available resources. Nutrition Counselling and Childcare Sessions (NCCS) were conducted in ICDS or Anganwadi centres, where caregivers of malnourished children obtained hands-on training (learning by doing) over 12 days relating to the best local childcare practices from mothers of PD children. Attention was also paid to related health issues such as immunization, vitamin A supplementation, hand washing practices, diarrhea management, prevention of low birth weight, early registration of pregnancy, antenatal care. The behaviour change messages were then practiced for the next 18 days by recipient mothers. The cycle continued for 6–9 months. The PD strategy also mobilized the community around the positive deviance approach through participatory processes; for example setting up village committees, ensuring convergence and partnership between the service providers, administration and NGOs involved in implementation and building capacity of childcare functionaries and the community using the "triple A" approach (assessment, analysis, action).

*The Impact* was evident from the case study of the district of Dakhin Dinajpur. This district was one of the first ones that had adopted the PD strategy, and it recorded a reduction in moderate and severe malnutrition from 25 per cent to 5 per cent in two years in 168 ICDS centres. Some factors explaining the impact include: extensive use of resource maps and community growth charts; mothers regularly contributing food for NCCS sessions; preponderance of girl children at the entry stage; 'ripple effect' resulting in improvement of nutrition status of siblings.

### 39.7.3 ICDS-III (World Bank Assisted) Project: 1999–2006

In the ICDS-III project, which operated in over 10 states of India, Information, Education and Communication (IEC) was one of the major interventions in the project and it had a major BCC focus for ensuring appropriate child caring practices in the households. It sought to primarily address the needs of under-3s through family based interventions instead of centre-based interventions [22]. A family-based approach involved extensive outreach and one-to-one contact through home visits as opposed to centre based approach wherein beneficiaries were expected to come to the health centre or anganwadi to avail the services.

Significant improvements in household behaviors regarding IYCF practices were seen when the Baseline Survey (BLS) results were compared to the Endline survey (ELS):

- Proportion of children under 3 years who were breastfed within 2 hours of birth
  (37% in BLS to 51% in ELS)
- Proportion of children age 6–9 months receiving complementary feeding
  (38% in BLS to 64% in ELS)
- Proportion of children age 6–36 months consuming vitamin A rich food
  (53% in BLS to 71% in ELS)

The states adopted various strategies for implementing the IEC with a BCC focus:

- Interpersonal communication through home visits and NHE sessions;

- Social mobilization through door-to-door contacts, rallies, mobile video van, *gramin mela* (rural fair), exhibitions, special campaign days;
- Print/electronic/audio–visual media such as brochures, ICDS newsletter, booklets and guidelines, flip-books, leaflets, pamphlets, calendars, hoardings & boards, audio jingles, TV spots, wall paintings and documentary films.
- Many states did not limit the IEC interventions to the ICDS blocks under the project, but covered the entire state.

A key factor also contributing to this impact was a marked improvement in *quality of implementation of services by AWWs* such as regular growth monitoring of under-3 children and weighing newborn at birth. Awareness of infant breastfeeding practices among the AWWs also improved. Experiences such as these contributed insights which helped formulate recommendations for strengthening the BCC component of the ICDS programme (Box 39.3).

### Box 39.3 Nutrition and health education and ICDS

Health and nutrition education is one of the six important components of the Integrated Child Development Services (ICDS) Programme. However, it remains a very weak component. A per NFHS-3 [23], only 10.9 percent pregnant mothers and 8.3 percent lactating mothers, even under the ICDS project, received health and nutrition education. Recognising the significance of this component, Government of India, in the XI Five Year Plan (2007–2012) made several recommendations, for "*Strengthening Nutrition and Health Education*". The Working Group (sub group – ICDS and nutrition) report for the XIth Plan [24] points out that the fundamental objective of Education in Nutrition is to help individuals to establish food habits and practices that are consistent with nutritional needs of the body and adapted to the cultural pattern and food resources of the area in which they live. While recommending that States develop specific IEC strategies for their own regions, it emphasizes that Behavior Change Communication (BCC) needs to go beyond the traditional printed materials and should involve identification of local communications' needs, use of multiple channels including folk media and mass media in addition to inter-personal communication (IPC) through AWWs and community level volunteers. Considering the fact that home visits are important for effective inter-personal communication (IPC), a welcome recommendation in the Plan is the suggestion that a Home Visit planner be introduced to help AWW to prioritize and plan home visits to households at critical periods of life cycle.

To strengthen the NHE function of ICDS, the Plan also recommends the redesigning of *mahila mandals* to enable these to become a more comprehensive parenting support initiative involving both mothers and fathers and not mothers alone. In addition to continuous NHE in ICDS, the Plan suggests inclusion of a fixed day in a month ('Mother & Child Day' or MCD) – in place of Nutrition & Health Day (NHD) – wherein AWWs, ANMs and supervisors would monitor sessions on health and nutrition issues both for the mothers and children; encourage participation of parents, local PRI members, NGOs and *mahila mandals* and particularly carry out one to one counseling for behavior change on infant feeding practices and improved care.

### 39.7.4 Community-based Maternal and Child Health Nutrition (MCHN) Project Uttar Pradesh – Interpersonal Counseling and BCC

The MCHN project implemented in four districts of UP was a multi-sectoral project and involved the Health–Family Welfare Department, ICDS, Panchayati Raj Institutions (PRI) and Department of Social and Preventive Medicine (PSM) of the medical colleges [25, 26]. In order to reduce child malnutrition and micronutrient deficiencies of iron, iodine and vitamin A, among the key strategies adopted were:

- Influence behavioural care practices (maternal–child health, nutrition, sanitation and hygiene) at family level with the help of the *Bal Parivar Mitra* (community based trained mobilizers).
- Establish a community based intervention and monitoring system for improving maternal and child health and nutrition.

*The MCHN Project* resulted in a significant decline of 43% among severely malnourished children; with this decline being slightly higher in case of female children in comparison to their male counterparts. Overall, the positive shift in nutritional status could be primarily attributed to adoption of practices pertaining to infant feeding (early initiation of breastfeeding and colostrum feeding), use of safe drinking water and other hygiene practices; as well as special attention given to children presenting with clinical signs of protein energy malnutrition.

From a communications perspective, some of the features leading to success of this project were:

- Sound planning of MCHN project which was a positive attribute that helped methodical execution of all the envisaged activities.
- Mobilizing community volunteers that is, BPMs (*Bal Parivar Mitra*) meaning 'friends of families' (mostly women) who made regular contacts with the target groups, helped increase correct knowledge and practices among households.
- Developing a pictorial monitoring format for the use of non-literate BPMs; this also served the purpose of IEC material as it carried uniform messages and pictorially illustrated all the activities using 'life cycle approach'.
- Defining the target audience, as 'risk-families' proved to be a time-efficient approach which enabled early identification of the population segments that were to be reached and counseled urgently. In other words, reaching the right message to the right recipient at the right time.
- Employing 'Inter-Personal Counseling (IPC)' as a major approach to communicate with largely non-literate community on MCHN issues.

### 39.7.5 Improving infant feeding project in Haryana

An infant feeding project in Haryana [27] aimed to assess the impact on prevalence of diarrhea and physical growth, of a community based intervention to promote exclusive breastfeeding until age 6 months and complementary feeding thereafter. The project focused on development of communication skills as well as clarity of messages. The study was a cluster randomized controlled trial in communities which implemented an intervention primarily based on nutrition–education–communication and built on existing health and nutrition services, with involvement of local NGOs. In four intervention and four control pair-matched communities, newborns (552 in intervention and 473 in control) were followed up every 3 months to the age of 18 months.

For the communication component: health and nutrition workers were trained in the intervention communities to counsel mothers for exclusive breastfeeding –complementary feeding at multiple opportunities. The training was based on the Integrated Management of Childhood Illness (IMNCI) approach which places major emphasis on communication skills. Among the factors which influenced feeding practices, an important one was increase in frequency of contact with households at multiple opportunities – immunization sessions, home visits, weighing sessions – which in particular facilitated contact with the target group soon after birth and thereafter. Enhanced clarity of messages and communication skills also contributed to the success of the intervention. For example, replacing '4–6 months' in the message with '6 months' of exclusive breast feeding was important, resulting in a large proportion of the infants in the intervention group starting complementary feeding at appropriate age.

Results showed that as compared to control communities, exclusive breastfeeding rates at 3 months were significantly higher in the intervention communities (79% versus 48%) – and the 7-day diarrhea prevalence was significantly lower – at 3 months and 6 months. The intervention promoted recognition of malnutrition as a problem, complementary feeding initiation at 6 month of age, optimal meal frequency, portion size and food density, and active feeding practices. Hygiene practices also improved – mothers reported washing their own and their child's hands before feeding the child.

Further, energy intakes from complementary foods overall were significantly higher in the intervention group children at 9 months and 18 months. However, the improvement in physical growth was less than that expected from the substantial increases in energy intakes perhaps because several inter-related factors (including maternal malnutrition) influence child growth, including birth weight and child morbidity.

It was concluded that in this pragmatic and educational intervention, the promotion of exclusive breastfeeding until age 6 months through existing primary health-care services was feasible, effective and potentially sustainable; it reduced the risk of diarrhea, and did not lead to growth faltering; particularly in low-birth weight infants. An important recommendation (emerging from the subtle gender discrimination seen in this project) was that interventions aiming for behavior modification toward improving child feeding practices must pay greater attention to gender bias in communication.

It is evident from these examples that NHE with a BCC focus had a significant measurable impact within a limited time frame and within the existing social and economic constraints of the environment; provided NHE is accorded a high priority and is effectively implemented.

## References


1. KANANI S (2002). Effective Nutrition Education and Communication: Issues and Challenges in Government Health Systems. *Medico Friend Circle Bulletin.* pp. 292–293, 6–9,
2. ZEITLIN MF (1988). The potential impact of nutrition education In: *Effective Communications for Nutrition in Primary Health Care.* Andersen JE and Valyasevi A, (eds). Report of the Asian Regional Workshop, Bangkok, Thailand, 3–7, 1983. The United Nations University.
3. Population Reports (2008). *Communication for Better Health.* Info Project: Centre for Communication Programs. John Hopkins Bloomberg School of Public Health.
4. KOTLER P and ZALTMAN G (1971). Social marketing: an approach to planned change. *Journal of marketing*, **35**, pp. 3–12.
5. RASMUSON MR, SEIDEL RE, SMITH WA, BOOTH EM (1988). Communication for Child Survival. Academy for Educational Development. *HEALTHCOM Project. AED.*
6. Health Canada. Broader Nutrition Education and Health Behavior Change Research: www.hc-sc.gc.ca/fn-an/label-etiquet/nutrition/educat/
7. ISRAEL RC, FOOTE D, TOGNETTI J (1987). Operational guidelines for social marketing project in public health and nutrition. Nutrition education series issue 14 UNESCO, ED – 87 / WS / 52.
8. KANAL K, HALLEN JB, SFORZA TC, CRAPE B, SMITASIRI S (2005). Cambodian weekly iron folic acid program team. Weekly iron folic acid supplements to prevent anaemia among Cambodian women in three settings: process and outcomes of social marketing and community mobilisation. *Nutrition Reviews*, **63**(12), pp. S126–S133.
9. GARCIA J, BARRETT ED, DIZON M (2005). Industry experience in promoting weekly iron folic acid supplementation in the Philippines. *Nutrition Reviews*, **63**(12), pp. S146–S151.
10. SMITASIRI S, ATTIG GA, VALYASEVI A, DHANAMITTA S, TONTISIRIN K (1993). Social marketing of vitamin rich foods in Thailand – A model nutrition communication for behaviour change process, *UNICEF and Institute of Nutrition*, Mahidol University, ISBN 974-587-516-3.
11. FAO/WHO (1996). *Preparation and use of food-based dietary guidelines.* Report of a joint consultation, Nicosia, Cyprus, FAO/WHO, Geneva.
12. Food-Based Dietary Guidelines. Food and Agriculture Organization of the United Nations. www.fao.org/ag/humannutrition/nutritioneducation/fbdg/49850/en/ind/

13. UNICEF (1992). *Care and Nutrition.* Theme Paper for International Conference on Nutrition by Engle P. United Nations Children's Food, New York.
14. HUBLEY J (1993). *Communicating Health:* An Action guide to Health Education and Health Promotion. The Macmillan Press Ltd., London and Basingstoke.
15. KANANI S, DAXINI M, SHARMA M (2006). *Behavior Change Communication Guidelines,* Supported by UNICEF (Gujarat). Department of Foods and Nutrition, The Maharaja Sayajirao University of Baroda, Vadodara, India.
16. KANANI S (1998). BEHAVIOUR Change Trials for Better Nutrition Of Pregnant And Lactating Women in Angarah Block, Bihar. A Report for the Linkages Project of Academy of Educational Development. CARE – BIHAR. *Department of Foods & Nutrition,* the Maharaja Sayajirao University of Baroda, Vadodara, India.
17. ACADEMY FOR EDUCATIONAL DEVELOPMENT (1996). *Final Report NCP: Nutrition Communication Project: Nutrition Education and Social Marketing Field Support Project.* (Funded by the US Agency for International Development). AED, Washington, D.C.
18. ZEITLIN M, GHASSEMI H, MANSUR M (1990). Positive Deviance in Child Nutrition with Emphasis on Psychosocial and Behavioral Aspects and Implications for Development. *Food and Nutrition Bulletin,* Supplement No. 14, United Nations University.
19. BOLLES K, SPERAW C, BERGGREN G, GUY LAFONTANT J (2002). Ti Foyer (hearth) community-based nutrition activities informed by the positive deviance approach in Leogane, Haiti: A programmatic description. *Food and Nutrition Bulletin,* **23**(4), pp. 9–15.
20. CORE: Child Survival Collaborations and Resources Group (2002). *Positive Deviance/Hearth for Nutrition.* Technical Advisory Group Meeting, Washington, DC..
21. MUSTAPHI P (2005). Addressing Malnutrition through Surveillance and Innovative Community based Strategies. UNICEF: Knowledge Community on Children in India.
22. GOVERNMENT OF INDIA (2006). *Implementation Completion Report of World Bank assisted ICDS-III / WCD Project Borrower's Evaluation Report,* GOI.
23. National Family Health Survey (NFHS)-3 (2005–06). International Institute of Population Sciences, Mumbai.
24. GOVERNMENT OF INDIA, PLANNING COMMISSION (2008). *Eleventh Five Year Plan (2007–2012). Volume II.* Social Sector. Oxford University Press, New Delhi.
25. GOVERNMENT OF UTTAR PRADESH and UNICEF (2006). *Community Based Maternal & Child Health Nutrition (MCHN) Project (MCHN) Project. Evaluation Report.* Submitted to GoUP (Directorate of FW & Directorate of ICDS) and UNICEF, Lucknow. ORG Centre for Social Research (A Division of ACNielsen ORG-MARG Private Limited), Lucknow.
26. VIR S, JAIN A, SINGH R (2006). Mission Poshan – Project to redesigning state programme for addressing malnutrition in under threes in Uttar Pradesh. In: Report of the Nutrition Foundation of India on "late infancy and early childhood (6–24 months)".
27. BHANDARI N, MAZUMDER, BAHL R, MARTINES J, BLACK RE, BHAN MK (2004). An Educational Intervention to Promote Appropriate Complementary Feeding Practices and Physical Growth in Infants and Young Children in Rural Haryana, India and other members of the Infant Feeding Study Group. *J. Nutr.,* **13**(4), pp. 2342–2348.

# 40

# From research to programs: Applying knowledge to improve nutrition outcomes

*Purnima Menon*

**Purnima Menon**, Phd, is a Research Fellow in IFPRI's Poverty, Health and Nutrition Division. Among other projects, she leads the monitoring and evaluation of *Alive and Thrive*, a Bill and Melinda Gates Foundation-supported initiative to improve infant and young child feeding and child nutrition, at scale, in Bangladesh, Vietnam and Ethiopia. Prior to joining IFPRI, Dr. Menon was a Research Associate in the Division of Nutritional Sciences at Cornell University (2006–07), a consultant to IFPRI (2001–06), and a Scientific Officer with the Nutrition Foundation of India (1994–95). Menon is Ph.D. in International Nutrition from Cornell University, a M.Sc. in Nutrition from Lady Irwin College (University of Delhi) and a B.Sc. in Nutrition from the University of Madras.

## 40.1 Introduction

Evidence-based decision-making for programs and policies has emerged as a critical ingredient for effective programs and policies. Evidence-based decision-making has been well integrated now into clinical medical practice overseas, but has entered the realm of public health programming only recently [1]. High quality research should be the basis for generating evidence for program and policy decision-making. However, the question of what types of research are most relevant to program decision-making is still often debated. Traditional public health specialists continue to defer to randomized controlled trials (RCTs) as the definitive evidence-base for decision-making about interventions. This is increasingly, however, being viewed as inadequate for effective decision-making, largely because RCTs often only yield information on "what" interventions are most efficacious, but not on "how" interventions had their impact [2]. Relying only on evidence from RCTs, without consideration of context and impact pathways, then, can be misleading and lead to lowered effectiveness in non-optimal program circumstances. Broadening the scope of the type of research, therefore, is important to consider when developing programs [3].

This chapter describes the different types of research that are relevant to the process of decision-making about programs. It does so by using a framework that demonstrates the links between different types of research and programmatic decision-making for the reader. First, however, it is useful to explain the concept of "program theory", which forms the backbone for how research links to programs.

## 40.2 Program theory

"Program theory" refers to the definition of the processes by which a program is intended to achieve its intended impact [4]. It is by now well accepted in the field of program evaluation that evaluations should be theory-driven to the extent possible as this allows for the best understanding of whether, why and how programs achieve, or do not achieve, their intended impacts [5].

Usually, program theory includes impact theory (which specifies the impact pathways) and two elements of process theory (which specifies the operational and utilization plans). *Impact theory* is intended to lay out the steps through which a given intervention in a program is expected to have an impact on the desired outcomes of interest. In effect, it specifies the causal pathways through which impacts are to be achieved, and forms the basis for any social program. It is important in specifying such impact theory to also define some of the conditions that need to be in place to achieve the intended impacts and some of the assumptions being made in statements about how the program will achieve the stated impacts. *Process theory* lays out the steps through which an intervention or program is implemented and includes steps related to the organization plan for delivering interventions as well as a service utilization plan for ensuring use of the program services and interventions.

Of particular importance at an early stage in development of a program, or the planning of an evaluation of program, is the development of program theory. An example of a program theory pathway for behavior change communications programs is shown in Fig. 40.1. The program theory developed at an early stage in program planning should be expanded, clarified and refined as various components of program strategies get further developed. This allows program implementers and researchers to articulate pathways of possible impact of program investments, to clarify which barriers are outside the scope of program plans, and to highlight where inputs from other stakeholders, programs, and initiatives will have to be leveraged to achieve desired impacts [6]. Most critically, it helps identify critical points on which research is needed to identify how best to move forward with program design, implementation or program refinement. Program theory also helps define the best approach for estimating program costs by identifying factors in program inputs and operations or program utilization that need to be mapped and the cost estimated.

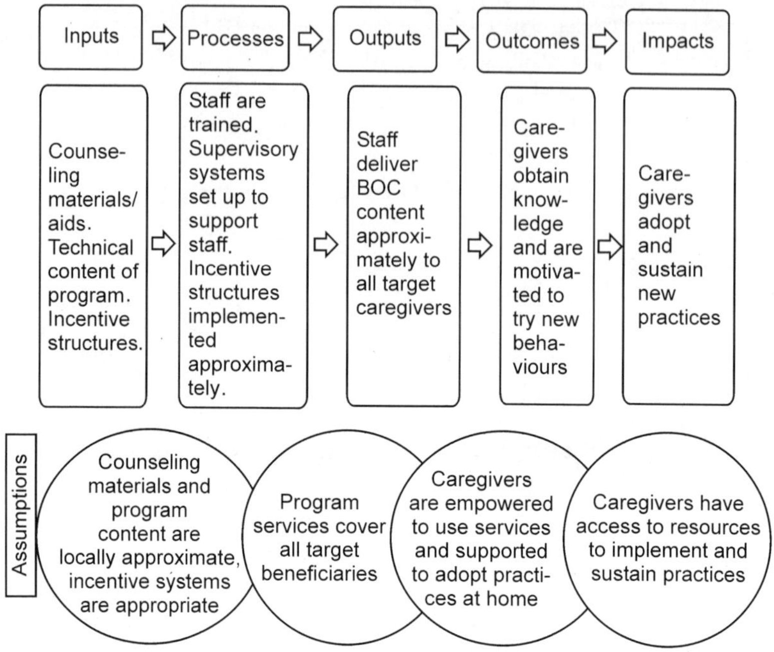


*40.1* Example of program theory of a behavior change communications programme.

## 40.3 Framing the links between research and programs

The framework (Figure 40.2) shows the types of research studies that have application to programs. As depicted in the framework, the program process itself consists of multiple stages, which are interlinked. They flow from early program decisions about intervention choice and operational designs, to later decisions on program scale-up, sustenance or even program termination. There is a role for program-oriented research to support each of these phases of program and policy-decision making. Figure 40.2 also shows the links between different types of research, and the different program decisions.

Building strong and meaningful links between program decision-making and program-oriented research is not straightforward. It requires vision on the part of program planners, policy-makers and donors, who must commission research to answer questions that are most relevant to the problems they are trying to solve. It also requires a creative and skilled set of researchers and research institutions who can either respond to the needs of a program, or who have the vision to invest in program-oriented research as part of their core research areas. More importantly, it requires that

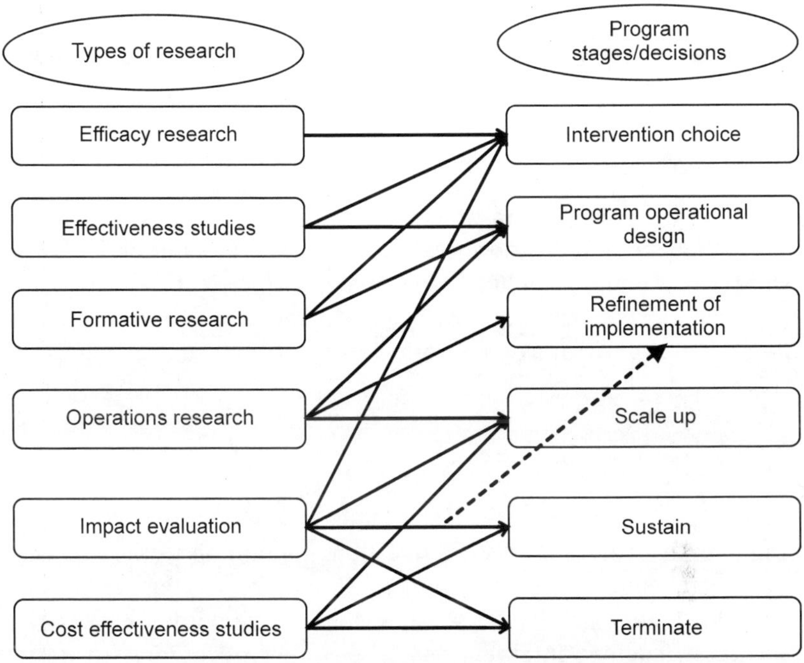


*40.2* Framing the links between research and program stages/decisions.

program managers, bureaucrats and policymakers, including politicians, to often accept programmatic findings that are at odds with their perceptions about the value of certain policy investments or programs.

There are few examples of the institutionalization of a program-oriented research focus within governments and national research programs; those countries that have invested in such links, however, have demonstrated improvements in the quality and scale of programs as well as the impacts of programs. An excellent example of this is the link between the nutrition and poverty alleviation program in Mexico (Progresa/Oportunidades) and the types of research studies commissioned by the government of Mexico. These studies spanned the gamut of the types of research shown in the Fig. 40.2 and each piece of research contributed to specific program decisions, from intervention choice (such as the choice of iron fortificant) to program targeting and scale-up [7, 8]. This approach to program-focused research has been largely absent in India. Even though many of the design and implementation bottlenecks in the Integrated Child Development Services (ICDS) – programme of India and other nutrition programs have been well-documented, there has not been a systematic effort to conduct research to identify effective solutions to these bottlenecks (Box 40.5).

Major types of program-oriented research, with the primary goal of providing an overview of the different types of research, rather than providing an in-depth methodological orientation is presented in the chapter. The reader is referred to the references in each of the sections for further reading.

## 40.4 Categories of program-oriented research

The major types of program-oriented research and their contributions to program decisions are described below, using the example of various nutrition interventions, including multiple micronutrient powders (MNPs) to reduce anemia among young children, and behavior change communication to improve infant and young child feeding (IYCF) practices.

### 40.4.1 Efficacy and effectiveness research

Clinical or community based efficacy studies use highly controlled research methods to answer very specific questions pertaining to the efficacy of certain treatment regimens or certain preventive interventions on nutritional or functional outcomes. These research studies often provide the basis for choosing efficacious interventions to include in programs to improve nutrition. It should be taken as an essential prerequisite that interventions chosen for inclusion in large scale nutrition programs meet basic standards of proven efficacy. In the case of MNPs for reducing anemia, first, efficacy trials tested the efficacy of using the MNPs against other iron supplements for reducing anemia; studies also tested MNPs in different dosages [9, 10, 11]. Following this set of basic research in controlled community based studies, a set of effectiveness studies that examined the impact of MNPs on anemia under less controlled, and "real life" program settings provided the evidence that this approach to reducing anemia had impact even in programs [12, 13]. Taken together, this set of studies provided the basis for inclusion of this approach in large scale national programs [14], and this innovative approach to reducing anemia is now being embraced in a variety of programs globally.

### 40.4.2 Formative research

Formative research is a basic prerequisite for introducing new programs or new program elements in communities. With origins in social marketing and behavior change communication, formative research is essential to tailoring program choices, key behavior change messages and approaches, and communication strategies to local contexts. It is particularly important where public health outcomes are dependent on behaviors that vary widely from place to place, because of differences in social and cultural context.

This is particularly true for nutrition-related behaviors such as infant and young child feeding [15, 16]. Formative research can either be used to design new content for behavior change communications programs [17, 18], or to adapt existing global or national technical materials to local requirements, as in adaptations to the counseling materials developed under the Integrated Management of Childhood Illness (IMCI) and Control of Diarrheal Diseases at WHO [19]. In the case of the IMCI counseling materials, the World Health Organization developed a set of basic counseling materials related to infant and young child feeding as part of the overall IMCI package of tools and materials. Along with this, recognizing that infant and young child feeding is strongly influenced by local context, available foods and resources, and cultural beliefs, WHO also developed a formal guidebook for how to adapt the IMCI counseling materials to the local context.

Formative research uses primarily qualitative methods such as in-depth interviews, focus group discussions, unstructured observations, case study as well as structured ethnographic methods [20]. The use of qualitative research for formative research, however, should be rigorous, and should follow all principles of strong qualitative research [21]. Sampling for formative research is usually purposive, as the goal should be to capture the range of expected variability in implementation contexts, e.g. in socio-cultural, religious, economic, rural versus urban, etc.

### Box 40.1 Hallmarks of good qualitative research

- Clear research protocol is developed.
- Sampling, even where purposive, is well thought through, and ideally, linked with sampling used in quantitative research (where mixed methods are used).
- Question guides are well-developed, pre-tested and refined.
- Data collection methods include detailed interview notes, taped transcripts of interviews and field notes describing context of interviews.
- Analysis methods include use of qualitative data analysis software to code text data; where software is not used, analysis methods include explicit procedures to code data, ensure reliability of codes (through multiple coders and debriefing techniques).
- Write-up of qualitative research findings aim to convey majority tendencies as well as minority tendencies, as well as the richness of data.

Quantitative data is also invaluable for formative research, but the use of the term 'formative research' largely implies the use of qualitative methods. However, with the increasing availability of large scale survey data such as the National Family Health Surveys (NFHS) in India, and the Demographic and Health Surveys (DHS) for other countries, on the internet, it is now possible to use these data to understand patterns, trends, and determinants of undernutrition before embarking on program strategy development. These data are often representative at the national and state/

regional level only, however, and therefore provide little information on more localized contexts. They are extremely useful for understanding the broad context, and comparing results from local formative research studies using qualitative methods. Still, quantitative analysis of large scale data sets should not substitute for rigorous qualitative field-based research, which is fundamental to the success of many programs that need adaptation of key health and nutrition messages, counseling approaches, or service delivery mechanisms.

The literature on behavior change communication for nutrition, in particular, is unequivocal in stressing that building nutrition communication programs, but also advocacy strategies and health systems strengthening strategies, should be based on a sound base of knowledge about the existing context and the major influences on behaviors. The major contribution of formative research is in developing this base of knowledge, and enabling the crafting of program strategies that are well-grounded in the contexts that the programs must operate in.

**Box 40.2 Methods for assessing impact and operational pathways**

*Quantitative methods*

- Facility assessments,
- Staff and client knowledge assessments
- Skill assessments
- Exit interviews on service use
- Structured observations
- Knowledge-trial-adoption surveys

*Qualitative methods*

- Focus group discussions
- In-depth narrative interviews
- Participant observation
- Event analysis
- Process tracing

### 40.4.3 Operations research

Operations research is a process that culminates with the effective use of applied programmatic research information for action. It is also particularly useful when embedded with impact evaluations, in which case it might also be referred to as a "process evaluation". However, here, the term "operations research" is used here to encompass both operations research and process evaluation since the difference between the two is most often in what the information from the research process is used for. In both, data is gathered on program implementation and utilization, and the results are used either to provide feedback to program implementers and improve program implementation quality [22], or to document the process of program implementation and utilization as part of an impact evaluation [23, 24].

Gathering data on intermediate processes using operations research contributes to impact evaluation since it provides information on potential explanations for differences in program impact between comparison groups [25, 26], and is particularly relevant where an expected impact is not found [27]. In many cases, lack of impact could be because the program, as implemented, was quite different from the program as intended. Problems in implementation, therefore, compromise the ability of impact evaluations to determine the true effectiveness of nutrition and public health programs. Since problems in implementation are usually due to various factors upstream of the actual implementation (e.g., logistical arrangements and resources, supervisory structures, staff technical skills, etc.), it is optimal if these factors are also assessed as part of the operations research conducted during an impact assessment [28].

From the point of view of scaling up a program, detailed information on implementation and factors influencing implementation are needed to plan the scaling up process. Of particular importance is information that can help identify and prioritize key infrastructural and staff level factors that need to be addressed for optimal impact of a specific intervention when implemented at a large scale. Key infrastructural factors include resource needs and the logistical arrangements for delivery of an intervention. Staff level factors include staff skills and capacity, supervisory systems and staff incentive structures, all of which directly impact optimal implementation of a program at the frontline level [29].

A variety of methods can be used when conducting operations research and process evaluations. These are described in Box 40.2. Ideally, operations research should rely on mixed research methods – using both qualitative and quantitative methods of research. It should also be based on program theory (described above), such that the set of research methods used is able to bring together insights from different perspectives and different stakeholders on the processes through which a program or intervention is being delivered and used by its intended beneficiaries. The methods used in operations research come from the fields such as quality assurance in health systems [30], medical anthropology, organizational behavior, and the policy sciences, among others. The primary requirement for conducting high quality operations research, however, is not disciplinary training in any of these disciplines; rather it is the ability to map and identify the critical impact and process pathways for different program components or interventions. Once such pathways are mapped, it is possible to then develop a protocol of research methods for understanding and elucidating these pathways using a variety of operations research methods. Table 40.1 depicts an example of the kinds of steps to be assessed when assessing the

*Table 40.1* Mapping research methods to steps in program theory [24]

| Steps in program pathway | Types of methods | Sample |
|---|---|---|
| Program staff distributes adequate amounts of micronutrient powders | Exit interviews at distribution points | Caregivers/children at distribution points |
| Program staff possess adequate knowledge to educate mothers about use of micronutrient powders | Knowledge assessments of program staff | Program staff who deliver behavior change comm.-unication messages |
| Program staff are able to incorporate micronutrient powder component activities into their routine activities in the integrated program | Qualitative group or individual interviews with program staff | Program staff who deliver behavior change communication messages and undertake supply-related activities for MNPs. |
| Mothers possess adequate knowledge about use of micronutrient powders | Knowledge assessments with mothers | Mothers of children targeted by the program |
| Mothers use micronutrient powders for children as advised | Qualitative group interviews to understand barriers to use<br>Surveys include questions on use patterns and barriers to use | Mothers of children targeted by the program |

feasibility of incorporating an MNP distribution into an ongoing maternal, child health and nutrition program and illustrates how specific research methods can inform different elements of a program pathway [24].

## 40.4.4 Impact evaluations

Impact evaluations, including evaluations of pilot projects, should be used for decision-making about scaling-up or replication of public health programs. They are the mechanism for providing evidence (or the lack thereof) of the effectiveness of mechanisms of using public health and nutrition services to improve health and wellbeing [31]. In spite of this understanding, impact evaluations are not invested in as much as they should be by donors and policymakers. However, with many recent international initiatives focusing on impact evaluation, there is increasing emphasis for the development and use of solid impact evaluations for decision making in the global health and development arena.

A variety of study designs can be used in impact evaluations, and often are, but it is useful to place these methods in relation to the level of rigor each approach to evaluation offers. The most rigorous designs are called

### Box 40.3 Case study: Use of formative, operations and impact evaluation research on the use of micronutrient powders (MNPs) to improve childhood anemia in Haiti

As part of the design of an intervention to improve child nutrition in Haiti, a formative research study, using mostly ethnographic methods [20] was conducted to understand the facilitators and barriers to moving from non-optimal to optimal recommended infant and young child feeding practices. The results of one component of the formative research demonstrated that the particularly salient nutrient gaps for infants and young children in this part of Haiti were gaps in iron and zinc [20]. Based on this, a rigorous cluster-randomized trial was designed to investigate the potential of MNPs for reducing childhood anemia in this population. The design of messages to ensure appropriate use of the MNPs was based on initial pretests of the use of the MNPs, and the communications on the use of the MNPs was integrated into the overall communications strategy of the program. A baseline assessment was conducted as part of the impact evaluation, and demonstrated very high levels of anemia among infants and young children (above 45% anemia), thus strengthening the findings from the formative research on the dietary gaps in iron. Implementation of the MNP intervention through an established integrated MCHN program commenced shortly after the baseline assessment. Operations research methods, including a variety of qualitative and quantitative methods were used to document the process of program implementation and of utilization of the MNPs by mothers of children in the program. The operations research methods used included structured observations at different program delivery points, structured and semi-structured interviews with stakeholders and focus group discussions with program staff. Two impact assessments were conducted; the first assessment was 3 months after the start of implementation, and covered intervention and comparison groups, and demonstrated that anemia was halved in the intervention group. The MNPs were then rolled out into the comparison areas. Following this, about 7 months after the MNPs were first distributed to the intervention group, anemia was re-assessed in the intervention group alone. This second assessment demonstrated that anemia had dropped from 53% at baseline to 14% at the second assessment in the intervention group. The series of research in this case culminated in the demonstrated effectiveness of MNPs for reducing childhood anemia in this part of Haiti [12] as well as the demonstrated feasibility of integrating MNPs and accompanying behavior change communication into an existing maternal and child health and nutrition [24]. Concurrent with these studies, the roll-out of the sales of MNPs through social marketing has led to the sustained sales and scale-up of MNPs to many other parts of the country. The rigorous effectiveness study also contributed to the Lancet Nutrition Series review of MNPs and the recommendation to include MNPs as an effective strategy for reducing anemia among infants and young children.

'probability' designs and enable evaluators to assign a probability level to the impact seen and attribute causality to the intervention or program using rigorous study designs such as randomization. Less rigorous designs include 'plausibility' designs, which are not set up to assign causality to the intervention. Rather, through use of a combination of statistical methods to control for confounding factors, and detailed data on mediating processes, plausibility evaluation designs aim to make it possible to assess the impact of the program with a high level of confidence but not assign causality to the program. The least rigorous of evaluation designs are called 'adequacy' designs; these designs usually include only before–after assessments which aim to assess progress against benchmarks, with no comparison group and little data on mediating or confounding factors. The choice of evaluation design must, ideally, be made in consultation with organizations and individuals who will use the results of the evaluation for decision-making. The level of rigor and the extent of data collected on different program steps should be made based on interactions with evaluation funders and program teams on the nature of decisions to be made based on results of the evaluation [32].

Planning for impact evaluations should begin as early as when intervention choice and program design/re-design are being contemplated, rather than as an afterthought to the program design and planning process. This is important because impact evaluation planning requires substantial discussion between evaluation/research teams and program implementation teams about evaluation goals, as well as decisions related to timing of baseline assessments, geographic scope of the evaluation, timing of end line assessments, and choice of impact indicators, among other issues.

In this chapter, given recent trends in the field of impact evaluation, the most rigorous of the impact evaluations designs have been described i.e., probability designs with program impact pathway documentation are described, to enable the reader to appreciate the requirements for an impact evaluation that unequivocally attributes impact in certain outcomes to a specific program or intervention. This can only be done with impact evaluation designs that are rigorous enough to rule out all other explanations for impacts seen on target populations. In such a rigorous quantitative assessment of the impact of any program/intervention, the design needs clearly attribute and rule out the impact seen to the interventions/programs. It is necessary for the design to compare outcomes for recipients of the program interventions to what those outcomes would have been had the program not been implemented at all. Two essential ingredients for achieving are (a) the double difference approach and (b) finding an appropriate comparison group that is not exposed to the program. Other features of high quality evaluations are mentioned in Box 40.4; many of these aspects are also covered in other sections of this chapter.

Two issues that relate to the rigor of impact evaluations are the use of a double-difference approach and the selection of a comparison group. These are described below.

(a) *Double difference approach* – The difference-in-differences (or double-difference) method is a central component of any rigorous impact evaluation. This method relies on baseline data collected in intervention and comparison areas before interventions are implemented and follow-up data (an end-line survey) collected as close as possible to the end-date

**Box 40.4 Characteristics of a high quality impact evaluation**

- Double difference method is used, i.e. before-after assessments with a comparison group
- Comparison group is valid and unbiased (ideally selected using randomization)
- Adequate data are gathered as part of baseline and endline assessments to ensure other explanations for impact are ruled out
- Data are gathered on intervention mediating factors as well as contextual factors
- Solid operations research/process evaluation component is included, and appropriate methods are used
- Mixed methods are used where appropriate, particularly to understand program impact pathways and operational pathways
- Attention is paid to the kinds of decisions that will be made based on results of the evaluation
- Stakeholders who must use the information are engaged from the planning stages of the evaluation

of the project to develop a "before/after" comparison. Unfortunately a majority of program evaluations, even today, use simple before–after assessments only in intervention communities, without comparison groups, making it impossible to make inferences about the specific impacts of the intervention activities or the program. For a rigorous double-difference approach to program evaluation, data need to be collected from areas covered by the intervention or program and those that are not covered by the program (the "comparison" group). The difference between the change in the outcomes for intervention and comparison groups in the baseline and end-line surveys will provide the difference-in-differences impact estimates [33, 34].

(b) *Identifying an appropriate comparison group* – Identifying an appropriate comparison group for individuals exposed to the interventions being evaluated is central to the application of the double-difference method, and of any rigorous impact evaluation. To isolate the impact of the intervention, it is important that intervention and comparison groups be identical in all characteristics, except for being exposed to the intervention/program such that the only plausible explanation for differences in stunting and IYCF practices between groups is the intervention.

A major problem with identifying an appropriate comparison group that is not exposed to the selected interventions is selection bias (e.g., areas chosen for coverage with the intervention could be fundamentally different from comparison areas in ways that bias the outcomes and impacts). For some programs, another challenge could be that very rapid scale-up can limit the number of areas in the country that are not covered by the program, thus eliminating many areas from being comparison areas. This is often the case in large scale national programs.

Options for establishing an appropriate comparison group include randomization of areas or individuals to the interventions. If holding back programming in comparison areas is not feasible for the entire duration of a project, another appropriate way to randomize in the context of large-scale programs is the randomized stepped-wedge approach. In this approach the staging of program roll-out is done using a random selection of areas for different phases of roll-out. Another approach is to set up comparison groups where certain program elements are absent or where interventions are delivered with differing intensities, and the choices of where to hold back program elements or to scale back on intensity are made randomly rather than purposefully. Randomization is considered the gold standard for impact evaluation, is simpler to analyze and communicate results, and therefore, should be a first choice for evaluating the impact of new programs or interventions, particularly those that are not being scaled up immediately to large areas. Where randomization is not feasible at all, options for establishing valid comparison groups include quasi-experimental designs, which involve choosing comparison groups based on certain criteria. Other options also include matching using econometric methods such as propensity score matching (PSM) or nearest neighbour matching (NNM) [35].

An important consideration for rigorous impact evaluations is that the surveys that generate the data for the double-difference analyses should gather adequate information on exposure to the interventions as well as on other relevant factors that might influence the impact of the interventions. This is important regardless of whether the evaluation design uses randomized methods or other approaches to identify comparison groups but is particularly important where randomized designs are not possible and where additional data are needed on program performance and on coverage, utilization and confounding factors to enable analyses that can build the case for plausibility.

Unfortunately, most impact evaluations do not gather detailed information on implementation and factors influencing implementation that are actually needed to provide the evidence base for scaling up to a full scale program, or for replicating a program in another setting. This is necessary both from the point of view of how evaluation results are used for scaling up pilot programs and from the point of view of interpretation of impact evaluation [2, 27]. The section on operations research above has more details on approaches and methods that can be used to understand program implementation and utilization processes.

Last, but not least, it is critical to consider the time it takes to assure that program implementation is of high quality and has achieved the desired scale and coverage in the interventions, before investing in the endline survey. Undertaking endline surveys to assess impact without assessing and assuring implementation scale or quality is not useful. The forms of research that can help assess whether programs are well designed and well implemented are described in the sections on formative and operations research.

## 40.4.5 Cost-effectiveness research

For policymakers and donors, assessing whether a program or intervention is cost-effective is a prime concern. Research on cost-effectiveness, therefore, is of critical importance in relation to programs. Most often, cost effectiveness research is embedded in program impact evaluations. Impact evaluations yield data on the effectiveness of an intervention, either in terms of decreased prevalence of undernutrition or improved nutritional status outcomes. Data on program costs are usually derived from a combination of sources, including program accounting systems, operations research, as well as baseline and endline surveys. It is important to consider a variety of costs when compiling data on program costs – the types of costs to consider include program operational costs as well as costs to program users. Different methods have been used to calculate program costs in the past; these include the CHOICE method developed by the World Health Organization [35], which is mainly input-based, as well as a more recently used approach known as "activity-based costing" [37]. Input-based costing is more "top down" in that broad financial inputs into programs are estimated mainly based on program financial accounting systems. These then are combined with information from surveys on the costs to beneficiaries of using program services to yield an overall cost figure. Although this sounds simple, it is quite complex and time-consuming. It requires a separation of costs by categories that are meaningful for the program inputs (e.g., technical, staffing, supplies, etc.) to be able to estimate the costs of "fixed" inputs versus of "variable" inputs. Fixed costs are costs that are often incurred in program start-up phases, and relate to the costs of capital investments, infrastructure, major equipment, etc. Variable costs, on the other hand, are the costs of operations such as training, supervision and monitoring, IEC and supplies such as medicines, nutrient supplements, etc., that are driven substantially by the level of use of the program by beneficiary populations.

Activity-based costing is a method of costing that is considered more "bottom-up" and is based on an approach that breaks a program down into the smallest activities and attempts to assign costs to each activity. It has been used successfully in the past [38, 39]. It is substantially more burdensome to compile program costs based on an activity-based costing approach even though this approach can be more meaningful in terms of identifying the most and least costly operational aspects of a program.

Regardless of the costing approach chosen, as with operations research and impact evaluations, it is useful to plan activities related to cost studies early in the program design and implementation process. This ensures that cost data are compiled from the start of a program and that total costs related to operations and utilization of a program are well-captured. Once both impact and cost data are available for a program and for non-program areas, it is then possible to calculate the cost-effectiveness of a program or an intervention. High quality impact evaluations that include a comparison group almost always also include cost studies as part of the evaluation design.

**Box 40.5 India's nutrition-related programs: some important programmatic research questions**

It is useful to consider the current status of research in informing the design and evolution of nutrition and other programs in India. India's flagship nutrition program is the Integrated Child Development Services (ICDS) program. Other programs that can have impact on nutrition through direct and indirect routes, include the Reproductive and Child Health (RCH) program that is part of the National Rural Health Mission (NRHM), water and sanitation programs, the National Rural Employment Guarantee Scheme (NREGS) and a variety of other food-entitlement programs intended to improve either individual or household food security.

Most of the programmatic research in India, as it applies to nutrition, has been done on the ICDS program, with many other aspects of research on programs to improve nutrition being largely neglected. Questions remain, therefore, on issues such as the following (among others):

- What is the potential to use the Reproductive Child Health (RCH)/ National Rural Health Mission (NRHM) platforms to improve nutrition outcomes for women and young infants and children?
- What is the nature of the links between the National Rural Employment Guarantee Act (NREGA) and nutrition? How can the implementation of the NREGA be improved to also address nutrition outcomes?
- How can water and sanitation programs in India be optimized to be able to deliver critical interventions for nutrition (such as hand-washing and hygiene interventions)?
- How should agricultural programs be conceived of and implemented so as to ensure that nutrition improvements are achieved?
- What gender-related aspects constrain the use of interventions for nutrition?

For the ICDS program specifically, some of the key design and implementation bottlenecks in the ICDS and other programs have been well-documented. At the same time, there has not been much investment in conducting research on how changing design features and/or implementation modalities can yield improvements in program performance and program effectiveness. Many studies are continuously being conducted on many aspects of the programs. However, there is no mechanisms known to coordinate program-oriented research in relation to the national and state level programs to address direct and indirect determinants of nutrition (questions such as those posed above) or to align the different pieces of research, and ensure that high quality research that is responsive to the program needs is routinely commissioned, funded, and implemented. More importantly, the process of integration of the existing global and national evidence on nutrition interventions is slow. Attention to these issues is critical if research is to play an important part in yielding program benefits in the Indian context.

*Conclusions*

This chapter has provided an overview of the links between research and programs, with a focus on introducing the reader to different types of research that are essential to inform different aspects of decision-making about programs. It is not intended to be an exhaustive chapter on the various methods of research but primarily an introduction to the kinds of research that can be, and should be, undertaken to improve programs and lead to better public health outcomes. It is encouraging to note where donors and governments have invested in programmatic research, there is a clear movement towards evidence-based decision-making about program strategies and intervention choices, both of which are important in an environment of limited funding for public health, nutrition and social assistance programs. Additional references provided along with this chapter provide resource materials on study examples that have used such research methods, as well as to textbook and toolkits/manuals for applying these research methods.

*Acknowledgements*

Jean-Pierre Habicht and Gretel Pelto at Cornell University and Marie Ruel at IFPRI are deeply acknowledged for their decade-plus of mentoring on program research. The author also acknowledges numerous colleagues at IFPRI for discussions and insights about program evaluation and applied programmatic research.

## References

1. FIELDING JE and BRISS PA (2006). Promoting evidence-based public health policy: can we have better evidence and more action? *Health Affairs*, **25**(4), pp. 969–978.
2. VICTORA CG, HABICHT JP, BRYCE J (2004). Evidence-Based Public Health: Moving Beyond Randomized Trials. *American Journal of Public Health*, **94**(3), pp. 400–405.
3. HABICHT JP, PELTO GH, LAPP J (2008). Methodologies to Evaluate the Impact of Large Scale Nutrition Programs, Washington DC, World Bank (in press). http://web.worldbank.org/WBSITE/EXTERNAL/TOPICS/EXTPOVERTY/EXTISPMA0,menuPK:384336~pagePK:149018~piPK:149093~theSitePK:384329,00.html#doingIE
4. ROSSI PH, LIPSEY MW, FREEMAN HE (2004). *Evaluation: A Systematic Approach*, 7th edn. Thousand Oaks, CA: Sage.
5. WHITE H. "*Theory-Based Impact Evaluation*". 3ie Working Paper 3, June 2009 (available at: http://www.3ieimpact.org/temp2.php?path=pdfs_papers/48.pdf&name=Theory Based%20Impact%20Evaluation%20by%20Howard%20White).
6. ROBERFROID D, PELTO GH, KOLSTEREN P (2007). Plot and see! Maternal comprehension of growth charts worldwide. *Tropical Medicine and International Health*, **12**(9), pp. 1074–1086.

7. LEVY S. Progress against poverty: sustaining Mexico's Progresa-Oportunidades Program. Brookings Inst Press. Washington, DC.
8. LEROY JL, VERMANDERE H, NEUFELD LM, BERTOZZI S (2008). Improving Enrollment and Utilization of the Oportunidades Program in Mexico Could Increase Its Effectiveness. *J. Nutr.*, **13**(8), pp. 638–641.
9. ZLOTKIN S, ARTHUR P, ANTWI KY, YEUNG G (2001). Treatment of anemia with microencapsulated ferrous fumarate plus ascorbic acid supplied as sprinkles to complementary (weaning) foods. *American Journal of Clinical Nutrition*, **74**, pp. 791–795.
10. ZLOTKIN S, ARTHUR P, SCHAUER C, ANTWI KY, YEUNG G, PIEKARZ A (2003). Home-fortification with iron and zinc sprinkles or iron sprinkles alone successfully treats anemia in infants and young children. *The Journal of Nutrition*, **133**, pp. 1075–1080.
11. GIOVANNINI M et al (2006). Double-blind, placebo-controlled trial comparing effects of supplementation with two different combinations of micronutrients delivered as sprinkles on growth, anemia, and iron deficiency in Cambodian infants. *Journal of Pediatrics Gastroenterology and Nutrition*, **42**, pp. 306–12.
12. MENON P et al (2007) Micronutrient Sprinkles Reduce Anemia among 9- to 24-month old Children When Delivered through an Integrated Health and Nutrition Program in Rural Haiti. *The Journal of Nutrition*, **137**, pp. 1023–1030.
13. HYDER SM, HASEEN F, RAHMAN M, ZLOTKIN S (2004). Delivery of microencapsulated iron Sprinkles in rural poor through female health workers: Lessons learnt at BRAC in Bangladesh. Abstract. Presented at INACG, Peru.
14. WORLD VISION MONGOLIA (2005). Report on the Effectiveness of Home-Based Fortification with Sprinkles in an Integrated Nutrition Program to Address Rickets and Anemia. *World Vision Mongolia*, Ulaanbaatar.
15. PELTO G, LEVITT E, THAIRU L (2003). Improving feeding practices: current patterns, common constraints, and the design of interventions. WHO Global Consultation on Complementary Feeding. *Food and Nutrition Bulletin*, **24**, pp. 43–82.
16. KANASHIRO HC, FUKOMOTO M, BENTLEY ME, JACOBY E, VERZOSA C, BROWN KH (1991). Use of recipe trials and anthropological techniques for the development of a home-prepared weaning food in the Central Highlands of Peru. *Journal of Nutrition Education,* **23**(1).
17. BENTLEY ME, DICKIN KL, MEBRAHTU S, KAYODE B, ONI GA, VERZOSA CC, BROWN KH, IDOWU JR (1991). Development of a nutritionally adequate and culturally appropriate weaning food in Kwara State, Nigeria: An interdisciplinary approach. *Social Science and Medicine* **33**(10), pp. 1103–1111.
18. DICKIN K, GRIFFITHS M, PIWOZ E (1997). Designing by Dialogue. A program planners' guide to consultative research for improving young child feeding. Washington, DC: *Manoff Group & The Academy for Educational Development.*
19. WHO (WORLD HEALTH ORGANIZATION) (1994). *Focused Ethnographic Study of Diarrhoeal Disease Manual.* Division for the Control of Diarrhoeal and Respiratory diseases. World Health Organization, Geneva
20. MENON P, RUEL MT, LOECHL C, PELTO G (2003). From research to program design: use of formative research in Haiti to develop a behavior change communication program to prevent malnutrition. Food Consumption and Nutrition Division Discussion paper #170. Washington, D.C.: *International Food Policy Research Institute.*
21. BERNARD HR (2006). *Research Methods in Anthropology: Qualitative and Quantitative Approaches.* Newbury Park, CA: Sage Publications.

22. LOECHL CU, RUEL MT, PELTO G, MENON P (2005). The use of operations research as a tool for monitoring and managing food-assisted maternal/child health nutrition (MCHN) programs: an example from Haiti. Food Consumption and Nutrition Division Discussion Paper 187. *International Food Policy Research Institute (IFPRI)*: Washington DC.

23. BONVECCHIO A, PELTO GH, ESCALANTE E, MONTERRUBIO E, HABICHT JP, NAVA F, VILLANUEVA MA, SAFDIE M, RIVERA JA (2007). Maternal knowledge and use of a micronutrient supplement was improved with a programmatically feasible intervention in Mexico. *J Nutr*, **137**(2), pp. 440–446.

24. LOECHL C, MENON P, ARIMOND M, RUEL MT, PELTO G, HABICHT JP, MICHAUD L (2009). Using programme theory to assess the feasibility of delivering micronutrient Sprinkles through a food-assisted maternal and child health and nutrition programme in rural Haiti. *Maternal and Child Nutrition*, **5**(1), pp. 33–48.

25. BONVECCHIO A, PELTO GH, ESCALANTE E, MONTERRUBIO E, HABICHT JP, NAVA F, VILLANUEVA MA, SAFDIE M, RIVERA JA (2007). Maternal knowledge and use of a micronutrient supplement was improved with a programmatically feasible intervention in Mexico. *J Nutr.*, **137**(2), pp. 440–6.

26. DICKIN KL, DOLLAHITE JS, HABICHT JP (2005). Nutrition Behavior Change among EFNEP Participants Is Higher at Sites That Are Well Managed and Whose Front-Line Nutrition Educators Value the Program. *The Journal of Nutrition*, **13**(5), pp. 2199–205.

27. RYCE J, VICTORA CG, HABICHT JP, BLACK RE, SCHERPBIER RW (2005). MCE-IMCI Technical Advisors. Programmatic pathways to child survival: Results of a multi-country evaluation of integrated management of childhood illness. *Health Policy and Planning* **20**(1), pp. i5–i17.

28. MENON P, MBUYA M, HABICHT JP, PELTO G, LOECHL CU, RUEL MT (2008). Assessing supervisory and motivational factors in the context of a program evaluation in rural Haiti. *Journal of Nutrition*, **138**(3), pp. 634–637.

29. BHATTACHARYYA K, WINCH PJ, LEBAN K, TIEN M (2001). Community health worker incentives and disincentives: how they affect motivation, retention, and sustainability. Arlington, *VA: BASICS II (USAID).*

30. NICHOLAS DD, HEIBY JR, HATZELL TA (1991). The Quality Assurance Project: Introducing quality improvement to primary health care in less developed countries. *Quality Assurance in Health Care* **3**(3), pp. 147–165.

31. Evaluation Gap Working Group (2006). When will we ever learn? Improving lives through impact evaluation. Washington, *DC: The Center for Global Development.*

32. HABICHT JP, VICTORA CS, VAUGHAN J (1999). Evaluation designs for adequacy, plausiblity and probability of public health programme performance and impact. *International Journal of Epidemiology*, **28**, pp. 10–18.

33. MALUCCIO J and FLORES R (2005). Impact evaluation of a conditional cash transfer program: The Red de Protección Social. Research Report 141. Washington, D.C.: *International Food Policy Research Institute.*

34. SKOUFIAS E (2005). PROGRESA and its impacts on the welfare of rural households in Mexico. Research Report 139. Washington, D.C.: *International Food Policy Research Institute.*

35. DONEGAN S, MALUCCIO JA, MYERS CK, MENON P, RUEL MT, HABICHT JP (2010). Two food assisted maternal and child health nutrition programs helped mitigate the impact of economic hardship on child stunting in Haiti. Forthcoming. *Journal of Nutrition.*

36. EDEJER, TESSA TAN-TORRES and WORLD HEALTH ORGANIZATION (2003). Making choices in health: WHO guide to cost-effectiveness analysis. Geneva, *World Health Organization.*
37. FIEDLER JL (2003). A cost analysis of the Honduras Community-Based Integrated Child Care Program. Washington, DC: The World Bank.
38. FIEDLER JL and CHUKO T (2008). The cost of Child Health Days: a case study of Ethiopia's Enhanced Outreach Strategy (EOS). *Health Policy and Planning*, **23**, pp. 222–233.
39. WATERS H, PENNY ME, CREED-KANASHIRO H, ROBERT R, NARRO N, WILLIS J, CAULFIELD L, BLACK RE (2006). The cost-effectiveness of a child nutrition education programme in Peru. *Health Policy and Planning*,. doi:10.1093/heapol/czl010.

# 41

# Research methods in public health nutrition: Critical factors

*Arun K. Nigam* and *Padam Singh*

**Arun K. Nigam** is currently the Executive President of Institute of Applied Statistics & Development Studies (IASDS). Nigam obtained his MSc degree in Mathematical Statistics in 1962 followed by PhD in 1970. He has taught at postgraduate level for nearly thirty years at Banaras Hindu University, Indian Agricultural Statistics Research Institute (IASRI) and Lucknow University, India.

**Padam Singh** holds a PhD degree in Statistics from Delhi University, India. He has been Member National Statistical Commission Government of India. He has held many important positions such as Director of the National Institute of Medical Statistics, Indian Council of Medical Research (ICMR), Additional Director General of ICMR, Joint Advisor Planning Commission of Government of India and Professor Indian Agricultural Statistics Research Institute (IASRI). He is presently Head, Research & Evaluation EPOS Health India and President, Institute of Applied Statistics and Development Studies (IASDS).

## 41.1 Introduction

Research is a serious and determined bid to investigate an issue through a systematic and planned methodology. Systematically planned research involves a sequence of steps as presented in Fig. 41.1.

Knowledge generated by good and relevant research generally finds applications. The criteria for a good research are as follows:

- *Reproducibility* – The results obtained should be reproducible under similar conditions.
- *Replicability* – The results and findings should be replicable in other areas as well.
- *Generalisation* – The results and findings should allow for generalization.
- *Standardisation* – The research should have been completed following the standard research protocol.

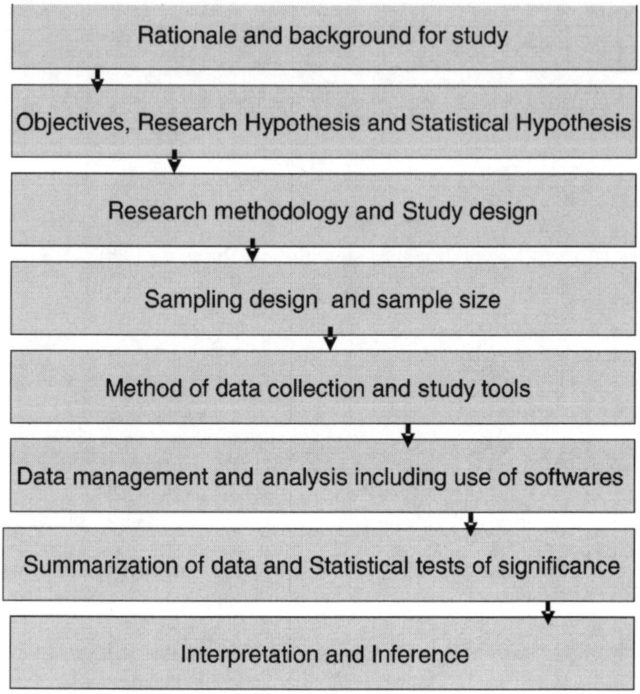


*41.1* Steps in systematically planned research.

Most research studies aim to answer fairly simple questions like

- What is the prevalence of anemia among under-3 children?
- What should be the RDA for Indians according to age, sex occupation categories?
- What should be the reference standards for Indians categorizing them as undernourished and normal?
- What is the nutritive value of traditional foods consumed by primitive tribes?
- What is the dietary intake of adolescents?
- Assessing the nutritional status of a programme.

A researcher is faced with a number of queries. Some of the frequently asked questions in a research study are as follows:

(i) Why this study?
   - Generate new information
   - Proof for a hypothesis: investigate what, why and how?

(ii) Where or in which areas, the study will be carried out?
   - Community based
   - School based

- Hospital based
- National or regional level

(iii) How much material or how many cases will be needed?
- Few based on availability of resources
- Adequate and scientifically planned
- Large countrywide

(iv) What is the basis of the selection?
- Purposive
- Scientific
- Particular target group

(v) What techniques of gathering data will be adopted?
- Interview method
- Anthropometric measurements
- Biochemical measurements
- 24 Hour recall method
- Actual weighment method

(vi) What method of analysis will be used?
- Software
- High level of statistical analysis
- Simple summarization and test of significance

The following sections will address all these issues.

## 41.2 Designing a research study – critical factors

Rationale of a study is based on undertaking a detailed review and identifying the gap as well as highlighting the dire need for undertaking the study including its relevance to national or regional priorities. The overall objective and the specific objectives need to be clearly defined. Formulation of relevant hypotheses is a pre-requisite to any research study. The two components of research objectives and hypothesis are interlinked and both of these must be clear, unambiguous and specific. An appropriate research design, which is relevant for studying the objectives, is then chosen. The adequacy of sample size is critical and should be determined on a scientific basis taking into account the desired precision, confidence level as well as nature of character to be studied, expected/likely outcomes and extent of variability. An appropriate choice of the sampling design is imperative for obtaining efficient and valid estimates

Questionnaires have to be designed to elicit information from the respondents through direct or indirect probing. The data collected through such a survey should be adjusted for non-sampling errors, depending upon their type and magnitude. Relevant estimates are then developed allowing for standard errors. While, the type and coverage of questionnaires is an important deciding factor about the quality of the data collected, any ill-conceived questionnaire may lead to substantive non-response and also to incorrect and evasive responses. At times questionnaires are unduly lengthy or contain many questions which are not relevant to the study, or one too short to provide a satisfactory coverage. A lengthy and clumsy questionnaire not only increases the cost of the survey but also makes management and supervision work, as well as editing and cleaning of data, much more cumbersome. Similarly, a questionnaire with insufficient coverage leads to loss in efficiency, because of the failure to collect some vital information. Each question must be unambiguous and non-overlapping, and the spirit of the question and possible response(s) must be clear to both the interviewer and the respondent.

It is for these reasons that pre-testing of the tools (questionnaires) is considered an important step toward finalization of tools. Through effective pre-testing more than half the battle is won and the follow-up checks and corrective measures go a long way in improving not only the quality of data generated but also is critical for making the emerging estimates much more relevant to the objectives of the study.

A pre-requisite to good quality data is effective training of the field staff as well as data editors/cleaners, and data analysts on the information sought along with all possible responses. Sufficient time should be given for field practice and the training should be evaluated. During field work there should be effective and quality monitoring. Even at 'Data Entry Level' there should be data validation employing range check, valid value check as well as internal consistency checks.

Analysis and tabulation plan should be consistent with the objectives and the hypothesis. It is important to mention that the 'Sample Size' is determined only for analyzing the data at the aggregate level but invariably there is an attempt to present disaggregated analysis in terms of related socio-economic, demographic, housing or household characteristics. This leads to decomposition of sample size according to these disaggregated groups and to invalid estimates, with unduly large standard errors.

For impact assessment studies, comparison of key indicators in the pre and post stage of the project is essential. The pre stage determination of key indicators is often done through a baseline survey carried out in the project area and even some times in a neighboring (control) area having similar features as the project area. One finds that many of the projects are implemented without any valid baseline survey. Further for making valid comparisons between findings of end line and baseline surveys one has to ensure that these are comparable. Usually simple difference in value/percentage of the two stages is compared, though such comparisons should be relative in the intervention area *versus* control area after adjustment for baseline differences in two areas. Many evaluation surveys give emphasis merely on process indicators, rather than outcome indicator(s) directly related to the main objective.

## 41.3 Hypothesis testing and P value

Every research has an objective which could be translated into a research hypothesis. Importantly the research hypothesis has to be converted into a "Statistical Null Hypothesis". A hypothesis is called the Null Hypothesis (HO) if it specifies that the effect of interest is zero; this statistical null hypothesis is often the negation of the research hypothesis. It proposes no difference or no relationship (significant one) in the variable under study for the groups. On the other hand, an "an alternative hypothesis" (H1), implies that the effect of interest is not zero i.e. there exists a significant difference (positive or negative) in the variable between the groups under investigation. Alternate hypothesis is true when null hypothesis is false.

*Example 41.1*

Research hypothesis: Adolescent girls are more anemic than adolescent boys.

Null hypothesis: Anemia level is same in adolescent girls and boys, i.e. there is no significant difference between the anemia levels of adolescent girls and boys.

$P_b = P_g$, where,
$P_b$ = Proportion of anemic boys (P1) and
$P_g$ = Proportion of anemic Girls (P2)

Generally, the Alternate hypothesis is anemia level is not the same among adolescent girls and boys.

Mathematically, $P_b \# P_g$

Anemia level is more among adolescent girls than boys; this could also be an Alternative hypothesis for testing.

Mathematically, $P_g > P_b$

The Alternative hypothesis could also be if anemia level is less among adolescent girls than boys.

Mathematically, $P_g < P_b$

*Example 41.2*

Another example could be comparing two groups of children receiving fortified food under ICDS programme or receiving usual non-fortified food under ICDS.

In this case the Null hypothesis is $P_f = P_U$, where

$P_f$ = Proportion of severely malnourished children among those receiving fortified food.

$P_U$ = Proportion of severely malnourished children among those receiving usual non-fortified food.

In this case the Alternate hypothesis would be that: Proportion of severely malnourished children is less among those receiving fortified food as compared to those receiving usual non fortified food.

Mathematically, $P_f < P_U$

In general,

Null hypothesis ($H_0$): Any hypothesis under test implying null ness/ negation.

$$H_0: P_1 = P_2$$

*Example*: There is no difference in the prevalence of anemia among adolescent boys and girls. Here

P1 = Prevalence of anemia among adolescent girls
P2 = Prevalence of anemia among adolescent boys

Alternate hypothesis ($H_1$): The competing hypothesis with the null hypothesis. The Alternative Hypothesis could be one of the following

Two-tailed $H_1$: $P_1$ # $P_2$

*Example*: There is difference in the prevalence of anemia among adolescent girls and boys

One Tailed $H_1$: $P_1 > P_2$

*Example*: The prevalence of anemia is higher among adolescent girls than boys

One Tailed $H_1$: $P_1 < P_2$

*Example*: The prevalence of anemia is lower among adolescent girls than boys interpretations on hypothesis ($H_0$ or $H_1$) are subject to sample fluctuations and as a result, two types of errors can occur. Below Table 41.1 indicates possible errors in drawing statistical inferences while testing the Null hypothesis.

*Table 41.1* Possible errors in drawing statistical inferences while testing the Null hypothesis

| In Actual | Inference | |
|---|---|---|
| | Accept $H_0$ | Reject $H_0$ |
| $H_0$ True | √ – Confidence level (1 – α) | Type-1 error α |
| $H_0$ False | Type 2 error β | √-Power (1 – β) |

Wrongly rejecting a $H_0$ is called type-1 error.

*Example*: When in reality there is no difference in the prevalence of anaemia among adolescent girls and boys, ($H_0$ is true) but on the basis of a sample we draw the inference in rejecting the above. This is type-1 error.

Here, *level of significance* α = Probability of type-1 error

Confidence level of the test 1 – α = Probability of accepting Null hypothesis when it is True.

The probability of this error is commonly known as P value. The maximum P value allowed in a study/problem is called level of significance or α level.

The level of significance is generally fixed at 5%. When we say that a difference is statistically significant at 5% level of significance all that we mean is that the observed difference could have occurred by chance in only 5% of the occasions or less. However, the level of significance could be 10% when only the leads are explored through exploratory study. But in case of introduction of new drugs or an intervention dealing with humans the level of significance has to be fixed as low as 0.1% to ensure safety.

Type-2 error is failure to accept $H_1$ when it is true, i.e. interpreting $H_0$ is true when it is not.

*Example*: When in reality there is difference in the prevalence of anemia among adolescent girls and boys, ($H_0$ is false) but on the basis of a Sample we draw the inference in accepting the Null hypothesis. This is type-2 error.

Here β = Probability of type-2 error and

Power of the test 1 – β = Probability of rejecting Null hypothesis when it is False.

The probability of this error is β error. The complementary of type-2 error is power of test i.e. 1 – β. The power of a test is the probability of correctly accepting $H_1$ when it is true, i.e. it is the probability of getting statistically significant result. The power of test is high if it is able to detect small differences in variable under study between groups.

## 41.4 Cut-off levels for different levels of significance in one-tailed and two-tailed test

While accepting or rejecting a Null hypothesis the decision is based on the value of the Test Statistic falling in the 'Acceptance Region' or 'Rejection Region'. If the value of Test Statistic falls in the 'Rejection Region' the Null hypothesis is rejected. Conversely, if the value of the Test Statistic falls in the 'Acceptance Region' the Null hypothesis is accepted. The size of the Rejection/Critical region is related to level of significance. That is if the level of significance is 0.05, the Critical region will correspond to the area under the assumed distribution as 5%.

All tests of significance assume normality. The cut-off values based on normal deviates (z α) corresponding to desired level of significance for one tailed and two tailed tests are summarized in the table below.

| α | Zα one-tailed | Zα two-tailed |
|---|---|---|
| 0.01 | 2.327 | 2.575 |
| 0.05 | 1.645 | 1.960 |
| 0.10 | 1.281 | 1.645 |
| 0.20 | 0.841 | 1.281 |

In a two-tailed test the rejection region is located in both the tails. If we are testing a hypothesis at 5% level of significance, the size of the rejection region is 0.025 on both sides of the tails. If we consult the table of areas under the normal curve we find this corresponds to 1.96 on each side. If the sample mean falls into the area beyond 1.96 S.E., the hypothesis is rejected. For one tailed test at 5% level of significance the Rejection Region would correspond to the value of Standard Normal Deviate beyond 1.645 on one side of the tail.

## 41.5 Research designs

There are different types of research designs which could be used in a given situation depending upon the objectives of the study. Some of the important research designs are as under:

- Observational or experimental
- Prospective or retrospective
- Longitudinal or cross-sectional

In an observational study the researcher collects information on the attributes or measurements of interest, but does not influence events. Observational studies are often descriptive. An example would be a study of prevalence of anemia among children. Observational studies include surveys. By contrast, in an experimental study the researcher deliberately influences events and investigates the effects of the intervention. Experimental studies are usually carried out to make comparisons between groups. Experimental studies include clinical trials. In general stronger inferences can be made from experimental studies than from observational studies. For example, the effect of Iron–folic acid (IFA) supplementation to pregnant women versus anemia level could be studied in an experimental situation or through intervention study. However, many times data collected in the cross sectional surveys are also analyzed for the same objective by analyzing the anemia levels according to consumption of IFA. But the inference drawn from intervention study will be more stronger than observation study.

In prospective studies, data is collected forwards in time from the start of the study. Cohort studies are prospective. Experimental studies are also prospective. In retrospective studies, data refer to past events. Case-control studies are retrospective. Cross-sectional studies are those in which individuals are observed only once. Observational studies are mainly cross-sectional. Most surveys are also cross-sectional.

Longitudinal studies are those which investigate changes over a period of time, in relation to an intervention. Observations are taken on more than one occasion. Clinical trials are longitudinal because we are interested in the effect of treatment commencing at one time point on outcome which is measured at a later time.

## 41.6 Sampling

A sample is a part of a population, called the 'universe', 'reference' or 'parent' population. Sampling is the process or technique of selecting a sample. Appropriate sample selection is very critical element of design set up for carrying out the research.

The reference population may be populations of people who process a particular attribute cases of a certain disease, clients of a clinic, acceptors of a certain programme, residents of a geographical area, workers in a certain occupation, recipients of a specified treatment, or people exposed to a certain intervention. The population is the aggregate of the elements or the sampling units. Listing of the sampling units with identification according to certain specifications is called the 'sampling frame'.

### *Sampling procedures*

Random sampling ensures chance of selection to every unit in the population. Simple random sampling guarantees that each member of the population has an equal chance of being included in the sample. The common methods of random sampling are lottery and use of random numbers.

The lottery method assigns numbers to the population; these number are then thoroughly mixed and a sufficient number drawn at random (without replacement) to provide the desired sample size. Tables of random numbers are used after numbers (e.g. sequential counts) have been assigned to members of the study population.

One can start anywhere in the random number table and continue selecting numbers until the desired sample size is reached. Digits of currency notes could also be used as a substitute of random number table.

### *Systematic sampling*

In systematic sampling, the first unit is chosen at random and then other units for the sample are chosen in a systematic way with an interval for example, every fifth household in the reference population.

### *Stratified sampling*

In stratified sampling population is divided into homogeneous groups (or strata) according to certain common characteristics; then a random sample is drawn from each stratum. For example, a population might be divided according to social class, race, sex or age. Appropriate estimation procedure has to be used with proper weighting. There is an important issue of allocation of sample to different strata.

### *Cluster sampling*

Cluster sampling involves choosing groups of units or clusters at random. The information relating to all the units in each cluster are collected. This method is operationally simpler and is less expensive than simple random sampling.

### *Multistage sampling*

Many times the frame of ultimately observable units is not available. In such a case sample is selected using different stages. For example in a survey for a district on nutritional status of children stages could be:

1st stage : village
2nd stage : household
3rd stage : child

*Probability proportional to size*

In probability proportional to size (PPS) sampling the probabilities to different units are assigned in proportion to their size.

**Box 41.1 30 Cluster WHO Methodology for coverage evaluation surveys (CES)**

In a 30 cluster survey, the sample of 30 villages is selected by PPS method and the sample of mothers of children with index child is selected is as follows:

- Prepare a rough sketch and identify a center.
- Draw all lanes/sub lanes from the centre as under-presented below:

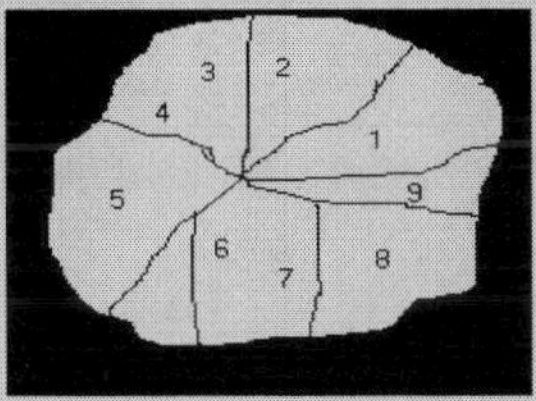


- Select one of the lanes/sub lanes randomly using digits of currency note. Let the lane so selected is 5th.
- In the selected lane walk across from the center till the end and count the steps say 'L'.
- Then select a random number from 1 to L using the digits of currency note and let the number so drawn is 'r'.
- Again walk from the center and stop at step 'r'.
- The House on your left is the randomly selected house. Enquire whether there is a child in the age group 12 to 23 months. If Yes collect the information about the child on the immunization status else proceed to next house following right hand rule. Continue till 7 children are selected.
- This is to be followed in all the 30 selected villages.

## 41.7 Determination of sample size

It is imperative that the sample size be sufficient to be dependable and to allow tests of statistical significance to be applied to the data collected. Unfortunately, there is no thumb rule or magic formula for determining the sample size without some knowledge or assumptions. Such as the prevalence of the condition or characteristic to be studied, the variability between different sampling units, the desired level of statistical significance and the magnitude of sampling errors.

The determination of Sample Size to situations that is (a) estimating average/proportion; or (b) in testing significance of two proportions/ averages are presented in the following sections.

*(a) In estimating average or proportion*

- The parameter (Hb level, prevalence of anemia) to be estimated;

- The degree of precision required;
- The desired confidence level; and
- The estimated degree of variability of observation, i.e. standard deviation.

Sample size: The formula for calculating sample size (n) is as follows:

$$n = (z\alpha^2 \, pq)/d^2$$

p = Likely value of the parameter
q = 1 – p; d = permissible margin of error; and
$z_\alpha$ = value of standard normal deviate corresponding to level of significance.

For 95% confidence level, this formula can be simplified as follows:

$$n = 4 \, pq/d^2$$

The term 'd' in above formula is the absolute margin of error. It is desirable to compute sample size with relative margin of error especially in situation where prevalence is low.

Expressing,

d = Ep, Where E = relative permissible margin in error, the formula simplifies to $n = z_\alpha^2 q / pE^2$,

Thus, n α 1/p; higher will be n for lower value of p [rare diseases].

Further, n α 1/ $E^2$; Higher will be n for lower value of E [Higher Precision], and n α $Z_\alpha^2$; Higher will be n for higher confidence level.

For estimating prevalence of anemia level among preschool children the computation of sample size is explained as under

p = 0.70 (70%), q = 0.30 and E = 0.10 (10% of P)

For α = 0.05 the value of $z_\alpha = 1.96$

In this case,

$n = z_\alpha^2 q / pE^2 = ((1.96*1.96)*0.30)/(0.70*0.10*0.10) = 165$

Table sample size

| p | E | n |
|---|---|---|
| 0.50 | 0.10 | 400 |
| | 0.20 | 100 |
| 0.05 | 0.10 | 7600 |
| | 0.20 | 1900 |
| 0.005 | 0.10 | 80,000 |
| | 0.20 | 20,000 |
| 0.0005 | 0.10 | 8,00,000 |
| | 0.20 | 2,00,000 |

The Sample sizes for some typical values of p (likely value of parameter) and E (relative permissible margin in the error) are given in the above Table for a = 0.05.

This sample size has to be multiplied by Design Effect, which is the ratio of statistical efficiency of the sampling design used to that of simple random sampling.

*(b) In testing for significance between two averages or proportions: intervention studies, Experimental Group versus Control Group*

The information required in arriving at the sample size is as follows:

- The amount of difference between two means (or proportions) that is to be regarded as practically important;
- The size of $\alpha$-error and $\beta$-error; and
- The estimated degree of variability of observation (i.e. standard deviation).

*Example:*

- The approximate value of the parameter/proportion for control group (e.g. 70%)
- Difference in the proportions (between the control and the experimental group) regarded as of practical importance (e.g. 20%).
- Level of significance required (usually 5% level, in a 2-sided test).
- How high should the probability of obtaining a significant result ("power") be (e.g. 90%)?

One may calculate the (reduced) power for detecting the difference of interest (e.g. 20%) or the (larger) difference that can be detected with 90% power.

The sample size is calculated using the formula:

$$n = 2[(Z_\alpha + Z_\beta)/K]^2$$

Where $K = D/\sigma$; $D = p_1 - p_2$; $\sigma^2 = pq$, p = Average of $p_1$ and $p_2$

Sample sizes per group for two-tailed test on proportions are presented in Tables 41.2 and 41.3.

The above examples are for proportions. The formulae for computation of sample size for averages are as under:

One sample situations (with usual notations)

$$n = \frac{Z_\alpha^2 \sigma^2}{d^2}$$

*Table 41.2* Sample sizes per group for two-tailed test on proportions

P1 = 0.60

| P2 | ALPHA | POWER 0.99 | 0.95 | 0.90 | 0.80 |
|---|---|---|---|---|---|
| 0.65 | 0.01 | 4580 | 3416 | 2867 | 2268 |
| 0.65 | 0.02 | 4133 | 3033 | 2518 | 1960 |
| 0.65 | 0.05 | 3519 | 2513 | 2047 | 1549 |
| 0.65 | 0.10 | 3032 | 2106 | 1683 | 1237 |
| 0.65 | 0.20 | 2516 | 1682 | 1309 | 923 |
| 0.70 | 0.01 | 1127 | 847 | 714 | 569 |
| 0.70 | 0.02 | 1019 | 754 | 629 | 494 |
| 0.70 | 0.05 | 870 | 628 | 515 | 395 |
| 0.70 | 0.10 | 752 | 529 | 427 | 319 |
| 0.70 | 0.20 | 627 | 426 | 336 | 243 |
| 0.75 | 0.01 | 489 | 370 | 314 | 252 |
| 0.75 | 0.02 | 443 | 330 | 278 | 220 |
| 0.75 | 0.05 | 379 | 276 | 229 | 178 |
| 0.75 | 0.10 | 329 | 234 | 191 | 145 |
| 0.75 | 0.20 | 276 | 190 | 152 | 112 |
| 0.80 | 0.01 | 266 | 203 | 173 | 140 |
| 0.80 | 0.02 | 241 | 182 | 154 | 123 |
| 0.80 | 0.05 | 207 | 153 | 127 | 100 |
| 0.80 | 0.10 | 180 | 130 | 107 | 83 |
| 0.80 | 0.20 | 152 | 107 | 86 | 65 |

Suppose an estimate is desired of the average retail price of twenty tablets of a commonly used tranquillizer. A random sample of retail pharmacies is to be selected. The estimate is required to be within 10 paisa of the true average price with 95% confidence. Based on a small pilot study, the SD = 85 paisa. How many pharmacies should be randomly selected?

$$n = \frac{4\ (0.85)\ (0.85)}{(0.10)\ (0.10)} = 277.56$$

Two Sample Situations (with usual notations)

$$n = \frac{\sigma^2 \left(Z_\alpha + Z_\beta\right)^2}{\left(\mu_1 - \mu_2\right)^2}$$

*Example*: A survey had indicated that the average weight of men over 55 years of age with newly diagnosed CHD was 90 kg. It is suspected that the average weight of such men is now somewhat lower.

How large a sample would be necessary to test, at 5% level of significance with power of 90%, that the average weight is decreased to 85 kg, with an estimated SD of 20 kg?

$$\sigma = 20;\ \alpha = 0.05;\ \beta = 0.90;\ \mu_1 = 90;\ \mu_2 = 85$$

$$n = \frac{(20)^2 (1.64 + 1.28)^2}{(90-85)^2} = 137$$

*Table 41.3* Sample sizes per group for two-tailed test on proportions

P1 = 0.70

| P2 | ALPHA | POWER 0.99 | 0.95 | 0.90 | 0.80 |
|---|---|---|---|---|---|
| 0.75 | 0.01 | 3907 | 2917 | 2450 | 1940 |
| 0.75 | 0.02 | 3527 | 2591 | 2153 | 1678 |
| 0.75 | 0.05 | 3005 | 2149 | 1753 | 1330 |
| 0.75 | 0.10 | 2590 | 1803 | 1443 | 1064 |
| 0.75 | 0.20 | 2151 | 1443 | 1125 | 796 |
| 0.80 | 0.01 | 935 | 704 | 595 | 476 |
| 0.80 | 0.02 | 846 | 627 | 525 | 414 |
| 0.80 | 0.05 | 723 | 524 | 431 | 332 |
| 0.80 | 0.10 | 626 | 442 | 358 | 269 |
| 0.80 | 0.20 | 523 | 358 | 283 | 206 |
| 0.85 | 0.01 | 393 | 299 | 254 | 205 |
| 0.85 | 0.02 | 356 | 267 | 225 | 180 |
| 0.85 | 0.05 | 306 | 224 | 186 | 146 |
| 0.85 | 0.10 | 266 | 191 | 156 | 120 |
| 0.85 | 0.20 | 223 | 156 | 125 | 94 |
| 0.90 | 0.01 | 206 | 158 | 136 | 111 |
| 0.90 | 0.02 | 187 | 142 | 121 | 98 |
| 0.90 | 0.05 | 161 | 120 | 101 | 80 |
| 0.90 | 0.10 | 141 | 103 | 85 | 67 |
| 0.90 | 0.20 | 119 | 85 | 69 | 53 |

## 41.8 Analysis

General issues of analysis of data revolve round the following:

- Data entry and management.
- Data cleaning and validation.
- Choice of analytical techniques for obtaining valid estimates and inferences.
- Choice of appropriate software.

It is observed that at times objectives are not clearly spelt out and are simply the statement of intentions. Further the objectives are too ambitious to be covered in a single research effort. Also the associated hypotheses are sometimes complex and consequently difficult to be tested. In such situations, one simply ends up with generation of tables without any linking with objective or hypothesis. Further the inferences may be erroneous, misleading having serious policy implications.

There are ways for controlling errors, bridging data gaps and improving the quality of data. These are applicable at different stages, viz. handling of data, sample selection and estimation. Every survey encounters the problem of missing data or data with inconsistencies. The problem of missing data occurs when some, or all of the responses, are not collected for a sample element, or when some responses are deleted because they fail to satisfy certain edit checks. Inconsistencies in data may also occur due to a variety of reasons, such as errors in tabulation, data entry or even in copying from a secondary source. In all such cases, it is a norm to treat it as missing data and handle it accordingly. Whereas total non-response, i.e., when all of the responses on a unit are not available, is handled by some form of weighting adjustment techniques, item non-responses are taken care of by imputation.

Imputation is a technique to handle non-responses by replacing each missing value with a real value. A number of imputation procedures are now available for assigning values for missing responses. These are deductive imputation, overall and class-mean imputations, random imputation, hot-deck imputation and imputation based upon regression.

Among the commonly used analytical tools are *t, F and chi-square* tests of significance. While t test is carried out to test the difference between two treatments (intervention *vs.* control), F test is used in analysis of variance for testing more than two treatments. Chi-square test is used to test the association between two or more categorical variables.

*Examples:*

*t* test: Testing the difference of anemia among boys and girls based on small samples .

*F* test: Testing the difference of anemia among scheduled caste, scheduled tribe and others (for more than 2 groups).

*Chi-Square test*: Testing the association of female literacy/education on infant feeding practice.

Among other commonly used statistical tools are regression. Of particular interest is the logistic regression for identifying risk factors in any causal factor analysis. For instance, one can determine risk factors along with their loading factors associated with undernutrition.

*Disaggregated analysis*

Most studies are planned to provide aggregated results but many times disaggregated results are desired for identifying the target groups and areas requiring special focus. The disaggregated/subgroup analysis can sometimes be more revealing.

*Example* 1: The map of UP given below provides pattern of underweight children in UP in 17 districts of UP from a survey based study carried in 1995 for UNICEF. On mapping the district-wise prevalence of underweight incidence (DWCD, UP, 1999) of <50 per cent, 50–69 per cent and ≥70 per cent, a distinct geographical pattern was observed (Figure 41.2). Highest incidence of malnutrition was observed in the waterlogged Tarai area bordering Nepal, followed by Central belt comprising the entire tract of Gangetic plains, and the lowest underweight percentages were observed in the Vindhyachal ranges which also include the dry Bundelkhand region.

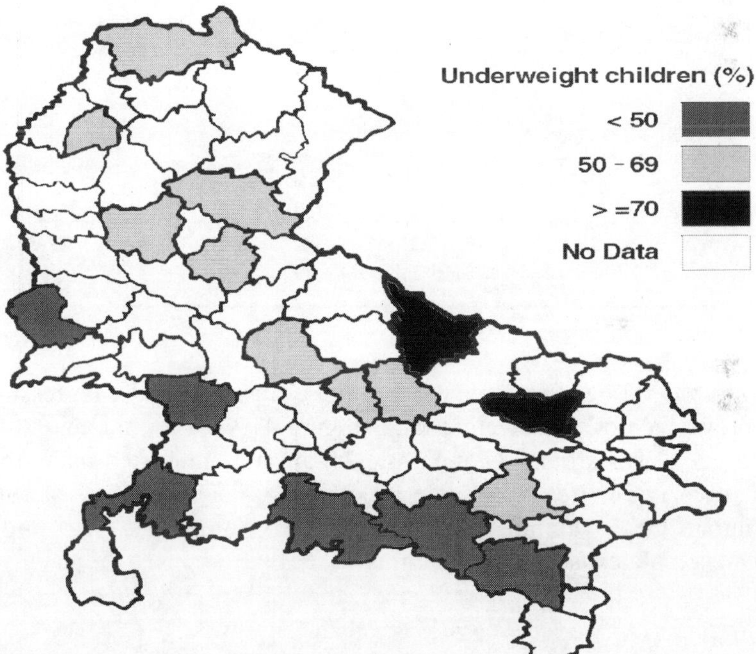


*41.2* Pattern of underweight children in UP.

This distribution of underweight in the state was not in concurrence with the common belief that the highest incidence of malnutrition in the state was in the poorer socio-economic region of Bundelkhand. Higher incidence of under nutrition was in fact noted in the waterlogged eastern region and in the wet Gangetic belt. This can be attributed to possibly higher occurrence of diarrhoea, infection and worm infestation which adversely affect the nutritional status of children.

*Example* 2: Analysis of underweight pattern through age groups of unequal widths 0–6, >6–11, 12–23, 24–35, 36–59 months indicated maximum underweight in children occurring between 12 and 24 months (Figure 41.3 present the usual bar diagram with reference). However, analysis of data on prevalence was undertaken at equal intervals (month wise) and it showed that the maximum underweight is attained at 11 months with the plateau beginning at 12 months itself (Figure 41.3), instead of 24 months, as was reported by earlier workers [2].

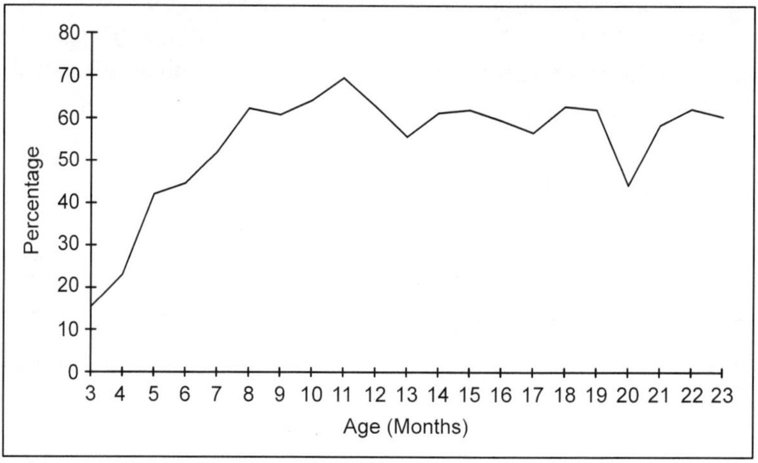


*41.3* Usual bar diagram with reference.

This was further substantiated through a fitted quadratic regression to the prevalence of underweight data (Figure 41.4). The maximum of the fitted curve was around 12 months. The analysis indicated malnutrition sets in early in life and accelerates during 8–11 months. Maximum malnutrition prevalence is attained already under one year and the prevalence plateaus at 12–35 months.

### *Small area statistics*

'Small area estimation' is a statistical technique which makes it possible to enhance the precision of subgroup estimates. The technique uses the idea of 'borrow strength' from similar other areas to develop more accurate estimates for a given area.

There has been a growing demand for reliable small area estimates both from the public and private sectors. In our country, with such large variations, there is an increasing concern about issues of distribution, equity

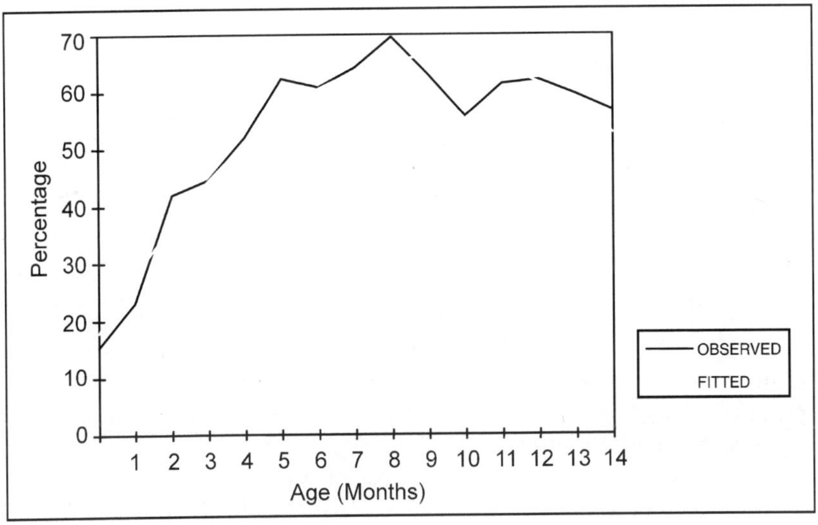


*41.4* Fitted quadratic regression to the prevalence of underweight data.

and disparity. There may exist sub-groups that are far below the average in certain respects and need upgrading.

Deep stratification or nested stratification (stratification within stratification), is very useful tool, if appropriately used. The technique provides a sampling design which requires a much smaller sample size and is intuitively more efficient than the conventional stratified design using only one stratification variable. Deep stratification is a tool which automatically controls variability according to disaggregated groups and even simple random sampling within each stratum usually leads to self weighting design, which is easy to analyse and interpret.

There are some concerns with reference to efficacy of surveys with regard to relative margin of error, particularly for sub-group estimates. The subgroups could be related socio-economic, demographic, housing or household characteristics, or even classifications like grades of anemia or undernutrition (mild, moderate and severe).

Sample size is usually determined for the overall indicator, keeping in mind the desired precision, complexity of the design and expected non-response. The subgroup indicator estimates as above mostly suffer from inadequacy of sample size. The inadequate sample size for each subgroup leads to highly imprecise and unreliable estimates for these subgroups. Disaggregated analysis by subgroups with inadequate sample size leads to erroneous inference. There could be situations where results based on such analysis find place in formulating policies, which may often have far reaching implications.

## 41.9 Softwares

SPSS (originally, Statistical Package for the Social Sciences) was released in its first version in 1968. It is among the most widely used programs for statistical analysis in social sciences. Statistics included in the base software:

- *Descriptive statistics*: Cross-tabulation, Frequencies, Descriptives, Explore, Descriptive Ratio Statistics
- *Bivariate statistics*: Means, t-test, ANOVA, Correlation (bivariate, partial, distances), Non-parametric tests
- Prediction for numerical outcomes – Linear regression
- Prediction for identifying groups – factor analysis, cluster analysis (two-step, K-means, hierarchical), discriminate functions
- Add-on modules provide additional capabilities. The available modules are as follows:
- SPSS Data Validation (added in version 14) – It allows programming of logical checks and reporting of suspicious values.
- SPSS Regression Models – Logistic regression, ordinal regression, multinomial logistic regression, and mixed models.
- SPSS Advanced Models – Multivariate GLM and repeated measures ANOVA (removed from base system in version 14).
- SPSS Classification Tree – It creates classification and decision trees for identifying groups and predicting behaviour.
- SPSS Table – It allows user-defined control of output for reports.
- SPSS Exact Test – It allows statistical testing on small samples.
- SPSS Categories
- SPSS Trends
- SPSS Conjoint
- SPSS Missing Value Analysis – It is simple regression-based imputation.
- SPSS Map
- SPSS Complex Samples (added in Version 12) – It adjusts for stratification and clustering and other sample selection biases.
- Epi Info is public domain statistical software for epidemiology developed by Centers for Disease Control and Prevention (CDC) in Atlanta, Georgia (USA).
- Epi Info has been in existence for over 20 years and is currently available for Microsoft Windows.
- Cranes Software International Ltd. (Cranes), a company that provides Enterprise Statistical Analytics and Engineering Simulation Software Products and Solutions across the globe, announced the launch of SYSTAT 13, the latest version of its flagship statistical software package.

SYSTAT 13 introduces the following new statistical methods:

- ARCH & GARCH Models in Time Series
- Best Subsets Regression
- Confirmatory Factor Analysis
- Environment Variables in Best Statistics
- Polynomial Regression
- Enhancements to existing methods such as ANOVA, Bootstrapping, Cross-tabulation, Fitting Distributions, Hypothesis Testing and more!
- SYSTAT, a proprietary product from the Cranes® Group of Companies, integrates both basic and advanced statistical tools with dazzling accompanying graphics.
- Additionally, SYSTAT has newly partnered with Cytel – a 20-year leader in the design and analysis of clinical trials – to bring you SYSTAT 13 with Exact Tests, a new SYSTAT product that contains Cytel's famous exact-inference testing procedures.

## References

1. VIR SC (2001). Nutritional status of children in Uttar Pradesh, *NFI Bulletin*, January 2001.
2. NIGAM AK (2001). Analysis of malnutrition data - Revisited. Invited talk at the International Conference on Statistics, Combinatorics and Related Areas held at Wollongong, Australia.

# 42

# Reducing malnutrition: An analysis of the Integrated Child Development Services (ICDS) scheme

*Deepika N. Chaudhery*

**Deepika N. Chaudhery**, PhD, is the Deputy Regional Director for Asia, Micronutrient Initiative (MI), Asia. Earlier, Dr Chaudhery as Coordinator Programs, MI, Asia, worked in close consultation with country governments in the development, delivery and quality assurance of micronutrient programs in six Asian countries – Afghanistan, Bangladesh, Indonesia, India, Nepal and Pakistan. Prior to this, Dr Chaudhery provided technical and programme management support to micronutrient India programmes as the Chief Executive Officer at the Micronutrient Initiative India Trust. Additionally, she has a vast experience in the field of reproductive and child health, HIV/AIDS and nutrition programmes as CARE India officer and as project officer, Nutrition, with UNICEF (India Country Office) based at Hyderabad.

## 42.1 Background

Even after 61 years of independence and reforms, under nutrition continues to remain a chronic public health problem in India. According to the most recent National Family and Health Survey (NFHS-3) 2005–06 [1], about 45% children less than 3 years of age are stunted (low weight-for-height) and 40% are underweight (low weight-for-age). Marginal improvement in nutritional status of children between NFHS-3 and NFHS-2 conducted in 1998–99 [2] has been disappointing.

Malnutrition, both undernutrition and micronutrient deficiencies, restricts the growth and development of children, resulting in a substantial dip in productivity levels in adulthood. This has a cumulative negative effect on the health parameters and hence the country's economic development.

Among the programs and initiatives which are meant to combat undernutrition is India's largest community-based outreach program for vulnerable children and women called the Integrated Child Development Services (ICDS) program. A key mandate of ICDS has been to improve nutritional and health standards of children below 6 years of age.

This chapter provides an overview of the ICDS program; tracks its contribution in improving nutrition and health outcomes; identifies limitations and outlines a way forward.

Sections 42.2, 42.3, 42.4 and 42.5 present program design and implementation framework, evolution and current reach. Section 42.6 provides an analysis of limitations and Section 42.7 outlines how nutrition and health outcomes were impacted when innovative approaches were implemented. Section 42.8 proposes a strategy and actions to improve the effectiveness of ICDS as it moves towards universalisation.

## 42.2 Program background: design and implementation framework

The Department of Women and Child Development (DWCD), Ministry of Human Resource Development (Mo HRD), Government of India (GoI) was rechristened as Ministry of Women and Child Development in 2006. Under the aegis of the MoHRD, the ICDS scheme was launched in 1975. It was introduced in 33 blocks with the objective of contributing to goals of the National Policy for Children and has significantly expanded since then.

This Section presents an outline of the design of the ICDS program – its objectives, package of services, infrastructure, human resources, and delivery mechanisms. It is important to note that the ICDS as described in this Section is the envisioned "program design". What the program actually looks like in different operational contexts is described in Sections 42.2 and 42.3.

Key participants of the scheme are children below 6 years, pregnant and lactating mothers and women in the 15–45 years age group. By 2006, ICDS covered about 6118 projects[1] across the country. Poised for universal coverage, as per GoI estimates of 2008 services are being provided to about 562.2 lakh (56.2 m) participants of which 467.2 lakh (46.7m) are children (0–6 years) and 95 lakh (9.5 m) are pregnant and lactating mothers, through a network of about 7.48 lakh (0.75 m) *anganwadi* centers [3] across the country.

### 42.2.1 Key objectives of ICDS [4]

- Improve nutritional and health status of children below 6 years of age;
- Build a foundation for the child's physical, psychological and emotional development;

1. ICDS project comprises 100 anganwadi centers, one for every village with 1000 population.

- Reduce incidence of mortality, morbidity, malnutrition and school dropouts;
- Enhance capability of the mother to look after health, nutritional and development needs of the child through proper community education; and
- Achieve effective coordination of policy and implementation among various departments to promote child development.

### 42.2.2 Basket of services under ICDS

- *Nutrition* – Supplementary feeding, growth monitoring and promotion, nutrition and health education;
- *Early care and stimulation* – For children under 3 years of age and *preschool education* for children 3–6 years of age;
- *Health* – Immunization, support in micronutrient supplementation (vitamin A, iron, folic acid), health check-ups, referral services, and treatment of minor illnesses;
- *Convergence* – Of other supportive services such as safe drinking water, environmental sanitation, women's empowerment, non-formal education and adult literacy.

Nutrition and early childhood care and preschool education related services are the primary responsibility of the Ministry of Women & Child Development whereas health related services fall under the direct purview of the Department of Health & Family Welfare. The *anganwadi* is the focal point for the delivery of services at the community level, located within the village or slum area it caters to. The *anganwadi* center (AWC) is expected to serve as a convenient meeting place for women's groups that create awareness and mobilize joint action for child growth and development.

### 42.2.3 Composition of the ICDS Team

The *anganwadi* worker (AWW) who as per policy is recommended to be a local resident of the village, is the nodal frontline worker of the ICDS program. The AWW, assisted by *anganwadi* helper, operate at the village level. The Supervisor, Child Development Project Officer (CDPO) and District Project Officer (DPO) are at the sector (20 to 25 AWCs), project (a project being about 100 villages/blocks and in rural areas is often an entire block) and district levels, respectively. In larger rural and tribal projects, there is an Additional Child Development Project Officer (ACDPO). The onus of implementing ICDS program activities lies with this team of ICDS functionaries.

Functionaries of the Department of Health include Auxiliary Nurse Midwife (ANM) and male health workers at village level, Lady Health Visitors (LHVs) at sector level, medical officer-in-charge (MOIC) at block level and Chief Medical officer (CMO) at district level. ANM's unit of operation is the sub-center that caters to 5,000–8,000 people. The Primary Health Center (PHC) established for every 30,000–50,000 population is managed by the PHC's MO. The health team works with the ICDS team to deliver services (Fig. 42.1).

An AWC was initially meant to cater to a population of 1,000 but now in actual practice ends up servicing 1500 persons or more. In a large village of about 3,000–3,500 population, there are about 2–3 AWCs. Presently, there are an average 125–150 AWCs per project/block, since additional AWCs have been sanctioned, based on increased village and block population. However, in tribal areas the number of AWCs per project is about 700.

**Box 42.1 Roles and responsibilities of ICDS project staff [15]**

| AWW | Supervisor | CDPO |
|---|---|---|
| • Village mapping. | • Preparing quarterly action plan. | • Recruiting and training staff. |
| • Conducting community survey twice a year and enlisting beneficiaries. | • Supervising service delivery and monitoring day-to-day AWC activities. | • Supervising daily activities of AWC including periodic field visits. |
| • Delivering services – growth monitoring and promotion; preschool education; distributing supplementary nutrition; assisting health staff in immunization and heath check-ups.<br>• Providing information and counseling to families/ communities during home visits and group meetings.<br>• Promoting community participation.<br>• Preparing Monthly Progress Report (MPR).<br>• Maintaining the AWC.<br>• Liaising with *panchayat*, primary schools, *mahila mandals*. | • Planning and organizing induction training of AWWs and helpers.<br>• Supervising and providing continuing education to AWWs during home visits.<br>• Planning and organizing sectoral meetings.<br>• Analyzing skills and performance of AWWs.<br>• Compiling/reviewing MPRs and interpreting data.<br>• Assessing shortfalls in achievements; sugges-ing corrective action.<br>• Coordinating with PHC, CHC and different departments (Education, Information & Broad-asting). | • Conducting monthly meetings with Superviors to discuss progress and problems.<br>• Convergence between ICDS, Health, Panchayati Raj Institution (PRI) and local leaders<br>• Maintaining records and registers – MPR; quar-erly/annual progress reports<br>• Procuring, storing and maintaining equipment and supplies.<br>• Procuring and distributing supplementary nutrition.<br>• Guiding and continuing education of project staff.<br>• Promoting community participation. |

The integrated ICDS package of services is intended to enhance impact of various nutrition, health and child development interventions. The package is delivered by the AWW with support from the helper. The AWW

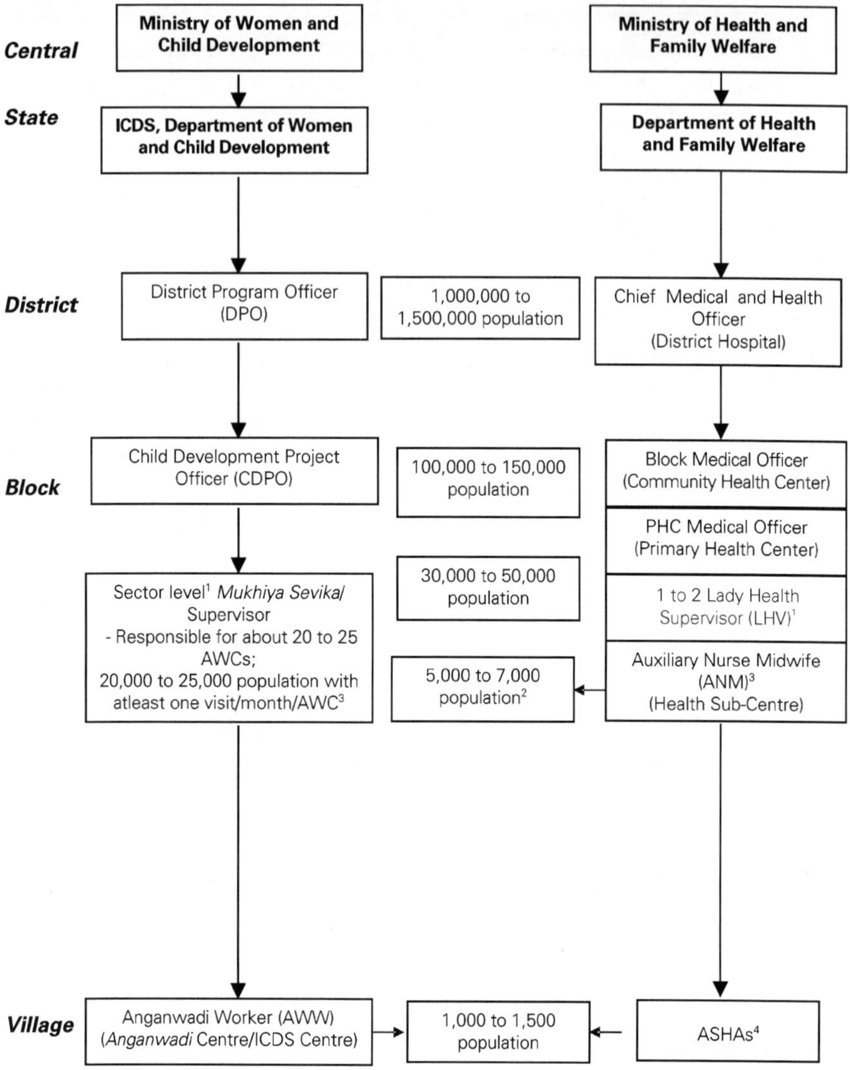


*42.1* ICDS and Health Systems': from Central to Village .

1 Villages covered by Lady Health Supervisor (LHV) and Mukhiya Sevika/ Supervisor are not necessarily the same

2 Health sub-centre is recommended to cover about 5,000 population.

3 ANM's monthly visit to villages is normally based on microplan prepared for immunization coverage - atleast one visit/village/month on the days fixed for immunization.

4 Accredited Social Health Activist (ASHAs)

needs to survey all families in the community to identify children below 6 years, pregnant and nursing mothers and adolescent girls in the catchment area. To enhance outreach of services and ensure better service utilization, the AWW needs to mobilize community support.

## 42.3 Key nutrition, early childcare and preschool education and health related services

### 42.3.1 Nutrition component under ICDS

*Supplementary feeding* – Under the ICDS program, children less than 6 years of age are expected to be given supplementary food (often referred to as supplementary nutrition) which provides 300 calories and 8–10 grams of protein while pregnant and lactating mothers and adolescent girls are to be provided food with 500 calories and 20–25 grams of protein to meet the calorie and protein deficits in Indian diets consumed by poor populations. Children who are severely malnourished are recommended to be provided double the quantity of food. This amounts to 600 calories and 16–20 grams of protein. Supplementary food consists of local grains, oil, and in some areas Ready-To-Eat (RTE) foods. In case of RTE foods, children less than 3 years are given Take-Home Rations (THR) and 3–6 year olds are served on-the-spot. As per the Supreme Court directives, Hot Cooked Meals (HCM) are being provided in many states. In addition, the GoI has recommended that the ICDS supplementary nutrition needs to be fortified with essential micronutrients comprising iron, calcium, vitamin A, thiamin, riboflavin, niacin, folic acid and vitamin C at 50% of the recommended dietary allowance per day [5]. Details are presented in Table 42.1.

Besides serving as a nutrition supplement, supplementary food is viewed to serve as an incentive and contact opportunity to attract mothers and their children to avail other nutrition, health and preschool education related services. This food is meant for the child/pregnant/lactating mother and adolescent girls and is not a substitute for home food.

*Growth monitoring and promotion* – Children below 3 years are weighed once a month and those between 3–6 years are weighed quarterly. It is mandated that weights of all children below 6 years be recorded on growth charts at the AWC. This helps to assess the growth pattern of an individual child, detect growth faltering and determine nutritional status. Therefore, each child's nutritional status is evaluated, gaps identified and remedial steps suggested.

Counseling for breastfeeding, complementary feeding and other health care needs is expected to be provided subsequent to the weighing. Counseling on feeding practices is central to "Growth Monitoring and Promotion" for achieving desired impact.

*Table 42.1* Recommended Dietary Allowances, nutrient intakes and gaps [5]

| | Age group 1–3 years | | | Age group 1–3 years | | | Pregnant women | | | Lactating women | | |
|---|---|---|---|---|---|---|---|---|---|---|---|---|
| | RDA[1] | Intake | Gap | RDA | Intake | Gap | RDA | Intake | Gap | RDA | Intake | Gap |
| Energy (kcal) | 1240 | 687 | 553 | 1690 | 978 | 712 | 2175 | 1654 | 521 | 2425 | 1852 | 573 |
| Protein (g) | 22 | 18.6 | 3.4 | 30 | 26.5 | 3.5 | 65 | 45 | 20 | 75 | 46.7 | 28.3 |
| Iron (mg) | 12 | 4.3 | 7.7 | 18 | 6.8 | 11.2 | 38 | 12 | 26 | 30 | 11.8 | 18.2 |
| Vitamin A (mg) | 400 | 56 | 344 | 400 | 66 | 334 | 600 | 111 | 489 | 950 | 107 | 843 |
| Calcium (mg) | 400 | 161 | 239 | 400 | 66 | 334 | 1000 | 352 | 648 | 1000 | 320 | 680 |
| Thiamin (mg) | 0.6 | 0.4 | 0.2 | 0.9 | 0.6 | 0.3 | 1.1 | 1.0 | 0.1 | 1.2 | 1.2 | 0 |
| Riboflavin (mg) | 0.7 | 0.3 | 0.4 | 1.0 | 0.3 | 0.7 | 1.3 | 0.5 | 0.8 | 1.4 | 0.6 | 0.8 |
| Niacin (mg) | 8.0 | 4.7 | 3.3 | 11.0 | 7.4 | 3.6 | 14.0 | 12.4 | 1.6 | 16 | 14.4 | 1.6 |
| Vitamin C (mg) | 30 | 9 | 21 | 40.0 | 15.0 | 25 | 40 | 26 | 14 | 80 | 28 | 52 |
| Free Folic Acid (mg) | 30 | 18 | 12 | 40 | 26 | 14 | 400 | 48 | 352 | 150 | 53 | 97 |

[1] RDA – Recommended Dietary Allowance

Mothers, caregivers and families of children who are growth faltered are to be provided support via appropriate information; extra counseling through increased number of home visits; ensuring access to basic health services such as immunization by ANM; and those found severely malnourished are given special care through therapeutic supplementary nutrition (referred as "double ration") and referral to a health facility.

The concept of community-based nutrition surveillance has also been introduced in ICDS projects of selected states. A community chart for nutritional status monitoring is maintained at AWCs since this reflects nutritional status of all children registered with the *anganwadi* at any point in time and is a useful tool for community dialogue.

*Nutrition and health education (NHE)* – The primary objective is to build the capacity of women in the 15–45 years age group to enable them to take care of their own health, nutrition and development needs as also to their children and families. NHE comprises of basic nutrition and health information related to child care and development including infant and young child feeding practices and environmental sanitation. It is built on local knowledge, attitude, practices and resources to cover all women. Home visits, mother's meetings, events such as Nutrition and Health Day, immunization sessions, growth monitoring days, and local festivals/ gatherings are contact points to deliver NHE with or without the use of Information Education and Communication (IEC) materials. "Growth promotion" is viewed as a critical component of the larger NHE.

### 42.3.2 Early childhood care and preschool education (ECCE)

As envisaged in ICDS, ECCE focuses on total development of the child (0–6 years). It includes promotion of early stimulation of under-3s through interventions with mothers/caregivers. It's program for 3–6 year olds in the *anganwadi* is directed towards providing and ensuring a stimulating environment, with emphasis on necessary inputs for optimal growth and development. Child-centered play-way activities, which build on local culture and practices, using local support materials developed by the AWW, are promoted.

Early learning component provides sound foundation for cumulative lifelong learning and development. It prepares children for primary schooling and offers substitute care to younger siblings, freeing older children, especially girls, to attend school. Local level coordination between the AWC and primary schools via convenient timings, location and supportive linkages between the AWW and primary school teacher is promoted [2].

### 42.3.3 Health

Health related services include immunization, delivery of micronutrient supplements, health check-ups, referral services and treatment of minor illnesses. These are provided by functionaries of the Health Department. ICDS provides support for the operationalization of the National Nutritional Anemia Control Program (NNACP) [6] and the National Policy on Management of Vitamin A Deficiency [7] under the purview of the Department of Health & Family Welfare. In coordination with the AWW, the ANM provides these services at the village level.

The NNACP aims at decreasing prevalence and incidence of anemia in young children and women in the reproductive age group, especially pregnant and lactating women. The program focuses on promotion of regular consumption of foods rich in iron, provision of IFA supplements in the form of tablets to "high-risk groups" and identification and treatment of severely anemic cases. The supplementation component recommends IFA in liquid formulation containing 20 mg elemental iron and 100 µg folic acid per day [8] for children aged 6–60 months; 1 big IFA tablet (100 mg elemental iron and 500 µg folic acid) a day for 100 days for pregnant and lactating mothers after the first trimester of pregnancy and 2 big tablets a day for minimum 100 days for severely anemic pregnant mothers and women who are 15–45 years old.

The National Policy for Management of Vitamin A Deficiency [7] promotes consumption of Vitamin A rich foods by pregnant and lactating women and by children under 5 years of age, promotion of colostrum feeding, exclusive breastfeeding for the first 6 months of life and continued breastfeeding until at least 2 years of life and administering massive doses of vitamin A. The massive dose component includes 9 mega doses of vitamin A supplement (VAS) for children 6 months to 5 years; first dose of 100,000 IU of vitamin A is recommended to be administered with measles vaccination at 9 months and subsequent 8 doses of 200,000 IU each at every 6 months interval. In the past five years, a biannual service delivery approach is being institutionalised to improve coverage of the 2nd to the 9th dose of VAS.

## 42.4 Training in ICDS

Training infrastructure includes the National Institute of Public Cooperation and Child Development (NIPCCD) at the national level, its regional centers located at Lucknow, Bangalore, Indore and Guwahati, 18 Mid Level Training Centers (MLTCs) and 283 *Anganwadi* Training Centers (AWTCs). While CDPOs are trained at NIPCCD, Supervisors' training is conducted at MLTCs and that of AWWs at AWTCs.

The curriculum for all levels of functionaries covers a wide range of nutrition, health and child development aspects and includes gender and community mobilization. AWWs are provided induction training for 15 days followed by a job course training and subsequent refresher programs. Job course training for CDPO's, supervisors and AWWs is for 30 days. Out of the 26 working days 23 days are for institutional training with practical and mock sessions while 3 days are allocated for supervised practice. Participatory techniques are used and classroom teaching is supported by role play, demonstration and exercises (9-11).

With the launch of "Udisha" project in 1999 (Box 42.2) under the ICDS, training of functionaries was redefined. "Udisha" was conceptualized as a dynamic and responsive human resource development program with a vibrant training and communication package [8]. It was supported by the World Bank during 1999–2004 and its three main components included regular training, innovative and area specific training and IEC.

## 42.5 Program evolution

This Section describes program evolution in terms of coverage and monetary investment by government and development partners. The ICDS program has evolved over the last 33 years. An expenditure of about Rs 1,190 crore[2] was incurred during the first 17 years, following which the government increased spending from Rs 2,271 crore[2] under the Eighth Five-Year Plan to Rs 4,557 crore[2] under the Ninth Five-Year Plan. The program has been supported by donors, including UNICEF, CARE, World Food Program and the Norwegian Agency for Development Cooperation [12]. The proposed outlay for the Eleventh Five-Year Plan is Rs 41764.80 crores[2] [13]. It is proposed that the financial assistance under the program will be on 85:15 sharing between the central and State governments during the Eleventh Five Year Plan followed by 75:25 sharing during the 12th Plan and 50:50 sharing thereafter.

World Bank supported ICDS in overlapping phases from 1990 to 2006. This includes Tamil Nadu Integrated Project (TNIP), ICDS – phases I, II and III and ICDS – Andhra Pradesh Economic Restructuring Project with International Development Assistance of about US$ 700 million [3].

### 42.5.1 World Bank assisted ICDS Phases I, II and III

- *ICDS Phase I* – Support was provided to the Tamil Nadu Integrated Project (TINP I and TINP II) as an alternative to the standard ICDS program; TINP I was implemented between 1980 and 1989 covering

[2] 1 crore = 10 million (Rs. 45 = One US $).

6 districts. TINP II was operationalised between 1991 and 1998 covering 24 districts in the state of Tamil Nadu.

### Box 42.2 Udisha - background and key features

Udisha was a national initiative for quality improvement in training of ICDS functionaries and caregivers. Udisha was based on a vision that all functionaries of ICDS should be developed into agents of social change.
The Department of Women and Child Development conducted a review of the entire training component of ICDS. This review was conducted over a period of two years and focused on training needs assessment, methodologies, syllabus, training resources, procedures, systems and program strategies. From this process 'emerged' the basic challenges which were attempted to be addressed by Udisha.

**Key features**

- *Revision of syllabus*

The revised syllabus under Udisha focused on AWW as a communicator, facilitator and a mobiliser and consisted of modules based on participatory methodologies and experiential learning. All modules focussed on a life cycle approach.

- *Training based on area/region specific needs*

About 75% of the core syllabus was common for the entire country, and 25% of the syllabus was based on area specific needs. This was developed by individual states to reflect the training needs for functionaries working in that region/area. Training need's assessment formed an integral part of the process.

- *Integration and coordination of training*

For better coordination amongst the various players such as trainees as well as trainers/institutions and to avoid duplication and overlapping, task forces were set up at National and State levels to facilitate the process of planning and training in states. The states in turn formulated State Training Action Plan and Training Calendars. The process focused on who, what, where, how and when to be trained.

- *Technical support and institution building*

Udisha encouraged NIPCCD to develop into a center of excellence and a premier institute of child development. It also envisaged a dynamic collaboration with India's leading institutes such as the National Institute of Nutrition, the National Center for Education, Research and Training and the National Institute of Health and Family Welfare.

- *Monitoring*

Udisha focused on improving the skills of the ICDS project managers and functionaries in collection, analysis, interpretation and use of data at the community level.

- *ICDS Phase II* – Support was extended to the standard government ICDS program and to additional activities. It operated in 461 new blocks in the states of Bihar, Jharkhand, Madhya Pradesh and Chhattisgarh between 1993 and 2002.
- *ICDS Phase III* – Primary emphasis shifted from expanded coverage to improving quality of services. Operations extended to 318 projects in Kerala, Maharashtra, Rajasthan, Tamil Nadu and Uttar Pradesh between the years 1999 and 2006. In addition, a restructured component included coverage of the erstwhile ICDS-II projects between the years 2002 and 2004 and expansion to Orissa and Uttrakhand.

- *ICDS Phase IV* – A five year phase four is planned to be implemented in 8 states - Bihar, Chhattisgarh, Jharkhand, Madhya Pradesh, Maharashtra, Rajasthan, Uttar Pradesh and Andhra Pradesh with support from the World Bank. Objectives of the project are to reduce child malnutrition and improve early child development outcomes among children 3–6 years of age [14]. Following a targeted approach, the project envisages covering 158 high-burden districts from these states for intensive implementation.

As coverage increased, more states and more districts or blocks within states were given sanctions for AWCs and additional staff. During the expansion phase there were innovations supported the World Bank, UNICEF and NGOs, e.g. CARE and the Micronutrient Initiative to increase coverage of nutrition and health related services and behaviors.

Under the Eleventh Five Year Plan – to comply with directions of the Supreme Court and to implement the National Common Minimum Program of the Government, the ICDS scheme has been expanded to cover 466 new projects and 188,168 additional AWCs. Based on revised population norms, recommended by the Inter-Ministerial Task Force, the states have given a requirement of 173 additional projects, 107,274 additional AWCs and 25,961 mini-AWCs [13].

## 42.6 Evidence from program evaluations and program limitations

Evidence from large scale program evaluations, including some select studies that were undertaken to measure impact of ICDS in improving nutrition and health services and behaviors of the target population are described in the Section. This Section also presents program limitations which have impeded progress.

### 42.6.1 Evidence from large-scale evaluations

Three large scale evaluations of the ICDS program were undertaken – two evaluations by NIPCCD, i.e. 1992–93 [15] and 2005–06 evaluation [3] and one by National Council of Applied Economic Research (NCAER) in 2001 [16]. While these showed improvement on some health, nutrition and preschool outcomes, significant gaps were identified in program implementation. Key recommendations were to have on-the-job training that incorporated innovative methods of imparting refresher training; strengthening supervision; focusing on NHE; intensifying implementation of the preschool education component; and improving community participation (Box 42.3).

**Box 42.3 Gaps and recommendations: NIPCCD program evaluation**

- Need to upgrade the physical infrastructural facilities of AWCs. Semi-permanent anganwadi structures need to be progressively replaced by permanent and pucca buildings and handpumps should be installed within the premises wherever possible. Categorical instructions may be issued not to locate AWCs in the areas predominantly inhabited by upper class and upper caste population, as it hinders utilization of services by the lowest castes and poor beneficiaries.
- Need to experiment with some innovative methods of imparting refresher training. The possibility of involving academic and technical institutions in strengthening continuing education needs to be explored.
- It should be mandatory for the Project Officers to organize frequent training workshops at the project level. The concept of establishing a resource centre at CDPO's office needs consideration and a policy decision.
- Supervision needs be strengthened. No Supervisor should have more than 20 AWCs under charge. A double or additional charge is detrimental for the supportive role. There is need therefore, to create a post of a substitute Supervisor in every project.
- Participation of ANMs in providing referral services, health check-up, home visits and NHE session needs to be promoted further. Both AWW and ANM should work in close collaboration in taking care of health needs of women and children.
- Coverage of children under supplementary nutrition, and particularly that of under-threes, should be improved through door-to-door surveys, encouraging consumption of food at the anganwadi and enhancing mothers' awareness about appropriate feeding practices.
- Implementation of NHE was found to be far below the desired level. It is suggested that Supervisors should be given the responsibility to hold formal NHE sessions regularly in AWCs under their charge. Rigorous monitoring by CDPOs and active participation of health functionaries can improve implementation of this component. For group formation and collecting women at one place for NHE sessions, locally popular social/recreational events may be organised. Utilisation of folk media such as nautanki, kathputli, etc, need to be included in the training curricula of functionaries to strengthen their skills in imparting NHE effectively.
- There is need for improving the implementation of pre–school education (PSE) component. Non-availability of material for play and learning is one of the major constraints. Efforts are needed to provide a minimum set of appropriate educational aids and material at every AWC.
- Irregular supply of equipment, food items, play material and medicine kits is one of the major problems in implementation of ICDS. The State Governments should take appropriate measures to streamline supplies for smoother implementation of the program.
- Community participation is a very weak link of the ICDS programme. It is imperative that community representatives should be involved right from the preparatory stage of initiating a project. Effective ways of augmenting participation need to be evolved. AWWs apparently do not have the requisite skills for promoting participation. CDPOs and Supervisors should take appropriate initiative in this regard.
- It was observed that coverage and outreach of services need to be improved in tribal areas, keeping in view the topographical factors. In urban areas also, the services provided were minimal and the situation was worse than that in tribal and rural areas. Steps need to be taken urgently to improve the situation in urban slums.

(*Source*: National Institute of Public Cooperation & Child Development. National Evaluation of the Integrated Child Development Services. New Delhi, 1992)

Based on 1992–93 and 1998–99 NFHS data, it was initially found that ICDS had significant and positive effect on nutritional outcomes, but on more rigorous exploration, little effect was found when children in ICDS villages were compared to children in non-ICDS villages [17].

NFHS 2005–06 [18] assessed utilization of services under ICDS. Key findings are as follows:

- 81% children under age six living in enumeration areas covered by an AWC, only 28.4% received any services.
- Most common services included receiving supplementary food (26% children < 6 years of age, 20.5% pregnant women and 16.5% lactating mothers); preschool education (23% for children 3–6 years of age); receiving health check ups (15.8% children under age six, 12.3% pregnant women and 8.5% lactating mothers) and 20% and 18% of children received immunization and growth monitoring services, respectively;
- Only 10.9% pregnant women and 8.3% lactating mothers received nutrition and health education.
- Children between 2 and 3 years were more likely to be taken to an AWC than younger and older children;
- Mothers with no education were least likely to take advantage of services offered by an AWC; and
- Only 50% of the age eligible children from scheduled tribes in areas covered by an AWC received some kind of service.

These findings clearly indicate a sub-optimal utilization of services under a program that has been operational for several years.

### 42.6.2 Select studies

In addition to large scale evaluations, numerous studies were conducted to assess different aspects of the program. Highlights from few studies over the last decade are given below.

Findings reported are variable. On 18 years of completion of ICDS, Ghandhi et al [19] concluded that the program benefited all sections of communities including backward and minorities. There was significant decrease in the prevalent of severely malnourished children from 21% in 1976 to 7% in 1990. Contrary to this, there are assessments which show limited impact of ICDS on the nutritional status of children [20, 21]. Nutritional status of 1286 pre-school children residing in urban, rural and slum areas of Chandigarh revealed that the prevalence of undernutrition was significantly higher among the ICDS beneficiaries (53.8%) than non-ICDS beneficiaries (46.9%) [20]. In another report between the years 1981 and 1991, the proportion of children with severe protein energy malnutrition living in the same 6 villages of Garhi tribal block of South Rajasthan declined from 14.6% to only 11.3% [21].

In a study conducted in Agra district of Uttar Pradesh, supplementary food was received by 20–48% of the pregnant mothers and 35–53.7 % of children and coverage with IFA tablets was in the range of 24–30 % indicating a clear need to strengthen service utilization [22].

An assessment indicated benefit of nutrition supplement provided by ICDS during latter part of pregnancy to undernourished pregnant women in maternal weight gain and birth weight. The ICDS supplemented mothers gained 100 grams more in pregnancy and the birth weight was higher by 58 g ($p < 0.05$) as compared to un-supplemented ICDS mothers. Birth weight in un-supplemented ICDS areas was 25 grams higher as compared to non ICDS area [23]. An assessment of the impact of non-formal preschool education on mental and cognitive development of rural and urban children showed positive findings [24]. Mean test scores among rural ICDS attendees aged 3–4 years were 73.77 compared to 67.33 for non-attendees. The scores for rural ICDS attendees 4–5 years old was 95.60 compared to 82.20 for non-attendees.

## 42.6.3 Program Limitations

This section analyses program limitations under key areas of program mandate i.e., coverage, capacity, training and supervision, linkage with the health sector, monitoring and community engagement.

*Program mandate*

ICDS has six objectives which cover a large program mandate making the scope of work for program functionaries extensive and diverse in nature. Moreover, objectives with reference to nutritional status are not stated in terms of measurable goals. In many cases, efforts have not been rigorous enough to improve coverage with services and changing behaviors. This has contributed to limited impact of ICDS on weight and height of children.

ICDS has not adequately focused on right age groups i.e. below 2 years with appropriate evidence based interventions that could improve nutritional status of young children. Emphasis has been on supplementary feeding and the 3–6 years age group. The understanding of links between key services and behaviors, and program impact has not been adequately communicated to district, block and sector levels. There has been little attempt to examine whether the program was moving towards impact or not.

While a key focus area of ICDS is to address malnutrition, most of the efforts were directed towards providing supplementary food and addressing severe undernutrition through not a comprehensive approach but only by the double ration approach. Child care and feeding practices were given very little attention. Efforts to streamline identification of beneficiaries and ensuring supply and consumption of supplementary food were far from satisfactory. Linkage with the health sector for provision of micronutrient supplements and referral of severely malnourished child has remained poor since the roles of ICDS functionaries were often not clearly defined for these services.

AWW was viewed by the government as a worker who would focus on activities to prevent malnutrition and promotive behaviors such as promoting and supporting breastfeeding and complementary feeding. Field observations reveals that she is often busy with supply of supplementary food as well as is drawn into different activities in the village – from conducting surveys for various departments to undertaking work during election duties, preventing her from focusing on her core responsibilities.

*Coverage*

Universalization of ICDS is the goal but this remains to be achieved in most states. Many existing AWCs currently cover more than 1000 population and reach of ICDS among urban slums and resettlement colonies continues to be patchy. There is limited flexibility at state and district levels for responding to population redistribution and new settlements. Focus has been essentially on increasing number of projects and AWCs with insufficient attention paid to identifying and reaching excluded families (due to geography and caste) even within current coverage areas.

*Infrastructure and human resources*

There are many ICDS projects which report inadequate infrastructure in terms of buildings to house an AWC and equipment such as weighing scales, records and registers. Human resources are also often not as per sanctions. It has been observed that the ICDS Supervisor positions in many states lie vacant for long periods.

*Staff expertise and capacity*

A key reason for inadequate focus and sharpness in ICDS efforts in improving nutritional status and child development outcomes is the absence of adequate technical and managerial expertise at various levels. Most ICDS officials and staff come from general academic backgrounds (and hence there are only a few who have received training in nutrition and child development and related disciplines including management) has been a contributory factor.

Many senior ICDS managers like DPOs and CDPOs think that undernutrition can be overcome by merely "supplementary feeding". This concept has percolated up to the AWW worker level.

*Training*

The ICDS training content and methodology in many cases is not designed in a manner that can help a field functionary to systematically plan for prevention and management of malnutrition in a community. ICDS functionary is not trained to be a good planner and manager of the day to day activities. Village survey is often completed systematically and the data is seldom used as a planning tool. She is therefore often not aware of the number of pregnant mothers and children <6 years in the village. In fact, there is a gap in her understanding of roles and responsibilities for achievement of the objectives. There are no protocols for prevention and treatment of malnutrition in routine ICDS training. However, within the Integrated Management of Neonatal Care Childhood Illnesses (IMNCI), training effort has been made to introduce this concept by health sector in select areas. Training programs provide the same content to all staff, not taking into account capacity and needs. Ongoing training and capacity building through supervisory visits and reviews is inadequate.

As a results of training gaps, the AWWs skills in counseling for growth promotion are found to be sub optimal. The AWW is provided with different IEC materials to support growth promotion and disseminate information on ICDS services, however their use is inadequate for reasons that vary from IEC not being well integrated with the training component to some materials having too much of information. Simple tools and job-aids required to guide day-to-day work are usually missing.

*Supervision*

Several evaluations on ICDS noted supervision as a missing link in the program. Training has not equipped supervisors to guide and mentor AWWs to achieve each of the objectives. Supervisors's role has focused primarily on supply and distribution of supplementary nutrition, attendance of children at AWCs and preschool education. Problem seeking and problem solving approach in supervision is inadequate. Limited mobility of supervisory staff restricts their ability to complete even mandatory field visits. Delayed payments of travel allowance to supervisory staff compounds the issue.

*Monitoring*

ICDS monitoring indicators and system do not track process outcomes critical to impact nutritional status and early childhood education. Due to the pressure of reporting information against various indicators listed in the monitoring format, it is not analyzed at either AWC or project level for program management and decision making. There is no system to check data entry of denominators and numerations and capacity to look at the most critical indicators continues to be weak.

*Linkage with health sector*

Three of the six objectives of ICDS are related to health services. However, linkages with the health system are not at the desirable level. In areas, where NGOs such as CARE or others are working to support the ICDS system, these linkages are found to be effective. Operationalisation of biannual vitamin A strategy has also addressed the issue of defining roles and responsibilities of ICDS and health sectors and linking the two systems effectively for achieving the goal. The health system has not been able to accord priority to some critical nutrition interventions such infant and young child feeding. Sector boundaries of ICDS and health are not co-terminus which often prevents in the formation of joint sector level operational plans and reviews involving AWWs, ANMs and supervisors of Health and ICDS.

*Community engagement*

This is not implemented as envisioned in the program. Mothers' groups and community volunteers have been tried in some contexts but there is insufficient experience and evidence to indicate if there are approaches that will work in different contexts. Role of Panchayati Raj Institutions (PRIs) in implementing and monitoring ICDS is not clearly defined and their involvement has been sporadic. It is important to recognize these limitations to be able to make modifications as the program moves forward.

## 42.7 Contribution of ICDS in improving nutrition and health services and behaviors of children and women: evidence from innovative approaches within ICDS

The recognition of the program limitations has been an ongoing process. State Governments with support from agencies such as the World Bank, UNICEF, CARE and the Micronutrient Initiative, through innovative approaches and program variations, have addressed many of these gap areas (highlighted in Section 42.6) to improve program effectiveness. The potential of ICDS to improve nutritional and health outcomes and thereby nutritional status is well demonstrated through these innovative approaches. Particularly the "what and how" which led to positive shifts in nutrition and health outcomes as described in this Section. Recently, the Micronutrient Initiative conducted a study of "Best Practices in ICDS" for the World Bank with one of the key objectives to inform the ICDS Reforms/ ICDS IV design. Many of the approaches described in this chapter are reflected in that analysis [25].

Successful innovations characterized by operating at reasonable scale covering a minimum of 100,000 population and resulting in positive nutrition services and behaviors including improvement in nutritional status[3] include the Tamil Nadu Integrated Nutrition Project-phase II, Dular, Integrated Nutrition and Health Project-phase II, *Keno Parbo Na, Anchal Se Agan Tak*, Community Based Maternal and Child Health Nutrition (MCHN) Project, ICDS phase-III, and fortification of supplementary food in West Bengal. These innovations have not addressed the preschool education component of the program. There are innovations under the District Primary Education Program to improve early childhood education which are not covered in this chapter.

### 42.7.1 Tamil Nadu Integrated Nutrition Project (TINP-I and II)

The evolution of the Tamil Nadu Integrated Nutrition Project (TINP) supported by the World Bank in 1980 went beyond supplementary feeding and focused on improving home based caring practices, in order to achieve an impact on moderate levels of undernutrition. There was a steady drop in malnutrition rates for all ages included. The mean weight at 6 months and 36 months in 1990 compared to 1982 was 360 grams (6.5% gain in weight) and 650 grams (6.2% gain in weight) heavier, respectively. These differences were significant in all monthly ages between 6 and 36 months. Percentage of children malnourished (-2SD of NCHS) decreased by 10.12 percentage points between 1982 and 1990. Evaluations indicated a decrease in underweight prevalence of about 1.5 percentage points per year in participating districts, twice the rate of non-participating ones [26]. The success of the TINP-I was founded on several factors including: selective feeding, careful focus on supplementing

---

[3] In ICDS Program, Nutritional status is also described as normal, Grades I, II, III and IV malnutrition. ICDS used Indian Academy of Paediatrics (IAP) classification is on the basis of Harvard growth standards where: normal – >80% of standard weight-for-age; Grade 1 – 71–80%; Grade II – 61–70%; Grade III – 51–60% and Grade IV – <50%.

Malnutrition is expressed in standard deviation units (Z-scores) from the median of the reference population in all innovations described in Section 42.4 with the exception of Community Maternal & Child Health & Nutrition Project which uses the IAP classification.

the dietary intake of young children when their growth faltered and until their growth resumed; favourable worker–Supervisor ratios; clear job descriptions; and a well-focused monitoring system.

Based on the experiences of TINP I, TINP-II launched in 1991 was implemented in 318 of the state's 385 rural blocks.

*Objective and implementation approaches*

TINP II modified the strategy to make significant reduction in high prevalence of children suffering from moderate undernutrition, by shifting towards a more preventive focus. Core strategies were regular growth monitoring and promotion, nutrition education and health checks for all children, therapeutic supplementary feeding for moderately and severely underweight children who presented with growth faltering, and high risk pregnant and lactating women. There was more emphasis on training ICDS workers, building supervision and monitoring and creating an efficient management and information system. Information was analyzed and fed back into project implementation. Community participation was enhanced and members were trained to promote growth recording, monthly weighing and spot feeding.

*Results*

The program halved the prevalence of severe malnutrition in villages where it was implemented [27] though it did not fully meet the objective of reducing moderate malnutrition. It was suggested that TINP interventions must include greater focus on home level actions and proactive integration with health systems for better results.

### 42.7.2 Dular

This initiative was undertaken in Bihar in 1999 and in Jharkhand in 2001 in collaboration with UNICEF to complement ICDS and build upon its infrastructure [28].

*Objectives and implementation approaches*

Improving prenatal attendance as well as promoting breastfeeding, colostrum feeding and appropriate complementary feeding practices for decreasing malnutrition were key objectives. One of the major goals of this program was to capitalize and develop community resources at the grassroots level. Dular established a community-based tracking system of the health status of women and of children 0–36 months of age by neighbourhood-based local resource persons (LRPs). Dular's approach seeks to ensure that girls and women of reproductive age have access to adequate nutrition, health care, and information about child care throughout their lives – especially while they are pregnant and nursing their young children. See Box 42.4 on implementation approaches.

**Box 42.4 Implementation strategy of the Dular program**

- Dular trains local resource groups (LRGs), which comprise of local resource persons (LRPs) (approximately one for every 10 to 15 households), who assist the AWWs in providing services to pregnant women and mothers of newborns in their homes.
- Focus is on promoting safe delivery, breastfeeding, immunization, and other essential care practices during pregnancy and early childhood.
- The Dular program is initially introduced to a village through the village contact drive (VCD).
  - This event consists of 2 days of training and advocacy, during which the objectives of the strategy are discussed with the community members and information is gathered regarding local beliefs and practices (for example, one of the most problematic common practices in tribal areas is the so-called hell-fasting, a fasting period for the mother commencing just after giving birth) related to women and children's health.
  - This information is used to plan project activities appropriate to local conditions that are maintained over a consistent period.
- LRPs identified during the village contact drive collectively form a LRG, which meets weekly with the AWW to review program progress.

*Results*

An impact evaluation of 744 women and children in Jharkhand showed that women in Dular villages were 4 times more likely to feed their newborns with colostrum than those in non-Dular villages. There was a significant difference in the proportion of women breastfeeding their infants before giving them other foods and liquids between the Dular and non-Dular villages (adjusted probabilities 41.4% and 17.1%, respectively). Young children in *Dular* areas had 45% lower prevalence of severe malnutrition than those in non-Dular villages.

## 42.7.3 Integrated Nutrition and Health Project (INHP) – Phase II

CARE India implemented a large-scale INHP II in partnership with Ministries of Women and Child Development and the state Health and Family Welfare Departments, local NGOs and Community Based Organizations from October 2001 to September 2006. INHP II was implemented in approximately 95,572 AWCs in 747 ICDS projects across 78 districts in 9 states – Andhra Pradesh (AP), Bihar, Chhattisgarh, Jharkhand, Madhya Pradesh (MP), Orissa, Rajasthan, Uttar Pradesh (UP) and West Bengal.

*Objectives and interventions*

The objectives of this project was to reduce child malnutrition and infant mortality by providing an integrated and comprehensive approach to supporting ICDS and Reproductive and Child Health (RCH) programs of the GoI. INHP supported a subset of national program interventions that effectively reduce child malnutrition, including antenatal care; home-based newborn care; infant and young child feeding; providing vitamin A supplements for children, supplementary nutrition and child immunization. These services reached around 102 million people including pregnant and lactating women and children less than 2 years of age [29].

*Implementers*

ICDS and RCH functionaries and volunteers[4] (in 40% of program areas), were supported by local NGO workers. There was one CARE officer for every 3–4 blocks, supporting and guiding ICDS, RCH and NGO staff on technical/ operational issues.

*Implementation approaches*

See Box 42.5

*Results*

An evaluation research was conducted in 2 intervention districts with controls in the two of the nine CARE supported states i.e. states of AP and UP to provide diverse socio-demographic contexts to assess "net impact" of the interventions package. Results from this research are presented in Table 42.2. There were improvements in early initiation of breast feeding, exclusive breastfeeding, timely introduction, quantity, quality and frequency of complementary feeding, responsive feeding, coverage with vitamin A and IFA supplements and contacts by service providers during the critical life cycle periods.

There was marked improvement in UP as compared to AP. While the program did not reduce underweight and stunting in the study populations, in UP, the intervention clearly had an effect on wasting. INHP interventions

---

4 Volunteers are active, interested members of their communities, who serve as promoters and monitors of nutrition and health practices and are called Change Agents. Each change agent accepts responsibility for reaching 15-20 families in his/her neighborhood on a voluntary basis. Each anganwadi center has 5-6 such change agents who act as a link between families and service providers in facilitating change and promoting local problem solving.

**Box 42.5 Implementation approaches in INHP-II**

It was recognized that malnutrition was near universal and increased between the 6 and 18 months period and only less than 10% infants in this age group were eating even half the recommended quantities of complementary foods in most states. This led to the development and adoption of an Essential Nutrition Action Framework which included guidance on how to deliver these actions at district, block, sector and village levels; a 3-step counseling guide and age specific feeding recommendations.

Critical elements of the overall INHP II implementation approach included:

- Mechanism to minimize exclusion (social map to include all eligibles, modified registers for tracking of services and behaviors).
- Home visits by AWW, volunteers and ANM during the critical period of pregnancy till the child is at least 2 years of age, more between 6 and 11 months to help establish adequate complementary feeding including use of simple tools, e.g. home visit planner to help prioritize these visits and their content (simple calculations showed that this could be accomplished with about 1-2 home visits on a working day by an AWW and the role of the ANM was to reinforce messages during her visits and/or immunization sessions).
- Strengthen fixed day/fixed site services where AWW and ANM deliver a package of nutrition and health services. This included immunization, antenatal care, distribution of Vitamin A and IFA, nutrition and health education and supplementary nutrition as Take Home Rations (THR) at the AWC and was referred to as Nutrition and Health Day.
- Strengthened supervisory processes and tools for focused implementation particularly, supervisory checklist, sector meeting checklist which provided guidance on content and processes to be monitored.
- District and block level planning and joint reviews conducted with participation from ICDS, Health and PRI.
- Ongoing capacity building on critical interventions and tasks to achieve the desired outcomes and impact.
- Use of data locally and efforts for Behaviour Change Communication (print and folk media in addition to interpersonal communication) and community mobilization.

protected against wasting among the following groups – all children, boys, infants 0–5 and 6–11 months. Anemia levels decreased slightly (from 88.6% to 86.7%) in intervention areas in UP while in control areas anemia increased (83.1% to 87.4%; $p < 0.05$) suggesting a protective effect of the intervention [30].

In addition, a program-wide evaluation across 8 states showed an eight percentage point reduction in underweight in children 12–23 months of age from 61% to 53 % over a period of 5 years.

## 42.7.4 Keno Parbo Na

Building on the ICDS infrastructure, an innovative initiative based on Positive Deviance (PD) approach was initiated in 2001 in a phased manner, with UNICEF support, in 4 districts including South 24 Paraganas, Dakshin Dinajpur, Murshidabad and Purulia of West Bengal.

*Table 42.2* Changes in selected infant and young child feeding behaviours, Nutrition Evaluation Research in CARE's Integrated Nutrition and Health Project - II

| ***Breastfeeding behaviours (0–5 months old)*** | Intervention (Karimnagar, AP) | | | Comparison (Rangareddy, AP) | | | Diffe-rence of Change | Intervention (Barabanki, UP) | | | Comparison (Unnao, UP) | | | Diffe-rence of change |
|---|---|---|---|---|---|---|---|---|---|---|---|---|---|---|
| | Baseline | Endline | Change | Baseline | Endline | Change | | Baseline | Endline | Change | Baseline | Endline | Change | |
| **Breastfeeding initiated 1 hour after delivery** | | | | | | | | | | | | | | |
| n[1] | 614 | 545 | | 591 | 610 | | | 789 | 741 | | 711 | 658 | | |
| % | 22.3 | 36.5 | **14.2** | 16.9 | 18.9 | **2.0** | **12.2**[1] | 4.6 | 59.0 | **54.4** | 2.1 | 10.5 | **8.4** | **46.0**[1] |
| **Prelacteal feeds** | | | | | | | | | | | | | | |
| n[1] | 614 | 545 | | 591 | 611 | | | 789 | 750 | | 711 | 661 | | |
| % | 61.7 | 49.2 | **–12.5** | 69.0 | 67.6 | **–1.4** | **–11.1**[1] | 91.8 | 44.4 | **47.4** | 96.1 | 93.2 | **–2.9** | **–44.5**[1] |
| **Exclusive breastfeeding** | | | | | | | | | | | | | | |
| n[1] | 614 | 549 | | 591 | 616 | | | 789 | 758 | | 712 | 679 | | |
| % | 77.0 | 70.7 | **–6.3** | 86.8 | 77.0 | **9.8** | **3.5** | 63.5 | 78.5 | **15.0** | 62.8 | 70.7 | **7.9** | **7.1**[1] |

***Complementary feeding Behaviours (6–23 months old)***

| | Intervention (Karimnagar, AP) | | | Comparison (Rangareddy, AP) | | | Diffe-rence of Change | Intervention (Barabanki, UP) | | | Comparison (Unnao, UP) | | | Diffe-rence of change |
|---|---|---|---|---|---|---|---|---|---|---|---|---|---|---|
| | Baseline | Endline | Change | Baseline | Endline | Change | | Baseline | Endline | Change | Baseline | Endline | Change | |
| **Introduction of solids at 6–8 months** | | | | | | | | | | | | | | |
| n[1] | 1746 | 2012 | | 1831 | 2034 | | | 1643 | 1650 | | 1666 | 1624 | | |
| % | 30.4 | 49.5 | **19.1** | 24.6 | 35.7 | **11.1** | **8.0**[1] | 22.1 | 52.8 | **30.7** | 26.8 | 56.5 | **29.7** | **1.0** |
| **Recommended complementary feeding frequency amongst breastfed children** | | | | | | | | | | | | | | |
| n[2] | 1620 | 1893 | | 1702 | 1901 | | | 1447 | 1476 | | 1445 | 1473 | | |
| 6–3 months (2–times/day) | 34.5 | 56.1 | **21.6** | 11.4 | 35.5 | **24.1** | **–3.5** | 2.3 | 25.4 | **23.1** | 3.2 | 18.2 | **15.0** | **8.1**[1] |
| 9–11 months | | | | | | | | | | | | | | |

| | | | | | | | | | | | | | | |
|---|---|---|---|---|---|---|---|---|---|---|---|---|---|---|
| (3 + times/day) | 12.9 | 28.3 | **15.4** | 7.6 | 17.3 | **9.7** | **5.7** | 3.1 | 23.9 | **20.8** | 4.6 | 11.3 | **6.7** | **14.1**[1] |
| 12–23months | | | | | | | | | | | | | | |
| (3 + times/day) | 15.5 | 42.4 | **26.9** | 9.6 | 40.9 | **31.3** | **–4.4** | 8.8 | 37.8 | **29.0** | 15.9 | 31.3 | **15.4** | **13.6**[1] |
| **Consumption of at least half the recommended quantity of solids** | | | | | | | | | | | | | | |
| $n^2$ | 1746 | 2012 | | 1831 | 2034 | | | 1643 | 1650 | | 1666 | 1624 | | |
| 6–8 months | | | | | | | | | | | | | | |
| (100+ g) | 26.7 | 43.2 | **16.5** | 16.0 | 27.6 | **11.6** | **4.9** | 1.0 | 6.0 | **5.0** | 0.8 | 1.3 | **0.5** | **4.5**[1] |
| 9–11 months | | | | | | | | | | | | | | |
| (150+ g) | 18.0 | 36.6 | **18.6** | 8.3 | 23.2 | **13.9** | **4.7** | 0.5 | 6.0 | **5.5** | 2.4 | 1.0 | **–1.4** | **6.9**[1] |
| 12–23months | | | | | | | | | | | | | | |
| (200+ g) | 20.1 | 44.8 | **24.7** | 10.3 | 35.7 | **25.4** | **0.7** | 1.5 | 6.9 | **5.4** | 2.1 | 3.2 | **1.1** | **4.3**[1] |
| **Consumption of 3 or more food groups in the past 24 hours** | | | | | | | | | | | | | | |
| $n^2$ | 1746 | 2012 | | 1831 | 2034 | | | 1643 | 1650 | | 1666 | 1624 | | |
| 6–8 months | 5.1 | 8.2 | **3.1** | 0.8 | 3.9 | **3.1** | **0.0** | 2.4 | 22.4 | **20.0** | 2.8 | 10.9 | **8.1** | **11.9**[1] |
| 9–11 months | 8.2 | 14.7 | **6.5** | 2.9 | 6.6 | **3.7** | **2.8** | 9.4 | 39.2 | **29.8** | 14.4 | 32.9 | **18.5** | **11.3**[1] |
| 12–23months | 15.0 | 22.1 | **7.1** | 4.6 | 16.3 | **11.7** | **–4.6**[1] | 25.6 | 53.4 | **27.8** | 31.1 | 43.7 | **12.6** | **15.2**[1] |
| **Fed from a separate plate** | | | | | | | | | | | | | | |
| $n^2$ | 1746 | 2012 | | 1831 | 2034 | | | 1643 | 1650 | | 1666 | 1624 | | |
| 6–8 months | 61.1 | 67.6 | **6.5** | 38.2 | 52.2 | **14.0** | **–7.5**[1] | 5.1 | 41.2 | **36.1** | 7.4 | 21.8 | **14.4** | **21.7**[1] |
| 9–11 months | 75.5 | 81.9 | **6.4** | 63.0 | 69.9 | **6.9** | **–0.5** | 19.8 | 44.7 | **24.9** | 19.2 | 26.7 | **7.5** | **17.4**[1] |
| 12–23months | 77.8 | 81.4 | **3.6** | 70.4 | 74.4 | **4.0** | **–0.4** | 37.0 | 57.8 | **20.8** | 45.4 | 49.9 | **4.5** | **16.3**[1] |

$n^1$ = Total no. of children 0–5 months; $n^2$ = Total no. of children 6–23 months; [1]Significant at 95% confidence level]

*Objectives and implementation approaches*

The objective was to reduce and prevent malnutrition among children under 3 years, by focusing on local solutions, resources and practices [31]. This included training of childcare workers; weighing children and determining their nutritional status; identifying pockets of high malnutrition; having discussions/brainstorming sessions to identify best care practices in the community; motivating families to adopt them through participatory learning during Nutritional Counseling and Child Care Sessions. See Box 42.6 for key elements of the strategy.

**Box 42.6 Keno Parbo Na - key elements of the program strategy**

- Community mobilisation around the Positive Deviance Approach through participatory processes, which involve the formation of village committees and pro-active dialogues between social groups and institutions, using cultural methods such as village picnics, fairs, etc.
- Convergence and partnership between the service providers, administration and NGOs involved in implementation.
- Capacity building of childcare functionaries and the community using the "triple A" approach through regular review of activities.
- Community based management of malnutrition through Nutritional Counselling and Care Sessions (NCCS), emphasizing positive behavioral changes in childcare practices (12 days of spot feeding and 18 days of Take Home Rations for children in grades II, III and IV children)
- Hands-on training of mothers or caregivers over a 12 day period, on infant feeding like exclusive breast feeding, complementary feeding, healthcare, hygiene, and psycho-social care practices followed by practice sessions at home for a further 18 days. The cycle extends over 6-9 months within which period mothers/caregivers start showing behaviour change.
- There is also emphasis on vitamin A supplementation, hand washing practices, diarrhoea management, prevention of low birth weight (LBW), early registration of pregnancy, and antenatal care.
- Action-oriented, realistic and time-bound indicators.

*Results*

An evaluation utilizing a case control design showed a positive effect on key behaviors and services particularly exclusive breastfeeding, timely initiation and frequency of complementary foods and Vitamin A coverage (Table 42.2). Higher percentage of mothers in PD area (69%) received health and nutrition education by AWW mostly at AWCs compared to 27% in control areas. The prevalence of underweight and stunting (45.6% and 25.2%, respectively) was significantly ($p<0.01$) lower in the PD area compared to control area (63.2% and 37.4%, respectively) in children aged 12–17 months. No gender differentials were observed in underweight or wasting between both groups, though prevalence of stunting reduced significantly among girls in the PD area compared to the control area.

## 42.7.5 Anchal Se Agan Tak (ASAT)

### *Objective and implementation approaches*

A comprehensive strategy to prevent and treat malnutrition was implemented in Rajasthan in 2005 [32]. Enhanced ICDS structures in terms of capacities to deliver quality services and community support at various levels were developed. At the village level, community volunteers called the *Gram Sampark Samooh* interfaced with families and systems to generate demand for services.

*Table 42.3* Key outcome indicators under the Positive Deviance project in West Bengal

| Indicators | Positive Deviance areas | Non-Positive Deviance areas |
|---|---|---|
| *Breastfeeding practices* | | |
| Percentage distribution of mothers of <12 months children according to breastfeeding practices | | |
| Time of initiation of breastfeeding <3 hours | 76.4 | 44.1** |
| Pre-lacteal feeds given | | |
| Percentage distribution of children of <12 months according to breastfeeding practices by current age | 22.1 | 65.4** |
| 4–5 months – solely breast fed | 69.7 | 61.3* |
| *Complementary feeding practices* | | |
| Percentage distribution of mothers of 12–23 month children by feeding practices | | |
| Age of initiation of complementary feeding in months | | |
| 6 | 44.0 | 28.8** |
| ≥7 | 40.5 | 50.2* |
| Frequency of other complementary feeds/day | | |
| 2–3 | 21.1 | 60.8** |
| 4–5 | 52.1 | 32.9** |
| ≥6 | 26.8 | 6.3** |
| *Immunization and vitamin A coverage* | | |
| Percentage distribution of children (12–23 months) completely immunized | 85.9 | 68.2** |
| Percentage distribution of children (18–35 months) who received massive dose of vitamin A supplementation | | |
| One dose | 34.2 | 40.7* |
| Two doses | 50.2 | 33.0** |

Positive deviance (intervention areas); Non-Positive Deviance (control areas).
*p<0.05, **p<0.01

A block support team was established in project blocks to assist staff at block and village level to implement the program. In project districts, a District Mobile Monitoring Training Team was constituted to monitor progress and provide on-the-job guidance to the village team. A District Support Team was constituted to improve coordination between sectors, review overall progress, and ensure effective implementation across the district. In addition, a state-level training and monitoring unit was formed. The program focused on household counseling, having a Maternal and Child Health and Nutrition (MCHN) Day, and a fixed Weighing and Counseling Day which was organised a week prior to the MCHN Day.

- Household counselling on various issues related to health and nutrition.
- *Maternal and Child Health and Nutrition (MCHN) Day*: A state-wide monthly fixed day event. It focused on immunization, vitamin A supplementation (twice a year), weighing of pregnant women, provision of IFA tablets to pregnant women and adolescent girls, salt testing and counselling on maternal and child issues. It was held at the AWC and was facilitated by the ANM and AWW with assistance from the *Sahyogini* (village volunteer) and the *anganwadi* helper.
- *Fixed Weighing and Counselling Day*: A state-wide initiative (initiated in February 2006) on a fixed day one week prior to the MCHN Day. All children in the village less than six years of age were weighed. The AWW and *Sahyogini* facilitate the process.
- Special Plan of Action (SPOA) initiated in 2005 in 14 blocks. The goal of SPOA was to manage child malnutrition through support of ICDS by training ICDS functionaries, adopting WHO standard protocols, strengthening referral services and counselling families. The strategy focused efforts on interventions and capacity building at the 3 levels: family, community and district hospitals.
- Training tools and modules were developed to train all functionaries in systematic training sessions.

*Results*

A survey utilizing a case control design was undertaken in 2006 to assess program impact. A higher percentage of women fed the newborn colostrum (47%) in ASAT project areas compared to control areas (18%). Weighing efficiency, exclusive breast feeding rates, timely initiation of complementary feeding were higher in ASAT areas compared to control areas. Diarrhoea episodes were less frequent in ASAT areas compared to control areas. There was more contact of the mothers with AWW and community volunteers in ASAT areas (59.7%) compared to control areas

(46.8%). There was marginal difference in prevalence of underweight in ASAT areas (50%) compared to control areas (56%). However, stunting was significantly higher in control areas in comparison to the ASAT group (45% compared to 35% in control areas; $p<0.01$). Factors contributing to success of ASAT include counseling focused on nutrition and health interventions, training and skill building of functionaries to prevent and treat malnutrition and enhanced ICDS structures, e.g. block and district teams.

### 42.7.6 Community-based Maternal and Child Health Nutrition Project (MCHN Project)

This 4-year project (2001–2005) was implemented in 8 blocks of 4 districts in Uttar Pradesh covering a population of 1.33 million in collaboration with UNICEF (Jhansi, Allahabad, Agra, Varanasi, 2 blocks per district). It was based on a multisectoral approach involving Health and ICDS as also Panchayati Raj Institution (PRI) for water and sanitation. The Departments of Social and Preventive Medicine of the Medical colleges provided coordination and technical support [33].

*Objectives*

The aim was to reduce underweight in children less than 2 years by 20%; improve coverage of children with vitamin A supplementation to 80%; ensure 60% women consume minimum 100 IFA tablets and 100% households use iodized salt. The target group referred to as "at risk families" comprised families with children below 2 years, pregnant, lactating women and newly weds and children below 6 years with severe malnutrition.

*Implementation approaches*

See Box 42.7.

*Results*

A baseline survey was undertaken in 2000 and an endline in 2005. There was a positive shift in behaviors and services. The practice of initiating breastfeeding within an hour of birth increased 5-fold (baseline 4.6%; endline 21.9%); percentage of infants introduced to semi-solid food between 6 and 9 months increased from 18% in baseline to 63% in endline; women receiving more than 90 IFA tablets during index pregnancy increased from 6% to 61% and consumption increased from 9% to 22%. For health, nutrition, water, hygiene and sanitation education as well as

## Box 42.7 Implementation approaches in Community-based Maternal and Child Health Nutrition (MCHN) Project

*Block officers*

- Two block level officers, designated as Block Trainer cum Monitor (BTMs), were appointed in each block for overseeing the overall implementation of project in their respective blocks.
- They, along with ANM and AWW were involved in identifying community based volunteers; providing support in organising and conducting pre-service and in-service training of a team of trainees comprising community volunteers, health worker (ANM) and ICDS worker (AWW) as well as in organizing quarterly monitoring meetings at the health sub-centre level (comprising 5–7 villages).

*Community volunteers*

- Community volunteers, referred as Community Health Nutrition Sanitation Mobilisers (CHNSMs) or in local language Bal Parivar Mitra (BPMS) meaning "friend of families with young children" were selected and assigned the tasks of reaching the "at risk families" at least once a fortnight.
- For the selection of the community volunteers, a social map of each village was prepared by ICDS workers with the help of BTMs and the community members.
- Three to five primary community clusters were identified on the basis of religion, caste or creed in a village with 1000–1500 population. In each village, effort was made to have a volunteer or a BPM selected from each of the clusters jointly by the ICDS and health frontline workers with the help of BTM and participation of community members.
- Volunteers with positive attitude on influencing social issues pertaining to women and children and who were vocal, dynamic and respected were selected.
- Each BPM was responsible for a cluster of 50–60 households but was expected to be working at a time with identified 15–20 "at risk families" in the cluster.
- The primary responsibility of these volunteers was to visit homes of identified families and counsel them on adoption of appropriate maternal and child care and feeding practices such as promotion of early initiation of breastfeeding, exclusive breastfeeding with emphasis on "no water" for first six months, complementary feeding, increasing food and rest during pregnancy, following appropriate hygiene and sanitation care, use of safe source of drinking water, use of iodised salt. The latter included salt and water testing.
  - Right advice at the right time to the right recipient or family was the principle applied in the interpersonal counseling sessions to be organized by BPMs with the selected risk family. These community volunteers were also responsible for undertaking monitoring and for maintaining records of actions taken.
  - Community volunteers were also in-charge of informing the "at risk families" of the importance of reproductive and child health and nutrition services such as antenatal care, routine immunization to children and vitamin A supplement administration. BPMs also mobilized the "at risk families" to avail of these services which were provided free of charge by frontline workers of primary health care centre and the ICDS.
- For rehabilitation of severely malnourished, special attention was directed at rapid screening by observation and follow up of severely malnourished children by BPMs. The volunteers were trained to screen severely malnourished children.
- Imparting training to BPMs was the most critical component of the project implementation since they were the primary persons reaching the "at risk families". Considering low levels of literacy of BPMs, a three-day intensive and easy to understand case-study based training was imparted. Focus was on development of skills for counseling, screening of severely malnourished

by observation and linking with service providers. In-service training continued during monitoring sessions.

- BPMs were given no monetary compensation but social recognition such as a badge to wear, a large name plate to be put on the doors of their house, a cloth bag for carrying monitoring forms and training manual as well as a certificate following completion of training.

Factors that contributed to the success of MCHN:

- Emphasis on under 2 years and "at risk families".
- Emphasis on correct advice to selected "risk families".
- Community mobilisers were incharge of only 15–20 "risk families"
- Supplies of IFA tablets and ORS ensured
- Trainings completed using pictorial monitoring card with emphasis on life cycle approach
- Monitoring by community mobilisers using pictorial cards
- A system to link with health established
- Technical core group established
- Project facilitator positioned at block levels and district levels

nutritional health services, Community Volunteers referred as *Bal Parivar Mitras* (BPMs) were the main contact points for counselling "at risk" families, followed by ANM and AWW. There was no emphasis on growth monitoring and promotion but on "right advice at right time to right receipient". There was considerable decline in percentage of severely malnourished children (baseline: 25%; endline: 14%) as per IAP classification and percentage of children with normal nutritional status improved marginally from 25% to 28%.

## 42.7.7 ICDS Phase III

Phase III of the World Bank assisted ICDS, originally in five states viz. Kerala, Uttar Pradesh, Rajasthan, Maharashtra and Tamil Nadu was expanded to six additional states of Madhya Pradesh, Bihar, Chhattisgarh, Jharkhand, Orissa and Uttaranchal in 2003. It also strengthened the ICDS program in all 35 states/union territories, by improving quality of training of ICDS functionaries through project Udisha [34].

### *Objectives and approaches*

The project aimed at accelerating improvement of nutrition status of children 0–6 years and women. It provided additional inputs over and above inputs admissible in the ICDS Scheme, viz. construction of civil works, hardware inputs for better service delivery (adult weighing scales, display boards, outdoor play materials), quality improvement (study tours, Free Expression for Quality Improvement (FREQI)[5], training for IEC etc) and

[5] Formation of quality circles to encourage better interaction among AWWs so that they could exchange notes freely, bring them to the notice of the supervisory staff and with their support achieve higher quality of service delivery.

monitoring and evaluation activities (development of computerized Monitoring Information Systems (MIS), social assessment, operational research studies, baseline/endline surveys). There was emphasis on introducing an Adolescent Girls Scheme to address the life cycle issue of malnutrition.

*Results*

Pre-post evaluation (baseline in 2000, endline in 2006) was conducted in five states. Percentage of children under 3 years who were breastfed within 2 hours of birth increased from 37% during baseline to 51% in endline. Only 21% children under 6 months were reported to have been exclusively breastfed which declined from 28% in baseline. Percentage of children 6–9 months receiving solid or semi-solid food and breast milk increased from 38% to 64% and percentage of children between 6 and 36 months who consumed vitamin A rich food increased from 53% to 71%.

There was significant improvement in services related to antenatal care of pregnant women, immunization, de-worming and treatment of diarrhoea. Impact of IEC and training led to increased awareness of infant feeding practices among AWWs though knowledge transfer from AWWs to women remained a cause of concern. Overall, underweight significantly decreased from 44.5% to 36%. Malnutrition rates decreased in each state: Kerala 11.1% to 3.5%; Maharashtra 51.8% to 42.6%; Rajasthan 43% to 35.4%; Tamil Nadu 50.9% to 39.5%; and UP 58.1% to 44.7%.

### 42.7.8 Fortification of supplementary food in West Bengal

In 2005, the Department of Women and Child Development in West Bengal with support from the Micronutrient Initiative supported the fortification of the supplementary food (comprising *khichdi*, a rice and dal mixture) with a premix called *vitashakti*[6] containing iron, vitamin A and folic acid. The key objective of this approach was of increasing iron and vitamin A stores and decreasing the prevalence of iron deficiency, anemia, and vitamin A deficiency. Introduced in the South 24 Parganas district, this approach has now been up-scaled to the entire state by the Government of Bengal.

*Implementation*

The premix is added to the cooked food (*khichdi*) by a spoon measuring 1.25 grams for 5 beneficiaries. The premix is initially mixed with water

[6] 14 mg microencapsulated ferrous fumerate, vitamin A 500 IU, folic acid 0.05 mg per 0.25 g serving.

and then added to the cooked food after it is removed from fire. The premix cost for each beneficiary is only Rs. 0.03/per day. Half-kg packets in a plastic container are provided to the AWCs and each packet can cater to 2000 beneficiaries. It is given to children from the age of 3 to 6 years, pregnant and lactating women.

*Results*

A cluster, randomized, double-blind, controlled trial was undertaken in 30 AWCs in the South 24 Parganas district [35]. Children in the age group of 36–66 months were randomly assigned to receive either a fortified or a non-fortified *khichdi* for a period of 24 weeks. Hemoglobin, serum ferritin, and serum retinol were measured. Prevalence of anemia decreased from 19.1% to 4.1%; mean serum ferritin levels showed a marked increase from 25.1 to 35.5 μg/l and prevalence of iron deficiency anemia showed a decrease from 4.9 to 0.4%. There were no significant differences in serum retinol concentrations or in the prevalence of vitamin A deficiency between the fortified- and non-fortified-khichdi groups. Overall, the prevalence rates of anemia, iron deficiency and iron deficiency anemia were significantly lower in the fortified group compared to the non-fortified group. This demonstrated that fortifying supplementary food can be effective at increasing iron stores and reducing the prevalence of iron deficiency and anemia at the community level. This assumes great importance in a country where about 70% children aged, 6–59 months and 55.3 % of women in the age group of 15–49 years, are suffering from anemia [1].

Common elements cutting across these projects contributing to positive outcomes were focused on:

- Critical age group of 0–3 years for achieving nutritional impact;
- Evidence based interventions;
- Strengthened capacity and structures at all levels in terms program content and operational "know-how";
- Supportive supervision (supervisors guiding and problem solving, use of checklists and frameworks);
- Implementation approaches (home visits during critical periods of the life cycle; allocation of Nutrition and Health days for service improvement); and
- Outcome-based monitoring system to track most critical behaviors and services.

Evidence described in this section clearly indicated that with renewed focus and strengthened capacity, the ICDS program can effectively deliver nutrition and health services.

## 42.8 Moving forward: revisit and refine key strategies

ICDS is one of the largest programs for child development not just in India but in the Asian sub-continent. Contributions that the program has made in improving nutrition and health outcomes in children and women have been discussed in Section 42.7. As ICDS moves towards universalization, it is critical that it revisits its design and implementation strategies by incorporating lessons learned from various innovation effects. Refinements around specific components are essential to achieve higher impact on nutritional status of children.

### 42.8.1 Recommendations

*Define objectives and interventions*

ICDS must clearly state which objectives will it hold itself accountable for. Currently it has a diverse mandate, from early childhood development, reducing child malnutrition, mortality, morbidity; improving adolescent health and nutrition to women's empowerment. These overlap with objectives of other government departments.

*Expand coverage*

Allocate resources needed to ensure that population norms are followed for establishing AWCs. There should be one AWC for 1,000 population with provision for increase. They should take into account special groups and areas (migrants, slums in small towns and isolated hamlets).

*Focus on younger children for nutrition impact*

The program should improve nutrition outcomes for under-3s particularly under-2s and strengthen the early childhood education component for 3–6 year olds.

*Prioritize "doable" evidence-based interventions*

Nutrition impact can be achieved through a package of "doable" interventions which includes early and exclusive breastfeeding, age appropriate complementary feeding including initiation at 6 months, age specific frequencies and quantities for children 6–24 months old, responsive feeding and feeding during and after illness, vitamin A supplementation, pediatric IFA supplementation beginning 6 months or home-based fortification to address iron deficiency anemia, use of iodized salt, zinc as adjuvant to oral rehydration salts in treatment of diarrhoea and linkages with health facilities for treatment of infections.

*Focus on effective operational approaches*

Ensure home visits with "appropriate content" to households at critical periods of the life cycle – on registration of marriage and pregnancy, newborn and infants on first day, first week, 6–8 months, 9–11 months and 12–18 months including contacts during and after sickness on a priority basis. Behavior Change Communication (BCC) support through interpersonal communication, and social mobilisation through print and mass media for transmitting key messages, at an optimal frequency to saturate the system is critical.

*Develop simple protocols for prevention/management of malnutrition*

Based on various innovative approaches supported by CARE, UNICEF, and the World Bank, essential nutrition action package (see Box 42.8 for age-specific feeding recommendations) [36] needs to be developed and adapted for use by the AWWs. AWWs need be accorded status of "community nutrition professionals".

While treatment of severe malnutrition is important, equally critical is that it is complemented with intensive program efforts on prevention of malnutrition. Mortality risk is highest in severely malnourished children, but at the same time it must be appreciated that the number of total children who are at risk of death in mild to moderate malnutrition is several times higher than in normally nourished. The prevention strategy must be centered around reducing incidence of low birth weight and not allowing the near 70% of children who are normal in early infancy to become undernourished by focusing on children <2 years and promoting and ensuring appropriate behaviors and services.

*Institutionalize a system for linkage with health system*

Roles and responsibilities of ICDS functionaries and management staff must be spelt out clearly with reference to immunisation, antenatal care, management of severe malnutrition and, micronutrient supplements. ICDS needs to play a significant role in undertaking the routine biannual survey, identifying all newborns, children <2 years and pregnant mothers. In addition, ICDS could play a significant role in mobilising community to seek health services and referrals. A system to bring the two sectors (ICDS and Health) for working as a team for achieving nutrition and health outcomes is critical.

*Training*

Create strong linkages between training and implementation. Build capacity to focus on how to achieve specific program objectives. While training

**Box 42.8 Age-specific feeding recommendations**

| Pregnancy | Up to 6 months of age | 6 to 8 months | 9 to 11 months | 12 months to 2 years |
|---|---|---|---|---|
| • Eat one additional meal<br>• Eat different types of food available in the house (meat, fish, eggs, milk, curd; fruits and vegetables; *dal* and cereals with added oil)<br>• Eat food received from the AWC<br>• Eat at least one IFA tablets daily for 100 days<br>• Rest for 1 to 2 hours during the day | *For child*<br>• Breastfeed within 1 hour of birth<br>• Only breastfeed; do not give water, other fluids, honey water, *ghutti,* or food<br>• Breastfeed frequently on-demand day and night<br>• For a newborn who does not feed vigorously; provide expressed breast milk with a clean small *katori* or cup as long as breastfeeding is not adequately vigorous<br>• Provide frequent feeding for a small newborn every 1–2 hours<br>• Contact the AWW/ANM immediately if your infant is not able to breastfeed | • Continue frequent, on-demand breastfeeding, day and night<br>• Introduce home foods by feeding little at a time 1–2 teaspoons to gradually increasing the quantity and consistency after a first few days<br>• Feed soft mashed or thick, pasty home foods 1 small *katori* at 2 times per day such as mixed rice and *dal, khichri*, *dalia*, rice *kheer*, *suji kheer*. Add 1/4 to 1/2 teaspoon of oil in each meal<br>• In addition give small potato/mashed banana/carrot/papaya/egg/meat/fish<br>• Feed child yourself, interact with child, feed from a separate bowl to assess how much the child has | • Continue frequent, on-demand breastfeeding, day and night.<br>• Feed soft mashed or thick, pasty home foods 1 small *katori* 3 times a day such as rice, *dal*, mashed *chapati* in *dal* with vegetables (potatoes, carrots, pumpkin, etc.), green leafy vegetables. Add 1/2 teaspoon of oil in each meal. Give curd, eggs, meat, fish, if available.<br>• In addition give seasonal fruits such as papaya, mango, banana, etc.<br>• Feed child yourself, interact with child, feed from a separate bowl to assess how much the child has eaten. Do not force feed, but use gentle | • Continue frequent, on-demand breastfeeding, day and night.<br>• Feed soft mashed or in small pieces home foods equal to 1 small *katori* 4 times per day such as rice, *dal, chapatti,* with vegetables (potatoes, carrots, pumpkin, etc.), green leafy vegetables. Add 1 to 2 teaspoon of oil in each meal. Give curd, eggs, meat, fish, if available.<br>• In addition give seasonal fruits such as papaya, mango, banana, etc.<br>• Feed child yourself, interact with child, feed from a separate bowl to assess how much the child has eaten. Do not force feed, but use gentle |

| | | | | |
|---|---|---|---|---|
| | • Increase frequency of breastfeeding during and after illness<br>• The infant should gain about 700 g per month<br>• Mother and baby undergo changes at around 3 months but continue giving only breastmilk<br>*For mother*<br>• Eat one additional meal<br>• Eat different types of food available in the house<br>• Eat food received from the AWC<br>• Avoid separation from your infant for more than 2–3 hours at a time | eaten. Do not force feed, but use gentle persuasion, with stories, songs and toys to keep the baby's attention.<br>• Increase frequency of breastfeeding during illness<br>• After illness, feed child 1 small *katori* of food 3 times until the child regains weight; encourage the child to eat more<br>• The infant should gain about 500 g per month | persuasion, with stories, songs and toys to keep the baby's attention.<br>• Increase frequency of breastfeeding during illness<br>• After illness, feed child 1 small *katori* of food 4 times until the child regains weight; encourage the child to eat more<br>• Seek first dose of Vitamin A (1 lakh IU) at 9 months with measles vaccination<br>• The child should gain about 300 g per month | persuasion, with stories, songs and toys to keep the baby's attention<br>• Increase frequency of breastfeeding during illness<br>• After illness, feed child 1 small *katori* of food 5 times until the child regains weight; encourage the child to eat more<br>• Seek second dose of Vitamin A (2 lakh IU) at 18 months and third dose at 24 months<br>• Give pediatric iron tablets (one tablet daily, crushed with food for 100 days each year)**<br>• The child should gain about 200 g per month |

For katori size we can assume an average size of 100 ml. However, katori sizes are not uniform. Health workers should estimate volumes of locally used utensils.

(Adapted from material developed by WHO, UNICEF, CARE would facilitate in appreciating each others role and in achieving the objectives.)

centers continue to undertake induction training, bulk training to be on-the-job by supervisors and CDPOs who are responsible for delivering results. Joint training with health sector for achieving specific objectives has proved to be effective.

*Strengthening supervision*

This should be a priority. Provide flexibility in appointments of supervisors to minimize vacancies and ensure mobility and village level support to the AWW. Holding supervisors responsible for specific results, ensuring intensive training of supervisors, and recognizing good performance will bring better results.

*Monitoring system and related capacities*

Revisit monitoring system of the ICDS and evolve it around tracking program outcomes. Institute periodic independent assessments for outcomes such as for feeding, caring (exclusive breastfeeding and appropriate complementary feeding), health-seeking behaviors and nutritional status. Use data generated by this system for program management and decision making at different levels. Provide support to the AWW to generate and use information locally, with tools like the home visits planner. Enhance capacities to gather, analyze, interpret and use data at block and district levels by CDPOs and DPOs. Joint review of data with health sector is considered critical for achieving the nutrition and health objectives.

*Community engagement*

Explore and build concrete mechanisms to engage civil society and communities. Involve local government (PRI) representatives in review forums of ICDS at block and district levels and build accountability mechanisms for AWWs and Supervisors to PRI members for delivery of services, availability of supplies, home visits and supervisory visits. Form people's committees for management of AWC functions.

Some of these recommendations are being integrated in ICDS Reforms which are underway. The five-year ICDS-IV Project, referred earlier, is planned to be implemented in 8 states with support from the World Bank. Objectives of the project are to reduce child malnutrition through expansion of utilization of nutrition services and awareness and adoption of appropriate feeding and caring behaviors by households of children 0–6 years of age; and improve early child development outcomes and school readiness among children 3–6 years of age [14].

Key reform principles proposed in the ICDS Reforms/ICDS-IV project include better targeting, flexibility in terms of management and program implementation with focus on maintaining quality in service delivery, simplified, evidence and outcome-based program design, stronger convergence at the operational level and strong monitoring and evaluation with focus on an outcome-based results framework.

In a country where high levels of malnutrition persist, utilizing ICDS program platform effectively to address the serious public health problem of malnutrition is critical. In every village, under the ICDS umberalla, delivery of appropriate evidence-based interventions through effective mechanisms by the AWWs with support from ANMs and ASHAs (Accredited Social Health Activists) of the National Rural Health Mission, and members of community groups will prevent a large majority of children from becoming malnourished.

## References


1. INTERNATIONAL INSTITUTE FOR POPULATION SCIENCES (IIPS) and ORC MACRO (2000). National Family Health Survey (NFHS-2). India. Mumbai: IIPS. 1998–99.
2. INTERNATIONAL INSTITUTE FOR POPULATION SCIENCES (IIPS) and MACRO INTERNATIONAL (2007). *National Family Health Survey (NFHS-3).* India, Volume 1, Mumbai: IIPS. 2005–06.
3. Integrated Child Development Services program website. Available at: http://wcd.nic.in/icds.htm. Accessed 10 October 2008.
4. INTEGRATED CHILD DEVELOPMENT SERVICES. Department of Women and Child Development, *Ministry of Human Resource Development*, GoI, New Delhi.
5. F.No. 5-9/2005/ND/Tech Vol(II) dated 24 February 2009. Revised nutritional and feeding norms of supplementary nutrition in the ICDS scheme. *Ministry of Women and Child Development,* Government of India.
6. Policy on Control of Nutritional Anemia (1991). National Nutritional Anemia Control Program. *Ministry of Health & Family Welfare*, GoI.
7. Policy on Management of Vitamin A Deficiency (1991). National Program for Prophylaxis Against Blindness in Children Due to Vitamin A Deficiency. *MoHFW*, GoI.
8. Letter no. Z.28020/50/2003-CH dated 23rd April, 2007, issued by Assistant Commissioner, Child Health, MoHFW, GoI.
9. Syllabus for job training of AWW (2006). Training Division, National Institute of Public Cooperation & Child Development, Ministry of Women & Child Development, GoI.
10. Syllabus for job training course of supervisors (2006). Training Division, National Institute of Public Cooperation & Child Development, *Ministry of Women & Child Development*, GoI.
11. Syllabus for job training course of Child Development Project Officers/ Additional Child Development Project Officers (2006). Training Division, National Institute of Public Cooperation & Child Development, *Ministry of Women & Child Development,* GoI.
12. GRAGNOLATI M, SHEKAR M, DAS GUPTA M, BREDENKAMP C, LEE Y (2005). India's Undernourished Children: A Call for Reform & Action. Washington, *DC: World Bank.*

13. Working Group on Development of Children for the Eleventh Five Year Plan (2007–2011), *Ministry of Women and Child Development,* GoI, Shastri Bhavan, New Delhi.
14. ICDS IV Project (2007). 2008–09 to 2012–13. Handbook. Central Project Management Unit. *Ministry of Women & Child Development*, GoI.
15. Syllabus for job training of AWW, Supervisor and CDPO (2006). Training Division, National Institute of Public Cooperation & Child Development, *Ministry of Women & Child Development,* GoI.
16. NATIONAL INSTITUTE OF PUBLIC COOPERATION & CHILD DEVELOPMENT (1992). National Evaluation of the Integrated Child Development Services. New Delhi.
17. NATIONAL COUNCIL OF APPLIED ECONOMIC RESEARCH (2001). Concurrent Evaluation of Integrated Child Development Services. New Delhi.
18. LOKSHIN M, DAS GUPTA M, GRAGNOLATI M, IVANSCHENKO O (2005). Improving child nutrition: Integrated Child Development Services in India. *Development & Change*, **36**, pp. 613–640.
19. INTERNATIONAL INSTITUTE FOR POPULATION SCIENCES AND MACRO INTERNATIONAL (2007). National Family Health Survey (NFHS-3). India : Key findings. Mumbai: IIPS. 2005–06.
20. GANDHI N, TANDON B, KRISHNAMURTHY KS (1995). Integrated Child Development Services Scheme & Nutritional Status of Indian children. *Journal of Tropical Pediatrics*, **41**, pp. 123–128.
21. BHANDARI B, GUPTA AP, MANDOWARA SL, SAHARE P, SINGHAL M (1993). Decadal Changes in Nutritional and Immunization Status of ICDS Beneficiaries. *Indian Journal of Maternal & Child Health*, **4**, pp. 9–10.
22. SWAMI HM, THAKUR JS, BHATIA SP, BHATIA V (2001). Nutritional Status of Pre-school Children in an Integrated Child Development Service Block of Chandigarh. *Journal of Indian Medical Association*. **99**, pp. 554–556.
23. NAYAR D, KAPIL U, NANDAN D (1998). Status of Receipt of ICDS Package of Services by Under 3 children & pregnant women in district Agra. *Indian Pediatrics*, **35**, pp. 459–462.
24. AGARWAL KN, AGARWAL DK, AGARWAL A, RAO S, PRASAD R, AGARWAL S, SINGH TB (2000). Impact of ICDS on Maternal Nutrition & Birth Weight in Rural Varanasi. *Indian Pediatrics*, **37**, pp. 1321–1327.
25. RAIZADA N, SACHAR RK, BHATIA RC, SEHGAL R, SONI RK (1993). Impact of Preschool Education Component of ICDS on Mental & Cognitive Development of Children. *Indian Journal of Maternal Health,* **4**, pp. 4–8.
26. A Review of "Best Practices" in ICDS (2007). *Micronutrient Initiative.* For the World Bank.
27. HEAVER R (2002). India's Tamil Nadu Nutrition Program. Lessons and Issues in Management & Capacity. *Health, Nutrition and Population Discussion Paper*. World Bank, Washington.
28. SHEKAR M (1991). The Tamil Nadu Integrated Nutrition Project: A Review of the Project with Special Emphasis on the Monitoring and Information System. Cornell Food and Nutrition Policy Program, Working Paper No. 14. *Ithaca*, New York: Cornell University.
30. DUBOWITZ T, LEVINSON D, PERTERMAN JN, VERMA G, JACOB S, SCHULTINK W (2007). Intensifying Efforts to Reduce Child Malnutrition in India: Evaluation of *Dular* program in Jharkhand, India. *Food & Nutrition Bulletin*, **28**, pp. 226–273.
31. CARE INDIA (2007). Reproductive & Child Health & Nutrition & HIV/AIDS (RACHNA) Program 2001–2006: Summary of Approaches and Results.

32. DREYFUSS M, LI Y, CHAUDHERY D, SINGH V (2006). Evaluation Research of Nutrition Interventions in INHP II Areas of CARE India: Final Evaluation Report. CARE India, King Georges Medical University and Johns Hopkins Bloomberg School of Public Health.
33. Impact Evaluation of Positive Deviance Program in West Bengal (2007). National Institute of Nutrition. *ICMR*, Hyderabad.
34. *Anchal Se Angan Tak* (ASAT) Strategy Evaluation (2006). Tufts University, *Friedman School of Nutrition Science & Policy.* Draft Report.
35. Community Based Maternal & Child Health Nutrition Project (2006). Evaluation. ORG Centre for Social Research (division of AC Nielsen ORG-MARG Pvt. Ltd.), Lucknow,
36. Implementation Completion Report for ICDS-III/WCD project (IDA Credit IN-N042) (2006). Borrower's Evaluation Report. Central Project Management Unit, *Ministry of Women & Child Development,* GoI.
37. VARMA JL, DAS S, SANKAR R, MANNAR MGR, LEVINSON FJ, HAMER DH (2007). Community-level micronutrient fortification of a food supplement in India: a controlled trial in preschool children aged 36–66 months. *American Journal of Clinical Nutrition,* **85**, pp. 1127–33.
38. Strengthening a package of Essential Nutrition Actions in Integrated Child Development Services and Reproductive and Child Health programs (2006). *CARE*, India.
37. ICDS DIRECTORATE. Accreditation in ICDS. Karnataka and Andhra Pradesh.

# 43

# National Rural Health Mission

*Deoki Nandan*

**Deoki Nandan**, MD, FAMS, FIPHA, FIAPSM, FISCD, is currently the Director of the National Institute of Health & Family Welfare, New Delhi. He has worked as Principal/Dean and Chief of hospital, S N Medical College, Agra. He has been actively working in the field of public health for more than 30 years and during this period has been associated as an advisor as well as consultant with many international organizations. He is also a member of many state-level committees and National Technical Expert Committees, specifically for AIDS, IMNCI and Child Health.

## 43.1 Introduction

The National Rural Health Mission (NRHM) was launched on 12th April 2005 throughout India with a commitment of the government to carry out the necessary architectural corrections in the basic health care delivery system. NRHM covers the entire country but has a special focus on eighteen states (of these 8 are EAG states), identified to have weak public health indicators and/or weak health infrastructure. These focused states are Arunachal Pradesh, Assam, Bihar, Chhattisgarh, Himachal Pradesh, Jharkhand, Jammu & Kashmir, Manipur, Mizoram, Meghalaya, Madhya Pradesh, Nagaland, Orissa, Rajasthan, Sikkim, Tripura, Uttaranchal and Uttar Pradesh. While all the Mission activities are the same for all the states/UTs in the country, the high focus states have the following additional support:

(i) An Accredited Social Health Worker (ASHA) in all villages with a population of 1000.
(ii) Project Management Support at the state and district level.

## 43.2 The vision of the mission

The mission seeks to provide effective health care to rural population

# Empowered Action Group (EAG) refers to the following 8 states – Bihar, Chattisgarh, Jharkhand, Madhya Pradesh, Orissa, Rajasthan, Uttaranchal and Uttar Pradesh.

throughout the country with special focus on 18 identified focused states [1]. Further, NRHM seeks to:

- Raise public spending on health from 0.9% to 2–3% of GDP, with improved arrangement for community financing and risk pooling.
- Undertake architectural correction of the health system to enable it to effectively handle increased allocations and promote policies that strengthen public health management and service delivery in the country.
- Revitalize local health traditions and mainstream Ayurveda, Yoga, Unani, Siddha and Homeopathy (AYUSH) into the public health system.
- Integrate the health concerns effectively through decentralized management at the district, with determinants of health like sanitation and hygiene, nutrition, safe drinking water, gender and social concerns.
- Addressed inter-state and inter-district disparities, especially among the 18 high focus states, including unmet needs for public health infrastructure.
- Ensure achievement of time bound goals and report the progress publicly.
- Improve access of rural people, especially poor women and children to equitable, affordable, accountable and effective primary health care.

## 43.3 The objectives of the mission

- Reduction in child and maternal mortality.
- Universal access to public health care services for food and nutrition, sanitation and hygiene with emphasis on services addressing women's and children's health and universal immunization.
- Prevention and control of communicable and non-communicable diseases, including locally endemic diseases.
- Access to integrated comprehensive primary health care.
- Population stabilization, gender and demographic balance.
- Revitalize local health traditions and mainstream AYUSH.
- Promotion of healthy life styles.

## 43.4 The expected outcomes from the mission as proposed for reflection in statistical data

- Infant Mortality Rate (IMR) reduced to 30/1000 live births by 2012.
- Maternal mortality reduced to 100/100,000 live births by 2012.

- Total Fertility Rate (TFR) reduced to 2.1 by 2012.
- Malaria Mortality Reduction Rate – 50% by 2010, additional 10% by 2012.
- Kala Azar Mortality Reduction Rate – 100% by 2010 and sustaining elimination until 2012.
- Filarial/Microfilaria Reduction Rate – 70% by 2010, 80% by 2012 and elimination by 2015.
- Dengue Mortality Reduction Rate – 50% by 2010 and sustaining at that level till 2012.
- Cataract operation – increasing to 46 lakhs by 2012.
- Leprosy Prevalence Rate – reduced from 1.8 per 10,000 in 2005 to less that 1 per 10,000 thereafter.
- Tuberculosis – DOTS services maintain 85% cure rate through entire mission period and also sustain planned case detection rate.
- Upgrading Community Health Centres to Indian Public Health Standards. Increase utilization of First Referral units from bed occupancy by referred cases of less than 20% to over 75%.
- Engaging 250,000 female Accredited Social Health Activists (ASHAs) in 18 states.

## 43.5 Goals, strategies and outcomes of the Mission

The mission seeks to provide universal access to equitable, affordable and quality health care services which is responsive to the needs of the people, reduction of child and maternal deaths, population stabilization, gender and demographic balance. In this process, the mission would help achieve goals set under the National Health Policy and the Millennium Development Goals. To achieve these goals NRHM will

- Facilitate increased access and utilization of quality health services by all.
- Forge a partnership between the Central, State and the Local governments.
- Set up a platform for involving the Panchayati Raj institutions and community in the management of primary health programmes and infrastructure.
- Provide an opportunity for promoting equity and social justice.
- Establish a mechanism to provide flexibility to the states and the community to promote local initiatives.
- Develop a framework for promoting inter-sectoral convergence for promotive and preventive health care.

### 43.5.1 The core strategies of the mission

The following core strategies have been adopted to achieve the goals of mission:

- Train and enhance the capacity of Panchayati Raj Institutions (PRIs) to own, control and manage public health services.
- Promote access to improved health care at household level through the female-health activist (ASHA).
- Health plan for each village through village-health committee of the panchayat.
- Strengthening sub-centre through better human resource development, clear quality standards, better community support and an untied fund to enable local planning, action and induction of more Multi-Purpose Workers (MPWs).
- Strengthening existing primary health care centres (PHCs) through better staffing and human resource development policy, clear quality standards, better community support and an untied fund to enable the local management committee to achieve these standards.
- Provision of 30–50 bedded community health centres (CHC) per lakh population for improved curative care to a normative standard (Indian Public Health Standards – IPHS defining personnel, equipment and management standards, its decentralized administration by a hospital management committee and the provision of adequate funds and powers to enable these committees to function at optimum levels).
- Preparation and implementation of an inter-sector District Health Plan including drinking water, sanitation, hygiene and nutrition.
- Integrating vertical health and family welfare programmes at national, state, district and block levels.
- Technical support to national, state and district health mission, for public health management.
- Strengthening capacities for data collection, assessment and review for evidence-based planning, monitoring and supervision.
- Formulation of transparent policies for deployment and career development of human resource for health.
- Developing capacities for preventive health care at all levels for promoting healthy life style, reduction in consumption of tobacco and alcohol, etc.
- Promoting non-profit sector particularly in underserved areas.

### 43.5.2 Supplementary strategies

In addition to these core strategies, some of the supplementary strategies of the mission include:

- Regulation of private sector including the informal Rural Medical Practitioners (RMP) to ensure availability of quality service to citizens at reasonable cost.
- Promotion of public private partnerships for achieving public health goals.
- Mainstreaming AYUSH, revitalizing local health traditions.
- Reorienting medical education to support rural health issues including regulation of medical care and medical ethics.
- Effective and visible risk pooling and social health insurance to provide health security to the poor by ensuring accessible, affordable, accountable and good quality hospital care.

## 43.6 Institutional mechanisms in the National Rural Health Mission

The following institutional mechanisms have been created to strengthen functioning at various levels:

- Village health and sanitation samiti (at village level consisting of panchayat representative/s, ANM/MPW, anganwadi worker, teacher, ASHA, community health volunteers),
- Hospital Management Committee/Rogi Kalyan Samiti for community management of public hospitals.
- District Health Mission, under the leadership of Zila Parishad with District Health Head as Convener and all relevant departments, NGOs, private professionals and others represented on it.
- State Health Mission, chaired by Chief Minister and co-chaired by Health Minister and with the State Health Secretary as Convener representation of related departments, NGOs, private professionals and others.
- Integration of Departments of Health and Family Welfare, at national and state level.
- National Mission Steering Group chaired by Union Minister for Health & Family Welfare with Deputy Chairman Planning Commission, Ministers of Panchayat Raj, Rural Development and Human Resource Development and public health professionals as members, to provide policy support and guidance to the Mission.
- Empowered Programme Committee chaired by Secretary Health and family Welfare, to be the Executive Body of the Mission.

As a part of this strategy, the state and district missions have been set up in all the states and UTs (Figure 43.1). The Departments of Health and Family Welfare have been merged at the level of the Government of India

(GoI) and similar system is being followed up at state levels. State level NRHM activities have been designed taking into consideration the reform commitments expected by states including enhanced public spending on health, decentralization, promotion of district level planning, etc.

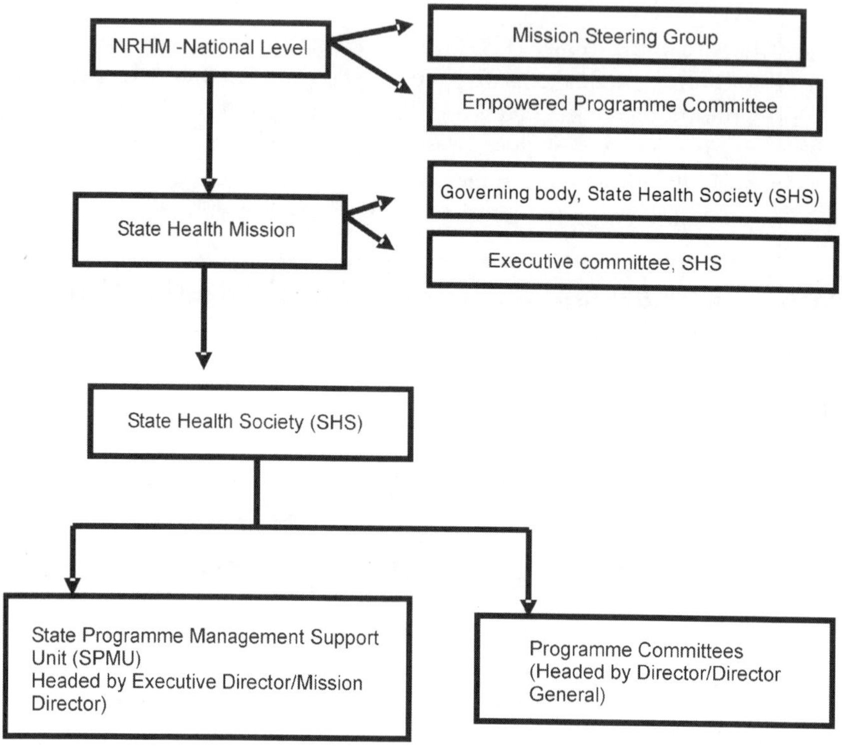


*43.1* Institutional Mechanisms under NRHM.

## 43.7 Accredited Social Health Activists (ASHA)

The core strategies envisaged to realize the objectives include improved access to health care at household level through local women in the age of 25–40 years known as Accredited Social Health Activist (ASHA). Every village/large habitat is to have an ASHA chosen by and accountable to the Panchayat. She is to serve as a bridge between the anganwadi workers, ANMs and community. As link between the community and the health facility, the ASHAs are expected to be the first person to call for any health related demand. Under the Framework of Implementation [2], it is proposed to have ASHAs in all the 18 high focus states and to support ASHAs in tribal districts of all the remaining states. One of the main approaches of NRHM involves large-scale transfer of knowledge and skills and health information to ASHAs. Each state is imparting trainings to them for 23 days in five episodes as per their state specific needs.

A set of guidelines have been developed to enable the states to develop and put in place a proper support mechanism for ASHA. These guidelines spell out the role of ASHA vis-à-vis Anganwadi Worker (AWW) of ICDS and the Auxiliary Nurse Midwives (ANM) of health sector [3]. She is to act as an interface between the community and the public health system. Working as an honorary volunteer, she receives performance-based compensation on specified services rendered by her.

The NRHM focuses on decentralization for planning at all levels; ASHA would facilitate preparation and implementation of the Village Health Plans along with anganwadi workers, ANMs, functionaries of other departments and self-help groups (SHGs) under the leadership of Village Health Committee of the *Panchayat* (elected village body). ASHA is also supplied with a drug kit containing generic AYUSH and allopathic formulations for common ailments, which is replenished, periodically.

Some of the roles and responsibilities of ASHA are

- To create awareness and provide information to community on determinants of health such as nutrition, basic sanitation and hygiene practices, healthy living and working conditions.
- To provide information on existing health services and the need for timely utilization of health and family welfare services.
- Counsel women on birth preparedness, RTIs/STDs (Reproductive Tract Infection / Sexually Transmitted Diseases).
- Mobilize community and facilitate them in accessing available health related services.
- Work with voluntary health and sanitation committee to develop a comprehensive village plan.
- Maintain drug kit to provide first aid facilities.

ASHA is viewed as a key person who would provide help to strengthen the services at the outreach level for a sub-centre, PHC or district health centre. In addition, ASHA is expected to provide data regarding the progress made by the village/community for the consolidation of report at PHC by the medical officer for the bi-monthly meetings.

The expected outcomes related to ASHAs at community level as envisaged in the Framework for Implementation (2005–2012) are as below:

- Availability of trained community level worker at village level, with a drug kit for generic ailments.
- Health and Nutrition Day at anganwadi level on a fixed day/month

for provision of immunization; Ante/post natal check ups and services related to mother and child health care, including nutrition.
- Availability of generic drugs for common ailments at sub-centre and hospital level.
- Access to good hospital care through assured availability of doctors, drugs and quality services at PHC/CHC level and assured referral–transport–communication systems to reach these facilities in time.
- Access to Universal Immunization improved through induction of auto disabled syringes, alternate vaccine delivery and improved mobilization services under the programme.
- Facilities for institutional delivery improved through provision of referral, transport, escort and improved hospital care subsidized under the Janani Surakshya Yojana (JSY) for the below-poverty-line families.
- Availability of assured health care at reduced financial risk through pilots of community health insurance under the mission.
- Availability of safe drinking water.
- Provisions for household toilets.
- Outreach services to medically under-served remote areas improved through mobile medical units.
- Awareness about preventive health including nutrition increased.

### 43.7.1 The integrated role of ASHA and organizing Village Health Nutrition Days

Health Days (referred also as Village Health and Nutrition Days or VHND) are organized every month at the anganwadi level in each village in which immunization, ante/post-natal check ups and services related to mother and child health care including nutrition are being provided. Space at each anganwadi centre (AWC) of ICDS (Integrated Child Development Services) is proposed to serve as the hub of health and nutrition activities in the village. The AWC space is also recommended to be utilized for dispensing out-patient services by any health provider and also serve as depot for medicines and contraceptives. It is proposed that NRHM will aim to establish a village level health institution co-located with AWC with a specific physical location.

The role of ASHAs under NRHM is very critical for child survival, child health and strengthening immune functions (Figure 43.2). A number of state governments have introduced innovative programmes related to various schemes under NRHM, where ASHAs play a central role such as vitamin A programme using the biannual administration strategy.

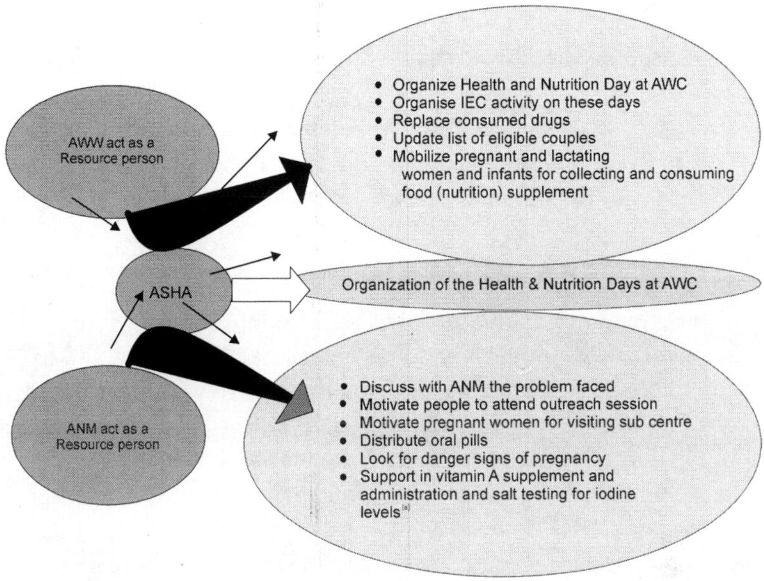


*43.2* Integrated role of ASHA.

[a]Task added by GoI in 2009 [4]

## 43.8 Implementation Framework and Plan of Action for NRHM

The inherent strength of NRHM lies in its implementation of various schemes with rigor and appropriate monitoring strategy. In order to achieve the goals of the NRHM, some of the key features identified in the Implementation Framework and the Plan of Action of the Mission are

- Making the public health delivery system fully functional and accountable to the community
- Human resources management
- Community involvement
- Decentralization
- Rigorous monitoring and evaluation against standards
- Convergence of health and related programmes from village level upwards
- Innovations and flexible financing and
- Interventions for improving the health indicators

### 43.8.1 Decentralization

In line with the above, the Mission seeks to adopt a convergent approach for interventions under the umbrella of the district plan which seeks to integrate all the related initiatives at the village, block and district levels. The District Health Action Plan is the main instrument for planning, inter-sectoral convergence, implementation and monitoring of the activities under the Mission. Based on the district plans, annual state plans are developed. The allocation of funds is as per these annual plans. It is also proposed to conduct periodic surveys on an annual basis to track the improvements in the facilities as well as in the reduction in health indicators. The state plans are approved by the Mission at the national level.

### 43.8.2 Convergent action on other determinants of health

One of the key components of NRHM is about effective integration of health concerns with determinants of health like sanitation and hygiene, nutrition and safe drinking water through a district plan for health. The status of health and related indicators depend on many factors such as drinking water, female literacy, nutrition, early childhood development, sanitation, women's empowerment along with hospitals and functional health systems. NRHM seeks to adopt a convergent approach for these key determinants for interventions under the umbrella of the district plan. Anganwadi Centre under the ICDS at the village level is proposed to be the principal hub for health action (Figure 43.3). The village committees constituted for drinking water, sanitation, ICDS etc. is envisaged to converge under one common village health committee to cover all these activities. Panchayati Raj Institutions (PRIs), the community level institutions are expected to be fully involved in this convergent approach so that the gains of integrated action can be reflected in district plans.

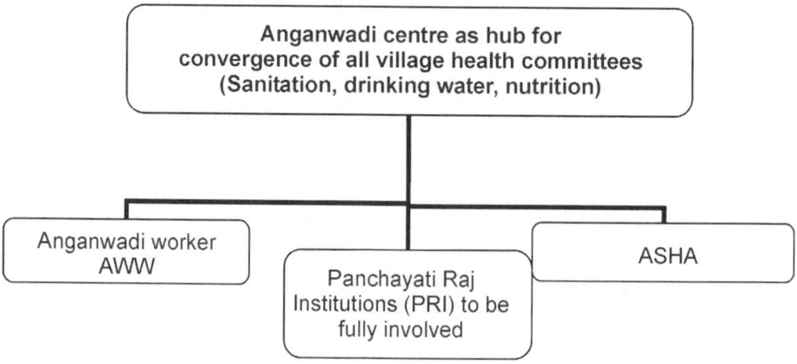


*43.3* Convergent action at village level.

Convergence is also envisaged at the level of the Mission Steering Group which has representation of all the concerned Ministries, such as Department of Women and Child Development, Department of Education and with AYUSH. The PRIs organizations (Self-help Groups, Schools, Water, Health and Sanitation Committee or Health, Nutrition and Sanitation Committees, Mahila Samakhya Groups, Zila Saksharta Samitis) are expected to provide an opportunity for seeking local levels accountability in the delivery of social sector programmes. There is a provision under the NRHM to provide for School Health Checkups and School Health Education in consultation with the states. As presented in Figures 43.3 and 43.4 (a, b), convergence of all programmes is at the village and facility levels.

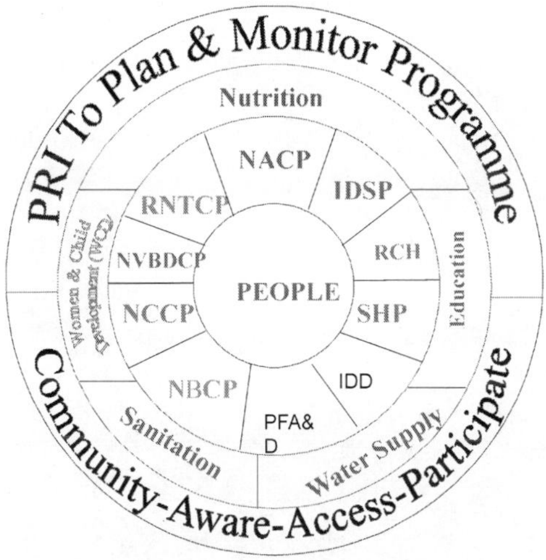


*43.4a* Intersectoral Convergence.

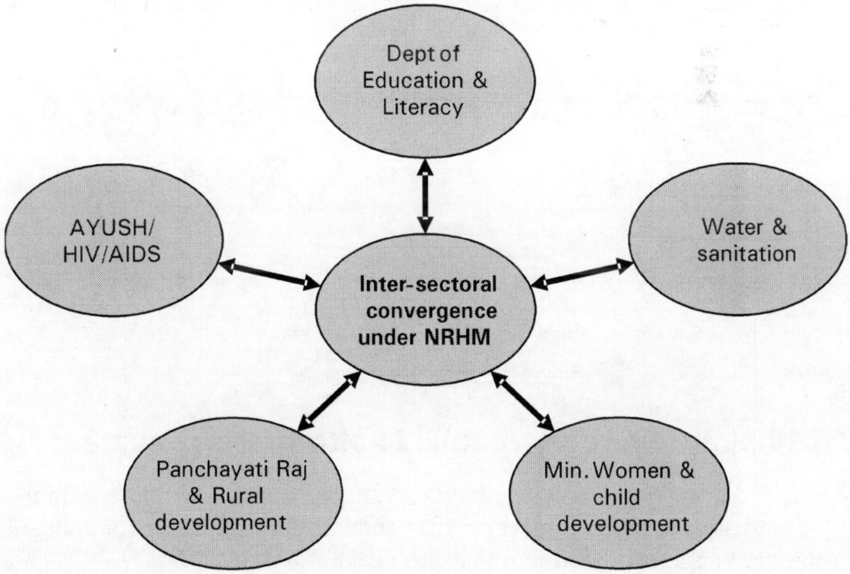


*43.4b* Intersectoral convergence under NRHM.

## 43.9 Nutrition: a determinant of health

NRHM has proposed service guarantee for health care at sub-health centre, primary health centre and community health centre. These include prevention and control of childhood diseases as well as malnutrition, vitamin A prophylaxis to the children, iron–folic acid to pregnant mothers and children and testing of iodine in salt. These nutrition services are proposed to be coordinated with the ICDS.

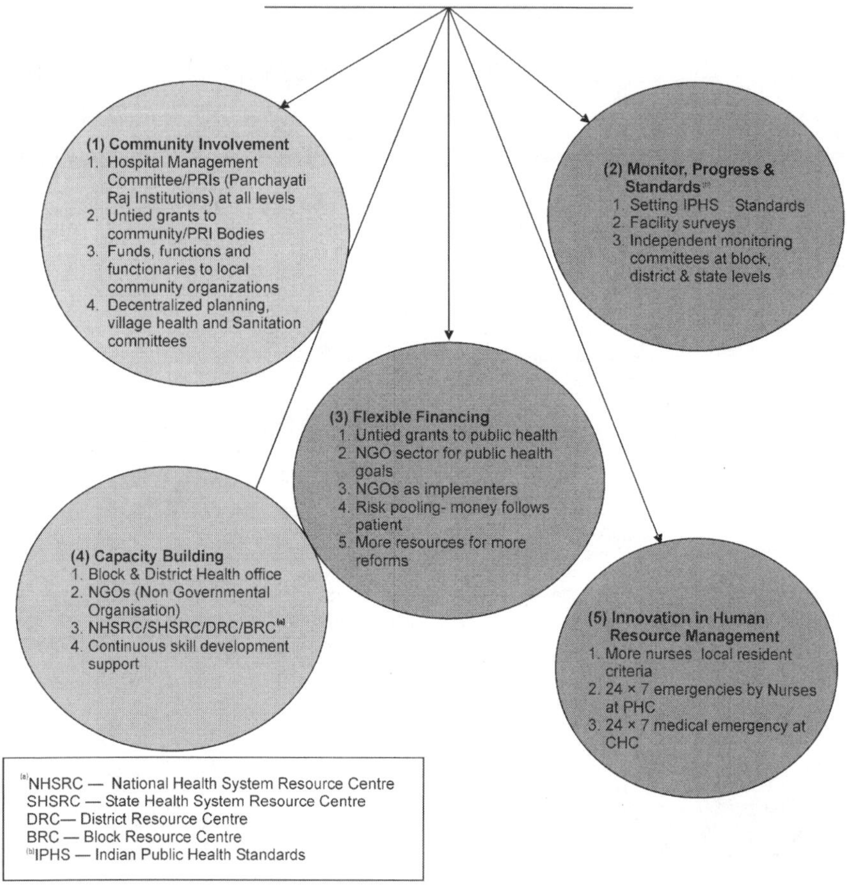


*43.5* NRHM – five main approaches.

## 43.10 Improving the public health delivery system

The status of public health infrastructure in the country, particularly in the EAG and north-east states is very weak and has been the cause for concern for many years. It is pertinent that providing the desired quality services especially in the EAG and the north-eastern states will not be possible till the infrastructure is sufficiently upgraded. Realizing this, the Mission seeks to establish functional health facilities in the public domain through revitalization of the existing infrastructure and fresh construction or renovation wherever required. The Mission also seeks to improve service delivery by putting in place enabling systems at all levels. This involves simultaneous corrections in manpower planning as well as infrastructure strengthening. The generic public health delivery system envisioned under NRHM from the village to the block level is presented in Fig. 43.6.

## 43.11 Indian Public Health Standards (IPHS)

The Indian Public Health Standards (IPHS) have been set up for all levels to ensure that quality in services is maintained throughout the delivery of health care services. Figure 43.7 presents the human resource requirements at various levels of health infrastructure under NRHM and Fig. 43.8 presents the details of IPHS.

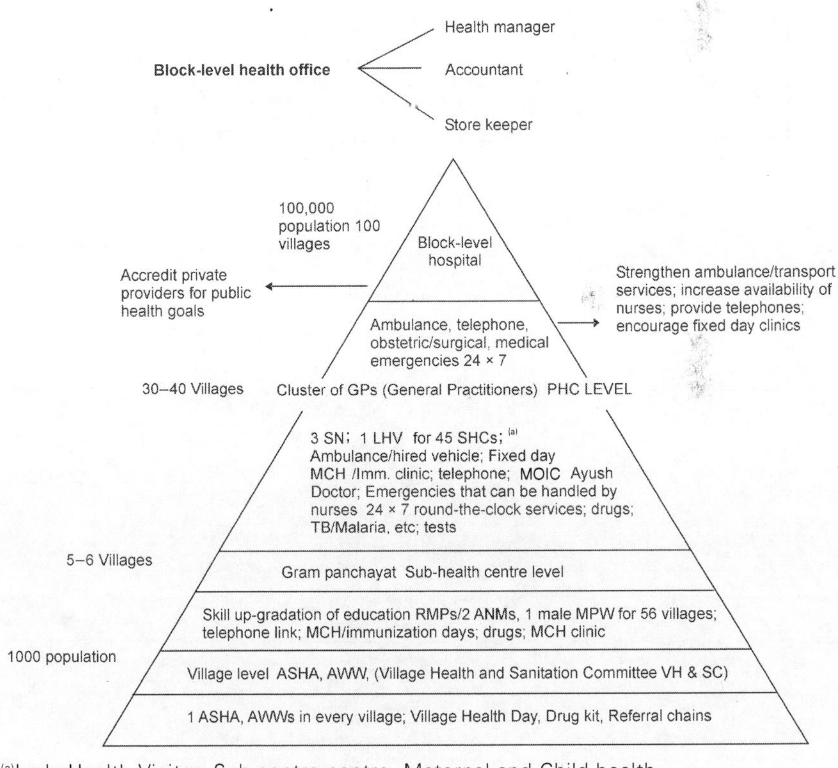


[a]Lady Health Visitor, Sub-centre centre, Maternal and Child health

*43.6* NRHM – Public Health Delivery Systems.

## 43.12 Public health infrastructure

Given the general observation that the health infrastructure is in poor condition in most of the states, NRHM has allocated the budget for

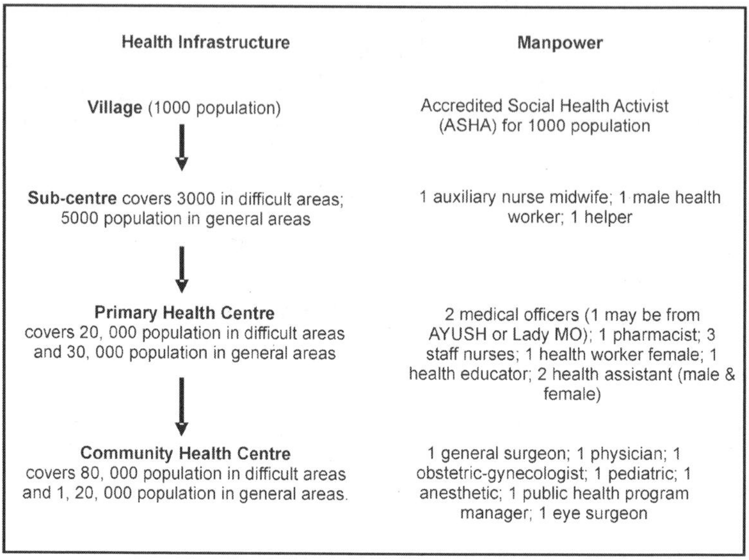


*43.7* Human resource requirements.

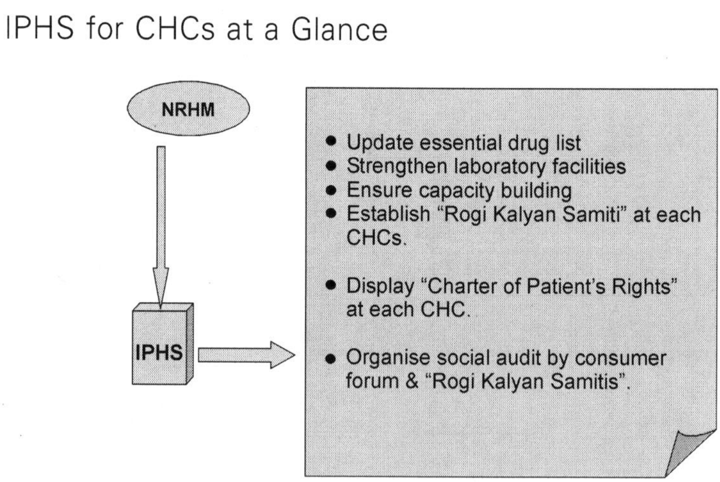


*43.8* Indian Public Health Standards (IPHS) at CHCs.

construction, subject to the condition that it should not be more than 33% of the total NRHM outlay in the case of high focus states and 25% in the case of non-high focus states.

In order to improve public health infrastructure, a number of initiatives have been put forth such as:

- Providing untied grants at sub-centre, PHC/CHC and district level.
- Provision for funds for taking up innovative schemes at district/state/ central level.
- Funds for *Rogi Kalyan Samitis* (welfare association for sick persons) for managing the health facilities.

The Mission seeks to ensure the availability of requisite equipment and drugs at all the public health care facilities and it is proposed to procure equipment and drugs progressively in a decentralized manner. It is also proposed to improve outreach activities in un-served and underserved areas specially inhabited by vulnerable sections through provision of Mobile Medical Units (MMU) in every district, which would cover anganwadi centres also.

## 43.13 Improving availability of critical manpower

The issues of availability of critical manpower in the rural areas is proposed to be addressed through initiatives like: (i) introduction of a trained voluntary community health worker (ASHA) in every village of the 18 high-focus states; (ii) an additional ANM at each sub-centre; (iii) three staff nurses at the primary health centres (PHC) to make them operational round the clock and additional specialists and paramedical staff at the community health centres (CHC).

In north-east States, keeping in view the difficulty in availing services of doctors and specialists, the emphasis is on recruitment, training and skill up-gradation of locally recruited ANMs, nurses, midwives and paramedics. Contractual appointment/local level engagement of medical and paramedical manpower, upgrading and multi-skilling of the existing medical personnel are some other options which are being planned to fill the critical gaps of manpower. A number of innovations like public-private partnership (PPP) for service provision, franchising of service providers, licensing and training of rural medical practitioners (RMP), rationalization of existing manpower are being explored. It is envisaged that stringent monitoring at all levels, involvement of the PRIs and monitoring by the *Rogi Kalyan Samitis* would ensure presence of doctors and paramedical in the rural areas. Besides compulsory posting of doctors in the rural areas, better cadre management and personnel policies would also help to improve manpower availability.

## 43.14 Capacity building

Capacity building at all levels in India has been a huge challenge and therefore various initiatives have been made under the Mission for capacity building of human resources. These are

(i) Programme Management Units (PMUs) at the state/district level – PMUs at the state/district level have been set up in order to provide managerial support for monitoring various activities under NRHM and also tracking of funds (Over 500 professionals have already been recruited). Additionally, the successful implementation of the Mission requires health sector reforms and development of human resources.
(ii) National Health System Resource Centre (NHSRC) – NHSRC at the Central and State levels (SHSRC) have been set up to provide technical support at the central and state government levels, respectively.
(iii) The NRHM also emphasizes the setting up of fully functional block and district level health management systems. Under NRHM, 70% of the resources would be utilized at block and below block levels while only 20% at the district level. Given the large army of ASHAs, ANMs, nurses, rural medical practitioners, the need of the hour is continuous development of the skills of these health personnel.
(iv) Strengthening nursing institutions and linking medical colleges – In order to provide skill development support to rural health workers, involving the voluntary sector in skill development, it is proposed to strengthen the nursing and medical institutions of our country.
(v) Strengthening of PRIs – It is proposed to gradually shift the central mechanism of the health facilities like sub-centres under the control of *panchayats* (elected village body) elicited community organization, with a view to make them more accountable.

## 43.15 Monitoring and review

One of the differences in the monitoring strategy of NRHM is to involve local communities in planning, implementing and monitoring. NRHM proposes an intensive accountability framework through a three pronged process of community based monitoring, external surveys and stringent internal monitoring. Role of Village Health Committees, PHC health monitoring and planning committees have been spelt out for ensuring monitoring at community level.

## 43.16 Flexible financing

One of the strengths of the Mission is to increase the share of central and state governments on health care from the current 20–80 to 40–60 sharing in the long run. While under X$^{th}$ Plan, 100% grants were planned to be provided to states, in the XI$^{th}$ Plan period the states are expected to contribute 15% to make the share of the Central Government 85%. This relative share of the centre and state is projected to be sustained at 75:25.

One of the practical problems experienced by the states has been the transfer of funds under different budget heads at different points of time vertically and for many programmes. Such a system has been found to often result in duplication of efforts, and wastage of scarce resources. The strength of Mission is recognised to lie in providing flexible financing options. The Mission attempts to bring all the schemes of the Ministry of Health and Family Welfare within the overarching umbrella of NRHM. From the XI$^{th}$ Plan onwards, the Framework of Implementation has proposed to have a single budget head for the activities under the Mission. The mechanism of flow of funds under the NRHM budget head is proposed through the Integrated Health Society at the state and the district levels.

### 43.16.1 Related financial mechanisms: provision of untied funds

In order to strengthen the sub-centres, each sub-centre will have an Untied Fund for local action at Rs 10,000 per annum. This fund will be deposited in a joint Bank account of the ANM and Sarpanch (Head of village committee or Panchayat ) and operated by the ANM, in consultation with the village health and sanitation committees. A revolving fund is to be set up at the village level for providing referral and transport facilities for emergency deliveries as well as immediate financial needs for hospitalization. The fund is to be operated by the village health and sanitation committee (VHSC). Such fund would also be made available to VHSC for various health activities including IEC, household survey, preparation of health register, organization of meetings at the village level, etc.

### 43.16.2 Financial Provisions under Janani Suraksha Yojana (JSY)

As per JSY, [5] cash assistance for institutional delivery is given to both mothers and ASHAs in the low- and high-performing states, on production of below poverty line (BPL) cards. All pregnant women delivering in the government health centre like sub-centre, PHC/CHC/FRU (First Re ferral Unit)/general wards of district hospitals and state hospitals or accredited private institutions are eligible to avail of this assistance. In the low-performing states, the assistance is Rs. 1400/- (about US $ 30) for a pregnant woman while in the high-performing states, the assistance is fixed at Rs. 700/- (about $ 15). The JSY has shown significant progress since its inception with a sharp increase in institutional deliveries.

## 43.17 NRHM progress made

The Mission has shown progress in many states in the past three to four year's time. More than 0.6 million ASHAs have been selected and are at various stages of selection and training. A total of 13,358 (additional PHCs) APHCs, PHCs, CHCs, and other sub-district facilities have been made 24 × 7 functional. The state of Bihar has reported that the average number of patients visiting a PHC every month has gone up from 39 in January 2006 to 3015 in August 2006. In Punjab, with the Alternate Health Delivery involving service providers under PRIs at 1310 subsidiary health centres, out-patient cases have gone up by 290% between June and October 2006. Regarding availability of medicines, states of UP and Jharkhand revised the per capita allocation for drugs in out-patient leading to better availability of drugs at health facilities [6].

Infant mortality rate is reduced to come to 55, down by 2 points in 2007 as compared to a point in earlier years (2003–06) [6]. Significant gains have also been reported in the rates of institutional deliveries which have increased by 66.4 % in MP, 50.2 % in Rajasthan, 47.3 % in Bihar, 43.8% in Orissa, 20.9% in Andhra Pradesh and 12.4% in Uttar Pradesh between District Level Household Survey DLHS-II (2004) and DLHS-III (2007). The status of full immunization has increased from 20.7% to 41.4% in Bihar, 25.7% to 54.1% in Jharkhand, 30.1% to 36.1% in MP, 53.5% to 62.4 % in Orissa, 23.9% to 48.8 % in Rajasthan and 25.8 % to 30.3 % in UP between DLHS II and DLHS III.

The success of NRHM depends to a large extent on many factors. One of these factors is the performance of ASHA or the link worker in the community and her linkages with the health system [3]. For the effective implementation of NRHM, each link worker must be fully aware of the facilities available in the area of operation and also what types of services are available at each facility. Support provided by the district and state nodal officers to immediately respond to local needs is another factor responsible for the successful functioning of NRHM, as the inputs provided by these officers include immediately responding to referrals made by ASHA, upgrading health facilities and infrastructure as per IPHS standards, timely provision of drugs and taking care of logistics as well as organizing campaigns and publicity activities with respect to availability of various services and schemes.

## References


1. National Rural Health Mission (2005–2012) Document, Ministry of Health and Family Welfare, Government of India.
2. Framework for Implementation (2005–2012). National Rural Health Mission-Meeting people's health needs in rural areas', Ministry of Health and Family Welfare, Government of India.
3. Guidelines for Operationalising Support Mechanism for ASHA. Department of Family Welfare. Ministry of Health & Family Welfare. Government of India. 2006.
4. TEWARI, B.K. State Level Awareness Meeting on NIDDCP, State Government of Chattisgarh, 31st October 2009, Raipur, Chhattisgarh.
5. JANANI SURAKSHA YOJANA (2006). Features & frequently asked questions & answers'. Government of India. http://mohfw.nic.in/dofw/JSY
6. NRHM-The Progress so far. http://mohfw.nic.in/nrhm
7. District Level Household and Facility Survey: Reproductive and Child Health Project. www.rchiips.org/ARCH-1.html

# Index